SANFORD GUIDE ®

W9-BFB-097

The Sanford Guide
To Antimicrobial Therapy
2016

46th Edition

THE SANFORD GUIDE TO ANTIMICROBIAL THERAPY 2016
46ᵀᴴ EDITION

Editors

David N. Gilbert, M.D.
Chief of Infectious Diseases
Providence Portland Medical Center, Oregon
Professor of Medicine, Oregon Health
Sciences University

Henry F. Chambers, M.D.
Professor of Medicine
Director, Clinical Research Services
UCSF Clinical and Translational Sciences Institute
University of California at San Francisco

George M. Eliopoulos, M.D.
Chief, James L. Tullis Firm,
Beth Israel Deaconess Hospital,
Professor of Medicine,
Harvard Medical School,
Boston, Massachusetts

Michael S. Saag, M.D.
Director, UAB Center for AIDS Research,
Professor of Medicine and Director,
Division of Infectious Diseases,
University of Alabama, Birmingham

Andrew T. Pavia, M.D.
George & Esther Gross Presidential Professor
Chief, Division of Pediatric Infectious Diseases
University of Utah, Salt Lake City

Contributing Editors

Douglas Black, Pharm. D.
Associate Professor
of Pharmacy,
University of Washington,
Seattle

Brian S. Schwartz, M.D.
Associate Professor
of Medicine
University of California
at San Francisco

David O. Freedman, M.D.
Director, Travelers Health Clinic,
Professor of Medicine,
University of Alabama,
Birmingham

Kami Kim, M.D.
Professor of Medicine, Microbiology & Immunology, Pathology
Albert Einstein College of Medicine
New York, NY

Managing Editor

Jeb C. Sanford

Memoriam

Jay P. Sanford, M.D.
1928-1996

Merle A. Sande, M.D.
1935-2007

Robert C. Moellering, Jr., M.D.
1936-2014

Publisher

Antimicrobial Therapy, Inc.

The Sanford Guides are updated annually and published by:

ANTIMICROBIAL THERAPY, INC.
P.O. Box 276, 11771 Lee Highway,
Sperryville, VA 22740-0276 USA
Tel 540-987-9480 Fax 540-987-9486
Email: info@sanfordguide.com   www.sanfordguide.com

Acknowledgements
Thanks to Ushuaia Solutions, SA, Argentina; Alcom Printing, Harleysville, PA and Fox Bindery, Quakertown, PA for design and production of this edition of the Sanford Guide.

Note to Readers
ce 1969, the Sanford Guide has been independently prepared and published. Decisions regarding the content of the Sanford Guide are solely those of the editors and the publisher. We welcome estions, comments and feedback concerning the Sanford Guide. All of your feedback is reviewed and taken into account in updating the content of the of the Sanford Guide.

ery effort is made to ensure accuracy of the content of this guide. However, current full prescribing ormation available in the package insert for each drug should be consulted before prescribing any duct. The editors and publisher are not responsible for errors or omissions or for any consequences m application of the information in this book and make no warranty, express or implied, with respect to the currency, accuracy, or completeness of the contents of this publication. Application of this information in a particular situation remains the professional responsibility of the practitioner.

For the most current information, subscribe to webedition.sanfordguide.com
or Sanford Guide mobile device applications

Printed in the United States of America
ISBN 978-1-930808-91-1
Pocket Edition (English)

QUICK PAGE GUIDE TO THE SANFORD GUIDE

—TABLE OF CONTENTS—

1

ABBREVIATIONS

3TC = lamivudine
AB,% = percent absorbed
ABC = abacavir
ABCD = amphotericin B colloidal dispersion
ABLC = ampho B lipid complex
AD = after dialysis
ADF = adefovir
AG = aminoglycoside
AIDS = Acquired Immune Deficiency Syndrome
AM-CL = amoxicillin-clavulanate
AM-CL-ER = amoxicillin-clavulanate extended release
AMK = amikacin
Amox = amoxicillin
AMP = ampicillin
Ampho B = amphotericin B
AM-SB = ampicillin-sulbactam
AP = atovaquone proguanil
APAG = antipseudomonal aminoglycoside
ARDS = acute respiratory distress syndrome
ASA = aspirin
ATS = American Thoracic Society
ATV = atazanavir
AUC = area under the curve
Azithro = azithromycin
bid = 2x per day
BL/BLI = beta-lactam/beta-lactamase inhibitor
BSA = body surface area
BW = body weight
CAS = culture & sensitivity
CAPB = carbapenem
CAPD = continuous ambulatory peritoneal dialysis
CDC = Centers for Disease Control
Cefpodox = cefpodoxime proxetil
Ceftaz = ceftazidime
Ceph = cephalosporin
CFB = cefoxitin
CFP = cefepime
Chloro = chloramphenicol
CIP = ciprofloxacin; **CIP-ER** = CIP extended release
Clarithro = clarithromycin, **ER** = extended release
Clav = clavulanate
Clinda = clindamycin
Clot = clotrimazole
CMV = cytomegalovirus
CO = chloroquine phosphate
Cobi = cobicistat
Ccr = creatinine clearance
CrCln = CrCl normalized for BSA
CRRT = continuous renal replacement therapy
C/S = culture & sensitivity
CSD = cat-scratch disease

CSF = cerebrospinal fluid
CXR = chest x-ray
d4T = stavudine
Dapto = daptomycin
DBPCT = double-blind placebo-controlled trial
dc = discontinue
ddC = zalcitabine
ddl = didanosine
DIC = disseminated intravascular coagulation
div = divided
DLV = delavirdine
DORI = doripenem
DOT = directly observed therapy
Doxy = doxycycline
DRSP = drug-resistant S. pneumoniae
DS = double strength
EBV = Epstein-Barr virus
EES = erythromycin ethyl succinate
EFZ = efavirenz
ELV = elvitegravir
EMB = ethambutol
ENT = entecavir
ER = extended release
ERTA = ertapenem
Erythro = erythromycin
ESBLs = extended spectrum β-lactamases
ESR = erythrocyte sedimentation rate
ESRD = endstage renal disease
Flu = fluconazole
Flucyt = flucytosine
FOS-APV = fosamprenavir
FTC = emtricitabine
G = generic
GAS = Group A Strep
Gati = gatifloxacin
GC = gonorrhea
Gemi = gemifloxacin
gm = gram
GNB = gram-negative bacilli
Griseo = griseofulvin
HEMO = hemodialysis
HIV = human immunodeficiency virus
HLR = high-level resistance
H/O = history of
HSCT = hematopoietic stem cell transplant
HSV = herpes simplex virus
IA = injectable agent/anti-inflammatory drugs
IDV = indinavir
IFN = interferon

IM = intramuscular
IMP = imipenem-cilastatin
INH = isoniazid
inv = investigational
IP = intraperitoneal
IT = intrathecal
Itra = itraconazole
IV = intravenous
IVDU = intravenous drug user
IVIG = intravenous immune globulin
Keto = ketoconazole
kg = kilogram
L-AB = liposomal ampho B
LCM = lymphocytic choriomeningitis virus
LCR = ligase chain reaction
Levo = levofloxacin
LP/R = lopinavir/ritonavir
µg (or mcg) = microgram
MDR = multi-drug resistant
MER = meropenem
Metro = metronidazole
Mino = minocycline
mL = milliliter
Moxi = moxifloxacin
MQ = mefloquine
MSM = men who have sex with men
MSSA/MRSA = methicillin-sensitive/resistant S. aureus
MTB = Mycobacterium tuberculosis
NAI = not FDA-approved (indication or dose)
NF = nitrofurantoin
NFR = nelfinavir
NNRTI = non-nucleoside reverse transcriptase inhibitor
NRTI = nucleoside reverse transcriptase inhibitor
NSAIDs = non-steroidal
NUS = not available in the U.S.
NVP = nevirapine
O Ceph 1, 2, 3 = oral cephalosporins
Oflox = ofloxacin
P Ceph 1, 2, 3, 4 = parenteral cephalosporins
P Ceph 3-AP = parenteral cephalosporins with antipseudomonal activity
PCR = polymerase chain reaction
PEP = post-exposure prophylaxis
PI = protease inhibitor
PIP-TZ = piperacillin-tazobactam
po = oral dosing
PO = primaquine
PRCT = Prospective randomized controlled trials
PTLD = post-transplant lymphoproliferative disease
Pts = patients
Pyri = pyrimethamine
PZA = Pyrazinamide

ABBREVIATIONS (2)

qid = 4x per day
QS = quinine sulfate
Quinu-dalfo = Q-D = quinupristin-dalfopristin
q[x]h = every [x] hours, e.g., q8h = every 8 hrs
q wk = dose weekly
R = resistant
RFB = rifabutin
RFP = rifapentine
Rick = Rickettsia
RIF = rifampin
RSV = respiratory syncytial virus
RTI = respiratory tract infection
RTV = ritonavir
rx = treatment
SA = Staph. aureus **sc** = subcutaneous
SD = serum drug level after single dose
Sens = sensitive (susceptible)

SM = streptomycin
SQV = saquinavir
SS = steady state serum level
STD = sexually transmitted disease
subcut = subcutaneous
Sulb = sulbactam
Sx = symptoms
Tazo = tazobactam
TBc = tuberculosis
TDF = tenofovir
TEE = transesophageal echocardiography
Teico = teicoplanin
Telithro = telithromycin
Tetra = tetracycline
tid = 3x per day
TMP-SMX = trimethoprim-sulfamethoxazole

TNF = tumor necrosis factor
Tobra = tobramycin
TPV = tipranavir
TST = tuberculin skin test
UTI = urinary tract infection
Vanco = vancomycin
VISA = vancomycin intermediately resistant S. aureus
VL = viral load
Vori = voriconazole
VZV = varicella-zoster virus
ZDV = zidovudine

ABBREVIATIONS OF JOURNAL TITLES

AAC: Antimicrobial Agents & Chemotherapy
Adv PID: Advances in Pediatric Infectious Diseases
AHJ: American Heart Journal
AIDS Res Hum Retrovir: AIDS Research & Human Retroviruses
AJG: American Journal of Gastroenterology
AJM: American Journal of Medicine
AJRCCM: American Journal of Respiratory Critical Care Medicine
AJTMH: American Journal of Tropical Medicine & Hygiene
AJT: American Journal of Transplantation
Aliment Pharmacol Ther: Alimentary Pharmacology & Therapeutics
Am J Hlth Pharm: American Journal of Health-System Pharmacy
Amer J Transpl: American Journal of Transplantation
AnEM: Annals of Emergency Medicine
AnIM: Annals of Internal Medicine
Ann Pharmacother: Annals of Pharmacotherapy
AnSurg: Annals of Surgery
Antivir Ther: Antiviral Therapy
ArDerm: Archives of Dermatology
AIM: Archives of Internal Medicine
ARRD: American Review of Respiratory Disease
BMJ: British Medical Journal
BMT: Bone Marrow Transplantation
Brit J Derm: British Journal of Dermatology
Can JID: Canadian Journal of Infectious Diseases
Canad Med J: Canadian Medical Journal
CCM: Critical Care Medicine
CCTID: Current Clinical Topics in Infectious Disease
CDBSR: Cochrane Database of Systematic Reviews
CID: Clinical Infectious Diseases
Clin Micro Inf: Clinical Microbiology and Infection
CMN: Clinical Microbiology Newsletter
Clin Micro Rev: Clinical Microbiology Reviews
CMAJ: Canadian Medical Association Journal
COID: Current Opinion in Infectious Disease

Curr Med Res Opin: Current Medical Research and Opinion
Derm Ther: Dermatologic Therapy
Dermatol Clin: Dermatologic Clinics
Dig Dis Sci: Digestive Diseases and Sciences
DMID: Diagnostic Microbiology and Infectious Disease
EID: Emerging Infectious Diseases
EJCMID: European Journal of Clin. Micro. & Infectious Diseases
Eur J Neurol: European Journal of Neurology
Exp Mol Path: Experimental & Molecular Pathology
Exp Rev Anti Infect Ther: Expert Review of Anti-Infective Therapy
Gastro: Gastroenterology
Hept: Hepatology
ICHE: Infection Control and Hospital Epidemiology
IDC No. Amer: Infectious Disease Clinics of North America
IDCP: Infectious Diseases in Clinical Practice
IJAA: International Journal of Antimicrobial Agents
Inf Med: Infections in Medicine
J AIDS & HR: Journal of AIDS and Human Retrovirology
J All Clin Immun: Journal of Allergy and Clinical Immunology
J Am Ger Soc: Journal of the American Geriatrics Society
J Chemother: Journal of Chemotherapy
J Clin Micro: Journal of Clinical Microbiology
J Clin Virol: Journal of Clinical Virology
J Derm Treat: Journal of Dermatological Treatment
J Hept: Journal of Hepatology
J Inf: Journal of Infection
J Med Micro: Journal of Medical Microbiology
J Micro Immunol Inf: Journal of Microbiology, Immunology, & Infection
J Ped: Journal of Pediatrics
J Viral Hep: Journal of Viral Hepatitis
JAC: Journal of Antimicrobial Chemotherapy
JACC: Journal of American College of Cardiology

JAIDS: JAIDS, Journal of Acquired Immune Deficiency Syndromes
JAMA: Journal of the American Medical Association
JAVMA: Journal of the Veterinary Medical Association
JCI: Journal of Clinical Investigation
JCM: Journal of Clinical Microbiology
JIC: Journal of Infection and Chemotherapy
JID: Journal of Infectious Diseases
JNeuro: Journal of Neurology
JTMH: Journal of Tropical Medicine and Hygiene
Ln: Lancet
LnID: Lancet Infectious Disease
Mayo Clin Proc: Mayo Clinic Proceedings
Med Lett: Medical Letter
Med Mycol: Medical Mycology
MMWR: Morbidity & Mortality Weekly Report
NEJM: New England Journal of Medicine
Neph Dial Transpl: Nephrology Dialysis Transplantation
OFID: Open Forum Infectious Diseases
Ped Ann: Pediatric Annals
Peds: Pediatrics
Pharmacother: Pharmacotherapy
PIDJ: Pediatric Infectious Disease Journal
QJM: Quarterly Journal of Medicine
Scand J Inf Dis: Scandinavian Journal of Infectious Diseases
Sem Resp Inf: Seminars in Respiratory Infections
SMJ: Southern Medical Journal
Surg Neurol: Surgical Neurology
Transpl Inf Dis: Transplant Infectious Diseases
Transpl: Transplantation
TRSM: Transactions of the Royal Society of Medicine

TABLE 1 – CLINICAL APPROACH TO INITIAL CHOICE OF ANTIMICROBIAL THERAPY*

Treatment based on presumed site or type of infection. In selected instances, treatment and prophylaxis based on identification of pathogens.
Regimens should be reevaluated based on pathogen isolated, antimicrobial susceptibility determination, and individual host characteristics. *(Abbreviations on page 2)*

ANATOMIC SITE/DIAGNOSIS/ MODIFYING CIRCUMSTANCES	ETIOLOGIES (usual)	SUGGESTED REGIMENS*		ADJUNCT DIAGNOSTIC OR THERAPEUTIC MEASURES AND COMMENTS
		PRIMARY	ALTERNATIVE†	
ABDOMEN: See Peritoneum, page 46; Gallbladder, page 17; and Pelvic Inflammatory Disease, page 26				
BONE: Osteomyelitis. Microbiologic diagnosis is essential. If blood culture negative, need culture of bone *(Eur J Clin Microbiol Infect Dis 33:371, 2014)*. Culture of sinus tract drainage not predictive of bone culture.				
Hematogenous Osteomyelitis *(see IDSA guidelines for vertebral osteo: CID July 29, 2015)*				
Empiric therapy—Collect bone and blood cultures before empiric therapy				
Newborn (<4 mos.)	S. aureus, Gm-neg. bacilli, Group B strep, Kingella kingae in children	MRSA possible: **Vanco + (Ceftaz or CFP)**	MRSA unlikely: (**Nafcillin** or **oxacillin**) + (**Ceftaz or CFP**)	Severe allergy or toxicity: (**Linezolid**^MM 10 mg/kg IV/po q8h + **aztreonam**).
Children (>4 mos.) — Adult: Osteo of extremity *(NEJM 370:352, 2014)*	S. aureus, Group A strep, Gm-neg. bacilli rare, Kingella kingae in children	MRSA possible: **Vanco 40 mg/kg/day div q6h**	MRSA unlikely: (**Nafcillin** or **oxacillin**) 150 mg/kg/day div q6h (max 12 gm)	Severe allergy or toxicity: **Clinda** or **TMP-SMX** or **linezolid**^MM. Adults: **ceftaz** 2 gm IV q8h, **CFP** 2 gm IV q12h. See Table 10B for adverse reactions to drugs.
Adult (>21 yrs) **Vertebral osteo ± epidural abscess** *(see IDSA guidelines for vertebral osteo: CID 61:859, 2015)*	S. aureus most common but variety other organisms. In Turkey: Brucella & M.TBc common	MRSA possible: **Vanco 15-20 mg/kg IV q 8-12h for trough of 15-20 µg/mL** (**Ceftriaxone** 2 gm q24h OR **CFP** 2 gm q8h OR **Levo** 750 mg q24h)	MRSA unlikely: **Nafcillin** OR **oxacillin** 2 gm IV q4h + (**Ceftriaxone** 2 gm q24h OR **CFP** 2 gm q8h OR **Levo** 750 mg q24h)	**Dx: MRI diagnostic test of choice, indicated to rule out epidural abscess.** For comprehensive review of vertebral osteomyelitis see NEJM 362:11, 2010. Whenever possible empirical therapy should be administered after cultures are obtained.
Blood & bone cultures essential				
Add **Ceftaz or CFP** if Gm-neg. bacilli on Gram stain Adult doses below.				
Specific therapy—Culture and in vitro susceptibility results known. See CID Jul 29, 2015 for IDSA Guidelines				
MSSA		**Nafcillin** or **oxacillin** 2 gm IV q4h or **cefazolin** 2 gm IV q8h	**Vanco** 15-30 mg/kg IV q 8-12h for trough of 15-20 µg/mL OR **Dapto** 6-8 mg/kg IV/day OR **Linezolid** 600 mg IV/po q12h	Other options if susceptible in vitro and allergy/toxicity issues **(see NEJM 362:11, 2010):** 1) **TMP-SMX** 8-10 mg/kg/d po/IV div q8h + **RIF** 300-450 mg po bid: limited data, particularly for MRSA (see AAC 53:2672, 2009); 2) **Levo** 750 mg po q24h) + **RIF** 600 mg po q24h; 3) **Fusidic acid** 500 mg IV q8h + **RIF** 300 mg po bid. *(CID 42:394, 2006)*; 4) **Ceftriaxone** 2 gm q24h
MRSA—See Table 6, page 82; IDSA Guidelines CID 52:e18-55, 2011; CID 52:285-92, 2011		**Vanco** 15-20 mg/kg IV q 8-12h for trough of 15-20 µg/mL) ± **RIF** 300-450 mg bid	**Linezolid** 600 mg q12h IV/po + **RIF** 300 mg po/IV bid OR **Dapto** 6 mg/kg q24h IV ± **RIF** 300-450 mg po/IV bid	*(CID 54:585, 2012)*(MSSA only). Duration of therapy 6 weeks, provided that epidural or paravertebral abscesses can be drained, consider longer course in those with extensive infection or abscess particularly if not amenable to drainage because of increased risk of treatment failure *(OFID Dec 5:1, 2014)* (although data are lacking that this approach improves efficacy versus a 6 wk course) and >8 weeks in patients undergoing device implantation.

TABLE 1 (2)

ANATOMIC SITE/DIAGNOSIS/ MODIFYING CIRCUMSTANCES	ETIOLOGIES (usual)	SUGGESTED REGIMENS*		ADJUNCT DIAGNOSTIC OR THERAPEUTIC MEASURES AND COMMENTS
		PRIMARY	**ALTERNATIVE§**	
BONE (continued)				
Hemoglobinopathy: Sickle cell/thalassemia	Salmonella, other Gm.-neg. bacilli	**CIP** 400 mg IV q12h OR **CIP** 750 mg PO bid	**Levo** 750 mg IV/PO q24h	Thalassemia: transfusion and iron chelation risk factors. Because of decreasing levels of susceptibility to fluoroquinolones among Salmonella spp. and growing resistance among other gram-negative bacilli, would add a second agent (e.g., third-generation cephalosporin) until susceptibility test results available. Alternative for salmonella is Ceftriaxone 2 gm IV q24h if nalidixic acid resistant
Contiguous Osteomyelitis Without Vascular Insufficiency				
Empiric therapy: Get cultures! Foot bone osteo due to nail through tennis shoe	P. aeruginosa	**CIP** 750 mg po bid or **Levo** 750 mg PO q24h	**Ceftaz** 2 gm IV q8h or **CFP** 2 gm IV q8h	See Skin—Nail puncture, page 56. Need debridement to remove foreign body.
Long bone, post-internal fixation of fracture	S. aureus, Gm.-neg. bacilli, P. aeruginosa	**Vanco** 15-20 mg/kg q8-12h IV for trough of 15-20 µg/mL + (**ceftaz** or **CFP**). See Comment	**Linezolid** 600 mg IV/po bid[NA] + (**ceftaz** or **CFP**). See Comment	Often necessary to remove hardware after union to achieve eradication. May need revascularization. **Regimens listed are empiric.** Adjust after culture data available. If susceptible Gm-neg. bacillus, **CIP** 750 mg po bid or **Levo** 750 mg po q24h. For other S. aureus options. See Hem. Osteo. Specific Therapy, page 4.
Osteonecrosis of the jaw	Probably rare adverse reaction to bisphosphonates	Infection may be secondary to bone necrosis and loss of overlying mucosa. Treatment: minimal surgical debridement, chlorhexidine rinses, antibiotics (e.g., PIP-TZ). Evaluate for concomitant actinomycosis, for which specific long-term antibiotic treatment would be warranted (CID 49:1729, 2009).		
Prosthetic joint	See prosthetic joint, page 33			
Spinal implant infection	S. aureus, coag-neg staphylococci, gram-neg bacilli	Onset within 30 days: culture, treat x 3 mos (CID 55:1481, 2012)	Onset after 30 days remove implant, culture & treat	See CID 55:1481, 2012
Sternum, post-op	S. aureus, S. epidermidis, occasionally, gram-negative bacilli	**Vanco** 15-20 mg/kg q8-12h IV for trough of 15-20 µg/mL recommended for serious infections.	**Linezolid** 600 mg po[NA][NB] bid	Sternal debridement for cultures & removal of necrotic bone. For S. aureus options: Hem. Osteo. Specific Therapy, page 4. If setting or gram stain suggests possibility of gram-negative bacilli, add appropriate coverage based on local antimicrobial susceptibility profiles (e.g. cefepime, PIP-TZ).
Contiguous Osteomyelitis With Vascular Insufficiency				
Most pts are diabetics with peripheral neuropathy & infected skin ulcers (see Diabetic foot, page 16)	Polymicrobic (Gm+ cocci (to include MRSA) (aerobic & anaerobic) and Gm-neg. bacilli (aerobic & anaerobic)	Debride overlying ulcer & submit bone for histology & culture. Select antibiotic based on culture results & treat for 6 weeks. **No empiric therapy unless acutely ill.** If acutely ill, see suggestions, Diabetic foot, page 16. Revascularize if possible.		**Diagnosis of osteo:** Culture bone biopsy (gold standard). Poor concordance of culture results between swab of ulcer and bone (CID 42:57, 63, 2008). Sampling by needle puncture inferior to biopsy (CID 48:888, 2009). Osteo more likely if ulcer >2 cm², positive probe to bone. ESR >70 & abnormal plain x-ray (JAMA 299:806, 2008). **Treatment:** (1) **Revascularize if possible;** (2) Culture bone; (3) Specific antimicrobial(s). Reviews: BMJ 339:b4905, 2006; Plast Reconstr Surg 117: (7 Suppl) 212S, 2006.
Chronic Osteomyelitis: Specific therapy By definition, implies presence of dead bone. **Need valid cultures**	S. aureus, Enterobacteriaceae, P. aeruginosa	**Empiric rx not indicated.** Base systemic rx on results of culture, sensitivity testing. If acute exacerbation of chronic osteo, rx as acute hematogenous osteo. Surgical debridement important.		**Important adjuncts:** removal of orthopedic hardware, surgical debridement, vascularized muscle flaps, distraction osteogenesis (Ilizarov) techniques. Antibiotic-impregnated cement & hyperbaric oxygen adjunctive measures. **NOTE: RIF** + (**vanco** or **β-lactam**) effective in animal model and in a clinical trial of S. aureus chronic osteo. The contribution of rifampin-containing regimens in this setting is not clear, however (AAC 53:2672, 2009).

Abbreviations on page 2.

*NOTE: All dosage recommendations are for adults (unless otherwise indicated) and assume normal renal function. PK, compliance, local/resistance, cost § Alternatives consider allergy, PK, compliance, local/resistance, cost

TABLE 1 (3)

ANATOMIC SITE/DIAGNOSIS/ MODIFYING CIRCUMSTANCES	ETIOLOGIES (usual)	SUGGESTED REGIMENS*		ADJUNCT DIAGNOSTIC OR THERAPEUTIC MEASURES AND COMMENTS
		PRIMARY	ALTERNATIVE†	
BREAST: Mastitis—Obtain culture; need to know if MRSA present. Review with definitions: BMJ 342:d396, 2011.				
Postpartum mastitis (Recent Cochrane Review: Cochrane Database Syst Rev 2013 Feb 28;2:CD005458; see also CID 54:71, 2012)				
Mastitis without abscess	S. aureus; less often S. pyogenes (Grp. A or B), E. coli, bacteroides species, maybe Corynebacterium sp. & selected coagulase-neg. staphylococci (e.g. S. lugdunensis)	**NO MRSA: Outpatient: Dicloxacillin** 500 mg po qid or **cephalexin** 500 mg po qid. **Inpatient: Nafcillin/oxacillin** 2 gm IV q4-6h	**MRSA Possible: Outpatient: TMP-SMX-DS** tabs 1-2 po bid or (if susceptible, **clinda** 300 mg po tid **Inpatient: Vanco** 1 gm IV q12h; if over 100 kg, 1.5 gm IV q12h.	If no abscess & controllable pain, ↑ freq of nursing may hasten response.
Mastitis with abscess				For painful abscess I&D is standard; needle aspiration reported successful. Resume breast feeding from affected breast as soon as pain allows. (Breastfeed Med 9:239, 2014)
Non-puerperal mastitis with abscess	S. aureus; less often Bacteroides sp., peptostreptococcus, & selected coagulase-neg. staphylococci	See regimens for Postpartum mastitis, page 6.		Smoking and diabetes may be risk factors (BMJ 342:d396, 2011). If subareolar & odoriferous, most likely anaerobes; need to **add metro** 500 mg IV/po tid. If not subareolar, staph. Need pretreatment aerobic/anaerobic cultures. Surgical drainage for abscess. **I&D standard.** Corynebacterium sp. assoc. with chronic granulomatous mastitis (JCM 53:2895, 2015). **Consider TB in chronic infections.**
Breast implant infection	Acute: S. aureus, S. pyogenes. Chronic: Look for rapidly growing Mycobacteria	Acute: **Vanco** 15-20 mg/kg IV q8-12h.	Chronic: Await culture results. See Table 12A for mycobacteria treatment.	Lancet Infect Dis 5:94, 462, 2005. Coag-negative staph also common (Aesthetic Plastic Surg 31:325, 2007).
CENTRAL NERVOUS SYSTEM				
Brain abscess				
Primary or contiguous source in 51 pts, 39 positive by standard culture using molecular diagnostics, 80 bacterial taxa & many polymicrobics (CID 54:202, 2012). Review: NEJM 371:447, 2014. Mild infection: NEJM 371:150, 2014.	Streptococci (60-70%), bacteroides (20-40%), Enterobacteriaceae (23-33%), S. aureus (10-15%), S. anginosus grp. Rare: Nocardia (below), Listeria. See S. aureus Comment	**P Ceph 3** [(**cefotaxime** 2 gm IV q4h or **ceftriaxone** 2 gm IV q12h) + (**metro** 7.5 mg/kg q6h or 15 mg/kg IV q12h)]	**Pen G** 3-4 million units IV q4h + **metro** 7.5 mg/kg q6h or 15 mg/kg IV q12h	If CT scan suggests cerebritis or abscesses <2.5 cm and pt neurologically stable and conscious, start antibiotics and observe. Otherwise, surgical drainage necessary. If blood cultures or other clinical data do not yield a likely etiologic agent, aspirate even small abscesses for diagnosis if this can be done safely.
		— Duration of rx unclear; usually 4-6 wks or until resolution by neuroimaging (CT/MRI) —		Experience with Pen G (HD) + metro without ceftriaxone or nafcillin/oxacillin has been good. We use ceftriaxone because of frequency of isolation of Enterobacteriaceae. **S. aureus is rare without positive culture;** if S. aureus, use vanco until susceptibility known. Strep. anginosus group esp. prone to produce abscess. Ceph/metro does not cover listeria
Post-surgical, post-traumatic. Review: NEJM 371:447, 2014.	S. aureus, Enterobacteriaceae	**For MSSA: Nafcillin or oxacillin** 2 gm IV q4h + (**ceftriaxone** or **cefotaxime**)	**For MRSA: Vanco** 15-20 mg/kg IV q 8-12h for trough of 15-20 mcg/mL + (**ceftriaxone** or **cefotaxime**)	Empirical coverage, de-escalated based on culture results. **Aspiration of abscess usually necessary for dx & rx. If P. aeruginosa suspected, substitute (Cefepime or Ceftazidime) for (Ceftriaxone or Cefotaxime).**
HIV-1 infected (AIDS)	Toxoplasma gondii	See Table 13A, page 156		

Abbreviations on page 2.   *NOTE: All dosage recommendations are for adults (unless otherwise indicated) and assume normal renal function. § Alternatives consider allergy, PK, compliance, local resistance, cost

TABLE 1 (4)

ANATOMIC SITE/DIAGNOSIS/ MODIFYING CIRCUMSTANCES	ETIOLOGIES (usual)	SUGGESTED REGIMENS* PRIMARY	SUGGESTED REGIMENS* ALTERNATIVE†	ADJUNCT DIAGNOSTIC OR THERAPEUTIC MEASURES AND COMMENTS
CENTRAL NERVOUS SYSTEM/Brain abscess *(continued)*				
Nocardia: Haematogenous abscess	N. farcinica, N. asteroides & N. brasiliensis See *AAC 58:795, 2014* for other species.	**TMP-SMX:** 15 mg/kg/day of TMP & 75 mg/kg/day of SMX, IV/po div in 2-4 doses + **Imipenem** 500 mg q6h IV. If multiorgan involvement some add **amikacin** 7.5 mg/kg q12h. After 3-6 wks of IV therapy, switch to po therapy. Immunocompetent pts: **TMP-SMX, minocycline** or **AM-CL** x 3+ months. Immunocompromised pts: Treat with 2 drugs x 1 yr.	**Linezolid** 600 mg IV or po q12h + meropenem 2 gm q8h.	**Linezolid** 600 mg po bid reported effective. For in vitro susceptibility testing: Wallace (+1) 903-877-7680 or U.S. CDC (+1) 404-639-3158. In vitro resistance to TMP-SMX may be increasing (*Clin Infect Dis 51:1445, 2010*), but whether this is clinically relevant is not known; Project: worse outcomes is not known; Project: TMP-SMX remains a drug of choice for CNS nocardia infection. If sulfonamide resistant or sulfa-allergic, **amikacin** plus one of: **IMP**, **MER**, **ceftriaxone** or **cefotaxime** N. farcinica is resistant to third-generation cephalosporins, which should not be used for treatment of infection caused by this organism. If TMP-SMX resistance reported, see *JCM 50:670, 2012* (before stopping TMP-SMX).
Subdural empyema: In adult 60-90% is extension of sinusitis or otitis media. Rx same as primary brain abscess. Surgical emergency: must drain. Review in *LnID 7:62, 2007.*				
Encephalitis/encephalopathy IDSA Guideline: *CID 47:303, 2008;* Intl diagnosis consensus: *CID 57:1114, 2013.* (For Herpes see *Table 14A, page 169* and for rabies, *Table 20B, page 233*)	H. simplex (42%), VZV (15%), Listeria (10%). Other: arboviruses, West Nile, rabies, Lyme, Parvo B19, Cat-scratch: Mycoplasma, EBV and others	Start IV **acyclovir** while awaiting results of CSF PCR for H. simplex. For amebic encephalitis see *Table 13A*. Start **Doxy** if setting suggests R. rickettsii, Anaplasma, Ehrlichia or Mycoplasma.		Review of all etiologies: *LnID 10:835, 2010.* **Anti-NMDAR** (N-Methyl-D-Aspartate Receptor) encephalitis: an autoimmune encephalitis; more common than individual viral etiologies as a cause of encephalitis in the California Encephalitis Project cohort (*CID 54:899, 2012*). Refs: *Chest 145:1143, 2014; J Clin Neuroscience 21:722 & 1169, 2014.*
Meningitis, "Aseptic": Pleocytosis of up to 100s of cells, CSF glucose normal, neg. culture for bacteria (see *Table 14A, page 166*) Ref: *CID 47:783, 2008*	Enteroviruses, HSV-2, LCM, HIV, other viruses, drugs [NSAIDs, metronidazole, carbamazepine, lamotrigine, TMP-SMX, IVIG, (e.g., detuximab), infliximab)]; rarely leptospirosis	For all but leptospirosis, IV fluids and analgesics. D/C drugs that may be etiologic. For lepto (**doxy** 100 mg IV/po q12h) or (**Pen G** 5 million units IV q6h) or (**AMP** 0.5-1 gm IV q6h). Repeat LP if suspect partially-treated bacterial meningitis. **Acyclovir** 5-10 mg/kg IV q8h sometimes given for HSV-2 meningitis (Note: distinct from HSV encephalitis where early rx is mandatory).		If available, PCR of CSF for enterovirus HSV-2 unusual without concomitant genital herpes (Mollaret's syndrome). For lepto, positive exposure epidemiologic history and concomitant hepatitis, conjunctivitis, dermatitis, nephritis. For list of implicated drugs: *Inf Med 25:331, 2008.*

Abbreviations on page 2.   *NOTE: All dosage recommendations are for adults (unless otherwise indicated) and assume normal renal function. § Alternatives consider allergy, PK, compliance, local resistance, cost

TABLE 1 (5)

ANATOMIC SITE/DIAGNOSIS/ MODIFYING CIRCUMSTANCES	ETIOLOGIES (usual)	SUGGESTED REGIMENS*		ADJUNCT DIAGNOSTIC OR THERAPEUTIC MEASURES AND COMMENTS
		PRIMARY	ALTERNATIVE†	
Meningitis, Bacterial, Acute. Goal is empiric therapy, then CSF exam within 30 min. If focal neurologic deficit, give empiric therapy, then head CT, then LP. (NEJM 354:44, 2006; Ln ID 10:32, 2010) **NOTE:** In children, treatment caused CSF cultures to be negative by 2 hrs when given with meningococcal & in partial response with pneumococci in 4 hrs (Peds 108:1169, 2001). For distribution of pathogens by age group, see NEJM 364:2016, 2011.				
Empiric Therapy—CSF Gram stain is negative—immunocompetent				
Age: **Preterm to <1 mo**	Group B strep 49%, E. coli 18% klebsiella 4%, misc. Gm-neg. 10%, misc. Gm-pos. 10%	AMP 100 mg/kg IV q6h + cefotaxime 50 mg/kg IV q6h	AMP 100 mg/kg IV q6h + gentamicin 2.5 mg/kg IV q8h	Regimens active vs. Group B strep, most coliforms, & listeria. If premature infant with long nursery stay, S. aureus, enterococci, and resistant coliforms potential pathogens, **optional empiric regimens (except for listeria): [nafcillin + (cefotaxime or ceftazidime)]. If high risk of MRSA, use vanco + cefotaxime. Alter regimen after culture/sensitivity data available.**
Age: **Preterm to <1 mo**		Intraventricular treatment not recommended.	Repeat CSF exam/culture 24–36 hr after start of therapy.	
Age: **1 mo–50 yrs** Hearing loss is 1st most common neurologic sequelae (Ln ID 10:32, 2010)	S. pneumo, meningococci, H. influenzae now uncommon, listeria unlikely in young adult & immunocompetent (add ampicillin if suspect listeria: 2 gm IV q4h)	Adult dosage: **((Cefotaxime 2 gm IV q4-6h OR ceftriaxone 2 gm IV q12h)) + vanco (dexamethasone)** For vanco dose, see footnote. **Dexamethasone:** 0.15 mg/kg IV q6h x 2-4 days. Give with, or just before, 1st dose of antibiotic (See Comment).** See footnote¹ for Vanco Adult dosage and¹ for ped. dosage	**((MER 2 gm IV q8h) (Peds: 40 mg/kg IV q8h)) + vanco (dexamethasone)** For severe pen. Allergy. **Dexamethasone:** 0.15 mg/kg IV q6h x 2-4 days to block TNF production (See Comment).	Value of **dexamethasone** shown in children with H. influenzae and adults with S. pneumoniae in some studies (NEJM 357:2431 & 2441, 2007; Ln ID 4:139, 2004). In the Netherlands, adoption of dexamethasone treatment in adult pneumococcal meningitis led to reduced mortality and hearing loss compared with historical control group (Neurology 75:1533, 2010). For patients with severe β-lactam allergy, see below (Empiric Therapy—positive gram stain and Specific Therapy) for alternative therapies.
Age: **≥50 yrs or alcoholism** or other debilitating assoc diseases or impaired cellular immunity	S. pneumo, listeria, Gm-neg. bacilli.	**(AMP 2 gm IV q4h) + (ceftriaxone 2 gm IV q12h or cefotaxime 2 gm IV q4-6h) + vanco ± IV dexamethasone** For vanco dose, see footnote.¹ 0.15 mg/kg IV q6h x 2-4 days, see Comment	**MER 2 gm IV q8h + vanco ± IV dexamethasone** For severe pen. Allergy. **Dexamethasone** dose: Give before, or concomitant with, 1st dose of antibiotic.	For patients with severe **β-lactam allergy**, see below (Empiric Therapy—positive gram stain and Specific Therapy) for alternative agents that can be substituted to cover likely pathogens. LP without CT for patients with altered level of consciousness and non-focal neurological exam associated with earlier treatment and improved outcome (CID 60:1162, 2015)
Post-neurosurgery Ventriculostomy/lumbar catheter; ventriculoperitoneal (VP) shunt[2] or Penetrating trauma w/o basilar skull fracture Ref: intraventricular therapy (J Micro Immunol & Infect 47:204, 2014)	S. epidermidis, S. aureus, P. acnes. Facultative and aerobic gram-neg bacilli, including: P. aeruginosa & A. baumannii (may be multi-drug resistant)	**Vanco** (to achieve trough level of 15-20 µg/mL) + **Cefepime or Ceftaz 2 gm IV q8h** — **If severe Pen/Ceph allergy,** substitute either: **Aztreonam** 2 gm IV q6-8h or **CIP** 400 mg IV q12h. **Intraventricular Rx if IV therapy inadequate or device not removed.** Intraventricular daily drug doses: Adult: **Vanco** 10-20 mg; **Gent** 4-8 mg; **Colistin** (base activity) 1.25 mg or 0.375 mg once a day; **Polymyxin B** 5 mg. Peds: Gent 1-2 mg; Polymyxin B 2 mg. See Comment	**Vanco** (to achieve trough level of 15-20 µg/mL) + **[MER 2 gm IV q8h]** **Vanco** + **If severe Pen/Ceph allergy,** for possible gram-negative bacilli or device removal/replacement. Adult: Vanco 5-20 mg; Gent 4-8 mg once daily; Colistin base activity 1.25 mg once daily; Polymyxin B 5 mg.	- Remove infected shunt and place external ventricular catheter for drainage or pressure control. - Intraventricular therapy used if the shunt cannot be removed or cultures fail to clear with systemic therapy. Logic for intraventricular therapy: achieve a 10-20 ratio of CSF concentration to MIC of infecting bacteria. Use only preservative-free drug. Clamp/close catheter for 1 hr after instillation of antibiotics into ventricles (CID 39:1267, 2004; CID 52:1858, 2010). - **Systemically ill patient:** systemic therapy once pathogen-directed intraventricular therapy once culture results are available. - **Not systemically ill,** indolent Gram-positive: can D/C systemic vanco/rifampin and treat with daily intraventricular therapy. - **Shunt reimplantation:** (1) coagulase-negative staphylococci or diphtheroids, or P. acnes may reimplant shunt after 3-4 days CSF cultures are negative, no further systemic therapy needed; (2) For Staph. aureus and Gram-negative bacilli, may internalize shunt after 3 serial CSF cultures are negative and then treat with systemic therapy for an additional week. Ref: N Engl J Med 362:146, 2010.
Trauma with basilar skull fracture	S. pneumoniae, H. influenzae, S. pyogenes	**Vanco** (to achieve trough level of 15-20 µg/mL) + **(Ceftriaxone** 50 mg/kg IV q6h; **cefriaxone** 50 mg/kg IV q12h; **vanco** 15 mg/kg IV q6h to achieve trough level of 15-20 µg/mL	**Vanco** (to achieve trough level of 15-20 µg/mL) + **(Cefriaxone** 2 gm IV q24h) + **[Dexamethasone** 0.15 mg/kg]	**Alternatives consider allergy, PK, compliance, local resistance, cost and clinical week.** Ref Clin Micro Rev 21:519, 2008.

¹ **Vanco adult dose:** 15-20 mg/kg IV q8-12h to achieve trough level of 15-20 µg/mL
² **Dosage of drugs used to treat children ≥1 mo of age: Cefotaxime** 50 mg/kg per day IV q6h; **ceftriaxone** 50 mg/kg IV q12h; **vanco** 15 mg/kg IV q6h to achieve trough level of 15-20 µg/mL

Abbreviations on page 2.

* **NOTE:** All dosage recommendations are for adults (unless otherwise indicated) and assume normal renal function.
† Alternatives consider allergy, PK, compliance, local resistance, cost
* Dosage of drugs used to treat children ≥1 mo of age.

See Clin Micro Rev 21:519, 2008.

TABLE 1 (6)

ANATOMIC SITE/DIAGNOSIS/ MODIFYING CIRCUMSTANCES	ETIOLOGIES (usual)	SUGGESTED REGIMENS* PRIMARY	SUGGESTED REGIMENS* ALTERNATIVE†	ADJUNCT DIAGNOSTIC OR THERAPEUTIC MEASURES AND COMMENTS
CENTRAL NERVOUS SYSTEM/Meningitis, Bacterial, Acute *(continued)*				
Empiric Therapy—Positive CSF Gram stain				
Gram-positive diplococci	S. pneumoniae	(**ceftriaxone** 2 gm IV q12h or **cefotaxime** 2 gm IV q4-6h) + **vanco** 15-20 mg/kg IV q8-12h (to achieve 15-20 µg/mL trough) + timed **dexamethasone** 0.15 mg/kg q6h IV x 2-4 days	**Alternatives: MER** 2 gm IV q8h or **Moxi** 400 mg IV q24h. **Dexamethasone** does not block penetration of vanco into CSF (CID 44:250, 2007).
Gram-negative diplococci	N. meningitidis	(**Cefotaxime** 2 gm IV q4-6h or **ceftriaxone** 2 gm IV q12h)	**Alternatives: Pen G** 4 mill. units IV q4h or **AMP** 2 gm IV q4h or **Moxi** 400 mg IV q24h or **chloro** 1 gm IV q6h (Chloro less effective than other alternatives; see JAC 70:979, 2015)
Gram-positive bacilli or coccobacilli	Listeria monocytogenes	AMP 2 gm IV q4h ± gentamicin 2 mg/kg IV loading dose then 1.7 mg/kg IV q8h	**If pen-allergic, use** TMP-SMX 5 mg/kg IV q6-8h or MER 2 gm IV q8h
Gram-negative bacilli	H. influenzae, coliforms, P. aeruginosa	(Ceftazidime or cefepime 2 gm IV q8h) ± gentamicin 2 mg/kg IV 1ˢᵗ dose then 1.7 mg/kg IV q8h (See Comment)	**Alternatives: CIP** 400 mg IV q8-12h; **MER** 2 gm IV q8h. **Aztreonam** 2 gm IV q6-8h. Consider adding intravenous **Gentamicin** to the β-lactam or **CIP** if gram-stain and clinical setting suggest P. aeruginosa or resistant coliforms.
Specific Therapy—Positive culture of CSF with in vitro susceptibility results available.				
H. influenzae	β-lactamase positive	**Ceftriaxone** 2 gm IV q12h (adult); 50 mg/kg IV q12h (peds)	**Pen. allergic: Chloro** 12.5 mg/kg IV q6h (max. 4 gm/day.) (Chloro less effective than other alternatives: see JAC 70:979, 2015); **CIP** 400 mg IV q8-12h; **Aztreonam** 2 gm IV q6-8h.
Listeria monocytogenes (CID 43:1233, 2006)		AMP 2 gm IV q4h ± **gentamicin** 2 mg/kg IV loading dose, then 1.7 mg/kg IV q8h	**Pen. allergic:** TMP-SMX 20 mg/kg per day div. q6-12h. **Alternative: MER** 2 gm IV q8h. Success reported with linezolid + RIF (CID 40:907, 2005) after AMP for brain abscess with meningitis.
N. meningitidis	Pen MIC 0.1-1 mcg per mL	**Ceftriaxone** or **cefotaxime** 2 gm IV q12h x 7 days (see Comment); if β-lactam allergic, **chloro** 12.5 mg/kg or 1 gm IV q6h (Chloro less effective than other alternatives. see JAC 70:979, 2015)	
S. pneumoniae	Pen G MIC			Rare isolates chloro-resistant. FQ-resistant isolates encountered.
	<0.1 mcg/mL	Pen G 4 million units IV q4h or **AMP** 2 gm IV q4h		
NOTES: 1. Assumes dexamethasone just prior to 1ˢᵗ dose & x 4 days 2. If MIC ≥1, repeat CSF exam after 24-48h. 3. Treat for 10-14 days	0.1-1 mcg/mL	**Ceftriaxone** 2 gm IV q12h or **cefotaxime** 2 gm IV q4-6h	**Vanco** 15-20 mg/kg IV q8-12h (15-20 µg/mL trough target) + (**ceftriaxone** or **cefotaxime** as above)	**Alternatives: Ceftriaxone** 2 gm IV q12h; **chloro** 1 gm IV q6h (Chloro less effective than other alternatives): see JAC 70:979, 2015)
	≥2 mcg/mL	**Ceftriaxone** 2 gm IV q12h or **cefotaxime** 2 gm IV q4-6h	**Vanco** 15-20 mg/kg IV q8-12h (15-20 µg/mL trough target) + (**ceftriaxone** or **cefotaxime** as above)	**Alternatives: Cefepime** 2 gm IV q8h or **MER** 2 gm IV q8h. **Alternatives: Moxi** 400 mg IV q24h
	Ceftriaxone MIC ≥1 mcg/mL			**Alternatives: Moxi** 400 mg IV q24h If MIC to ceftriaxone >2 mcg/mL, add RIF 600 mg po/IV 1x/day to **vanco** + (**ceftriaxone** or **cefotaxime**).
E. coli, other coliforms, or P. aeruginosa	Consultation advised— need susceptibility results	(Ceftazidime or cefepime 2 gm IV q8h) + gentamicin 2 mg/kg IV x 1 dose, then 1.7 mg/kg IV q8h x 21 days. Repeat CSF cultures in 2-4 days.		**Alternatives: CIP** 400 mg IV q8-12h; **MER** 2 gm IV q8h. If pos. CSF culture after 2-4 days, start intraventricular therapy; see Meningitis, Post-neurosurgery, page 8.
Prophylaxis for H. influenzae and N. meningitidis				
Haemophilus influenzae type B		**Children: RIF** 20 mg/kg po (not to exceed 600 mg) q24h x 4 doses		**Household:** If there is one unvaccinated contact age ≤4 yrs in the household, give prophylaxis to all (adults & children) in the home except pregnant women.
For 1st 24 hrs in a day care contact residing with index case or same day care facility as index case for 5-7 days before onset		**Adults (non-pregnant): RIF** 600 mg q24h x 4 days		**Child Care Facilities:** With 1 case, if attended by unvaccinated children ≤2 yrs, consider prophylaxis + vaccinate susceptible. If all contacts >2 yrs no prophylaxis. If ≥ 2 cases in 60 days & unvaccinated children attend, prophylaxis recommended for children & personnel (Am Acad Ped Red Book 2006, page 313).

Abbreviations on page 2.   *NOTE: All dosage recommendations are for adults (unless otherwise indicated) and assume normal renal function. § Alternatives consider allergy, PK, compliance, local resistance, cost

TABLE 1 (7)

ANATOMIC SITE/DIAGNOSIS/ MODIFYING CIRCUMSTANCES	ETIOLOGIES (usual)	SUGGESTED REGIMENS*		ADJUNCT DIAGNOSTIC OR THERAPEUTIC MEASURES AND COMMENTS
		PRIMARY	ALTERNATIVE[1]	
CENTRAL NERVOUS SYSTEM/Meningitis, Bacterial, Acute/Prophylaxis for H. influenzae and N. meningitides (continued)				
Prophylaxis for Neisseria meningitidis exposure (close contact) Pre-exposure **NOTE:** CDC reports **CIP-resistant group B meningococcus** from selected counties in N. Dakota & Minnesota. **Avoid CIP.** Use **ceftriaxone, RIF,** or single 500 mg dose of **azithro** (*MMWR 57:173, 2008*).		**Ceftriaxone** 250 mg IM x 1 dose (child <15 yrs 125 mg IM x 1) **OR [RIF** 600 mg po q12h x 4 doses. (Children ≥1 mo 10 mg/kg po q12h x 4 doses, <1 mo 5 mg/kg q12h x 4 doses) **OR** If not CIP-resistant, **CIP** 500 mg po x 1 dose (adult)		**Spread by respiratory droplets,** not aerosols, hence close contact req. ↑ risk if close contact for at least 4 hrs during wk before illness onset (e.g., housemates, day care contacts, cellmates) or exposure to pt's nasopharyngeal secretions (e.g., kissing, mouth-to-mouth resuscitation, intubation, nasotracheal suctioning).
Meningitis, chronic Defined as symptoms + CSF pleocytosis for ≥4 wks	MTB cryptococcosis, other fungal, neoplastic, Lyme, syphilis, Whipple's disease	Treatment depends on etiology. No urgent need for empiric therapy, but when TB suspected treatment should be expeditious.		Long list of possibilities: bacteria, parasites, fungi, viruses, neoplasms, vasculitis, and other miscellaneous etiologies—see *Neurol Clin 28:1061, 2010.* See *NEJM 370:2408, 2014* for diagnosis of neuroleptospirosis by next generation sequencing technologies.
Meningitis, eosinophilic *LnID 8:621, 2008*	Angiostrongyliasis, gnathostomiasis, baylisascaris	Corticosteroids	Not sure anthelmintic therapy works	1/3 lack peripheral eosinophilia. Need serology to confirm diagnosis. Steroid ref.: *LnID 8:621, 2008.* Automated CSF count may not correctly identify eosinophils (*CID 48:322, 2009*).
Meningitis, HIV-1 infected (AIDS) See *Table 11, SANFORD GUIDE TO HIV/AIDS THERAPY*	As in adults, >50 yrs: also consider cryptococci, M. tuberculosis, syphilis, HIV aseptic meningitis, Listeria monocytogenes	If etiology not identified: treat as adult >50 yrs + obtain CSF/serum crypto-coccal antigen (*see Comments*)	For crypto rx, *see Table 11A, page 127*	C. neoformans most common etiology in AIDS patients. H. influenzae, pneumococci, listeria, TBc, syphilis, viral, histoplasma & coccidioides also need to be considered. Obtain blood cultures.
EAR				
External otitis				
Chronic	Usually 2° to seborrhea	Eardrops: [**polymyxin B + neomycin + hydrocorti-sone** qid] + **selenium sulfide shampoo]**		Control seborrhea with dandruff shampoo containing selenium sulfide (Selsun) or [ketoconazole shampoo] + (medium potency steroid solution, triamcinolone 0.1%)].
Fungal	Candida species	**Fluconazole** 200 mg po x 1 dose & then 100 mg po x 3-5 days.		
"Necrotizing (malignant) otitis externa" Risk groups: Diabetes mellitus, AIDS, chemotherapy.	Pseudomonas aeruginosa in >95% (*Otol & Neurotology 34:620, 2013*)	**CIP** 400 mg IV q8h: 750 mg po q8-12h only for early disease	**PIP-TZ** 3.375 gm q4h or extended infusion 3.375 gm over 4 hrs q8h) + **Tobra**	Very high ESRs are typical. Debridement usually required. R/O osteomyelitis. CT or MRI scan. If bone involved, treat for 6-8 wks. Other alternatives if P. aeruginosa susceptible: **IMP** 0.5 gm q6h or **MER** 1 gm IV q8h or **CFP** 2 gm IV q12h or **Ceftaz** 2 gm IV q8h.
"Swimmer's ear"; occlusive devices (earphones); contact dermatitis, psoriasis	Acute infection usually 2° S. aureus (11%), other Pseudomonas (11%), Anaerobes (2%), S. epidermidis (46%), candida (8%)	Mild: eardrops: **acetic acid + propylene glycol + HC** (**Vosol HC**) 5 gtts 3-4x/day until resolved. Moderate-severe: Eardrops **CIP + HC** (**Cipro HC Otic**) 3 gtts bid x 7 days. Alternative: **Finafloxacin** 0.3% otic suspension 4 gtts q12h x 7d (for P. aeruginosa and S. aureus)		Rx includes gentle cleaning. Recurrences prevented (or decreased) by drying with alcohol drops (1/3 white vinegar, 2/3 rubbing alcohol) after swimming, then antibiotic drops or 2% acetic acid solution. Ointments should not be used in ear. Do not use neomycin or other aminoglycoside drops if tympanic membrane punctured.

*NOTE: All dosage recommendations are for adults (unless otherwise indicated) and assume normal renal function. § Alternatives consider allergy, PK, compliance, local resistance, cost

TABLE 1 (8)

ANATOMIC SITE/DIAGNOSIS/ MODIFYING CIRCUMSTANCES	ETIOLOGIES (usual)	SUGGESTED REGIMENS*		ADJUNCT DIAGNOSTIC OR THERAPEUTIC MEASURES AND COMMENTS
		PRIMARY	ALTERNATIVE†	
EAR (continued)				
Otitis media—infants, children, adults (Cochrane review: Cochrane Database Syst Rev. Jan 31;1:CD000219, 2013; *American Academy of Pediatrics Guidelines: Pediatrics 131:e964, 2013*)				
Acute Two PRDB trials indicate efficacy of antibiotic rx if age < 36 mos & definite AOM (*NEJM 364:105, 116 & 168, 2011*)				
Initial empiric therapy of acute otitis media (AOM) NOTE: **Treat children <2 yrs old.** If >2 yrs old, afebrile, no ear pain/less/ questionable exam, consider analgesic treatment without antimicrobials. Favorable results in mostly afebrile pts with waiting 48hrs before deciding on antibiotic use (*JAMA 296:1235, 1290, 2006*)	Overall detection in middle ear fluid: No pathogen 4% Virus 70% Bact. + virus 66% Bacteria 92% Bacterial pathogens from middle ear: S. pneumo 49%, H. influenzae 29%, M. catarrhalis 28%. Ref.: (*CID 43:1417 & 1423, 2006. Children 6 mos-3 yrs. 2 episodes AOM/yrs & 63% are virus positive (CID 46:815 & 824, 2008)*)	**If NO antibiotics in prior month:** Amox po HD[3] For dosage, *see footnotes*. **All doses are pediatric** **Duration of rx:** <2 yrs old x 10 days; ≥2 yrs x 5-7 days. Appropriate duration unclear. May be inadequate for severe disease (*NEJM 347:1169, 2002*) **For adult dosages, see** *Sinusitis, page 50, and Table 10A*	**Received antibiotics in prior month:** Amox·HD[3] or **AM-CL** extra-strength[4] or **cefdinir** or **cefpodoxime** or **cefprozil or cefuroxime axetil** For dosage, *see footnotes*. **All doses are pediatric**	**If allergic to β-lactam drugs?** If history unclear or rash, effective oral ceph OK; with eff & IgE-mediated allergy, e.g., anaphylaxis. High failure rate with **TMP-SMX** if etiology is DRSP or H. influenzae; azithro/clarithro have limited efficacy against S. pneumo and H. influenzae. **Spontaneous resolution occurred in:** 90% pts infected with M. catarrhalis, 50% with H. influenzae, 10% with S. pneumoniae; overall 80% resolve within 2-14 days (*Ln 363:465, 2004*). Risk of DRSP ↑ if age <2 yrs, antibiotics last 3 mos, &/or daycare attendance. Selection of drug based on (1) effectiveness against β-lactamase producing H. influenzae & M. catarrhalis, & (2) effectiveness against S. pneumo, inc. DRSP. **Cefaclor, loracarbef, & ceftibuten less active vs. resistant S. pneumo.** than other agents listed. No benefit of antibiotics in treatment of otitis media with effusion (*Cochrane Database Syst Rev. Sep 12;9:CD009163, 2012*). For persistent otorrhea with PE tubes, hydrocortisone/bacitracin/colistin eardrops[M15] & 5 drops tid x 7 d more effective than po AM-CL (*NEJM 370:723, 2014*).
Treatment for clinical failure after 3 days	Drug-resistant S. pneumoniae main concern	**NO antibiotics prior to last 3 days:** AM-CL high dose or **cefdinir** or **cefpodoxime** or **cefprozil** or **cefuroxime axetil** or **ceftriaxone** x 3 days. For dosage, *see footnotes*. **All doses are pediatric** Duration of rx as above	**Antibiotics in month prior to last 3 days:** ((IM) ceftriaxone) and/or (clindamycin) and/or (tympanocentesis) *See clindamycin Comments*	**Clindamycin** not active vs. H. influenzae or M. catarrhalis. S. pneumo usually also resistant to clindamycin. Definition of failure: no change in ear pain, fever, bulging TM or otorrhea after 3 days of therapy. Tympanocentesis will allow culture. **Newer FQs active vs. drug-resistant S. pneumo (DRSP), but not approved for use in children** (*PIDJ 23:390, 2004*). **Vanco is active vs. DRSP.**
After >48hrs of nasotracheal intubation	Pseudomonas sp., Klebsiella, enterobacter	Ceftazidime or CFP or IMP or MER or (PIP-TZ) or CIP. (*For dosages, see Ear, Necrotizing (malignant) otitis externa, page 10*)		With nasotracheal intubation >48 hrs, about ½ pts will have otitis media with effusion.

Abbreviations on page 2.

NOTE: All dosage recommendations are for adults (unless otherwise indicated) and assume normal renal function. § Alternatives consider allergy, PK, compliance, local resistance, cost

[3] **Amoxicillin UD or HD** = amoxicillin usual dose or high dose; **AM-CL HD** = amoxicillin-clavulanate high dose. Data supporting amoxicillin HD: *PIDJ 22:405, 2003.*
[4] **Drugs & peds dosage (all po unless specified) for acute otitis media: Amoxicillin HD** = 40 mg/kg per day div q12h or q8h. **Amoxicillin HD** = 90 mg/kg per day div q12h or q8h. **AM-CL HD** = 90 mg/kg per day div q12h. **Extra-strength AM-CL oral suspension** (Augmentin ES-600) available with 600 mg AM & 42.9 mg CL / 5 mL—dose 90 mg/kg per day div bid. **Cefuroxime axetil** 30 mg/kg per day div q12h. **Ceftriaxone** 50 mg/kg IM x 3 days. **Clindamycin** 20-30 mg/kg per day div qid (may be effective vs. DRSP but no activity vs. H. influenzae)
Other drugs suitable for drug (e.g., penicillin) - sensitive S. pneumo: TMP-SMX 4 mg/kg of TMP q12h. Erythro-sulfisoxazole 50 mg/kg per day of erythro div q6-8h; **Clarithro** 15 mg/kg per day div q12h. Other FDA-approved regimens: 10 mg/kg q24h on days 2-5. Other FDA-approved regimens: **azithro** 10 mg/kg per day x 1.8 then 5 mg/kg q24h on days 2-5; 30 mg/kg x 1 & 30 mg/kg q24h x 3 days & 30 mg/kg x 1. **Cefprozil** 15 mg/kg q12h. **cefpodoxime proxetil** 10 mg/kg per day as single dose; **cefaclor** 40 mg/kg per day q8h; **loracarbef** 15 mg/kg q12h. **Cefdinir** 7 mg/kg q12h or 14 mg/kg q24h.

TABLE 1 (9)

ANATOMIC SITE/DIAGNOSIS/ MODIFYING CIRCUMSTANCES	ETIOLOGIES (usual)	SUGGESTED REGIMENS* PRIMARY	ALTERNATIVE¹	ADJUNCT DIAGNOSTIC OR THERAPEUTIC MEASURES AND COMMENTS
EAR, Otitis Media (continued)				
Prophylaxis: acute otitis media *J Laryngol Otol 126:874, 2012*	Pneumococci, H. influenzae, M. catarrhalis, Staph. aureus, Group A strep (see Comments)	**Sulfisoxazole** 50 mg/kg po at bedtime or **amoxicillin** 20 mg/kg po q24h	**Use of antibiotics to prevent otitis media is a major contributor to emergence of antibiotic-resistant S. pneumo!** Pneumococcal protein conjugate vaccine decreases freq AOM due to vaccine serotypes. Adenoidectomy at time of tympanostomy tubes ↓ need for future hospitalization for AOM *(NEJM 344:1188, 2001).*	
Mastoiditis. Complication of acute or chronic otitis media. If chronic, look for cholesteatoma (Keratoma)				
Acute	*1st episode:* S. pneumoniae H. influenzae M. catarrhalis *If secondary to chronic otitis media:* P. aeruginosa S. aureus S. pneumoniae	Obtain cultures, then empiric therapy. 1st episode: **Ceftriaxone** 2 gm IV once daily OR **Levofloxacin** 750 mg IV once daily	Acute exacerbation of chronic otitis media. Surgical debridement of auditory canal, then [**Vancomycin** (dose to achieve tough of 15-20 mcg/mL) + **PIP-TZ** 3.375 gm IV q6h] OR [**Vancomycin** (dose as above) + **Ciprofloxacin** 400 mg IV q8h]	• Diagnosis: CT or MRI • Look for complication: osteomyelitis, suppurative lateral sinus thrombophlebitis, purulent meningitis, brain abscess • ENT consultation for possible mastoidectomy • S. aureus *(J Otolaryng Head Neck Surg 38:483, 2009).*
Chronic	As per 1st episode and: S. aureus P. aeruginosa Anaerobes Fungi	Generally not ill enough for parenteral antibiotics	Culture ear drainage. May need surgical debridement. Topical: Fluoroquinolone ear drops. ENT consult.	• Diagnosis: CT or MRI
EYE				
Eyelid: Little reported experience with CA-MRSA *(See Cochrane Database Syst Rev 5:CD005556, 2012)*				
Blepharitis	Etiol. unclear. Factors include Staph. aureus & Staph. epidermidis, seborrhea, rosacea, & dry eye	Lid margin care with baby shampoo & warm compresses q24h. Artificial tears if assoc. dry eye (see Comment).		Usually topical ointments of no benefit. If associated rosacea, add doxy 100 mg po bid for 2 wks and then q24h.
Hordeolum (Stye)				
External (eyelash follicle)	Staph. aureus	Hot packs only. Will drain spontaneously.		Infection of superficial sebaceous gland
Internal (Meibomian glands): Can be acute, subacute or chronic.	Staph. aureus, MSSA Staph. aureus, MRSA-CA Staph. aureus, MRSA-HA	Oral **dicloxacillin** + hot packs **TMP-SMX-DS,** tabs ii po bid **Linezolid** 600 mg po bid possible therapy if multi-drug resistant	I&D and culture. Rarely drain spontaneously, may need I&D and culture. Role of fluoroquinolone eye drops is unclear. MRSA often resistant to lower conc.; may be susceptible to higher concentration of FQ in ophthalmologic solutions of gati; levo or moxi.	Also called stye. Infection of superficial meibomianitis.
Conjunctivitis: *Review: JAMA 310:1721, 2013*				
Conjunctivitis of the newborn (**ophthalmia neonatorum**): by day of onset post-delivery—all dose pediatric				
Onset 1st day	Chemical due to silver nitrate prophylaxis	None		Usual prophylaxis is erythro ointment; hence, silver nitrate irritation rare.
Onset 2-4 days	N. gonorrhoeae	**Ceftriaxone** 25-50 mg/kg IV x 1 dose (see Comment), not to exceed 125 mg		Treat mother and her sexual partners. Hyperpurulent. Topical rx inadequate. **Treat neonate for concomitant Chlamydia trachomatis.**
Onset 3-10 days	Chlamydia trachomatis	**Erythro base or ethylsuccinate syrup** 12.5 mg/kg q6h x 14 days. No topical rx needed.		Diagnosis by NAAT. Alternative: **Azithro suspension** 20 mg/kg po q24h x 3 days. Treat mother & sexual partner.

NOTE: All dosage recommendations are for adults (unless otherwise indicated) and assume normal renal function. ¹Alternatives consider allergy, PK, compliance, local resistance, cost

TABLE 1 (10)

ANATOMIC SITE/DIAGNOSIS/ MODIFYING CIRCUMSTANCES	ETIOLOGIES (usual)	SUGGESTED REGIMENS* PRIMARY	ALTERNATIVE†	ADJUNCT DIAGNOSTIC OR THERAPEUTIC MEASURES AND COMMENTS
EYE/Conjunctiva (continued)				
Onset 2–16 days	Herpes simplex types 1, 2	Topical anti-viral rx under direction of ophthalmologist.		
Ophthalmia neonatorum prophylaxis: **erythro** 0.5% ointment × 1 or **tetra** 1% ointment^{AUS} × 1 application; effective vs gonococcus but not C. trachomatis				Also give Acyclovir 60 mg/kg/day IV div 3 doses *(Red Book online, accessed Jan 2011)*.
Pink eye (viral conjunctivitis). Usually unilateral	Adenovirus types 3 & 7 in children, 8, 11 & 19 in adults	No treatment. Artificial tears may help. (some studies show 2 day reduction of symptoms with steroids; not recommended)		Highly contagious. Onset of ocular pain and photophobia in an adult suggests associated keratitis—rare.
Inclusion conjunctivitis (adult) Usually unilateral & concomitant genital infection	Chlamydia trachomatis	**Azithro** 1 g once	**Doxy** 100 mg bid × 7 days	Oculogenital disease. Diagnosis NAAT. Urine NAAT for both GC & chlamydia. Treat sexual partner. May need to repeat dose of azithro.
Trachoma—a chronic bacterial keratoconjunctivitis linked to poverty	Chlamydia trachomatis	**Azithro** 20 mg/kg po single dose—78% effective in children; Adults: 1 gm po.	**Doxy** 100 mg po bid × minimum of 21 days or **tetracycline** 250 mg po qid × 14 days.	Starts in childhood and can persist for years with subsequent damage to cornea. Topical therapy of marginal benefit. Avoid doxy/tetracycline in young children. Mass treatment works *(NEJM 358:1777 & 1870, 2008; JAMA 299:778, 2008)*.
Suppurative conjunctivitis, bacterial: Children and Adults (Eyedrops speed resolution of symptoms: *Cochrane Database Syst Rev, Sep 12;9:CD001211, 2012)*	Staph. aureus, S. pneumoniae, H. influenzae, Viridans Strep, Moraxella sp.	FQ ophthalmic solns: **CIP** (generic), others expensive **Besi, Levo, Moxi**) All 1–2 gtts q2h while awake 1°–2 days, then q4–8h up to 7 days.	**Polymyxin B + trimethoprim** solution 1–2 gtts q3–6h x 7–10 days.	**FQs** best spectrum for empiric therapy. High concentrations ↑ likelihood of activity vs S. aureus—even MRSA. Polymyxin spectrum only Gm-neg bacilli. TMP active vs Gm-neg, prep of only **TMP**. Most S. pneumo resistant to **gent** & tobra.
Gonococcal (peds/adults)	N. gonorrhoeae	**Ceftriaxone** 25–50 mg/kg IV/IM (not to exceed 125 mg) as one dose in children; 1 gm IM/IV as one dose in adults		
Cornea (keratitis): Usually serious and often sight-threatening. Prompt ophthalmologic consultation essential for diagnosis, antimicrobial and adjunctive therapy! Herpes simplex most common etiology in developed countries; bacterial and fungal infections more common in underdeveloped countries.				
Viral				
H. simplex	H. simplex, types 1 & 2	**Trifluridine** ophthalmic soln, one drop q2h up to 9 drops/day until re-epithelialized. One drop 5 times per day while awake until corneal ulcer heals; then, one drop three times per day for 7 days. See Comment	**Ganciclovir** 0.15% ophthalmic gel. Indicated for acute herpetic keratitis. One drop 5 times per day while awake to 5x/day, for total not to exceed 21 days. **Vidarabine** ointment—useful in children. Use 5x/day for up to 21 days (currently listed as discontinued in U.S.).	Approx. 30% recurrence rate within one year: consider prophylaxis with acyclovir 400 mg bid for 12 months to prevent recurrences *(Arch Ophthal 130:108, 2012)*. Severe infection or immunocompromised host, consider adding **acyclovir** 400 mg po tid.
Varicella-zoster ophthalmicus	Varicella-zoster virus	**Famciclovir** 500 mg po tid or **valacyclovir** 1 gm po tid x 10 days	**Acyclovir** 800 mg po 5x/day x 10 days	Clinical diagnosis most common: dendritic figures with fluorescein staining in patient with varicella-zoster of ophthalmic branch of trigeminal nerve.

Abbreviations on page 2.   *NOTE: All dosage recommendations are for adults (unless otherwise indicated) and assume normal renal function.

Abbreviations on page 2.   *NOTE: All dosage recommendations are for adults (unless otherwise indicated) and assume normal renal function. § Alternatives consider allergy; PK; compliance, local resistance, cost

TABLE 1 (11)

ANATOMIC SITE/DIAGNOSIS/ MODIFYING CIRCUMSTANCES	ETIOLOGIES* (usual)	SUGGESTED REGIMENS*		ADJUNCT DIAGNOSTIC OR THERAPEUTIC MEASURES AND COMMENTS
		PRIMARY	ALTERNATIVE§	
EYE/Cornea (keratitis) *(continued)*				
Bacterial		**All treatment listed for bacterial, fungal, protozoan is topical unless otherwise indicated**		
Acute: No comorbidity	S. aureus, S. pneumo, S. pyogenes, Haemophilus sp.	**Moxi** 0.5%: ophthalmic 0.5%: 1 drop q1h for the first 48h then taper according to response	**CIP** 0.3% ophthal or **Levo** 0.5% ophthal 1-2 gtts/hr x 24-72 hrs, then taper	Regimens vary: some start rx by applying drops q5 min for 5 doses; some apply drops q15-30 min for several hours; some extend interval to q2h during sleep. In a clinical trial, drops were applied q1h for 48-72h, then q2h through day 6; then q2h during waking hours on days 7-9; then q6h until healing (Cornea 29:751, 2010). **Note:** despite high concentrations, may fail vs. MRSA. Prior use of fluoroquinolones associated with increased MICs (JAMA Ophthalmol. 131:310, 2013); high MICs associated with poorer outcome (Clin Infect Dis 54:1381, 2012).
Contact lens users	P. aeruginosa.	**CIP** 0.3% ophthalmic solution or **Levo** 0.5% ophthalmic solution 1-2 gtts hourly x24-72h, taper based on response.	**Gent** or **Tobra** 0.3% ophthalmic solution 1-2 gtts hourly x24h then taper based on clinical response.	Recommend alginate swab culture and susceptibility testing; refer to ophthalmologist. **Cornea abrasions:** treated with Tobra, Gent, or CIP gtts qid for 3-5 days; referral to ophthalmologist recommended cornea infiltrate or ulcer, visual loss, lack of improvement or worsening symptoms (Am Fam Physician. 87:114, 2013).
Dry cornea, diabetes, immunosuppression	Staph. aureus, S. epidermidis, S. pneumoniae, S. pyogenes, Enterobacteriaceae, listeria	**CIP** 0.3% ophthalmic solution 1-2 gtts hourly x24-72 hrs, then taper based on clinical response.	**Vanco** (50 mg/mL) + **Ceftaz** (50 mg/mL) hourly for 24-72h, taper depending upon response. See Comment.	Specific therapy guided by results of alginate swab culture.
Fungal	Aspergillus, fusarium, candida and others.	**Natamycin** (5%): 1 drop every 1-2 h for several days; then q3-4h for several days can reduce frequency depending upon response.	**Amphotericin B** (0.15%): 1 drop every 1-2 hours for 3 wks, then q2-3h for several days; can reduce frequency depending upon response.	Obtain specimens for fungal wet mount and cultures. Numerous other treatment options (1% topical Itra for 6 wks, oral Itra 100 mg bid for 3 wks, topical voriconazole 1% hourly for 2 wks, topical miconazole 1%, 5x a day, topical silver sulphadiazine 0.5-1.0% 5x a day) appear to have similar efficacy (Cochrane Database Syst Rev 2:004241, 2012)
Mycobacteria. Post-refractive eye surgery	M. chelonae, M. abscessus	**Moxi** eye drops: 1 gtt qid, probably in conjunction with other active antimicrobials		Alternative: systemic rx: Doxy 100 mg po bid + Clarithro 500 mg po bid (PLoS One 10:00/6236, 2015).
Protozoan Ref: contact lens users. CID 35:434, 2002.	Acanthamoeba, sp.	Optimal regimen uncertain. Suggested regimen: **Chlorhexidine** 0.02% or Polyhexamethylene biguanide (PHMB) 0.02% + (Propamidine isethionate 0.1%) (Brolene) or Hexamidine (Desmodine 0.1%)) drops. Apply one drop every hour for 48h, then one drop every hour only while awake for 72h, then one drop every two hours while awake for 3-4 weeks, then reducing frequency based on response (Ref: Am J Ophthalmol 148:487, 2009; Curr Op Infect Dis 23:590, 2010).		Uncommon. Trauma and soft contact lenses are risk factors. To obtain suggested drops: Leiters Park Ave Pharmacy (800-292-6773; www.leiterrx.com). Cleaning solution outbreak: MMWR 56: 532, 2007.

Abbreviations on page 2.   *NOTE: All dosage recommendations are for adults (unless otherwise indicated) and assume normal/renal function. § Alternatives consider allergy, PK, compliance, local resistance, cost

TABLE 1 (12)

ANATOMIC SITE/DIAGNOSIS/ MODIFYING CIRCUMSTANCES	ETIOLOGIES (usual)	SUGGESTED REGIMENS*		ADJUNCT DIAGNOSTIC OR THERAPEUTIC MEASURES AND COMMENTS
		PRIMARY	ALTERNATIVE†	
EYE/Cornea (keratitis) (continued)				
Lacrimal apparatus				
Canaliculitis	Actinomyces Staph., Strept. Rarely, Arachnia, fusobacterium, nocardia, candida	Remove granules & irrigate with **pen G** (100,000 mcg/mL). **Child: AM-CL or cefprozil or cefuroxime**.	If fungi, irrigate with **nystatin** approx. 5 mcg/mL: 1 gtt tid	Digital pressure produces exudate at punctum; Gram stain confirms diagnosis. Hot packs to punctal area qid. M. chelonae reported after use of intracanalicular plugs (*Ophth Plast Reconstr Surg* 24: 241, 2008).
Dacryocystitis (lacrimal sac)	S. pneumo, S. aureus, H. influenzae, S. pyogenes, P. aeruginosa	Often consequence of obstruction of lacrimal duct. Empiric systemic antimicrobial therapy based on Gram stain of aspirate—*see Comment*.		Need ophthalmologic consultation. Surgery may be required. Can be acute or chronic. Culture to detect MRSA.
Endophthalmitis: Endogenous (secondary to bacteremia or fungemia) and exogenous (post-injection, post-operative) types				
Bacterial: Haziness of vitreous key to diagnosis. Needle aspirate of both vitreous and aqueous humor for culture prior to therapy. Intravitreal administration of antimicrobials essential.				
Postocular surgery (cataracts) Early, acute onset (incidence 0.05%)	S. epidermidis 60%, Staph. aureus, streptococci, & enterococci each 5–10%, Gm-neg. bacilli 6%	**Immediate ophthal. consult.** If only light perception or worse, immediate vitrectomy + intravitreal vanco 1 mg & intravitreal ceftazidime 2.25 mg. No clear data on intravitreal steroid. May need to repeat intravitreal antibiotics in 2–3 days. Can usually leave lens in. Adjunctive systemic antibiotics (e.g., Vancomycin, Ceftazidime, Moxifloxacin or Gatifloxacin[4,6]) not of proven value, but recommended in endogenous infection.		
Low grade, chronic	Propionibacterium acnes, S. epidermidis, S. aureus (rare)	Intraocular **vanco**. Usually requires vitrectomy, lens removal.		
Post filtering blebs for glaucoma	Strep. species (viridans & others), H. influenzae	Intravitreal agent (e.g., **Vanco** 1 mg + **Ceftaz** 2.25 mg) and a topical agent. Consider a systemic agent such as **Amp-Sulb** or **Ceftriaxone or Ceftaz** (add **Vanco** if MRSA is suspected)		
Post-penetrating trauma	Bacillus sp., S. epiderm.	Intravitreal agent as above + systemic **clinda** or **vanco**. Use topical antibiotics post-surgery (tobra & cefazolin drops).		
None, suspect hematogenous	S. pneumoniae, N. meningitidis, Staph. aureus, Grp B Strep, K. pneumo	(**cefotaxime** 2 gm IV q4h or **ceftriaxone** 2 gm IV q24h) + **vanco** 30-60 mg/kg/day in 2-3 div doses to achieve target trough serum concentration of 15-20 mcg/mL, pending cultures. Intravitreal antibiotics as with early post-operative.		
IV heroin abuse	Bacillus cereus, Candida sp.	Intravitreal agent based on etiology and antimicrobial susceptibility.		
Mycotic (fungal): Broad-spectrum antibiotics, often corticosteroids, indwelling venous catheters	Candida sp., Aspergillus sp.	Intravitreal **ampho B** 0.005-0.01 mg in 1 mL. *Also see Table 11A, page 125 for concomitant systemic therapy. See Comment.*		Patients with Candida spp. chorioretinitis usually respond to systemically administered antifungals (*Clin Infect Dis* 53:262, 2011). Intravitreal amphotericin and/or vitrectomy may be necessary for those with vitritis or endophthalmitis (*Br J Ophthalmol* 92:466, 2008; *Pharmacotherapy* 27:1711, 2007).
Retinitis				
Acute retinal necrosis	Varicella zoster, Herpes simplex	IV **acyclovir** 10–12 mg/kg IV q8h x 5–7 days, then 800 mg po 5x/day x 6 wks		Strong association of VZ virus with atypical necrotizing herpetic retinopathy.
HIV+ (AIDS) CD4 usually <100/mm³	Cytomegalovirus	See *Table 14A, page 168*		Occurs in 5–10% of AIDS patients

Abbreviations on page 2.   *NOTE: All dosage recommendations are for adults (unless otherwise indicated) and assume normal renal function. § Alternatives consider allergy; PK: compliance, local resistance, cost

TABLE 1 (13)

ANATOMIC SITE/DIAGNOSIS/ MODIFYING CIRCUMSTANCES	ETIOLOGIES (usual)	SUGGESTED REGIMENS* PRIMARY	SUGGESTED REGIMENS* ALTERNATIVE†	ADJUNCT DIAGNOSTIC OR THERAPEUTIC MEASURES AND COMMENTS
EYE/Retinitis (continued)				
Progressive outer retinal necrosis	VZV, H. simplex, CMV (rare)	**Acyclovir** 10-12 mg/kg IV q8h for 1-2 weeks, then (**valacyclovir** 1000 mg po tid, or **famciclovir** 500 mg po tid, or **acyclovir** 800 mg po tid). Ophthalmology consultation imperative; approaches have also included intra-vitreal injection of anti-virals (foscarnet, ganciclovir implant). In rare cases due to CMV use **ganciclovir/valganciclovir** (see CMV retinitis, Table 14A).		Most patients are highly immunocompromised (HIV with low CD4 or transplantation). In contrast to Acute Retinal Necrosis, lack of intraocular inflammation or arteritis. May be able to stop oral antivirals when CD4 recovers with ART (Ocul Immunol Inflammation 15:425, 2007).
Orbital cellulitis (see page 54) for erysipelas, facial	S. pneumoniae, H. influenzae, M. catarralis, S. aureus, anaerobes, group A strep, occ. Gm-neg bacilli post-trauma	**Vancomycin** 15-20 mg/kg IV q8-12h (target **vancomycin** trough serum concentrations of 15-20 μg/mL) + **metro** ((**Ceftriaxone** 2 gm IV q24h) + **Metronidazole** 1 gm IV q12h) **PIP-TZ** 3.375 gm IV q6h		If penicillin/ceph allergy: **Vanco** + **levo** 750 mg IV once daily + **metro** IV. Problem is frequent inability to make microbiologic diagnosis. Image orbit (CT or MRI). Risk of cavernous sinus thrombosis. If vanco intolerant, another option for s. aureus is dapto 6 mg/kg IV q24h.
FOOT				
"Diabetic foot"—Two thirds of patients have triad of neuropathy, deformity and pressure-induced trauma. IDSA Guidelines CID 54:e132, 2012.				**General:** 1. Glucose control, eliminate pressure on ulcer 2. **Assess for peripheral vascular disease** 3. Caution in use of TMP-SMX in patients with diabetes, as many have risk factors for hyperkalemia (e.g., advanced age, reduced renal function, concomitant medications) (Arch Intern Med 170:1045, 2010). **Principles of empiric antibacterial therapy:** 1. Obtain culture; cover for MRSA in moderate, more severe infections pending culture data, local epidemiology. 2. Severe limb and/or life-threatening infections require initial parenteral therapy with predictable activity vs. Gm-positive cocci including MRSA, coliforms (& other aerobic Gm-neg. rods, & anaerobic Gm-neg. bacilli). 3. **NOTE:** The regimens listed are suggestions consistent with general principles. Other alternatives exist & may be appropriate for individual patients. 4. Is there an associated osteomyelitis? Risk increased if ulcer area > 2 cm², positive probe to bone, ESR > 70 and abnormal plain x-ray. Negative MRI reduces likelihood of osteomyelitis (JAMA 299:806, 2008). MRI is best imaging modality (CID 47:519 & 528, 2008).
Ulcer without inflammation	Colonizing skin flora	No antibacterial therapy.		
		Low strength evidence for improved healing with biologic skin equivalent or negative pressure wound therapy. Low strength evidence for platelet derived growth factor and silver cream (AVIM 159:532, 2013).		
Mild infection	S. aureus (assume MRSA), S. agalactiae (Gp B), S. pyogenes predominate	**Oral therapy:** Dicloxa or cephalexin or AM-CL (not MRSA) Doxy or TMP-SMX-DS (MRSA) CLINDA (covers MSSA, MRSA, strep) Dosages in footnote⁵		
Moderate infection	As above, plus coliforms possible	**Oral:** As above **Parenteral therapy:** [based on prevailing susceptibilities: (**AM-SB** or **PIP-TZ** or **ERTA** or other carbapenem) plus (**vanco** or alternative anti-MRSA drug as below)] until MRSA excluded]. Dosages in footnote⁶,⁷		
Osteomyelitis See Comment.				
Extensive local inflammation plus systemic toxicity.	As above, plus anaerobic bacteria. Role of enterococci unclear.	**Parenteral therapy: Vanco** plus [**β-lactam/β-lactamase inhibitor**] or (**vanco** plus [**DORI** or **IMP** or **MER**]). Other alternatives: 1. **Dapto** or **linezolid** for vanco 2. **CIP** or **Levo** or **Moxi** or **aztreonam** plus **metronidazole** for β-lactam/β-lactamase inhibitor Dosages in footnote⁷ **Assess for arterial insufficiency!**		

---

⁵ TMP-SMX-DS 1-2 tabs po bid, **minocycline** 100 mg po bid, **Pen VK** 500 mg po bid. (O Ceph 2, 3: **cefprozil** 500 mg po q12h; **cefuroxime axetil** 500 mg q12h; **cefdinir** 300 mg q12h or 600 mg po q24h; **cefpodoxime** 200 mg po q12h). **CIP** 750 mg po bid, **Levo** 750 mg po qd. **Diclox** 500 mg qid. **Cephalexin** 500 mg qid. **AM-CL** 875/125 bid. **Doxy** 100 mg bid. **CLINDA** 300-450 mg tid po q24h, **TMP-SMX-DS** 1-2 tabs po bid, **CIP** 750 mg po bid. **Levo** 750 mg po qd. **Moxi** 400 mg po q24h. **linezolid** 600 mg po bid

⁶ AM-CL-ER 2000/125 q12h, **(parenteral β-lactam/β-lactamase inhibitors: AM-SB** 3 gm IV q6h. **PIP-TZ** 3.375 gm IV q6h or 4.5 gm IV q8h or 4 hr infusion of 3.375 gm q8h; **carbapenems: Doripenem** 500 mg

⁷ **Vanco** 1 gm IV q12h, (**parenteral β-lactam/β-lactamase inhibitors: AM-SB** 3 gm IV q6h; **PIP-TZ** 3.375 gm IV q6h or 4.5 gm IV q8h or 4 hr infusion of 3.375 gm q8h; **carbapenems: Doripenem** 500 mg (1-hr infusion) q8h, **ERTA** 1 gm IV q24h, **IMP** 0.5 gm IV q6h, **MER** 1 gm IV q8h, **daptomycin** 6 mg per kg IV q24h, **linezolid** 600 mg IV q12h, **aztreonam** 2 gm IV q12h, **CIP** 400 mg IV q12h, **Levo** 750 mg IV q24h, **Moxi** 400 mg IV q24h, **metro** IV q24h, **metro** IV loading dose 1 gm, then 0.5 gm IV q6h.

Abbreviations on page 2. **NOTE:** All dosage recommendations are for adults (unless otherwise indicated) and assume normal renal function. § Alternatives consider allergy, PK, compliance, local resistance, cost

TABLE 1 (14)

ANATOMIC SITE/DIAGNOSIS/ MODIFYING CIRCUMSTANCES	ETIOLOGIES (usual)	SUGGESTED REGIMENS*		ADJUNCT DIAGNOSTIC OR THERAPEUTIC MEASURES AND COMMENTS
		PRIMARY	ALTERNATIVE[1]	
FOOT (continued)				
Onychomycosis: See Table 11, page 129, fungal infections				
Puncture wound: **Nail/Toothpick**	P. aeruginosa (Nail). S. aureus, Strept (Toothpick)	Cleanse. Tetanus booster. Observe.		See page 4. 1–2% evolve to osteomyelitis.
GALLBLADDER				
Cholecystitis, cholangitis, biliary sepsis, or common duct obstruction (partial: 2° to tumor, stones stricture). Cholecystitis Ref: NEJM 358:2804, 2008.	Enterobacteriaceae 68%, enterococci 14%, bacteroides 10%, Clostridium sp. 7%, rarely candida	**(PIP-TZ** or **AM-SB)** or If life-threatening: **IMP** or **MER** or **DORI**	**[P Ceph 3*** + **metro)** or **(Aztreonam*** + **metro)** or **(CIP*** + **metro)** or **Moxi**	In severely ill pts, antibiotic therapy complements adequate biliary drainage. 15–30% pts will require decompression: surgical, percutaneous or ERCP-placed stent. Gallbladder bile is culture pos in 40–60% (J Infect 51:128, 2005). No benefit to continuation of antibiotics after surgery in pts with acute calculous cholecystitis (JAMA 312:145, 2014).
		Dosages in footnote[*] on page 16. *** Add vanco for empiric activity vs. enterococci		
GASTROINTESTINAL				
Gastroenteritis—Empiric Therapy (laboratory studies not performed or culture, microscopy, toxin results NOT AVAILABLE)				
Premature infant with necrotizing enterocolitis	Associated with intestinal flora	Treatment should cover broad range of intestinal bacteria using drugs appropriate to age and local susceptibility patterns, rationale as in diverticulitis/peritonitis, page 22.		Pneumatosis intestinalis, if present on x-ray confirms diagnosis. Bacteremia-peritonitis in 30–50%. If Staph. epidermidis isolated, add vanco (IV). For review and general management, see NEJM 364:255, 2011.
Mild diarrhea (≤3 unformed stools/day, minimal associated symptomatology)	Bacterial (See Severe, below), parasitic (noro/virus), usually causes mild to moderate disease. For traveler's diarrhea, see page 20	Fluids only + lactose-free diet, avoid caffeine		**Rehydration: For po fluid replacement,** see Cholera, page 19. **Antimotility:** (Do not use if fever, bloody stools, or suspicion of HUS): Loperamide (Imodium) 4 mg po, then 2 mg after each loose stool to max. of 16 mg per day. Bismuth subsalicylate (Pepto-Bismol) 2 tablets (262 mg) po qid.
Moderate diarrhea (≥4 unformed stools/day &/or systemic symptoms)		Antimotility agents (see Comments) + fluids		**Hemolytic uremic syndrome (HUS):** Risk in **children** infected with E. coli O157:H7 is 8–10%. Early treatment with TMP-SMX or FQs ↑ risk of HUS.
Severe diarrhea (≥6 unformed stools/day, &/or temp ≥101°F, tenesmus, blood, or fecal leukocytes)	Shigella, salmonella, C. jejuni, Shiga toxin + E. coli, toxin-positive C. difficile, Klebsiella oxytoca, E. histolytica. For typhoid fever, see page 62	**FQ (CIP** 500 mg po q12h or **Levo** 500 mg q24h) times 3–5 days	**TMP-SMX-DS** po bid times 3–5 days. Campylobacter resistance to TMP-SMX common in tropics	**Norovirus:** Etiology of over 90% of non-bacterial diarrhea (± nausea/vomiting). Lasts 12–60 hrs. Hydrate. No effective antiviral. **Other potential etiologies:** Cryptosporidia—no treatment in immuno-competent host. Cyclospora—usually chronic diarrhea, responds to TMP-SMX (see Table 13A).
NOTE: **Severe afebrile bloody diarrhea should ↑ suspicion of Shiga-toxin E. coli O157:H7 & others** (MMWR 58 (RR-12):1, 2009).		If recent antibiotic therapy (C. difficile colitis possible): add: **Metro** 500 mg po tid times 10–14 days	**Vanco** 125 mg po qid times 10–14 days	Klebsiella oxytoca identified as cause of antibiotic-associated hemorrhagic colitis (cytotoxin positive): NEJM 355:2418, 2006.

Abbreviations on page 2.   *NOTE: All dosage recommendations are for adults (unless otherwise indicated) and assume normal renal function. § Alternatives consider allergy, PK, compliance, local resistance, cost

TABLE 1 (15)

ANATOMIC SITE/DIAGNOSIS/ MODIFYING CIRCUMSTANCES	ETIOLOGIES (usual)	SUGGESTED REGIMENS*		ADJUNCT DIAGNOSTIC OR THERAPEUTIC MEASURES AND COMMENTS
		PRIMARY	ALTERNATIVE†	
GASTROINTESTINAL				
Gastroenteritis—Specific Therapy (results of culture, microscopy, toxin assay AVAILABLE) (Ref.: *NEJM 370:1532, 2014*)				
If culture negative, probably **Norovirus** (Norwalk) other virus (*EID 17:1381, 2011*) — See Norovirus, page 174. **NOTE:** WBC > 15,000 suggestive of C. difficile in hospitalized patient.	**Aeromonas/Plesiomonas**	CIP 750 mg po bid x3 days.	TMP-SMX DS tab 1 po bid x 3 days	Although no absolute proof, increasing evidence for Plesiomonas as cause of diarrheal illness (*NEJM 361:1560, 2009*).
	Campylobacter jejuni History of fever in 53-83% of patients. Self-limited diarrhea in normal host.	Azithro 500 mg po q24h x 3 days.	Erythro stearate 500 mg po qid x 5 days or CIP 500 mg po bid (CIP resistance increasing).	**Post-Campylobacter Guillain-Barré:** assoc. 15% of cases (*Ln 366:1653, 2005*). Assoc. with small bowel lymphoproliferative disease, may respond to antimicrobials (*NEJM 350:239, 2004*). See *Traveler's diarrhea, page 20*.
	Campylobacter fetus Diarrhea uncommon. More systemic disease in debilitated hosts.	Gentamicin (See Table 10D)	AMP 100 mg/kg/day IV div q6h or IMP 500 mg IV q6h	**Reactive arthritis** another potential sequelae (*NEJM 352:239, 2004*). Draw blood cultures. In bacteremic pts, 32% of C. fetus resistant to FQs (*CID 47:790, 2008*). Meropenem inhibits C. fetus at low concentrations in vitro. Clinical review: *CID 58:1579, 2014*.
Differential diagnosis of toxin-producing diarrhea: • **C. difficile** • **Klebsiella oxytoca** • **S. aureus** • Shiga toxin producing **E. coli (STEC)** • Enterotoxigenic **B. fragilis** (*CID 47:797, 2008*) More on C. difficile: Treatment review: *CID 51:1306, 2010* SHEA/IDSA treatment guidelines: *ICHE 31:431, 2010; ESCMID guidelines: Clin Microbiol Infect 15:1067, 2009; AnIM 155:839, 2011* *(Continued on next page)*	**C. difficile** toxin positive antibiotic-associated colitis. po meds okay. WBC < 15,000; no increase in serum creatinine.	Metro 500 mg po tid or 250 mg po qid x 10-14 days	Vanco 125 mg po qid x 10-14 days Teicoplanin^(NUS) 400 mg po bid x10 days Fidaxomicin 200 mg po bid x 10 days	**D/C antibiotic. If possible: avoid antimotility agents, hydration, enteric isolation.** Recent reviews suggest antimotility agents can be used cautiously in certain pts with mild disease who are receiving rx (*CID 48: 598, 2009*). **Relapse in 10-20%.** Vanco superior to metro in sicker pts. Relapse in 10-20%. Fidaxomicin had lower rate of recurrence than Vanco for diarrhea with non-NAP1 strains (*NEJM 364:422, 2011*).
	po meds okay; Sicker; WBC >15,000; ≥ 50% increase in baseline creatinine	Vanco 125 mg po qid x 10-14 days. To use IV vanco, see Table 10A, page 107.		**Vanco taper** (tabs 125 mg po) – week 1 – qid, week 2 – q24h, then every 3rd day for 3 wks (*NEJM 359: 1932, 2008*). Another option: After initial Vanco, **rifaximin**^(NUS) 400-800 mg po daily divided (tid or bid) x 2 wks.
	Post-treatment relapse	1st relapse Metro 500 mg po tid x 10 days	2nd relapse Vanco 125 mg po qid x 10-14 days, then immediately start taper (See Comments)	**Fecal transplant** more efficacious than vancomycin (15/16 [93%] versus 7/26 [27%]) in curing recurrent C. difficile infection (*New Engl J Med: 368:407, 2013*). For vanco instillation in bowel, add 500 mg vanco to 1 liter of saline and perfuse at 1-3 mL/min to maximum of 2 gm in 24 hrs (*CID 690, 2002*). **Note: IV vanco not effective.** Indications for **IV tigecycline** IV to treat severe C. diff refractory to standard rx (*CID 48:1732, 2009*).
	Post-op ileus; severe disease with toxic megacolon (*NEJM 359:1932, 2008; CID 61:934, 2015*)	Metro 500 mg IV q6h + vanco 500 mg q6h via nasogastric tube (or naso-small bowel tube) + retrograde via catheter in cecum. See comment for dosage. No data on efficacy of Fidaxomicin in severe life-threatening disease.		C. diff reported successful use of tigecycline IV to treat severe C. diff refractory to standard rx (*CID 48:1732, 2009*).
	Enterohemorrhagic E. coli (EHEC). Some produce **Shiga toxin E. coli (STEC)** and cause **hemolytic uremic syndrome (HUS).** Strains: 0157:H7, 0104:H4 and others. Classically bloody diarrhea and afebrile	**Hydration:** avoid antiperistaltic drugs. 25% increased risk of precipitating HUS in children < age 10 yrs given TMP-SMX, beta lactam, metronidazole or azithromycin for diarrhea (*CID 55:33, 2012*). In uncontrolled study, antibiotic treatment of STEC outbreak, shorter excretion of E. coli, lower mortality (*BMJ 345:e4565, 2012*). If on empiric antibiotics, then Dx of STEC, reasonable to discontinue antibiotics. Avoid all antibiotics in children age < 10 yrs with bloody diarrhea until Dx of STEC excluded; azithromycin may be the safest choice (*JAMA 307:1046, 2012*).		**HUS** more common in children, 15% in age < 10; 6-9% overall. **Diagnosis:** EIA for Shiga toxins 1 & 2 in blood (*MMWR 58(RR-12), 2009*). **Treatment:** in vitro and in vivo data, that exposure of STEC to TMP-SMX (or other antibiotics) induces a burst of HUS toxin production as bacteria die (*JID 181:664, 2000*). **HUS bad disease:** 10% mortality, 50% some degree of permanent renal damage (*CID 38:1298, 2004*).

NOTE: All dosage recommendations are for adults (unless otherwise indicated) and assume normal renal function. § Alternatives consider allergy, PK, compliance, local resistance, cost

TABLE 1 (16)

ANATOMIC SITE/DIAGNOSIS/ MODIFYING CIRCUMSTANCES	ETIOLOGIES (usual)	SUGGESTED REGIMENS*		ADJUNCT DIAGNOSTIC OR THERAPEUTIC MEASURES AND COMMENTS
		PRIMARY	ALTERNATIVE§	
GASTROINTESTINAL/Gastroenteritis—Specific Therapy *(continued)*				
(Continued from previous page)				
	Klebsiella oxytoca— antibiotic-associated diarrhea	Responds to stopping antibiotic		Suggested that stopping NSAIDs helps.
	Listeria monocytogenes	Usually self-limited. Value of oral antibiotics (e.g., ampicillin or TmP-SMX) unknown, but their use might be reasonable in populations at risk for serious listeria infections. Those with bacteremia/meningitis require parenteral therapy: see pages 9 & 61.		Recognized as a cause of food-associated febrile gastroenteritis. Not detected in standard stool cultures. Populations at risk of severe systemic disease: pregnant women, neonates, the elderly, and immunocompromised hosts *(MMWR 57:1097, 2008)*.
	Salmonella, non-typhi—For typhoid (enteric) fever, see page 62. Fever in 71-91%, history of bloody stools in 34%	If asymptomatic or illness mild, antimicrobial therapy not indicated. If immunocompromised, if vascular grafts or prosthetic joints, hemoglobinopathy, or hospitalized with fever and severe diarrhea (see typhoid fever, page 62). **CiP** 500 mg bid) or **(Levo** 500 mg q24h) x 7-10 days (14 days if immunocompromised).	**Azithro** 500 mg po once daily x 7 days (14 days if immunocompromised).	**Treat** if age <1 y or >50 yrs, if immunocompromised, if vascular grafts or prosthetic joints, hemoglobinopathy, or hospitalized with fever and severe diarrhea (see typhoid fever, page 62). ↑ resistance to TMP-SMX and chloro. Ceftriaxone, cefotaxime usually active if IV therapy required (see footnote 11, page 25, for dosage). CLSI has established new interpretive breakpoints for susceptibility to CiP: susceptible strains, MIC < 0.06 µg/mL *(Clin Infect Dis 55:1107, 2012)*. **Primary treatment of enteritis is fluid and electrolyte replacement.**
	Shigella Fever in 58%, history of bloody stools 51%	**CiP** 750 mg bid x 3 days	**Azithro** 500 mg once daily x 3 days	Recommended adult CiP dose of 750 mg once daily for 3 days *(NEJM 361:1560, 2009)*. **Pockets of resistance (see Comment)** Peds doses: Azithro 10 mg/kg/day once daily x 3 days. For severe disease, ceftriaxone 50-75 mg/kg per day x 2-5 days. CiP suspension 10 mg/kg x 5 days. Benefit of treatment unclear. Susceptible to **metro.** **Immunocompromised children & adults:** Treat for 7-10 days. Pockets of resistance: S. flexneri resist to CiP & ceftriaxone *(MMWR 59:1619, 2010)*; S. sonnei resist to CiP in travelers *(MMWR 64:318, 2015)*; S. sonnei suscept to CiP but resist to azithro in MSM *(MMWR 64:597, 2015)*.
	Spirochetosis (Brachyspira pilosicoli)	Benefit of treatment unclear. Susceptible to metro, ceftriaxone, and Moxi		Anaerobic intestinal spirochete that colonizes colon of domestic & wild animals plus humans. Called enigmatic disease due to uncertain status *(Digest Dis & Sci 58:202, 2013)*.
	vibrio cholerae (toxigenic - O1 & O39) Treatment decreases duration of disease, volume losses, & duration of excretion	**Primary therapy is rehydration.** Select antibiotics based on susceptibility of locally prevailing isolates. Options include: **Doxycycline** 300 mg po single dose **OR Azithromycin** 1 gm po single dose **OR Tetracycline** 500 mg po qid x 3 days **OR Erythromycin** 500 mg po qid x 3 days.	**For pregnant women: Azithromycin** 1 gm po single dose **OR Erythromycin** 500 mg po qid x 3 days **For children: Azithromycin** 20 mg/kg po as single dose; for other age-specific alternatives, see CDC website http://www.cdc.gov/haitiichole ra/hcp_goingtohaiti.htm	**Antimicrobial therapy shortens duration of illness, but rehydration is paramount.** When IV hydration is needed, use Ringer's lactate. Switch to PO repletion with Oral Rehydration Salts (ORS) as soon as able to take oral fluids. ORS are commercially available for reconstitution in potable water. If not available, WHO suggests a substitute can be made by dissolving ½ teaspoon salt and 6 level teaspoons of sugar per liter of potable water *(http://www.who.int/cholera/technical/en/)*. CDC recommendations for other aspects of management developed for Haiti outbreak can be found at http://www.cdc.gov/haitiicholera/hcp_goingtohaiti.htm Isolates from this outbreak demonstrate reduced susceptibility to ciprofloxacin and resistance to sulfisoxazole, nalidixic acid and furazolidone.

*NOTE: All dosage recommendations are for adults (unless otherwise indicated) and assume normal renal function. § Alternatives consider allergy, PK, compliance, local resistance, cost

Ref.: *NEJM 355:2418, 2006*.

Abbreviations on page 2.

TABLE 1 (17)

ANATOMIC SITE/DIAGNOSIS/ MODIFYING CIRCUMSTANCES	ETIOLOGIES (usual)	SUGGESTED REGIMENS*		ADJUNCT DIAGNOSTIC OR THERAPEUTIC MEASURES AND COMMENTS
		PRIMARY	ALTERNATIVE§	
GASTROINTESTINAL/Gastroenteritis—Specific Therapy *(continued)*				
Vibrio parahaemolyticus, V. mimicus, V. fluvialis	Antimicrobial rx does not shorten course. Hydration.			Shellfish exposure common. Treat severe disease: **FQ, doxy, P Ceph 3**
Vibrio vulnificus	Usual presentation is skin lesions & bacteremia, life-threatening; treat early: **ceftaz + doxy** *—see page 54*; **Levo** or **CIP + ceftaz** or **ceftriaxone**. Ref: Epidemiol Infect. 142:878, 2014.			
Yersinia enterocolitica Fever in 68%, bloody stools in 26%	No treatment unless severe. If severe, combine **doxy** 100 mg IV bid + **tobra** or **gent** 5 mg/kg per day once q24h). **TMP-SMX** or **FQs** are alternatives.			Mesenteric adenitis pain can mimic acute appendicitis. Lab diagnosis difficult; requires "cold enrichment" and/or yersinia selective agar. Desferoxamine therapy increases severity, discontinue if pt on it. Iron overload states predispose to yersinia
Gastroenteritis—Specific Risk Groups–Empiric Therapy				
Anoreceptive intercourse	Herpes viruses, gonococci, chlamydia, syphilis *See Genital Tract, page 22*			
Proctitis (distal 15 cm only)				
Colitis	Shigella, salmonella, campylobacter, E. histolytica (see Table 13A)			See specific GI pathogens, Gastroenteritis, above.
HIV-1 infected (AIDS): >10 days diarrhea	G. lamblia			
	Acid fast: Cryptosporidium parvum, Cyclospora cayetanensis			
	Other: Isospora belli, microsporidia (Enterocytozoon bieneusi, Septata intestinalis)			
Neutropenic enterocolitis or "typhlitis" (CID 56:711, 2013)	Mucosal invasion by **Clostridium septicum**. Occasionally caused by C. sordellii or P. aeruginosa	Appropriate agents include PIP-TZ, IMP, MER, DORI plus bowel rest.		Tender right lower quadrant may be clue, but may be diffuse or absent in immunocompromised. Need surgical consult. Surgical resection controversial but may be necessary. **NOTE:** Resistance of clostridia to clindamycin reported. PIP-TZ, IMP, MER, DORI should cover most pathogens.
Traveler's diarrhea, self-medication. Patient often afebrile	**Acute.** 60% due to diarrheagenic E. coli, shigella, salmonella, campylobacter, C. difficile, amebiasis (see Table 13A). **If chronic:** cyclospora, cryptosporidia, giardia, isospora	**CIP** 750 mg po bid for 1-3 days **OR** **Levo** 500 mg po q24h for 1-3 days **OR** **Oflox** 300 mg po bid for 3 days **OR** **Rifaximin** 200 mg po tid for 3 days **OR** **Azithro** 1000 mg po once or 500 mg po q24h for 3 days **For pediatrics:** Azithro 10 mg/kg/day as a single dose for 3 days or Ceftriaxone 50 mg/kg/day as single dose for 3 days. Avoid FQs. **For pregnancy:** Use Azithro. Avoid FQs.		**Antimotility agent:** For non-pregnant adults with no fever or blood in stool, add loperamide 4 mg po x 1, then 2 mg po after each loose stool to a maximum of 16 mg per day. **Comments:** Rifaximin approved only for ages 12 and older. Works only for diarrhea due to non-invasive E. coli; do not use if fever or bloody stool. Ref: NEJM 361:1560, 2009; NOTE: Self treatment with FQs associated with acquisition of resistant Gm-neg bacilli (CID 60:837, 847, 872, 2015).
Prevention of Traveler's diarrhea	Not routinely indicated. Current recommendation is to take **FQ + Imodium** with 1st loose stool.			

*NOTE: All dosage recommendations are for adults (unless otherwise indicated) and assume normal renal function. § Alternatives consider allergy, PK, compliance, local resistance, cost

TABLE 1 (18)

ANATOMIC SITE/DIAGNOSIS/ MODIFYING CIRCUMSTANCES	ETIOLOGIES (usual)	SUGGESTED REGIMENS*		ADJUNCT DIAGNOSTIC OR THERAPEUTIC MEASURES AND COMMENTS
		PRIMARY	**ALTERNATIVE¹**	
GASTROINTESTINAL *(continued)*				
Gastrointestinal Infections by Anatomic Site: Esophagus to Rectum				
Esophagitis	Candida albicans, HSV, CMV	*See* SANFORD GUIDE TO HIV/AIDS THERAPY *and Table 11A.*		
Duodenal/Gastric ulcer; gastric cancer, MALT lymphomas (not C²NSAIDs) Comparative effectiveness & tolerance of treatment *(BMJ 351:4052, 2015)*	**Helicobacter pylori** *See* **Comment** Prevalence of pre-treatment resistance increasing	**Sequential therapy:** **Rabeprazole** 20 mg + **amox** 1 gm) bid x 5 days, then **rabeprazole** 20 mg + **clarithro** 500 mg + **tinidazole** 500 mg bid for another 5 days. Can modify by substituting Levo for Clarithro *(JAMA 309:578, 2013; Ln 381:205, 2013).* See footnote§	**Quadruple therapy (10-14 days):** bismuth subsalicylate 2 tabs qid + **metro** 500 mg qid + **tetracycline** 500 mg qid + **omeprazole** 20 mg bid.	**Comment:** In many locations: 20% failure rates with previously recommended triple regimens (**PPI + Amox + Clarithro**) are not acceptable. With 10 days of quadruple therapy (**omeprazole** 20 mg po twice daily) + (3 capsules po four times per day, each containing **Bismuth subcitrate potassium** 140 mg + **Tetracycline** 125 mg)), eradication rates were 93% in a per protocol population and 80% in an intention-to-treat population, both significantly better than with 7-day triple therapy regimen (PPI + Amox + Clarithro) *(Lancet 377:905, 2011).* Exercise caution regarding potential interactions with other drugs, contraindications in pregnancy and warnings for other special populations. **Dx: Stool antigen**—Monoclonal EIA >90% sens. & 92% specific. Other tests: If endoscoped, rapid urease &/or histology &/or culture; urea breath test, but some office-based tests underperform. Testing ref: *BMJ 344:44, 2012.* **Test of cure:** Repeat stool antigen and/or urea breath test >8 wks post-treatment. **Treatment outcome:** Failure rate of triple therapy 20% due to clarithro resistance. Cure rate with sequential therapy 90%.
		100% compliance/94% eradication rate reported: (**Pantoprazole** 40 mg + **Clarithro** 500 mg + **Amox** 1000 mg) po bid x 7 d *(AAC 58:5936, 2014)*. High cure rates reported in Taiwan with (**Rabeprazole** 20 mg + **Amox** 750 mg) po 4x/day x 14 days		
Small intestine: Whipple's disease: *NEJM 356:55, 2007; LnID 8:179, 2008).* Treatment: *JAC 69:219, 2014.* *See* Infective endocarditis, culture-negative, page 30.	Tropheryma whipplei	**Doxycycline** 100 mg po bid + **Hydroxychloroquine** 200 mg po tid x) x1 year, then **Doxycycline** 100 mg po bid for life Immune reconstitution inflammatory response (IRIS) reactions occur. Thalidomide therapy may be better than steroids for IRIS reaction *(J Infect 60:79, 2010)*		In vitro susceptibility testing and collected clinical experience *(JAC 69:219, 2014)*. In vitro resistance to TMP-SMX plus frequent clinical failures & relapses. Frequent in vitro resistance to carbapenems. Complete in vitro resistance to Ceftriaxone.

* Can substitute other proton pump inhibitors for omeprazole or rabeprazole–all bid: **esomeprazole** 20 mg po tabs: **lanzoprazole** 30 mg (FDA-approved), **pantoprazole** 40 mg (not FDA-approved for this indication).

§ **Bismuth preparations:** (1) In U.S., **bismuth subsalicylate (Pepto-Bismol)** 262 mg tabs; adult dose for helicobacter is 2 tabs (524 mg) qid. (2) Outside U.S., colloidal bismuth subcitrate (De-Nol) 120 mg chewable tablets; dose is 1 tablet qid. In the U.S., bismuth subcitrate is available in combination cap only (Pylera), each cap contains bismuth subcitrate 140 mg + Metro 125 mg + Tetracycline 125 mg), given as 3 caps po 4x daily for 10 days **together with a** twice daily PPI.

*NOTE: All dosage recommendations are for adults (unless otherwise indicated) and assume normal renal function. § Alternatives consider allergy, PK, compliance, local resistance, cost

TABLE 1 (19)

ANATOMIC SITE/DIAGNOSIS/ MODIFYING CIRCUMSTANCES	ETIOLOGIES (usual)	SUGGESTED REGIMENS*		ADJUNCT DIAGNOSTIC OR THERAPEUTIC MEASURES AND COMMENTS
		PRIMARY	ALTERNATIVE†	
GASTROINTESTINAL/Gastrointestinal Infections by Anatomic Site: Esophagus to Rectum (continued)				
Diverticulitis, perirectal abscess, peritonitis. Also see Peritonitis, page 46	Enterobacteriaceae, occasionally P. aeruginosa, Bacteroides sp., enterococci	**Outpatient rx—mild diverticulitis, drained perirectal abscess:** [(TMP-SMX-DS bid) or (CIP 750 mg bid or **Levo** 750 mg q24h)] + **metro** 500 mg q6h. All po x 7–10 days.	**AM-CL-ER** 1000/62.5 mg 2 tabs po bid x 7–10 days **OR Moxi** 400 mg po q24h x 7–10 days	Must "cover" both Gm-neg. aerobic & Gm-neg. anaerobic bacteria. **Drugs active only vs. anaerobic Gm-neg. bacilli:** clinda, metro. **Drugs active only vs. aerobic Gm-neg. bacilli:** APAG[10] P Ceph 2/3 (alternate Table 10A, page 102), aztreonam, PIP-TZ, CIP, Levo. **Drugs active vs. both aerobic/anaerobic Gm-neg. bacteria:** cefoxitin, cefotetan, TC-CL, PIP-TZ, AM-SB, ERTA, DORI, IMP, MER, Moxi, & tigecycline.
		Mild–moderate disease—Inpatient—Parenteral Rx: (e.g. focal periappendiceal peritonitis, peridiverticular abscess, endomyometritis) **PIP-TZ** 3.375 gm IV q6h **or** 4.5 gm IV q8h **or** **ERTA** 1 gm IV q24h **or** **MOXI** 400 mg IV q24h.	[(CIP 400 mg IV q12h) or (**Levo** 750 mg IV q24h)] + (**metro** 500 mg IV q6h or 1 gm IV q12h) **OR Moxi** 400 mg IV q24h	**Increasing resistance of B. fragilis group** Clinda Moxi Cefoxitin Cefotetan % Resistant: 42–80 34–45 48–60 19–35 Ref: Anaerobe 17:147, 2011; AAC 56:1247, 2012; Surg Infect 10:111, 2009. **Resistance (B. fragilis):** Metro, PIP-TZ rare. Resistance to FQ increased in enteric bacteria, particularly if any FQ used recently.
		Severe life-threatening disease, ICU patient: **IMP** 1 gm IV q8h **or DORI** 500 mg IV q8h (1-hr infusion).	**AMP + metro + (CIP** 400 mg IV q12h or **Levo** 750 mg IV q24h) **OR** [**AMP** 2 gm IV q6h + **metro** 500 mg IV q6h + **aminoglycoside**[10]	**Ertapenem** poorly active vs. P. aeruginosa/Acinetobacter sp. **Concomitant surgical management important,** esp. with moderate-severe disease. **Role of enterococci remains debatable.** Probably pathogenic in infections of biliary tract. Probably need drugs active vs. enterococci in pts with valvular heart disease.
			Severe penicillin/cephalosporin allergy: (aztreonam 2 gm IV q6h to q8h) + [**metro** (500 mg IV q6h) or (1 gm IV q12h)] **OR** [(**CIP** 400 mg IV q12h) or (**Levo** 750 mg IV q24h)] + metro	**Tigecycline: Black Box Warning:** All cause mortality higher in pts treated with tigecycline (2.5%) than comparators (1.8%) in meta-analysis of clinical trials. Cause of mortality risk difference of 0.6% (95% CI 0.1, 1.2) not established. Tigecycline should be reserved for use in situations when alternative treatments are not suitable (FDA MedWatch Sep 27, 2013).
		[See Table 10D, page 118.]	[See Table 10D, page 118.]	
GENITAL TRACT: Mixture of empiric & specific treatment. Divided by sex of the patient. For sexual assault (rape), see Table 15A, page 200. See CDC Guidelines for Sexually Transmitted Diseases, MMWR 64(RR-3):1, 2015.				
Both Women & Men:				
Chancroid	H. ducreyi	**Ceftriaxone** 250 mg IM single dose OR **azithro** 1 gm po single dose	**CIP** 500 mg po x 3 days OR **erythro base** 500 mg po tid x 7 days.	In HIV+ pts, failures reported with single dose azithro (CID 21:409, 1995). Evaluate after 7 days, ulcer should objectively improve. All patients treated for chancroid should be tested for HIV and syphilis. All sex partners of pts with chancroid should be examined and treated if they have evidence of disease or have had sex with index pt within the last 10 days.

10 Aminoglycoside = antipseudomonal aminoglycosidic aminoglycoside, e.g., amikacin, gentamicin, tobramycin

Aminoglycoside = antipseudomonal aminoglycosidic aminoglycoside, e.g., amikacin, gentamicin, tobramycin

*NOTE: All dosage recommendations are for adults (unless otherwise indicated) and assume normal renal function. § Alternatives consider allergy, PK, compliance, local resistance, cost

Abbreviations on page 2.

TABLE 1 (20)

GENITAL TRACT/Both Women & Men (continued) CDC Guidelines: MMWR 64(RR-3):1, 2015

ANATOMIC SITE/DIAGNOSIS/ MODIFYING CIRCUMSTANCES	ETIOLOGIES (usual)	SUGGESTED REGIMENS* PRIMARY	ALTERNATIVE§	ADJUNCT DIAGNOSTIC OR THERAPEUTIC MEASURES AND COMMENTS
Non-gonococcal or post-gonococcal urethritis, cervicitis **NOTE: Assume concomitant N. gonorrhoeae** (Chlamydia conjunctivitis, see page 12) Non-gonococcal urethritis: Mycoplasma genitalium	Chlamydia 50%, Mycoplasma genitalium (30%). Other known etiologies (10–15%): trichomonas, herpes simplex virus, see AJD 206:357, 2012. Ref: CID 61:S774, 2015. Mycoplasma genitalium Ref: CID 61:S802, 2015.	**Doxy** 100 mg bid po x 7 days) or (**azithro** 1 gm po as single dose). Evaluate & treat sex partner In pregnancy: **Azithromycin** 1 gm po single dose OR amox 500 mg po tid x 7 days **Azithro** 500 mg po x1 then 250 mg po once daily x 4 days	(**Erythro** base 500 mg bid po x 7 days) or (**Ofloxacin** 300 mg q12h po x 7 days) or (**Levo** 500 mg q24h x 7 days) In pregnancy: **Erythro** base 500 mg po qid for 7 days **Doxy & FQs contraindicated** **Moxi** 400 mg once daily x 10–14 days	**Diagnosis:** NAAT for C. trachomatis & N. gonorrhoeae on urine or cervix or urethra specimens (AnIM 142:914, 2005). Test all urethritis/cervicitis pts for HIV & syphilis. **In pregnancy, prefer doxy** x 7d (See Trans Dis 41:79, 2014). Azithromycin 1 gm was superior to doxycycline for M. genitalium male urethritis (CID 48:1649, 2009), but may select resistance leading to ↑ failure of multi-dose azithromycin retreatment regimens (CID 48:1655, 2009). Diagnosis by NAAT, if available. Doxy ineffective. No cell wall so beta-lactams ineffective. Cure with single dose Azithro only 67% (CID 61:S802, 2015). High failure rate of Azithro x 1 for M. genitalium (CID 56:934, 2013). Can try Moxi 400 mg once daily x 10 days (if Azithro failure (PLoS One 3:e3618, 2008). New FQ resistance in Japan (JAC 69:2376, 2014).
Recurrent/persistent urethritis	**C. trachomatis** (43%), **M. genitalium** (30%), **T. vaginalis** (13%) (CID 52:163, 2011).	**Metro** 2 gm po x 1 dose + **Azithro** 1 gm po x 1 dose	**Tinidazole** 2 gm po x 1 + **Azithromycin** 1 gm po x 1	
Gonorrhea. FQs no longer recommended for treatment of gonococcal infections (See CDC Guidelines MMWR 64(RR-3):1, 2015; CID 61:S785, 2015) **Cephalosporin resistance:** JAMA 309:163 & 185, 2013				
Conjunctivitis (adult)	N. gonorrhoeae	**Ceftriaxone** 1 gm IM or IV single dose + **Azithro** 1 gm po x 1		Consider one-time saline lavage of eye.
Disseminated gonococcal infection (DGI, dermatitis-arthritis syndrome)	N. gonorrhoeae	**Ceftriaxone** 1 gm IV q24h or **Cefotaxime** 1 gm q8h IV or **Ceftizoxime** 1 gm q8h IV) + **Azithro** 1 gm po x 1		Treat for a minimum of 7 days. Owing to high-level resistance to oral cephalosporins and fluoroquinolones in the community, "Step-down" therapy should be avoided unless susceptibilities are known and demonstrate full activity of cephalosporin or fluoroquinolone. **Treat presumptively for concomitant C. trachomatis. Treat presumptively** to cover resistant GC (usually tetra resistant, too) and C. trachomatis. Azithro now recommended to cover resistant GC (usually tetra resistant, too) and C. trachomatis. GC endocarditis may occur in the absence of concomitant urogenital symptoms (Infection 42: 425, 2014). Severe valve destruction may occur.
Endocarditis	N. gonorrhoeae	**Ceftriaxone** 1–2 gm IV q12–24 hours x 4 weeks + **Azithro** 1 gm po x 1		Ceftriaxone resistance in N. gonorrhoeae has been reported (AAC 55: 3538, 2011); determine susceptibility if any isolate recovered.
Pharyngitis Dx: NAAT	N. gonorrhoeae	**Ceftriaxone** 250 mg IM x 1 + **Azithro** 1 gm po x 1 **Alternative: Azithro** 2 gm po x 1.		Pharyngeal GC more difficult to eradicate. Repeat NAAT 14 days post-rx. **Spectinomycin**NUS not effective
Urethritis, cervicitis, proctitis (uncomplicated) For prostatitis, see page 27 **Diagnosis:** Nucleic acid amplification test (NAAT) on vaginal swab, urine or urethral swab. MMWR 64(RR-3):1, 2015	N. gonorrhoeae 50% of pts with urethritis, cervicitis have concomitant C. trachomatis — **treat for both even if NAAT indicates single pathogen.**	**Ceftriaxone** 250 mg IM x 1 + **Azithro** 1 gm po x 1 **Rx failure: Ceftriaxone** 500 mg IM x 1 + **Azithro** 2 gm po x 1; treat partner. NAAT for test of cure post-treatment. **Severe Pen/Ceph allergy:** (**Gent** 240 mg IM + **Azithro** 2 gm po x 1) OR (**Gem** 320 mg + **Azithro** 2 gm po x 1 dose) (CID 59:1083, 2014) (nausea in >20%) **Ceftriaxone** 250 mg IM x 1 + **Azithro** 1 gm po x 1.	Due to resistance concerns, **do not use FQs.**	**Screen for syphilis.** **After Rx for ALL of these approaches listed below):** • **Oral cephalosporin** use is no longer recommended as primary therapy owing to emergence of resistance, MMWR 61:590, 2012. • Other single-dose cephalosporins: cefixime 500 mg IM, cefotaxime 2 gm IM + probenecid 1 gm po.
Pregnancy				

*NOTE: All dosage recommendations are for adults (unless otherwise indicated) and assume normal renal function. § Alternatives consider allergy, PK, compliance, local resistance, cost

TABLE 1 (21)

ANATOMIC SITE/DIAGNOSIS/ MODIFYING CIRCUMSTANCES	ETIOLOGIES (usual)	SUGGESTED REGIMENS*		ADJUNCT DIAGNOSTIC OR THERAPEUTIC MEASURES AND COMMENTS
		PRIMARY	ALTERNATIVE†	
GENITAL TRACT/Both Women & Men (continued)				
Granuloma inguinale (Donovanosis)	Klebsiella (formerly Calymmatobacterium) granulomatis	**Azithro** 1 gm po q wk. x 3 wks	**TMP-SMX** one DS tablet bid x 3 wks **OR Erythro** 500 mg po qid x 3 wks **OR CIP** 750 mg po bid x 3 wks **OR Doxy** 100 mg po bid x 3 wks	Clinical response usually seen in 1 wk. **Rx until all lesions healed**, may take 4 wks. Treatment failures & recurrence seen with doxy & TMP-SMX. Relapse can occur 6–18 months after apparently effective rx. If improvement not evidence in first few days, some experts add gentamicin 1 mg/kg IV q8h.
Herpes simplex virus	See Table 14A, page 169			
Human papilloma virus (HPV)	See Table 14A, page 174			
Lymphogranuloma venereum Ref: CID 61:S865, 2015	Chlamydia trachomatis, serovars L1, L2, L3	**Doxy** 100 mg po bid x 21 days	**Erythro** 0.5 gm po qid x 21 days or **Azithro** 1 gm po qwk x 3 weeks (clinical data lacking)	Dx based on serology; biopsy contraindicated because sinus tracts develop. Nucleic acid ampli tests for C. trachomatis will be positive. In MSM, presents as fever, rectal ulcer, anal discharge (CID 39:996, 2004; Dis Colon Rectum 52:507, 2009).
Phthirus pubis (**pubic lice, "crabs"**) & scabies	Phthirus pubis & Sarcoptes scabiei	See Table 13A, page 161		
Syphilis Diagnosis: JAMA 312:1922, 2014; treatment: JAMA 312:1905, 2014; management: CID 61:S818, 2015.	T. pallidum NOTE: Test all pts with syphilis for HIV, test all HIV patients for latent syphilis.			
Early: primary, secondary or latent <1 yr. Screen with treponema-specific antibody or RPR/VDRL, see JCM 50:2, 2012; CID 58:1116, 2014.		**Benzathine pen G (Bicillin L-A)** 2.4 million units IM x 1 dose or **Azithro** 2 gm po x 1 dose (See Comment)	**Doxy** 100 mg po bid x 14 days) or **tetracycline** 500 mg po qid x 14 days) or **(ceftriaxone** 1 gm IM/IV q24h x 10-14 days). Follow-up mandatory.	If early or congenital syphilis, **quantitative VDRL at 0, 3, 6, 12 & 24 mos** after rx. If <2000 in early syphilis, VDRL should ↓ 4-fold by 12 mos, & 4 tubes 24 mos. Update on congenital syphilis MMWR 59:413, 2010. Early latent: 2 tubes (4x) at 12 mos. With 1°, 50% will be RPR seronegative at 12 mos, 24% neg. FTA/ABS at 2-3 yrs (AnIM 114:1005, 1991). If titers fail to fall, examine CSF; if CSF (+), treat as neurosyphilis; if CSF is negative, retreat with benzathine Pen G x 3 weekly x 3 wks. If no other options: **Azithro** 2 gm po x 1 dose equivalent to **benzathine Pen G** 2.4 M x 1 dose in early syphilis (J Infect Dis 201:1729, 2010). **Azithro-resistant syphilis** documented in California, Ireland, & elsewhere (CID 44:S130, 2007; AAC 54:583, 2010).
More than 1 yr's duration (latent of indeterminate duration, cardiovascular, late benign gumma).	For penicillin desensitization method, see Table 7, page 83 and MMWR 64 (RR-3):1, 2015	**Benzathine pen G (Bicillin L-A)** 2.4 million units IM x 3 = 7.2 million units total	**Doxy** 100 mg po bid 28 days or **tetracycline** 500 mg po x 28 days; **Ceftriaxone** 1 gm IV or IM q24h for 10-14 days MAY be an alternative (No clinical data, consult an ID specialist)	NOTE: Use of **benzathine procaine penicillin** is inappropriate! No data on efficacy of alternatives. **Indications for LP (CSC):** neurologic symptoms; treatment failure, any eye or ear involvement, other evidence of active syphilis (aortitis, gumma, iritis).
Neurosyphilis—Very difficult to treat. Includes ocular (retrobulbar neuritis). **All need CSF exam.**		**Pen G** 18-24 million units per day either as continuous infusion or as 3-4 million units IV q4h x 10-14 days	**(Procaine pen G** 2.4 million units IM q24h + **probenecid** 0.5 gm po qid) both x 10-14 days—See Comment	**Ceftriaxone** 2 gm (IV or IM) q24h x 14 days. 23% failure rate reported (AJM 93:481, 1992). For penicillin allergy, either desensitize to penicillin or obtain infectious diseases consultation. Serologic criteria for response to rx: **4-fold or greater ↓ in VDRL titer over 6-12 mos.**
HIV infection [AIDS] CID 44:S130, 2007.		Treatment same as HIV-uninfected with close follow-up. Treat early neurosyphilis if CD4 count: MMWR 56:625, 2007		Skin test for penicillin allergy. Desensitize if necessary. Parenteral pen G is only drug with documented efficacy.
Pregnancy and syphilis		Same as for non-pregnant, some recommend 2nd dose **benzathine pen G** (2.4 million units) 1 wk. after initial dose esp. in 3rd trimester or with 2° syphilis		Monthly quantitative VDRL or equivalent. If 4-fold ↓, re-treat. Doxy tetracycline contraindicated. Erythro not recommended because of high risk of failure to cure fetus

Abbreviations on page 2.

*NOTE: All dosage recommendations are for adults (unless otherwise indicated) and assume normal renal function. § Alternatives consider allergy, PK, compliance, local resistance, cost

TABLE 1 (22)

ANATOMIC SITE/DIAGNOSIS/ MODIFYING CIRCUMSTANCES	ETIOLOGIES (usual)	SUGGESTED REGIMENS* PRIMARY	ALTERNATIVE[1]	ADJUNCT DIAGNOSTIC OR THERAPEUTIC MEASURES AND COMMENTS
GENITAL TRACT/Both Women & Men (continued)				
Congenital syphilis: (Update on Congenital Syphilis: MMWR 64(RR-3):1, 2015)	T. pallidum	Aqueous crystalline pen G 50,000 units/kg per dose IV q12h x 7 days, then q8h for 10 day total	Procaine pen G 50,000 units/kg IM q24h for 10 days	Another alternative: Ceftriaxone ≤30 days old, 75 mg/kg IV/IM q24h (use with caution in infants with jaundice) or >30 days old 100 mg/kg IV/IM q24h. If symptomatic, ophthalmologic exam indicated. If more than 1 day of rx missed, restart entire course. **Need serologic follow-up!**
Warts, anogenital	See Table 14A, page 174			
Women:				
Amnionitis, septic abortion	Bacteroides, esp. Prevotella bivius; Group B, A strepto-cocci; Enterobacteriaceae; C. trachomatis. Rarely U. urealyticum.	[(Cefoxitin or DORI[NAI] or IMP or MER or AM-SB or ERTA or PIP-TZ) + doxy] OR [Clinda + (aminoglycoside or ceftriaxone)] Dosage: see footnote[††]		D&C of uterus. **In septic abortion,** Clostridium perfringens may cause fulminant intravascular hemolysis. **In postpartum patients** with enigmatic fever and/or pulmonary emboli, **consider septic pelvic vein thrombophlebitis** (See Vascular system, septic pelvic vein thrombophlebitis, page 68.) After discharge: doxy or clinda for C. trachomatis.
Cervicitis, mucopurulent Treatment based on results of nucleic acid amplification test	N. gonorrhoeae Chlamydia trachomatis	Treat for Gonorrhea, page 23 Treat for non-gonococcal urethritis, page 23		Criteria for diagnosis: 1) (muco) purulent endocervical exudate and/or 2) sustained endocervical bleeding after passage of cotton swab. >10 WBC/hpf of vaginal fluid is suggestive. Intracellular gram-neg diplococci are specific but insensitive. If in doubt, send swab or urine for culture. EIA or nucleic acid amplification test and treat for both.
		Note: In US and Europe, 1/3 of Grp B Strep resistant to clindamycin	Mycoplasma genitalium, less likely to respond to doxy than azithro.	
Endomyometritis/septic pelvic phlebitis				
Early postpartum (1st 48 hrs) (usually after C-section)	Bacteroides, esp. Prevotella bivius; Group B, A strepto-cocci; Enterobacteriaceae; C. trachomatis, M. hominis	[(Cefoxitin or ERTA or IMP or MER or AM-SB or PIP-TZ) + doxy] or [Clinda + (aminoglycoside or ceftriaxone)] Dosage: see footnote[††]		See Comments under Amnionitis, septic abortion, above
Late postpartum (48 hrs to 6 wks) (usually after vaginal delivery)	C. trachomatis, N. gonorrhoeae	Doxy 100 mg IV or po q12h times 14 days		Tetracyclines not recommended in nursing mothers; discontinue nursing. M. hominis sensitive to tetra, clinda, not erythro.
Fitz-Hugh-Curtis syndrome		Treat as for pelvic inflammatory disease immediately below.		Perihepatitis (violin-string adhesions). Sudden onset of RUQ pain. Associated with salpingitis. Transaminases elevated in < 30% of cases.
Pelvic actinomycosis; usually tubo-ovarian abscess	A. Israelii most common	AMP 50 mg/kg/day IV div 3-4 doses x 4-6 wks, then Pen VK 2-4 gm/day po x 3-6 mos.	Doxy or ceftriaxone or clinda	Complication of intrauterine device (IUD). Remove IUD. Can use **Pen G** 10-20 million units/day IV instead of **AMP** x 4-6 wks

[††] **P Ceph 2 (cefoxitin** 2 gm IV q6-8h, **cefotetan** 2 gm IV q12h; **cefuroxime** 750 mg IV q8h; **AM-SB** 3 gm IV q6h; **PIP-TZ** 3.375 gm IV q6h; **cefotaxime** 2 gm IV q8h, see Table 10D, page 118); **P Ceph 3 (cefotaxime** 2 gm IV q8h; **ceftriaxone** 2 gm IV q24h); 3.375 gm q8h; **doxy** 100 mg IV/po q12h; **clinda** 450-900 mg IV q8h; **aminoglycoside (gentamicin,** see Table 10D, page 118); **vanco** 1 gm IV q12h; **doripenem** 500 mg IV q8h (1-hr infusion); **IMP** 0.5 gm IV q6h; **ertapenem** 1 gm IV q24h; **MER** 1 gm IV q8h; **azithro** 500 mg IV/po q12h; **linezolid** 600 mg IV/po q12h; **vanco** 1 gm IV q12h

Abbreviations on page 2.   *NOTE: All dosage recommendations are for adults (unless otherwise indicated) and assume normal renal function. § Alternatives consider allergy, PK: compliance, local resistance, cost

TABLE 1 (23)

ANATOMIC SITE/DIAGNOSIS/ MODIFYING CIRCUMSTANCES	ETIOLOGIES (usual)	SUGGESTED REGIMENS*		ADJUNCT DIAGNOSTIC OR THERAPEUTIC MEASURES AND COMMENTS
		PRIMARY	ALTERNATIVE§	
GENITAL TRACT/Women *(continued)*				
Pelvic Inflammatory Disease (PID), salpingitis, tubo-ovarian abscess				
Outpatient rx: limit to pts with temp <38°C, WBC <11,000 per mm³, minimal evidence of peritonitis, active bowel sounds & able to tolerate oral nourishment *NEJM 372:2039, 2015;* *CDC Guidelines MMWR 64(RR-3):1, 2015*	N. gonorrhoeae, chlamydia, bacteroides, Enterobacteriaceae, streptococci, especially S. agalactiae Less commonly: G. vaginalis, Haemophilus influenzae, cytomegalovirus (CMV), M. genitalium, U. urealyticum	**Outpatient rx:** [(**ceftriaxone** 250 mg IM (√ x 1) (± **metro** 500 mg po bid x 14 days)) + (**doxy** 100 mg po bid x 14 days)]. **OR** (**cefoxitin** 2 gm IM both probenecid 1 gm po with as single dose) plus (**doxy** 100 mg po bid with **metro** 500 mg bid—both times 14 days)	**Inpatient regimens:** [(**Cefotetan** 2 gm IV q12h or **cefoxitin** 2 gm IV q6h) + (**doxy** 100 mg IV/po q12h)] **Clinda** 900 mg (IV q8h) + (**gentamicin** 2 mg/kg loading dose, then 1.5 mg/kg q8h or 4.5 mg/(kg once per day), then **doxy** 100 mg bid x 14 days	Another alternative parenteral regimen: **AM-SB** 3 gm IV q6h + **doxy** 100 mg IV/po q12h. Recommended treatments don't cover M. genitalium so if no response after 7-10 d consider M. genitalium NAAT and treat with Moxi 400 mg x 14 days. Remember: Evaluate and treat sex partner. FQs not recommended due to increasing resistance *MMWR 64(RR-3):1, 2015* & www.cdc.gov/std/treatment). Suggest initial patient evaluation/therapy for pts with tubo-ovarian abscess. For inpatient regimens, continue treatment until satisfactory response for ≥24-hr before switching to outpatient regimen. Improved routine testing for chlamydia and N. gonorrhoeae among outpatients resulted in reduced hospitalization and ectopic pregnancy rates (*J Adolescent Health 51:80, 2012*).
Vaginitis— *MMWR 64(RR-3):1, 2015*				
Candidiasis Pruritus, thick cheesy discharge, pH <4.5 *See Table 11A, page 125*	Candida albicans 80-90%. C. glabrata, C. tropicalis may be increasing—they are less susceptible to azoles	**Oral azoles: Fluconazole** 150 mg po x 1; **itraconazole** 200 mg po x 1 day. For milder cases, **Topical Therapy** with one of the over the counter preparations usually successful (e.g. clotrimazole, butoconazole, miconazole, or tioconazole) as creams or vaginal suppositories.	**Intravaginal azoles:** variety of strengths—from 1 dose to 14 days. Drugs available (all end in -azole): butocon, clotrim, micon, tiocon, tercon (doses: *Table 11A*)	Nystatin vag. tabs times 14 days less effective. Other rx for azole-resistant strains: gentian violet, boric acid. If recurrent candidiasis (≥4 or more episodes per yr): 6 mos. suppression with: fluconazole 150 mg po q week or itraconazole 100 mg po q24h or clotrimazole vag. suppositories 500 mg q week.
Trichomoniasis (*CID 61:S837, 2015*) Copious foamy discharge, pH >4.5 Treat sexual partners—see Comment	Trichomonas vaginalis **Dx:** NAAT & PCR available & most sensitive; wet mount not sensitive. Ref. *JCM 54:7, 2016*.	**Metro** 2 gm as single dose or 500 mg po bid x 7 days **OR** **Tinidazole** 2 gm po single dose **Pregnancy:** See Comment	**For rx failure:** Re-treat with metro 500 mg bid x 7 days; if 2nd failure: metro 2 gm po q24h x 3-5 days or **Tinidazole** 2 gm po q24h x 5 days	Treat male sexual partners (**2 gm metronidazole as single dose**). Nearly 20% men with NGU are infected with trichomonas (*JID 188:465, 2003*). For alternative option in refractory cases, see *CID 33:1341, 2001*. **Pregnancy:** No data implicating metro teratogenic or mutagenic. For discussion of treating trichomonas, including issues in pregnancy, see *MMWR 64(RR-3):1, 2015.*
Bacterial vaginosis (BV) Malodorous vaginal discharge, pH >4.5	Etiology unclear: associated with Gardnerella vaginalis, mobiluncus, Mycoplasma hominis, Prevotella sp., & Atopobium vaginae et al.	**Metro** 0.5 gm po bid x 7 days or **metro vaginal gel** (0.75%) 1 applicator intra-vaginally) 1x/day x 5 days **OR** **2% clinda vaginal cream** 5 gm intravaginally at bedtime x 7 days	**Clinda** 0.3 gm po bid x 7 days or **clinda ovules** 100 mg intravaginally at bedtime x 3 days.	Reported 50%† cure rate if abstain from sex or use condoms. *CID 44:213 & 220, 2007.* Treatment of male sex partner **not** indicated unless balanitis present. Metro extended release tabs 750 mg po q24h x 7 days available; no published data. **Pregnancy:** Oral **metro** or oral **clinda** 7-day regimens (see CDC STD Guidelines, *MMWR 64(RR-3):1, 2015*). If recurrent BV can try adding **boric acid** gelatin capsule 600 mg hs x 21 days, followed by Metro vaginal gel 2x/week x 16 weeks (*Sex Trans Dis 36:732, 2009*).

¹² 1 applicator contains 5 gm of gel with 37.5 mg metronidazole

Abbreviations on page 2.   *NOTE: All dosage recommendations are for adults (unless otherwise indicated) and assume normal renal function. § Alternatives consider allergy, PK, compliance, local resistance, cost

TABLE 1 (24)

ANATOMIC SITE/DIAGNOSIS/ MODIFYING CIRCUMSTANCES	ETIOLOGIES (usual)	SUGGESTED REGIMENS* PRIMARY	ALTERNATIVE§	ADJUNCT DIAGNOSTIC OR THERAPEUTIC MEASURES AND COMMENTS
GENITAL TRACT (continued)				
Men:				
Balanitis	Candida 40%, Group B strep, gardnerella	**Metro** 2 gm po as a single dose **OR Fluc** 150 mg po x1 OR **Itra** 200 mg po bid x 1 day.		Occurs in 1/4 of male sex partners of women infected with candida. Exclude circinate balanitis (Reiter's syndrome); (non-infectious) responds to hydrocortisone cream.
Epididymo-orchitis (CID 61:S770, 2015)				
Age <35 yrs	N. gonorrhoeae, Chlamydia trachomatis	**Ceftriaxone** 250 mg IM x 1 + **doxy** 100 mg po bid x10 days) + bed rest, scrotal elevation, analgesics.		Enterobacteriaceae occasionally encountered. Test all pts age < 35 yrs for HIV and syphilis.
Age >35 years or MSM (insertive partners in anal intercourse)	Enterobacteriaceae (coliforms)	**Levo** 500-750 mg IV/po once daily) OR (**Oflox** 300 mg po bid) or (400 mg IV twice daily) for 10-14 days. **AM-SB, P Ceph 3, PIP-TZ** (Dosage: see footnote page 25) for MSM can be mixed GC/chlamydia with enterics so treat with FQ AND Ceftriaxone 250 mg IM x1 Also: bed rest, scrotal elevation, analgesics		Midstream pyuria and scrotal pain and edema. NOTE: Do urine NAAT (nucleic acid amplification test) to ensure absence of N. gonorrhoeae with concomitant lack of FQ-resistant gonorrhoeae or of chlamydia if using adequate test with reliable activity. Other causes include: mumps, brucella, TB, intravesicular BCG, B. pseudomallei, coccidioides, Behçet's.
Non-gonococcal urethritis	See page 23 (CID 61:S763, 2015).			
Prostatitis—Review: CID 50:1641, 2010. See Guidelines 2015 http://onlinelibrary.wiley.com/doi/10.1111/bju.13101/epdf				
Acute	N. gonorrhoeae, C. trachomatis	**ceftriaxone** 250 mg IM x 1 then **doxy** 100 mg bid x 10 days.		FQs no longer recommended for gonococcal infections. Test for HIV. In AIDS pts, prostate may be focus of Cryptococcus neoformans.
Uncomplicated (with risk of STD; age < 35 yrs)	Enterobacteriaceae (coliforms)	**FQ** (dosage: see Epididymo-orchitis, >35 yrs, above) or **TMP-SMX** 1 DS tablet (160 mg TMP) po bid x 10-14 days (minimum). Some authorities recommend 4-6 wks therapy.	**TMP-SMX-DS** 1 tab po bid x 1-3 mos (Fostomycin, see Comment)	Treat as acute urinary infection, 14 days (not single dose regimen). Some recommend 3-4 wks therapy. If uncertain, do NAAT for C. trachomatis and N. gonorrhoeae. If resistant enterobacteriaceae, use ERTA 1 gm IV qd. If resistant pseudomonas, use IMP or MER (1gm IV q6 or q8 respectively).
Uncomplicated with low risk of STD	Enterobacteriaceae 80%, enterococci 15%, P. aeruginosa	**CIP** 500 mg po x 4 wks OR **Levo** 750 mg po q24h x 4 wks.		**With treatment failures** consider infected prostatic calculi. FDA approved dose of levo is 500 mg; editors prefer higher dose. Fosfomycin penetrates prostate; case report of success with 3 gm po q24h x 12-16 wks (CID 61:1141, 2015).
Chronic bacterial				
Chronic prostatitis/chronic pain syndrome	The most common prostatitis syndrome. Etiology is unknown.	**α-adrenergic blocking agents are controversial** (AnIM 133:367, 2000).		Pt has 5x of prostatitis but negative cultures and no cells in prostatic secretions. Rev.: JAC 46:157, 2000. In randomized double-blind study, CIP and an alpha-blocker of no benefit (AnIM 141:581 & 639, 2004)
HAND (Bites: See Skin)				
Paronychia				
Nail biting, manicuring	Staph. aureus (maybe MRSA)	Incision & drainage; culture	**TMP-SMX-DS** 1-2 tabs po bid while waiting for culture result.	See Table 6 for alternatives: Occasionally--candida, gram-negative rods.
Contact with saliva— dentists, anesthesiologists, wrestlers	Herpes simplex (Whitlow)	**Acyclovir** 400 mg po x 10 days	**Famciclovir** or **valacyclovir** see Comment	Gram stain and routine culture negative. Famciclovir/valacyclovir for primary genital herpes; see Table 14A, page 169
Dishwasher (prolonged water immersion)	Candida sp.	**Clotrimazole** (topical)		Avoid immersion of hands in water as much as possible.

*NOTE: All dosage recommendations are for adults (unless otherwise indicated) and assume normal renal function. §Alternatives consider allergy; PK, compliance, local resistance, cost

Abbreviations on page 2.

TABLE 1 (25)

ANATOMIC SITE/DIAGNOSIS/ MODIFYING CIRCUMSTANCES	ETIOLOGIES (usual)	SUGGESTED REGIMENS* PRIMARY	ALTERNATIVE§	ADJUNCT DIAGNOSTIC OR THERAPEUTIC MEASURES AND COMMENTS
HEART **Infective endocarditis— Native valve—empiric rx awaiting cultures—No IV illicit drugs** Valvular or congenital heart disease and no modifying circumstances. See Table 15C, page 204 for prophylaxis	**NOTE: Diagnostic criteria** include evidence of continuous bacteremia (multiple positive blood cultures), new murmur (worsening of old murmur) of valvular insufficiency, definite emboli, and echocardiographic (transthoracic or transesophageal) evidence of valvular vegetations, see Table 15C, page 204. For antimicrobial prophylaxis, see Table 15C, page 204. Viridans strep 30–40%, "other" strep 15–25%, enterococci 5–18%, staphylococci 20–35% (including coag-neg staphylococci-CID 46:232, 2008).	**Vanco** 15–20 mg/kg IV q8–12h (target trough conc of 15–20 μg/mL) + **Ceftriaxone** 2g q24h OR **Vanco** 15–20 mg/kg IV q8–12h (target trough conc of 15–20 μg/mL) + **Gent** 1 mg/kg q8h IV/IM	Substitute **Dapto** 6 mg/kg IV q24h (or q48h for CrCl < 30 mL/min) for **Vanco**	If patient not acutely ill and not in heart failure, wait for blood culture results. If initial 3 blood cultures neg. after 24–48 hrs, obtain 2–3 more blood cultures before empiric therapy started. Gent dose is for CrCl of 80 mL/min or greater; use low-dose Gentamicin for only a few days carries risk of nephrotoxicity (CID 48:713, 2009). Gent is used for synergy; peak levels need not exceed 4 μg/mL and troughs should be < 1 μg/mL. Coagulase-negative staphylococci can occasionally cause native valve endocarditis (CID 46:232, 2008). Modify therapy based on identification of specific pathogen as soon as possible to obtain best coverage and to avoid toxicities. **Surgery indications:** See NEJM 368:1425, 2013. Role of surgery in pts with left-sided endocarditis with large vegetation (NEJM 366:2466, 2012). No difference in 15 yr survival between bioprosthetic and mechanical valve (JAMA 312:1323, 2014).
Infective endocarditis—Native valve—IV illicit drug use ± evidence rt-sided endocarditis — empiric therapy	**S. aureus (MSSA & MRSA).** All others rare	**Vanco** 15–20 mg/kg IV q8–12h to achieve target trough concentrations of 15–20 mcg/mL recommended for serious infections.	**Dapto** 6 mg/kg IV q24h. Approved for right-sided endocarditis.	Target gent levels: peak 3 mcg/mL, trough < 1 mcg/mL. If very obese pt, recommend consultation for dosage adjustment. Infuse vanco over 2 hrs to avoid "red man" syndrome. **S. bovis suggests occult bowel pathology** (new name: *S. gallolyticus*).
Infective endocarditis—Native valve—culture positive Ref: Circulation 132:1435, 2015. Viridans strep, S. bovis (S. gallolyticus subsp. gallolyticus) MIC ≤0.12 mcg/mL		[(**Pen G** 12–18 million units/day IV, divided q4h) x 4 wks OR (**ceftriaxone** 2 gm IV q24h x 4 wks) OR (**Pen G** 12–18 million units/day IV, divided q4h x 2 wks) PLUS **gentamicin** IV 1 mg/kg q8h IV x 2 wks]	(**Ceftriaxone** 2 gm IV q24h x 4 wks) + **gentamicin** 1 mg/kg per IV q8h both x 2 wks). If allergy pen G or ceftriax, use **vanco** 15 mg/kg IV q12h x 4 wks. 2 gm/day max unless serum levels measured x 4 wks	Since relapse rate may be greater in pts for > 3 mos. prior to start of rx, the penicillin-gentamicin synergism theoretically may be advantageous in this group.
Viridans strep, S. bovis (S. gallolyticus) with penicillin G MIC >0.12 to ≤0.5 mcg/mL	Viridans strep, S. bovis, nutritionally variant streptococci (e.g. S. abiotrophia) tolerant strep	**Pen G** 18 million units/day IV (divided q4h) x 4 wks PLUS **gentamicin** 1 mg/kg IV q8h x 2 wks **NOTE: Low dose of Gent**	**Vanco** 15 mg/kg IV q12h to max. 2 gm/day unless serum levels documented x 4 wks	Can use cefazolin for pen G in pt with allergy that is not IgE-mediated (e.g., anaphylaxis). Alternatively, can use vanco. (See Comment above on gent and vanco).
For viridans strep or S. bovis with **pen G MIC >0.5** and enterococci susceptible to AMP/pen G, vanco, gentamicin (synergy positive) **NOTE: Inf. Dis. consultation suggested**	"**Susceptible" enterococci,** viridans strep, S. bovis, nutritionally variant streptococci (new names are: Abiotrophia sp. & Granulicatella sp.)	[(**Pen G** 18–30 million units per day IV, divided q4h x 4–6 wks) OR (**AMP** 12 gm/day IV, divided q4h + **gent** x 4–6 wks)]	**Vanco** 15 mg/kg IV q12h (to max of 2 gm/day unless serum levels measured PLUS **gentamicin** 1 mg/kg q8h IV x 4–6 wks **NOTE: Low dose of gent**	**It is necessary to remove infected valve & valve culture neg., 2 weeks antibiotic treatment post-op sufficient** (CID 41:187, 2005). 4 wks of rx if symptoms > 3 mos., 6 wks of rx if enterococci. Vanco for pen-allergic pts; do not use cephalosporins. Do not give gent once-q24h for enterococcal endocarditis. Target gent peak 20–50 mcg/mL, trough <1 mcg/mL. Vanco peak 5–12 mcg/mL. **NOTE:** Because of ↑ frequency of resistance (see below), all enterococci causing endocarditis should be tested in vitro for susceptibility to penicillin, gentamicin and vancomycin plus β lactamase production.

*NOTE: All dosage recommendations are for adults (unless otherwise indicated) and assume normal renal function. § Alternatives consider allergy, PK compliance, local resistance cost

TABLE 1 (26)

ANATOMIC SITE/DIAGNOSIS/ MODIFYING CIRCUMSTANCES	ETIOLOGIES (usual)	SUGGESTED REGIMENS*		ADJUNCT DIAGNOSTIC OR THERAPEUTIC MEASURES AND COMMENTS
		PRIMARY	ALTERNATIVE§	
HEART/Infective endocarditis—Native valve—culture positive		(continued) Ref. *Circulation* 132:1435, 2015.		
Enterococci: MIC streptomycin >2000 mcg/mL, MIC gentamicin >500-2000 mcg/mL, no resistance to penicillin	Enterococci, high-level aminoglycoside resistance. Esp with E. faecium, often concomitant resistance to Vanco	**E. faecium** (assumes Vanco-resistance): **Dapto** 8-12 mg/kg IV q24h + **Cefotaroline** 2 gm q8h OR **Ceftriaxone** 2 gm IV q12h; **AMP** 2 gm IV q4h x 6 wks (*CID* 56:1261, 2013 & AHA Guidelines).	**E. faecalis: Ceftriaxone** 2 gm q12h + **AMP** 2 gm IV q4h x 6 wks (*CID* 56:1261, 2013 & AHA Guidelines)	10-25% E. faecalis and 45-50% E. faecium resistant to high gent levels. May have to consider surgical removal of infected valve. Theory of efficacy of combination of Amp + Ceftriaxone: sequential blocking of PBPs 4&5 (Amp) and 2&3 (ceftriaxone).
Enterococci: Pen G MIC >16 mcg/mL; no gentamicin resistance	Enterococci, intrinsic pen G/AMP resistance (E. faecium or E. faecalis)	**E. faecium: Dapto** 8-12 mg/kg IV q24h + (**AMP** 2 gm IV q4h OR **Cefotaroline** 600 mg IV q8h) OR **Dapto** 8-12 mg/kg IV q24h + **Gent** 1 mg/kg q8h *(Curr Infect Dis Rep 16:431, 2014)*	**E. faecalis: Vanco** 15 mg/kg IV q12h + **Gent** 1 mg/kg IV q8h OR, if beta lactamase positive: **AM-SB** 3 gm IV q6h + **Gent** 1 mg/kg IV q8h	Target Vanco trough levels at 10-20 mcg/mL **Gentamicin** used for synergy; peak levels need not exceed 4 mcg/mL and trough should be <1.
Enterococci: Pen/AMP resistant + high-level gent/strep resistant + vanco resistant, usually VRE Consultation suggested	Enterococci, vanco-resistant, resistant to beta-lactams Common VRE pattern of susceptibilities	**E. faecium: Dapto** 8-12 mg/kg IV q24h + (**AMP** 2 gm IV q4h OR **Cefotaroline** 600 mg IV q8h) *(Curr Infect Dis Rep 16:431, 2014)*	**E. faecalis** (rare situation): **Dapto** 8-12 mg/kg IV q24h + **AMP** 2 gm IV q4h OR **Cefotaroline** 600 mg IV q8h *(Curr Infect Dis Rep 16:431, 2014)*	AMP or Cefotaroline lessens risk of developing Dapto resistance & reverses resistance if present. Quinu-dalfo 7.5 mg/kg IV (central line) q8h is alternative for E. faecium (IE: faecalis is resistant). Quinu-dalfo + AMP- see *Circulation 127:1810, 2013)* (success reported). Linezolid mono- or combo-therapy for both E. faecium / E. faecalis: variable success; bacteriostatic for enterococci *(Curr Infect Dis Rep 16:431, 2014)*.
Staphylococcal endocarditis Aortic &/or mitral valve infection—MSSA Surgery indications: see Comment page 28.	Staph. aureus, methicillin-sensitive	**Nafcillin** (oxacillin) 2 gm IV q4h x 4-6 wks	**Cefazolin** 2 gm IV q8h x 4-6 wks) OR **Vanco** 30-60 mg/kg/day in 2-3 divided doses to achieve trough of 15-20 mcg/mL x 4-6 wks	If IgE-mediated penicillin allergy. 10% cross-reactivity to cephalosporins *(AnM 141:16, 2004)*. **Cefazolin** and **Nafcillin** probably similar in efficacy and Cefazolin better tolerated *(AAC 55:5122, 2011)*
Aortic and/or mitral valve—MRSA	Staph. aureus, methicillin-resistant	**Vanco** 30-60 mg/kg per day in 2-3 divided doses to achieve target trough concentrations 15-20 mcg/mL recommended for serious infections.	**Dapto** 8-10 mg/kg IV q24h (NOT FDA approved for this indication or dose)	In clinical trial *(NEJM 355:653, 2006)*, high failure rate with both vanco and dapto in small numbers of pts. For other alternatives, see Table 6, pg 82. Cefotaroline references: *(JAC 68:936 & 2921, 2013.* Case reports of success with Telavancin *(JAC 65:1315, 2010; AAC 54:5376, 2010; (JAC vol B), 2011)* and ceftaroline *(JAC 67:1267, 2012; J Infect Chemo online 7/14/12)*.
Tricuspid valve infection (usually IVDUs): MSSA	Staph. aureus, methicillin-sensitive	**Nafcillin** (oxacillin) 2 gm IV q4h **PLUS gentamicin** 1 mg/kg IV q8h x 2 wks. **NOTE: low dose of gent.**	If penicillin allergy: **Vanco** 30-60 mg/kg/d in 2-3 divided doses to achieve trough of 15-20 mcg/mL x 4 wks OR **Dapto** 8-12 mg/kg IV q24h (avoid if concomitant left-sided endocarditis; 8-10 mg/kg IV q24h used in some cases, but not FDA approved	**2-week regimen not long enough** if metastatic infection (e.g. osteo) or left-sided endocarditis. If **Dapto** is used treat for at least 4 wks. **Dapto** resistance can occur de novo, after or during vanco, or after/during dapto therapy. Cefazolin 2 gm q8h also an option. Fewer adverse events and discontinuations vs nafcillin *(Clin Infect Dis 59:369, 2014)*.

Abbreviations on page 2.

*NOTE: All dosage recommendations are for adults (unless otherwise indicated) and assume normal renal function. § Alternatives consider allergy, PK, compliance, local resistance, cost

TABLE 1 (27)

ANATOMIC SITE/DIAGNOSIS/ MODIFYING CIRCUMSTANCES	ETIOLOGIES (usual)	SUGGESTED REGIMENS*		ADJUNCT DIAGNOSTIC OR THERAPEUTIC MEASURES AND COMMENTS
		PRIMARY	ALTERNATIVE†	
HEART/Infective endocarditis—Native valve—culture positive *(continued)*				
Tricuspid valve-MRSA	Staph. aureus, methicillin-resistant	**Vanco** 15-20 mg/kg q8-12h to achieve target trough concentrations of 15-20 mg/mL, recommended for serious infections **x 4-6 wks**	**Dapto** 6 mg/kg IV q24h x 4-6 wks equiv to **vanco** for rt-sided concentrations: both vanco & dapto did poorly lt-sided endocarditis (*NEJM 355: 653, 2006*). (See Comments & table 6, page 82)	**Linezolid:** Limited experience (see *JAC 58:273, 2006*) in patients with few treatment options; 64% cure rate; clear failure in 21%; thrombocytopenia in 31%. **Dapto** dose of 8-12 mg/kg may help in selected cases, but not FDA-approved
Slow-growing fastidious Gm-neg. bacilli–any valve	HACEK group *(see Comments)*	**Ceftriaxone** 2 gm IV q24h x 4 wks OR **CIP** 400 mg IV q12h or 500 mg po bid x 4 wks (Bartonella resistant – see below)	**AM-SB** 3 gm IV q6h x 4 wks or **CIP** (400 mg IV q12h or 500 mg po bid) x 4 wks	**HACEK** (acronym for **Haemophilus parainfluenzae, H. (aphrophilus) aggregatibacter, Actinobacillus, Cardiobacterium, Eikenella, Kingella**) Penicillinase-positive HACEK organisms should be susceptible to AM-SB + ceftriaxon!. Ref: *Circulation 111:e394, 2005.*
Bartonella species–any valve	B. henselae, B. quintana	(**Doxy** 100 mg IV/po bid + **RIF** 300 mg IV/po bid) x 6-8 wks		**Dx:** immunofluorescent antibody titer ≥1:800: blood cultures only occ. positive, or PCR of tissue from surgery. **Surgery:** Over 75% pts require valve surgery; relation to cure unclear. B. quintana transmitted by body lice among homeless
Infective endocarditis—"culture negative"	Fever, valvular disease, and ECHO vegetations ± emboli and neg. cultures.	Etiology in 348 patients studied by serology, culture, histoplasm, & molecular detection: C. burnetti 48%, Bartonella sp. 28%, and rarely (Abiotrophia elegans (nutritionally variant strep), Mycoplasma hominis, Legionella pneumophila, Tropheryma whipple—together 1%), *Mycoplasma* identified (most on antibiotic). See *CID 51:131, 2010* for approach to work-up. Chronic Q fever: *JCM 52:1637, 2014.*		
Infective endocarditis—Prosthetic valve—empiric therapy (cultures pending) S. aureus now most common etiology (*JAMA 297:1354, 2007*).				
Early (<2 mos post-op)	S. epidermidis, S. aureus, Rarely, Enterobacteriaceae, diphtheroids, fungi.	**Vanco** 15-20 mg/kg q8-12h + **RIF** 600 mg po q24h	**Gentamicin** 1 mg/kg IV q8h	Early surgical consultation advised especially if etiology is S. aureus, evidence of heart failure, presence of diabetes and/or renal failure, or concern for valve ring abscess (*JAMA 297:1354, 2007; CID 44:364, 2007*). Early valve surgery not associated with improved 1 year survival in patients with S. aureus prosthetic valve infection (*CID 60:741, 2015*).
Late (>2 mos post-op)	S. epidermidis, viridans strep, enterococci,S. aureus			
Infective endocarditis— Prosthetic valve—positive blood cultures Treat for 6 weeks, even if suspect Viridans Strep. **Surgical consultation advised:** Indications for surgery: severe heart failure, S. aureus infection, prosthetic dehiscence, resistant organism, emboli due to large vegetation (*JACC 48:e1, 2006*). See also, *Eur J Clin Micro Infect Dis 38:528, 2010.*	Staph. epidermidis	(**Vanco** 15-20 mg/kg q8-12h + **RIF** 300 mg po q8h) x 6 wks + **gentamicin** 1 mg/kg IV q8h x 14 days.		If S. epidermidis is susceptible to natcillin/oxacillin (in vitro not common), then substitute natcillin (or oxacillin) for vanco. Target vanco trough concentrations 15-20 μg/mL. Some clinicians prefer to wait 2-3 days after starting vanco/ gent before starting RIF, to decrease bacterial density and thus minimize risk of selecting rifampin-resistant subpopulations.
	Staph. aureus	Methicillin sensitive: (**Natcillin** 2 gm IV q4h + **RIF** 300 mg po q8h) **times 6 wks + gentamicin** 1 mg per kg IV q8h **times 14 days.** Methicillin resistant: (**Vanco** 15-20 mg/kg q8-12h to achieve a target trough of 15-20 mcg/mL) + **RIF** 300 mg po q8h **times 6 wks + gentamicin** 1 mg per kg IV q8h **times 14 days.**		In theory, could substitute CIP for aminoglycoside, but no clinical data and resistance is common. Select definitive regimen based on susceptibility
	Viridans strep, enterococci	See Infective endocarditis, native valve, culture positive, page 26 "feat for 6 weeks.		
	Enterobacteriaceae or P. aeruginosa	**aminoglycoside (tobra** (P. aeruginosa) + **PIP-TZ** (P. aeruginosa) or **an anti-pseudomonal Pen**) or **P Ceph 3 AP** or **P Ceph 4**		High mortality. Valve replacement plus antifungal therapy standard therapy but some success with antifungal therapy alone.
	Candida, aspergillus	*Table 11, page 122*		Select definitive regimen based on susceptibility. Can occur with native valves, also.

Abbreviations on page 2. *NOTE: All dosage recommendations are for adults (unless otherwise indicated) and assume normal renal function. § Alternatives consider allergy, PK, compliance, local resistance, cost

TABLE 1 (28)

ANATOMIC SITE/DIAGNOSIS/ MODIFYING CIRCUMSTANCES	ETIOLOGIES (usual)	SUGGESTED REGIMENS*		ADJUNCT DIAGNOSTIC OR THERAPEUTIC MEASURES AND COMMENTS
		PRIMARY	ALTERNATIVE§	
HEART *(continued)*				
Infective endocarditis—Q fever *LnID 10:527, 2010; NEJM 366:715, 2007.*	Coxiella burnetii	**Doxy** 100 mg po bid + **hydroxychloroquine** 600 mg/day for at least 18 mos *(Mayo Clin Proc 83:574, 2008). Pregnancy: Need long term* **TMP-SMX** *(see CID 45:548, 2007).*		**Dx:** Phase I IgG titer >800 plus clinical evidence of endocarditis. Treatment duration: 18 mos for native valve, 24 mos for prosthetic valve. Monitor serologically for 5 yrs
Pacemaker/defibrillator infections British guidelines: *JAC 70:325, 2015)*	S. aureus (40%), S. epidermidis (40%), Gram-negative bacilli (5%), fungi (5%).	**Device removal** + **vanco** 15-20 mg/kg IV q8-12h + **RIF** 300 mg po bid	**Device removal** + **dapto** 6 mg per kg IV q24h[NA] ± **RIF** *(no data)* 300 mg po bid	**Duration of rx after device removal:** For "pocket" or subcutaneous infection, 10-14 days; if lead-assoc. endocarditis, 4-6 wks depending on organism. Device removal and absence of valvular vegetation assoc. with significantly higher survival at 1 yr *(JAMA 307:1727, 2012)*.
Pericarditis, purulent— empiric therapy *Ref: Medicine 88: 52, 2009.*	Staph. aureus, Strep. pneumoniae, Group A strep, Enterobacteriaceae	**Vanco + CIP** *(Dosage, see footnote[4])*	**Vanco + CFP** *(see footnote[4])*	Drainage required if signs of tamponade. Forced to use empiric vanco due to high prevalence of MRSA.
Rheumatic fever with carditis *Ref: Ln 366:155, 2005*	Post-infectious sequelae of Group A strep infection (usually pharyngitis)	ASA, and usually prednisone 2 mg/kg po q24h for symptomatic treatment of fever, arthritis, arthralgia. May not influence carditis.		Clinical features: Carditis, polyarthritis, chorea, subcutaneous nodules, erythema marginatum. Proph: *see page 62*
Ventricular assist device-related infection *CID 57:1438, 2013*	S. aureus, S. epidermidis, aerobic gm-neg bacilli, Candida sp	After culture of blood, wounds, drive line, device pocket and maybe pump: **Vanco** 15-20 mg/kg IV q8-12h + (**Cefepime** 2 gm IV q12h) + **fluconazole** 800 mg IV q24h.	Can substitute **daptomycin** 10 mg/kg/d[AM] for **vanco, (CIP** 400 mg IV q12h or **Levo** 750 mg IV q24h) for cefepime, and (**vori, caspo, micafungin or anidulafungin**) for **fluconazole**. Modify regimen based on results of culture and susceptibility tests. Higher than FDA-approved Dapto dose because of potential emergence of resistance.	
JOINT—*Also see Lyme Disease, page 58*				
Reactive arthritis Reiter's syndrome *(See Comment for definition)*	Occurs wks after infection with C. trachomatis, Campylobacter jejuni, Yersinia enterocolitica, Shigella/Salmonella sp.	Only treatment is non-steroidal anti-inflammatory drugs		Definition: Urethritis, conjunctivitis, arthritis, and sometimes uveitis and rash. Arthritis: asymmetrical oligoarthritis of ankles, knees, feet, sacroiliitis. Rash: palms and soles—keratoderma blennorrhagica, circinate balanitis of glans penis. HLA-B27 positive predisposes to Reiter's
Poststreptococcal reactive arthritis *(See Rheumatic fever, above)*	Immune reaction after strep pharyngitis: (1) arthritis onset in <10 days, (2) lasts months, (3) unresponsive to ASA	Treat strep pharyngitis and then NSAIDs (prednisone needed in some pts)		A reactive arthritis after a β-hemolytic strep infection in absence of sufficient Jones criteria for acute rheumatic fever. Ref.: *Mayo Clin Proc 75:144, 2000.*

[4] **Aminoglycosides** *(see Table 10D, page 118),* **IMP** 0.5 gm IV q6h, **MER** 1 gm IV q8h, **natcillin** or **oxacillin** 2 gm IV q4h, **PIP-TZ** 3.375 gm IV q6h or 4.5 gm q8h, **AM-SB** 3 gm IV q6h, **P Ceph 1** (cephalothin 2 gm IV q4h or cefazolin 2 gm IV q8h), **CIP** 750 mg IV q12h, **vanco** 1 gm IV q12h, **RIF** 600 mg po q24h, **aztreonam** 1 gm IV q8h, **CFP** 2 gm IV q12h

Abbreviations on page 2.   ***NOTE:** All dosage recommendations are for adults (unless otherwise indicated) and assume normal renal function. § Alternatives consider allergy, PK, compliance, local resistance, cost*

TABLE 1 (29)

ANATOMIC SITE/DIAGNOSIS/ MODIFYING CIRCUMSTANCES	ETIOLOGIES (usual)	SUGGESTED REGIMENS*		ADJUNCT DIAGNOSTIC OR THERAPEUTIC MEASURES AND COMMENTS
		PRIMARY	ALTERNATIVE[1]	
JOINT (continued)				
Septic arthritis: Treatment requires both adequate drainage of purulent joint fluid and appropriate antimicrobial therapy. **There is no need to inject antimicrobials into joints.** Empiric therapy after collection of blood and joint fluid for culture; review Gram stain of joint fluid.				
Infants <3 mos (neonate)	Staph. aureus, Enterobacteriaceae, Group B strep	**If MRSA not a concern:** (Nafcillin or oxacillin) + P Ceph 3	**If MRSA a concern:** Vanco + P Ceph 3	Blood cultures frequently positive. Adjacent bone involved in 2/3 pts. Group B strep and gonococci most common community-acquired etiologies.
Children (3 mos–14 yrs)	S. aureus 27%, S. pyogenes & S. pneumo 14%, H. influ 3%, Gm-neg. bacilli 6%, other (GC, N. mening) 14%, unk 36%	**Vanco + (Cefotaxime, ceftizoxime or ceftriaxone)** until culture results available Steroids—see Comment		Marked ↓ in H. influenzae since use of conjugate vaccine. **NOTE:** Septic arthritis due to salmonella has no association with sickle cell disease, unlike salmonella osteomyelitis. 10 days of therapy as effective as a 30-day treatment course if there is a good clinical response and CRP levels normalize quickly (CID 48:1201, 2009).
Adults (review Gram stain): See page 58 for Lyme Disease and page 58 for gonococcal arthritis				
Acute monoarticular				
At risk for sexually-transmitted disease	N. gonorrhoeae (see page 23), S. aureus, streptococci, rarely aerobic Gm-neg. bacilli	**Gram stain negative: Ceftriaxone** 1 gm IV q24h or **cefotaxime** 1 gm IV q8h or **ceftizoxime** 1 gm IV q8h	If Gram stain shows Gm+ cocci in clusters: **vanco** 15-20 mg/kg IV q8-12h.	For treatment comments, see Disseminated GC, page 23
Not at risk for sexually-transmitted disease	S. aureus, streptococci, Gm-neg. bacilli	**All empiric choices guided by Gram stain**	**Vanco+** (CIP or Levo)	Differential includes gout and chondrocalcinosis (pseudogout). **Look for crystals in joint fluid.** **NOTE:** See Table 6 for MRSA treatment.
		Vanco + P Ceph 3	See Table 3, page 72	
		For treatment duration, see Table 2 & Table 3		
Chronic monoarticular	Brucella, nocardia, mycobacteria, fungi			
Polyarticular, usually acute	**Gonococci,** B. burgdorferi, acute rheumatic fever; viruses, e.g., hepatitis B, rubella vaccine, parvo B19	Gram stain usually negative for GC. If sexually active, culture urethra, cervix, anal canal, throat, blood, joint fluid, and then: **ceftriaxone** 1 gm IV q24h	See Table 12	If GC: usually associated petechiae and/or pustular skin lesions and tenosynovitis. Consider Lyme disease if exposure areas known to harbor infected ticks. See page 58. Expanded differential includes gout, pseudogout, reactive arthritis (HLA-B27 pos.)
Septic arthritis, post intra-articular injection	MSSE/MRSE 40% MSSA/ MRSA 20%, P. aeruginosa, Propionibacteria, AFB	**No empiric therapy.** Arthroscopy for culture/sensitivity, crystals, washout		Treat based on culture results x 14 days (assumes no foreign body present).

Abbreviations on page 2.

*NOTE: All dosage recommendations are for adults (unless otherwise indicated) and assume normal renal function. § Alternatives consider allergy, PK, compliance, local resistance, cost

TABLE 1 (30)

ANATOMIC SITE/DIAGNOSIS/ MODIFYING CIRCUMSTANCES	ETIOLOGIES (usual)	SUGGESTED REGIMENS* PRIMARY	ALTERNATIVE†	ADJUNCT DIAGNOSTIC OR THERAPEUTIC MEASURES AND COMMENTS
JOINT *(continued)*				
Infected prosthetic joint (PJI) • Suspect infection if sinus tract or wound drainage, acutely painful prosthesis, chronically painful prosthesis, or high ESR/CRP assoc. w/painful prosthesis. **Empiric therapy is NOT recommended.** Treat based on culture and sensitivity results. **3 surgical options:** 1) Debridement and prosthesis retention (if sx < 3 wks after implantation < 30 days): **IDSA Guidelines:** Data do not allow assessment of value of adding antibacterial cement to temporary joint spacers (CID 55:474, 2012). Evidence of systemic absorption of Tobra from antibiotic-impregnated cement spacers (CID 58:1783, 2014).	MSSA/MSSE	**Debridement/Retention:** [(**Nafcillin** 2 gm IV q4h or **Oxacillin** 2 gm IV q4h) or **Cefazolin** 2 gm IV q8h] + **Rifampin** 300 mg po bid x 2-6 weeks followed by [(**Ciprofloxacin** 750 mg po bid OR **Levofloxacin** 750 mg po q24h) + **Rifampin** 300 mg po bid for 3-6 months (shorter duration for total hip arthroplasty)] **1-stage exchange:** IV/PO regimen as above for 4-6 wks **2-stage exchange:** regimen as above for 4-6 wks	(**Daptomycin** 6-8 mg/kg IV q24h OR **Linezolid** 600 mg po/IV bid) + **Rifampin** 300 mg po bid	**Confirm isolate susceptibility to fluoroquinolone and rifampin:** for fluoroquinolone-resistant isolate consider using other active TMP-SMX, Doxy, Minocycline, Amoxicillin-Clavulanate, Clindamycin, or Linezolid Enterococcal infection: addition of aminoglycoside optional. • P. aeruginosa infection—consider adding aminoglycoside (but if this improves outcome unclear). Prosthesis retention most important risk factor for treatment failure (Clin Microbiol Infect 16:1789, 2010).
	MRSA/MRSE	**Debridement/Retention:** (**Vancomycin** 15 mg/kg IV q8-12h + **Rifampin** 300 mg po bid) x 2-6 weeks followed by [(**Ciprofloxacin** 750 mg po q24h) + **Rifampin** 300 mg po bid] for 3-6 months (shorter duration for total hip arthroplasty) **1-stage exchange:** regimen as above for 4-6 wks **2-stage exchange:** regimen as above for 4-6 wks	(**Daptomycin** 6-8 mg/kg IV q24h OR **Linezolid** 600 mg po/IV bid) + **Rifampin** 300 mg po bid	(Linezolid 600 mg + Rifampin 300 mg) may be effective as salvage therapy if device removal not possible (Antimicrob Ag Chemother 55:4308, 2011) If prosthesis is retained, consider long-term, suppressive therapy, particularly for staphylococcal infections; depending on in vitro susceptibility options include TMP-SMX, Doxycycline, Minocycline, Amoxicillin, Ciprofloxacin, Cephalexin. Amoxicillin, Ciprofloxacin, Cephalexin. Role of sonication of prosthesis for Dx (N Engl J Med 357:654, 2007). Other treatment consideration: Rifampin is bactericidal vs. biofilm-producing bacteria. Never use Rifampin alone due to rapid development of resistance. Rifampin 300 mg po/IV bid + Fusidic acid* 500 mg po tid is another option (Clin Microbiol Inf 12(S3):93, 2006). Watch for toxicity if Linezolid is used for more than 2 weeks of therapy.
	Streptococcus (Grps A, B, C, D, viridans, other)	**Debridement/Retention: Penicillin G** 20 million units IV continuous infusion q24h or in 4-6 divided doses OR **Ceftriaxone** 2 gm IV q24h x 4-6 weeks **1 or 2 stage exchange:** regimen as above for 4-6 wks	**Vancomycin** 15 mg/kg IV q12h	
	Enterococci	**Debridement/Retention: Pen-susceptible: Ampicillin** 12 gm IV OR **Penicillin G** 20 million units IV continuous infusion q24h or in 4-6 divided doses x 4-6 weeks **Pen-resistant: Vancomycin** 15 mg/kg IV q12h x 4-6 weeks **1 or 2 stage exchange:** regimen as above for 4-6 wks	**Daptomycin** 6-8 mg/kg IV q24h OR **Linezolid** 600 mg po/IV bid	
	Propionibacterium acnes	**Debridement/Retention: Penicillin G** 20 million units IV q24h OR **Ceftriaxone** 2 gm IV q24h x 4-6 weeks **1 or 2 stage exchange:** regimen as above for 4-6 wks	**Vancomycin** 15 mg/kg IV q12h OR **Clindamycin** 300-450 mg po/IV bid	
	Gm-neg enteric bacilli	**Debridement/Retention: Ertapenem** 1 gm q24h IV OR other beta-lactam (e.g., **Ceftriaxone** 2 gm IV q24h OR **Cefepime** 2 gm IV q12h, based on susceptibility) x 4-6 weeks **1 or 2 stage exchange:** regimen as above for 4-6 wks	**Ciprofloxacin** 750 mg po bid	
	P. aeruginosa	**Debridement/Retention: Cefepime** 2 gm IV q12h OR **Meropenem** 1 gm IV q8h + **Tobramycin** 5.1 mg/kg once daily x	**Ciprofloxacin** 750 mg po bid or 400 mg IV q8h	
Rheumatoid arthritis	**TNF inhibitors** (adalimumab, certolizumab, etanercept, golimumab, infliximab) and other anti-inflammatory biologics (tofacitinib, rituximab, tocilizumab, abatacept) ↑ risk of TBc, fungal infection, legionella, listeria, and malignancy. See Med Lett 55:1, 2013 for full listing.			Empiric MRSA coverage recommended if risk factors are present and in high prevalence areas. Immunosuppression, not duration of therapy, is a risk factor for recurrence. 7 days of therapy may be sufficient for immunocompetent patients undergoing one-stage bursectomy (J Antimicrob Chemo 65:1008, 2010).
Septic bursitis; Olecranon bursitis; prepatellar bursitis	Staph. aureus >80%, M. tuberculosis (rare), M. marinum (rare)	[**Nafcillin** or **oxacillin** 2 gm IV q4h or **Cefazolin** 2 gm IV q8h] if **MSSA**	[**Vanco** 15-20 mg/kg IV q8-12h or **linezolid** 600 mg po q12h] if **MRSA**	MSSA: Nafcillin/oxacillin 500 mg po qid or Cefazolin 2 gm IV q8h. If MRSA: **Daptomycin** 6 mg/kg IV q24h.

NOTE: All dosage recommendations are for adults (unless otherwise indicated) and assume normal renal function. § Alternatives consider allergy, PK, compliance, local resistance, cost

Abbreviations on page 2.   *NOTE: All dosage recommendations are for adults (unless otherwise indicated) and assume normal renal function.*

TABLE 1 (31)

ANATOMIC SITE/DIAGNOSIS/ MODIFYING CIRCUMSTANCES	ETIOLOGIES (usual)	SUGGESTED REGIMENS*		ADJUNCT DIAGNOSTIC OR THERAPEUTIC MEASURES AND COMMENTS
		PRIMARY	ALTERNATIVE¹	
KIDNEY & BLADDER				
Acute Uncomplicated Cystitis & Pyelonephritis in Women				
Cystitis Diagnosis: dysuria, frequency, urgency; suprapubic pain & no vaginal symptoms	E. coli (75-95%) K. pneumoniae S. saprophyticus	**TMP-SMX DS** 1 tab po bid x 3 days. Avoid if > 20% or more local E. coli are resistant	**Fosfomycin** 3 gm po x 1 dose	• Pyridium (phenazopyridine) may hasten resolution of dysuria • Other beta lactams are less effective • Nitrofurantoin & Fosfomycin active vs. ESBLs; however, if early pyelonephritis active go to low renal concentrations • On occasion vaginitis can mimic symptoms of cystitis
		Nitrofurantoin 100 mg po bid x 5 days	**Pivmecillinam** 400 mg po bid x 3-7 days	
	Presence of enterococci, Grp B streptococcus, other S. epidermidis suggests contamination	**CIP** 250 mg po bid OR **CIP-ER** 500 mg po once daily OR **Moxi** 400 g po once daily) x 3 days		
	Often no need for culture if uncomplicated			
Pyelonephritis Diagnosis: fever, CVA, pain, nausea/vomiting	Same as for Cystitis, above. Need urine culture & sensitivity testing	**Outpatient:** **Ceftriaxone** 1 gm IV, then (**CIP** 500 mg po bid OR **CIP-ER** 1000 mg po once daily OR **Levo** 750 mg po once daily) x 7 days Culture/sens results may allow **TMP-SMX DS** 1 tab po bid	**Inpatient:** Local resistance data important **Ceftriaxone** 1 gm IV q24hr OR (**CIP** 400 mg IV q12h OR **Levo** 750 mg IV once daily OR **Moxi** 400 mg IV once daily. If ESBLs & E. coli: **MER** 0.5-1 gm IV q8h	• When tolerating po fluids, can transition to oral therapy; drug choice based on culture/sens results • No need for follow-up urine cultures in pts who respond to therapy • If symptoms do not abate quickly, imaging of urinary tract for complications, e.g., silent stone or stricture • Avoid Fosfomycin, Nitrofurantoin, Pivmecillinam due to low renal concentrations
Pregnancy: Asymptomatic bacteriuria & cystitis Drug choice based on culture/ sensitivity results; do follow-up culture one week after last dose of antibiotic	E. coli (70%) Klebsiella sp. Enterobacter sp. Proteus sp. Grp B Streptococcus	**Nitrofurantoin** (but not in 1st trimester) 100 mg po q12h x 5-7 days OR **Amox-Clav** 500 mg po q8h x 3-7 days OR **Cephalexin** 500 mg po q6h x 7 days OR **TMP-SMX DS** 1 tab po bid	**TMP-SMX DS** (but not in 1st trimester or at term) 1 tab po q12h x 3 days OR **Cefpodoxime** 100 mg po q12h x 3-7 days	• Treatment recommended to avoid progression to cystitis or pyelonephritis • Untreated bacteriuria associated with increased risk of low birth wt, preterm birth & increased perinatal mortality • If post-treatment culture positive, re-treat with different drug of longer course of same drug • If documented failure after 2nd course, Nitrofurantoin 50 or 100 g po qhs x duration of pregnancy
Pregnancy: Acute pyelonephritis Diagnosis: CVA pain, fever, nausea/vomiting in 2nd/3rd trimester. See Comment	Same as for Cystitis, above. Regimens are empiric therapy (see Comment)	**Moderately ill: Ceftriaxone** 1 gm IV q24hr OR **Cefepime** 1 gm IV q12h. If Pen-allergic, **Aztreonam** 1 gm IV q8h (no activity vs. Gram-pos cocci)	**Severely ill: Pip-Tazo** 3.375 gm IV q6h IV OR **MER** 500 mg IV q8h OR **ERTA** 1 gm IV q24h	• Differential includes: placental abruption & infection of amniotic fluid • Try to avoid FQs and AGs during pregnancy • Switch to po therapy after afebrile x 48 hrs • Treat for 10-14 days
Recurrent UTIs in Women (2 or more episodes in 6 mos / 3 or more infections in 1 yr) Risk factors: family history, spermicide use, presence of cystocele, elevated post-void residual urine volume	Same as for Cystitis, above. Regimens are options for antimicrobial prophylaxis	**Continuous: (TMP-SMX SS** 40/200 mg OR **Cephalexin** 250 mg) po once daily	**Post-coital: (TMP-SMX SS** OR **Cephalexin** 250 mg) OR **CIP** 125 mg) 1 tab po	• If pyelo recurs, re-treat. Once asymptomatic continue suppressive therapy for duration of pregnancy. Nitrofurantoin 50-100 mg po qhs OR Cephalexin 250-500 mg po qhs • No strong evidence to support use of cranberry juice • Topical estrogen cream reduces risk of recurrent UTI in postmenopausal women • Probiotics need more study

Abbreviations on page 2.   *NOTE: All dosage recommendations are for adults (unless otherwise indicated) and assume normal renal function. **PK:** compliance, local resistance, cost

¹ Alternatives consider allergy, PK, compliance, local resistance, cost

TABLE 1 (32)

ANATOMIC SITE/DIAGNOSIS/ MODIFYING CIRCUMSTANCES	ETIOLOGIES (usual)	SUGGESTED REGIMENS*		ADJUNCT DIAGNOSTIC OR THERAPEUTIC MEASURES AND COMMENTS
		PRIMARY	ALTERNATIVE§	
KIDNEY & BLADDER/Acute Uncomplicated Cystitis & Pyelonephritis in Women				
Asymptomatic Bacteriuria in Women Defined: 2 consecutive clean catch urine cultures with ≥ 10⁵ CFU/mL of same organism	Same as for Cystitis, above	**Treatment Indicated:** pregnancy, urologic procedure causing bleeding from mucosa	**No treatment indicated:** non-pregnant premenopausal women, spinal cord injury pts, elderly women in/out of nursing home, prosthetic joint surgery	• Asymptomatic bacteriuria & pyuria are discordant. 60% of pts with pyuria have no bacteriuria and pyuria commonly accompanies asymptomatic bacteriuria.
Acute Uncomplicated Cystitis & Pyelonephritis in Men. Risk of uncomplicated UTI increased with history of insertive anal sex & lack of circumcision. See also, Complicated UTIs in Men & Women, below				
Cystitis	E. coli (75-95%) Rarely other enterobacteriaceae	**TMP-SMX DS** 1 tab po bid x 7-14 days	Low risk of MDR-GNB: (**CIP** 400 mg IV q12h OR **Levo** 750 mg IV once daily) x 7-14 days	• If recurrent, evaluate for prostatitis. • Cystitis plus symptoms of bladder outlet obstruction suggests concomitant acute bacterial prostatitis • Consider presence of STDs. Recommend NAAT for C. trachomatis & N. gonorrhoeae
Pyelonephritis		Low risk of MDR-GNB: (**CIP** 500 mg po bid OR **CIP-ER** 1000 mg po once daily OR **Levo** 750 mg po once daily) x 7-14 days	High risk of MDR bacilli: **MER** 0.5-1 gm IV q8h x 7-14 days	• Avoid Nitrofurantoin due to low renal concentration in prostate • If any hint of obstructive uropathy, image collecting system asap • Case report: Fostomycin 3 gm daily used for MDR gm-neg bacilli (CID 61:1141, 2015)
Acute Complicated UTIs in Men & Women				
Defined: UTI plus co-morbid condition that increases infection severity & risk of failure, e.g., diabetes, pregnancy, late diagnosis, chronic foley catheter, suprapubic tube, obstruction secondary to stone, anatomic abnormalities, immunosuppression	E coli or Other enterobacteriaceae plus: P. aeruginosa Enterococci S aureus Candida sp.	Prior to empiric therapy: urine culture & sensitivity. If hypotensive: blood cultures. If obstructive uropathy suspected, need imaging of urinary tract asap. See Comments Low risk of MDR GNB: **Ceftriaxone** 1 gm IV once daily OR **Cefepime** 1 gm IV q12h OR **Pip-Tazo** 3.375 gm IV q6h OR **Gent** 5 mg/kg IV Once daily. If Pen-allergic: **Aztreonam** 2 gm IV q8h	Risk of MDR GNB: **Levo** 750 mg IV once daily OR **MER** 0.5-1 gm IV q8h OR Risk of MDR GNB ≥ 20%: **Ceftolozane-tazobactam** 1.5 gm IV q8h OR **Ceftazidime-avibactam** 2.5 gm IV q8h	• Uncontrolled infection, esp. if obstruction, can result in emphysematous pyelonephritis, renal abscess, carbuncle, papillary necrosis or perinephric abscess • Due to co-morbidities & frequent infections, increased risk of drug-resistance pathogens • Due to high incidence of resistance and infection severity, Nitrofurantoin, Fostomycin & TMP-SMX should not be used for empiric therapy • If Enterococci confirmed, need to adjust therapy based on in vitro susceptibility • Duration of treatment varies with status of co-morbid conditions, need for urologic procedures & individualized pt clinical response

Abbreviations on page 2. *NOTE: All dosage recommendations are for adults (unless otherwise indicated) and assume normal renal function. § Alternatives consider allergy, PK, compliance, local resistance, cost

TABLE 1 (33)

ANATOMIC SITE/DIAGNOSIS/ MODIFYING CIRCUMSTANCES	ETIOLOGIES (usual)	SUGGESTED REGIMENS*		ADJUNCT DIAGNOSTIC OR THERAPEUTIC MEASURES AND COMMENTS
		PRIMARY	ALTERNATIVE†	
LIVER (for spontaneous bacterial peritonitis, see page 46)				
Cholangitis		See Gallbladder, page 17		
Cirrhosis & variceal bleeding	Esophageal flora	(Norfloxacin 400 mg po bid or CIP 400 mg IV q12h) x max. of 7 days	Ceftriaxone 1 gm IV once daily for max. of 7 days	Short term prophylactic antibiotics in cirrhotics with G-I hemorr. with or without ascites, decreases rate of bacterial infection & ↑ survival (Hepatology 46:922, 2007).
Hepatic abscess Klebsiella liver abscess ref.: Ln 12:881, 2012	Enterobacteriaceae (esp. Klebsiella sp.), bacteroides, enterococci, Entamoeba histolytica, Yersinia enterocolitica (rare), Fusobacterium necrophorum (Lemierre's). For echinococcus, see Table 13, page 160. For cat-scratch disease (CSD), see pages 45 & 57	Metro + (ceftriaxone or cefoxitin or PIP-TZ or AM-SB) or CIP or levo	Metro (for amoeba) + either IMP, MER or DORI	**Serological tests for amebiasis should be done on all patients;** if neg. surgical drainage or percutaneous aspiration. In pyogenic abscess, ½ have identifiable GI source or underlying biliary tract disease. If amoeba serology positive, treat with metro alone without surgery. Empiric metro included for both E. histolytica & bacteroides **Hemochromatosis** associated with Yersinia enterocolitica liver abscess, regimens listed are effective for yersinia. Klebsiella pneumonia genotype K1 associated ocular & CNS Klebsiella infections.
Hepatic encephalopathy	Urease-producing gut bacteria	Rifaximin 550 mg po bid (take with lactulose)		Refs: NEJM 362:1071, 2010; Med Lett 52:87, 2010.
Leptospirosis	Leptospirosis, see page 61			
Peliosis hepatis in AIDS pts	Bartonella henselae and B. quintana	See page 57		
Post-transplant infected "biloma"	Enterococci (incl. VRE), candida, Gm-neg. bacilli (P. aeruginosa 8%), anaerobes 5%	Linezolid 600 mg IV bid + CIP 400 mg IV q12h + fluconazole 400 mg IV q24h	Dapto 6 mg/kg per day + Levo 750 mg IV q24h + fluconazole 400 mg IV q24h	Suspect if fever & abdominal pain post-transplant. Exclude hepatic artery thrombosis. Presence of candida and/or VRE bad prognosticators.
Viral hepatitis	Hepatitis A, B, C, D, E, G	See Table 14E and Table 14F		
LUNG/Bronchi				
Bronchiolitis/wheezy bronchitis (expiratory wheezing)				
Infants/children (≤ age 5) Ref: RSV, Table 14A page 175 Ref: Ln 368:312, 2006	**Respiratory syncytial virus** (RSV) 50%, parainfluenza 25%, human metapneumovirus	Antibiotics not useful, mainstay of therapy is oxygen. Ribavirin for severe disease: 6 gm vial (20 mg/mL) in sterile H₂O by SPAG-2 generator over 18-20 hrs daily times 3-5 days.		RSV most important. Rapid diagnosis with antigen detection methods. For palivizumab (a humanized mouse monoclonal antibody), **palivizumab** See Table 14A, page 175. RSV immune globulin is no longer available. Guidance from the American Academy of Pediatrics recommends use of Palivizumab only in newborn infants born at 29 weeks gestation (or earlier) and in special populations (e.g., those infants with significant heart disease). (Pediatrics 2014;134:415–420)
Bronchitis				
Infants/children (≤ age 5)	< Age 2: Adenovirus; age 2–5: parainfluenza 3 virus, human metapneumovirus Usually viral: M. pneumoniae 5%, C. pneumoniae 5%. See Persistent cough (Pertussis)	**Antibiotics not indicated.** Antitussive ± inhaled bronchodilators. Throat swab PCR available for Dx of mycoplasma or chlamydia		Antibiotics indicated only with associated sinusitis or heavy growth on throat culture for S. pneumo., Group A strep, H. influenzae or no improvement in 1 week. Otherwise rx is symptomatic.
Adolescents and adults with acute tracheobronchitis (Acute bronchitis) Ref.: JAMA 312:2678, 2014				Purulent sputum alone not an indication for antibiotic therapy. Expect cough to last 2 weeks. If fever/rigors, get chest x-ray. **If mycoplasma documented, use either doxy over macrolides due to increasing macrolide resistance (JAC 68:506, 2013).**

Abbreviations on page 2.   *NOTE: All dosage recommendations are for adults (unless otherwise indicated) and assume normal renal function. § Alternatives consider allergy, PK, compliance, local resistance, cost

TABLE 1 (34)

ANATOMIC SITE/DIAGNOSIS/ MODIFYING CIRCUMSTANCES (continued)	ETIOLOGIES (usual)	SUGGESTED REGIMENS* PRIMARY	ALTERNATIVE[1]	ADJUNCT DIAGNOSTIC OR THERAPEUTIC MEASURES AND COMMENTS
LUNG/Bronchi/Bronchitis (continued)				
Persistent cough (>14 days), afebrile during community outbreak: Pertussis (whooping cough) 10–20% adults with cough >14 days have pertussis (Review: Chest 146:205, 2014)	Bordetella pertussis & occ. Bordetella parapertussis. Also consider asthma, gastroesophageal reflux, post-nasal drip, mycoplasma and also chlamydia.	**Peds doses: Azithro OR clarithro OR erythro estolate[15] OR erythro base[15] OR TMP-SMX** (doses in footnote[15])	**Adult doses: Azithro po 500 mg day 1, 250 mg q24h x 2–5 OR erythro estolate 500 mg po qid times 14 days OR TMP-SMX-DS 1 tab po bid times 14 days OR 1 gm ER q24h times 7 days**	**3 stages of illness:** catarrhal (1–2 wks), paroxysmal coughing (2–4 wks), and convalescence (1–2 wks). Treatment may abort or eliminate pertussis in catarrhal stage, but does not shorten paroxysmal stage. **Diagnosis:** PCR on nasopharyngeal secretions or ↑ pertussis-toxin antibody. **Rx assist at eradication at NP carriage.** In non-outbreak setting, likelihood of pertussis increased if post-tussive emesis or inspiratory whoop present (JAMA 304:890, 2010). Recommended by Am. Acad. Ped. Red Book 2006 for all household or close contacts, community-wide prophylaxis not recommended. (1) consider chest x-ray, esp. if febrile (JAMA 309:2223, 2013); (4) D/C tobacco
Pertussis: Prophylaxis of household contacts.		Drugs and doses as per treatment immediately above. Vaccination of newborn contacts.		
Acute bacterial exacerbation of chronic bronchitis (ABECB) adults (almost always smokers with COPD) Ref: NEJM 359:2355, 2008.	Viruses 20–50%, C. pneumoniae 5%, M. pneumoniae <1%, role of S. pneumo, H. influenzae & M. catarrhalis controversial. Tobacco use, air pollution contribute.	**Role of antimicrobial therapy is debated even for severe disease, but recent study of >80,000 patients shows value of antimicrobial therapy in patients hospitalized with severe disease (JAMA 303(20):2035, 2010). For mild or moderate disease, no antimicrobial treatment or maybe azithro, doxy FQs with enhanced activity vs. drug-resistant S. pneumo (Gemi, Levo, Moxi or Prulifloxacin). Duration varies with drug, range 3–10 days** x 1 modestly reduced frequency of acute exacerbations in pts with milder disease (NEJM 365:689, 2011). **Drugs & doses in footnote.**		**Severe ABECB =** 1 dyspnea, ↑ sputum viscosity/purulence &/or low O2 sat.; (2) inhaled anticholinergic bronchodilator; (3) antimicrobial use; (5) ↑ sputum volume. For severe ABECB: (1) O Ceph or AM-CL, azithro/clarithro, or O Ceph or FQs.
Fever, cough, myalgia during influenza season (See NEJM 360:2605, 2009 regarding novel H1N1 influenza A)	Influenza A & B	See Influenza, Table 14A, page 173.	See Influenza, Table 14A, page 173.	**Complications: Influenza pneumonia, secondary bacterial pneumonia.** Community MRSA and MSSA, S. pneumoniae, H. influenzae.
Bronchiectasis: Acute exacerbation	H. influ., P. aeruginosa, and rarely S. pneumo.	**Gemi, levo, or moxi** x 7–10 days. Dosage in footnote[15].		Many potential etiologies: obstruction, ↓ immune globulins, cystic fibrosis, dyskinetic cilia, tobacco, prior severe or recurrent necrotizing bronchitis e.g. pertussis.
Prevention of exacerbation	Not applicable	Two randomized trials of **Erythro 250 mg po bid** (JAMA 309:1260, 2013) or **250 mg po q24h** (JAMA 309:1251, 2013), x 1 year showed prolongation in the rate of acute exacerbations, with preservation of lung function, and better quality of life versus placebo in adults with non-cystic fibrosis bronchiectasis.		**Caveats:** higher rates of macrolide resistance in oropharyngeal flora, potential for increased risk of a) cardiovascular deaths from macrolide-induced QTc prolongation, b) liver toxicity, or c) hearing loss (see JAMA 309:1295, 2013). **Pre-treatment screening:** baseline liver function tests, electrocardiogram; assess hearing, sputum culture to exclude mycobacterial disease.
Specific organisms	Aspergillus (see Table 11), MAI (Table 12) and P. aeruginosa (Table 5A).			

[15] **ADULT DOSAGE: AM-CL** 875/125 mg po bid or 500/125 mg po q8h or 2000/125 mg po bid; **azithro** 500 mg po q24h x 4 days or 500 mg po q24h x 3 days; **cefaclor** 500 mg po q8h or 500 mg extended release 375 mg po q12h; **cefdinir** 300 mg po q12h or 600 mg po q24h; **cefditoren** 200 mg or 400 mg po q12h; **cefpodoxime proxetil** 200 mg po q12h; **cefprozil** 500 mg po q12h; **ceftibuten** 400 mg po q24h; **cefuroxime axetil** 250 or 500 mg po q12h; **clarithro** 500 mg po q12h; **clarithro extended release** 1000 mg po q24h; **doxy** 100 mg po bid; **erythro base** 40 mg/kg/day po div q6h; **erythro estolate** 40 mg/kg/day po div q6h; **FQs: CIP** 750 mg po q24h x 4 days; **gemi** 320 mg po q24h; **levo** 500 mg po q24h; **loracarbef** 400 mg po q12h; **moxi** 400 mg po q24h; **prulifloxacin** 600 mg po q24h (where available); **TMP-SMX** 1 DS tab po bid.

PEDS DOSAGE: azithro 10 mg/kg/day po on day 1, then 5 mg/kg/day po q24h x 4 days; **clarithro** 7.5 mg/kg po q12h; **erythro base** 40 mg/kg/day div q6h; **erythro estolate** 40 mg/kg/day div q8-12h; **TMP-SMX** (>6 mos. of age) 8 mg/kg/day (TMP component) div bid.

Abbreviations on page 2.　*NOTE: All dosage recommendations are for adults (unless otherwise indicated) and assume normal renal function. § Alternatives consider allergy, PK, compliance, local resistance, cost

TABLE 1 (35)

ANATOMIC SITE/DIAGNOSIS/ MODIFYING CIRCUMSTANCES	ETIOLOGIES (usual)	SUGGESTED REGIMENS*		ADJUNCT DIAGNOSTIC OR THERAPEUTIC MEASURES AND COMMENTS
		PRIMARY	ALTERNATIVE§	
LUNG/Bronchi (continued)				
Pneumonia: CONSIDER TUBERCULOSIS IN ALL PATIENTS: ISOLATE ALL SUSPECT PATIENTS				
Neonatal: Birth to 1 month	**Viruses:** CMV, rubella, H. simplex **Bacteria:** Group B strep, listeria, coliforms, S. aureus, P. aeruginosa **Other:** Chlamydia trachomatis, syphilis	**AMP + gentamicin ± cefotaxime**. Add **vanco** if MRSA a concern. For chlamydia therapy, **erythro** 12.5 mg per kg po or IV qid times 14 days.		Blood cultures indicated. Consider C. trachomatis if afebrile pneumonia, staccato cough. IgM >1:8. therapy with erythro or sulfisoxazole. If MRSA documented, **vanco**, **TMP-SMX**, & **linezolid** alternatives. **Linezolid** dosage from birth to age 11 yrs is **10 mg per kg q8h.**
Age 1-3 months Pneumonitis syndrome. Usually afebrile	C. trachomatis, RSV, parainfluenza virus 3, human metapneumovirus, Bordetella, S. pneumoniae, S. aureus (rare)	**Outpatient: po erythro** 12.5 mg/kg q6h x 14 days or po **azithro** 10 mg/kg x dose, then 5 mg/kg x 4 days.	**Inpatient: If afebrile erythro** 10 mg/kg IV q6h or **azithro** 2.5 mg/kg IV q12h (see Comment). **If febrile** add **cefotaxime** 200 mg/kg per day IV q8h	Pneumonitis syndrome: Cough, tachypnea, dyspnea, diffuse infiltrates, afebrile. Usually requires hospital care. Reports of hypertrophic pyloric stenosis after erythro under age 6 wks; not sure about azithro; bid azithro dosing theoretically might ↑ risk of hypertrophic pyloric stenosis. If lobar pneumonia, give AMP 200–300 mg per kg per day for S. pneumoniae. No empiric coverage for S. aureus, as it is rare etiology.
		For **RSV, see** Bronchiolitis CID 53:617, 2011).		
Infants and Children, age > 3 months (IDSA Treatment Guidelines CID 53-617, 2011.)				
Outpatient	RSV, human metapneumovirus, rhinovirus, influenza virus, adenovirus, parainfluenza virus, Mycoplasma, H. influenzae, S. pneumoniae.	**Amox** 90 mg/kg in 2 divided doses x 5 days	**Azithro** 10 mg/kg x 1 dose (max 500 mg), then 5 mg/kg (max 250 mg) x 4 days OR **Amox-Clav** 90 mg/kg (Amox) in 2 divided doses x 5 days	Antimicrobial therapy not routinely required for preschool-aged children with CAP as most infections are viral etiologies.
Inpatient	S. aureus (rare) As above	Fully immunized: **AMP** 50 mg/kg IV q6h Not fully immunized: **Cefotaxime** 150 mg/kg IV divided q8h	Fully immunized: **Cefotaxime** 150 mg/kg IV divided q8h	If atypical infection suspected, add **Azithro** 10 mg/kg x 1 dose (max 500 mg), then 5 mg/kg (max 250 mg) x 4 days. If community MRSA suspected, add **Vanco** 15-20 mg/kg q8-12h OR **Clinda** 40 mg/kg/day divided q6-8h. Duration of therapy: 10-14 days. Depending on clinical response, may switch to oral agents as early as 2-3 days.

Abbreviations on page 2.   *NOTE. All dosage recommendations are for adults (unless otherwise indicated) and assume normal renal function. § Alternatives consider allergy, PK, compliance, local resistance, cost

TABLE 1 (36)

ANATOMIC SITE/DIAGNOSIS/ MODIFYING CIRCUMSTANCES	ETIOLOGIES (usual)	SUGGESTED REGIMENS* PRIMARY	ALTERNATIVE§	ADJUNCT DIAGNOSTIC OR THERAPEUTIC MEASURES AND COMMENTS

LUNG/Bronchi/Pneumonia *(continued)*

Adults (over age 18) — IDSA/ATS Guideline for CAP in adults: *CID 44 (Suppl 2): S27–S72, 2007; NEJM 370:543, 2014; NEJM 371:1619, 2014*				
Community-acquired, empirical therapy for outpatient Prognosis prediction: CURB-65 (*Thorax 58:377, 2003*) C: confusion = 1 pt U: BUN > 19 mg/dl = 1 pt R: RR > 30/min = 1 pt B: BP <90/60 = 1 pt Age > 65 yr = 1 pt Total = 1, ok to treat as out-patient; ≥ 2 hospitalization recommended	S. pneumo, atypicals and mycoplasma in particular, Hemophilus, Moraxella, viral pathogens: up to 30% of cases (*BMC Infect Dis 15:89, 2015*) and co-infection, often viral, in ~20% of cases (*BMC Infect Dis 15:64, 2015.*)	**Azithro** 0.5 gm po day 1 then 250 mg daily day 2-5 OR **Clarithro** 500 mg po bid or **Clarithro-ER** 1 gm po q24h x 5-7 days OR **Doxy** 100 mg po bid x 5-7 days OR if Doxy unavailable **Minocycline** 200 mg po/IV x 1, then 100 mg po/IV bid	**Levo** 750 mg po q24h x 5 days OR **Moxi** 400 mg po q24h x 5 days OR **Amox-Clav (1000/62.5)** (Augmentin-XR) 2 tabs po bid or **Amox** 1 g po tid] + [**Azithro** or **Clarithro** x 7 days]	**Azithro/Clarithro:** active against atypical pneumonia agents, but S. pneumo resistance as high as 20-30%, **alternative regimen** (**Levo** or **Moxi**) recommended if high local prevalence of macrolide resistance or co-morbidities (e.g., COPD, alcoholism, CHF). **Moxi** has anaerobic activity and may be preferred over levo for post-obstructive pneumonia or aspiration. **Amox-Clav or Amox + Azithro or Clarithro** another alternative for patients with comorbidities, in setting of high prevalence of S. pneumo macrolide resistance, or if prior antibiotic in last 3 mo. Oral cephalosporins (cefdinir 300 mg q12h, cefpodoxime 200 mg q12h or cefprozil 500 mg q12h) can be substituted for Amox-Clav or Amox.
Community-acquired, empirical therapy for patient admitted to hospital, non-ICU (See *NEJM 370:543, 2014*)	As above + legionella, Gram-negative bacilli Post-Influenza: S. aureus, S. pneumo. No pathogen detected in majority of patients, viruses more common than bacteria (*NEJM 373:415, 2015*)	**Ceftriaxone** 1 g IV q24h + [**Azithro** 500 mg IV/po q24h or **Doxy** 100 mg IV/po q12h]	**Levo** 750 mg IV/po q24h OR **Moxi** 400 mg IV/po q24h or **Gati** 400 mg IV q24h (not available in US)	Administration of antibiotic within 6h associated with improved survival in pneumonia with severe sepsis (*Eur Respir J 39:156, 2012*) Duration of therapy 5-7 days. Improved outcome with β-lactam/macrolide combo vs β-lactam alone in hospitalized CAP of moderate- or high- but not low-severity (*Thorax 68:493, 2013*) Blood and sputum cultures recommended. Test for influenza during influenza season. Consider urinary pneumococcal antigen and urinary legionella for sicker patients. Add **vanco** 15-20 mg/kg IV q8-12h to cover MRSA for pneumonia with concomitant or precedent influenza or for pneumonia in an IVDU.
Community-acquired, empirical therapy for patient admitted to ICU	As above	As above + [**Vanco** 15-20 mg/kg IV q8-12h OR **Linezolid** 600 mg IV/PO q12h] **Procalcitonin:** Several clinical trials and meta-analyses indicate that normalization of procalcitonin levels can be used to guide duration of antibiotic therapy. Safe to discontinue antibiotics when procalcitonin level has decreased to 0.1-0.2 mcg/mL (*CID 55:651, 2012; JAMA 309:717, 2013*).	As above + [**Vanco** 15-20 mg/kg IV q8-12h OR **Linezolid** 600 mg IV/PO q12h]	**Ertapenem** could substitute for ceftriaxone; need azithro for atypical pathogens; do not use if suspect P. aeruginosa. **Legionella:** Not all legionella species detected by urine antigen; if suspicious do PCR on airway secretions. (*CID 57:1275, 2013*).

NOTE: All dosage recommendations are for adults (unless otherwise indicated) and assume normal renal function. §Alternatives consider allergy, PK, compliance, local resistance, cost

Abbreviations on page 2.

Abbreviations on page 2.

TABLE 1 (37)

ANATOMIC SITE/DIAGNOSIS/ MODIFYING CIRCUMSTANCES	ETIOLOGIES (usual)	SUGGESTED REGIMENS*		ADJUNCT DIAGNOSTIC OR THERAPEUTIC MEASURES AND COMMENTS
		PRIMARY	**ALTERNATIVE§**	
LUNG/Bronchi/Pneumonia/Adults over age 18 *(continued)*				
Health care or hospital-acquired, or ventilator-associated pneumonia	As above + MDR Gram-negatives	**Cefepime** 2 gm IV q12h or **PIP-TZ** 4.5 mg/kg q8h	**MERO** 1 gm IV q8h	For patients with early onset HAP or VAP, no recent prior hospitalization, low risk for MDR options include **ceftriaxone** 1 gm q24h, **erta** 1 gm q24h, or **levo** 750 mg IV/po q24h. For late-onset infections (> 5 days in the hospital, risk factors for MDR organisms) or risk factors for MRSA add **vanco** 15-20 mg/kg IV q8h or **linezolid** 600 mg IV/po q12h. If legionella suspected, add **levo** 750 mg IV/po or **Azithro** 500 mg to the regimen. If pseudomonas suspected, add **CIP** 400 mg IV q8h or **levo** 750 mg IV/po or **Tobra** 5 mg/kg q24h to increase likelihood that at least one drug will be active.
Pneumonia —Selected specific therapy after culture results (sputum, blood, pleural fluid, etc.) available. Also see Table 2, page 69				
Acinetobacter baumannii (See also Table 5A) Crit Care Med 43:1194 & 1332, 2015	Patients with VAP	Use **IMP** or **MER** if susceptible (See Comment)	If **IMP** resistant: **Polymyxin B** (preferred) OR **colistin** + **MER**. Colistin Dose: Table 10A, page 112.	Subactam portion of AM-SB often active; dose: 3 gm IV q6h. Polymyxin resistance may evolve. Treatment options: CID 60:1295 & 1304, 2015. Some add nebulized Colistin 75 mg q12h
Actinomycosis	A. Israelii and rarely others	**AMP** 50 mg/kg/day IV div in 3-4 doses x 4-6 wks, then **Pen VK** 2-4 gm/day po x 3-6 wks	**Doxy** or **ceftriaxone** or **clinda**	Can use **Pen G** instead of AMP: 10-20 million units/day IV x 4-6 wks.
Anthrax Inhalation (applies to oro-pharyngeal & gastrointestinal forms) Treatment (Cutaneous: See page 51) Ref: www.bt.cdc.gov; CDC panel recommendations for adults; Emerg Infect Dis 20(2), doi: 10.3201/eid2002.130687. American Academy of Pediatrics recommendations Pediatrics 133:e1411, 2014.	Bacillus anthracis To report possible bioterrorism event: 770-488-7100 Plague, tularemia: See page 42. Chest x-ray; mediastinal widening & pleural effusion	**Adults (including pregnancy):** CIP 400 mg IV q8h + (**Linezolid** 600 mg IV q12h) **Meropenem** 2 gm IV q8h (see comments) + **raxibacumab** 40 mg/kg IV over 2 hrs). Switch to po after 2 wks if stable: CIP 500 mg q12h or Doxy 100 mg q12h to complete 60-day regimen.	**Children:** CIP 10 mg/kg IV q8h (max 400 mg/dose) + (**Linezolid** 10 mg/kg IV q8h (age <12 yr) or **Linezolid** 15 mg/kg IV q12h (age >12 yr) (max 600 mg per dose)) + **Meropenem** 40 mg/kg IV q8h (max 2 gm per dose) (see comments) + **raxibacumab** 40-80 mg/kg IV over 2 hrs. Switch to po after 2 wks if stable: CIP 15 mg/kg q12h or Doxy 2.2 mg/kg q12h (<45 kg) or 100 mg q12h (>45 kg) q12h to complete 60-day regimen for oral dosage.	1. Meropenem if meningitis cannot be excluded.; Linezolid preferred over Clinda for meningitis. 2. Clinda + meningitis: **Linezolid** (adults) or 67,000 units/kg (children, max 4 million units per dose) IV q4h can be substituted for Meropenem for pen-susceptible strain. 3. For children ~8 years of age tooth staining likely with Doxy for 60 days. Alternatives for oral switch include Clinda 10 mg/kg q8h (max dose 600 mg) or Levo 8 mg/kg q12h for <50 kg, 500 mg q24h >50 kg or for pen-susceptible strains Amox 25 mg/kg (max dose 1 gm) q8h or Pen VK 25 mg/kg q8h. 4. Levo and Moxi are alternatives to CIP. 5. For complete recommendations see Emerg Infect Dis 20(2), doi: 10.3201/eid2002.130687 (adults) and Pediatrics 133:e1411, 2014 (children). 6. Anthrax immune globulin (Anthrasil) FDA approved for emergency use (U.S. strategic, national stockpile). 1. Consider alternatives to Doxy for pregnant adult 2. Alternatives include Clinda, Levo, Moxi, and for pen-susceptible strains Amox or Pen VK.
Anthrax, prophylaxis: See: Emerg Infect Dis 20(2), doi: 10.3201/eid2002.130687. 60 days of **antimicrobial prophylaxis** + 3-dose series of Biothrax Anthrax Vaccine Adsorbed.	Info: www.bt.cdc.gov	**Adults (including pregnancy):** CIP 500 mg po q12h or **Doxy** 100 mg po q12h x 60 days + 3-dose series of Biothrax Anthrax Vaccine Adsorbed	**Children:** CIP or Doxy (see above for dosing) x 60 days + 3-dose series of Biothrax Anthrax (not FDA approved, to be made available on investigational basis)	

*NOTE: All dosage recommendations are for adults (unless otherwise indicated) and assume normal renal function. § Alternatives consider allergy, PK, compliance, local resistance, cost

TABLE 1 (34)

ANATOMIC SITE/DIAGNOSIS/ MODIFYING CIRCUMSTANCES	ETIOLOGIES (usual)	SUGGESTED REGIMENS*		ADJUNCT DIAGNOSTIC OR THERAPEUTIC MEASURES AND COMMENTS
		PRIMARY	ALTERNATIVE†	
LUNG/Bronchi/Pneumonia: Selected specific therapy after culture results (sputum, blood, pleural fluid, etc.) available. *(continued)*				
Burkholderia (Pseudomonas) pseudomallei (etiology of melioidosis) Can cause primary or secondary skin infection. See NEJM 367:1035, 2012	Gram-negative	Initial parenteral rx: Ceftazidime 30-50 mg per kg IV q8h or IMP 20 mg per kg IV q8h. Rx minimum 10 days & improving, then po therapy → See Alternative column	Post-parenteral po rx: Adults (see Comment for children): TMP-SMX 5 mg/kg (TMP component) bid x 3 mos. Doxy 2 mg/kg bid x 3 mos.	**Children ≤8 yrs old & pregnancy:** For oral regimen, use **AM-CL-ER** 1000/62.5, 2 tabs po bid times 20 wks. Even with treatment, relapse rate is 10%. Max. daily ceftazidime dose: 6 gm. Tigecycline: No clinical data but active in vitro (AAC 50:1555, 2006)
Haemophilus influenzae	β-lactamase negative β-lactamase positive	AMP IV, amox po, TMP-SMX AM-CL, O Ceph 2/3, P Ceph 3, FQ	azithro/clarithro, doxy, FQ	25-35% strains β-lactamase positive: ↑ resistance to both TMP-SMX and doxy. See Table 10A, page 102 for dosages. High % of commensal H. hemolyticus misidentified as H. influenza (JID 195:81, 2007).
Klebsiella sp.—ESBL pos. & other coliforms[16]	β-lactamase positive	IMP or MER if resistant, Colistin + (IMP or MER)		ESBL inactivates all cephalosporins. β-lactam/β-lactamase inhibitor drug activ not predictable: co-resistance to all FQs & often aminoglycosides.
Legionella species Relative bradycardia common feature		Azithro 500 mg IV or Levo 750 mg IV or Moxi 400 mg IV See Table 10A, pages 108 & 111 for dosages. Treat for 7-14 days (CID 39:1734, 2004)		Legionella website: www.legionella.org. Two studies support superiority of Levo over macrolides (CID 40:794 & 800, 2005), although not FDA-approved. Meta-analysis favors a FQ (JAC 69:2354, 2014).
Hospitalized/ immunocompromised		AM-CL, O Ceph 2/3, P Ceph 2/3, macrolide[17], FQ, TMP-SMX		**Doxy** another option. See Table 10A, page 102 for dosages.
Moraxella catarrhalis	93% β-lactamase positive	TMP-SMX 15 mg/kg/day IV/po in 2-4 divided doses + Imipenem 500 mg IV q6h for first 3-4 weeks then TMP-SMX 10 mg/kg/day in 2-4 divided doses x 3-6 mos.	IMP 500 mg IV q6h + amikacin 7.5 mg/kg IV q12h x 3-4 wks & then po TMP-SMX	**Duration:** 3 mos. if immunocompetent; 6 mos. if immunocompromised. **Measure peak sulfonamide levels:** Target is 100-150 mcg/mL 2 hrs post dose.
Nocardia pneumonia Expert Help: Wallace Lab (+1) 903-877-7680; CDC (+1) 404-639-3158 Ref: Medicine 88:250, 2009.	N. asteroides, N. brasiliensis			**Linezolid** active in vitro (Ann Pharmacother 41:1694, 2007). In vitro TMP-SMX may be increasing (Clin Infect Dis 51:1445, 2010), but whether this is associated with worse outcomes is not known.
Pseudomonas aeruginosa Combination rx controversial: superior in animal model (AAC 57:2788, 2013) but no benefit in observational trials (AAC 57:1270, 2013; CID 57:208, 2013).		(PIP-TZ 3.375 gm IV q4h or prefer 4-hr infusion of 3.375 gm IV q8h) + Tobra 5 mg/kg IV once q24h (see Table 10D, page 118). Could substitute anti-pseudomonal cephalosporin or carbapenem (IMP, MER) for PIP-TZ if pt. strain is susceptible.		Options: CFP 2 gm IV q8h; CIP 400 mg IV q8h + PIP-TZ; IMP 500 mg IV q6h + CIP 400 mg IV q8h; if multi-drug resistant [Polymyxin B (preferred) OR Colistin] + (IMP or MER) + consider Colistin by inhalation 80 mg bid Expert Rev Antiinfect Ther 13:1237, 2015. Also available for inhalation rx: tobra and aztreonam
Q Fever Acute atypical pneumonia. See MMWR 62 (3):1, 2013.	Often ventilator-associated			
	Coxiella burnetii	No valvular heart disease: Doxy 100 mg po bid x 14 days	Valvular heart disease: (Doxy 100 mg po bid + hydroxychloroquine 200 mg tid) x 12 months (CID 57:836, 2013)	In pregnancy: TMP-SMX DS 1 tab po bid throughout pregnancy.

[16] Dogma on duration of therapy not possible with so many variables: i.e. certainty of diagnosis, infecting organism, severity of infection and number/severity of co-morbidities. Agree with efforts to de-escalate & shorten course. Treat at least 7-8 days. Need clinical evidence of response: fever resolution, improved oxygenation, falling WBC. Refs: AJRCCM 171:388, 2005; CID 43:375, 2006; COID 19:185, 2006.

[17] **Macrolide** = azithromycin, clarithromycin and erythromycin.

Abbreviations on page 2.   *NOTE: All dosage recommendations are for adults (unless otherwise indicated) and assume normal renal function. § Alternatives consider allergy, PK, compliance, local resistance, cost

TABLE 1 (39)

ANATOMIC SITE/DIAGNOSIS/ MODIFYING CIRCUMSTANCES	ETIOLOGIES (usual)	SUGGESTED REGIMENS*		ADJUNCT DIAGNOSTIC OR THERAPEUTIC MEASURES AND COMMENTS
		PRIMARY	ALTERNATIVE†	
LUNG/Bronchi/Pneumonia/Selected specific therapy after culture results (sputum, blood, pleural fluid, etc.) available. *(continued)*				
Staphylococcus aureus Duration of treatment: 2-3 wks if just pneumonia; 4-6 wks if concomitant endocarditis and/or osteomyelitis. IDSA Guidelines, CID 52 (Feb 1):1, 2011.	Nafcillin/oxacillin susceptible	Nafcillin/oxacillin 2 gm IV q4h	Vanco 30-60 mg/kg/d iv in 2-3 divided doses or linezolid 600 mg IV q12h	Adjust dose of vancomycin to achieve target trough concentrations of 15-20 mcg/mL. Some authorities recommend a 25-30 mg/kg loading dose (actual body weight) in severely ill patients (CID 49:325, 2009).
	MRSA	Vanco 15-20 mg/kg q8-12h IV in 2-3 divided doses or Linezolid 600 mg IV/po q12h	Dapto not an option; pneumonia developed during dapto rx (CID 49:1286, 2009). Ceftaroline 600 mg IV q8h. FQ (if susceptible in vitro)	Prospective trial for MRSA pneumonia: cure rate with Linezolid (58%), Vanco (47%), p = 0.042; no difference in mortality (CID 54:621, 2012). Telavancin 10 mg/kg IV x 60 min q24h another option. Perhaps lower efficacy if CrCl < 50mL/min (AAC 58:2030, 2014).
Stenotrophomonas maltophilia		TMP-SMX 15-20 mg/kg/day div q8h (TMP component)		Tigecycline only if no other option (J Chemother 24:150, 2012) but only if MIC < 2mcg/mL. Rarely may need to use polymyxin combination therapy.
Streptococcus pneumoniae	Penicillin-susceptible	AMP 2 gm IV q6h, amox 1 gm po tid, pen G IV,¹⁸ doxy, Ö Ceph 2 ² Ceph 2/3; may add Azithro 500 mg IV/po (JAC 69:1441, 2014). See Table 10A, page 102 for other dosages.		Treat until afebrile. (min. of 5 days) and/or until serum procalcitonin normal.
	Penicillin-resistant, high level	FQs with enhanced activity: Gemi, Levo, Moxi; P Ceph 3 (resistance rare); high-dose IV AMP, vanco IV — see Table 5A, page 87 for more data. If all options not possible (rx, allergy), linezolid active: 600 mg IV or po q12h. Dosages Table 10A. Treat until afebrile, 3-5 days (min. of 5 days). In CAP may add Ceftaroline 600 mg IV q12h superior to Ceftriaxone (CID 51:641, 2010).		
Francisella tularemia Treatment Ref: JAMA 285:2763, 2001 & www.bt.cdc.gov		Streptomycin 15 mg per kg IV bid or (gentamicin 5 mg per kg IV qd) times 10 days	Doxy 100 mg IV or po bid times 14-21 days or CIP 400 mg IV (or 750 mg po) bid times 14-21 days.	Pregnancy, as for non-pregnant adults. Tobramycin should work.
Postexposure prophylaxis		Doxy 100 mg po bid times 14 days	CiP 500 mg po bid times 14 days	Pregnancy. As for non-pregnant adults
Viral (interstitial) pneumonia suspected. See Influenza, Table 14A, page 173. Ref. Chest 133:1221, 2008.	Consider Influenza, adenovirus, coronavirus (MERS/SARS), hantavirus, metapneumovirus, parainfluenza virus, respiratory syncytial virus	Oseltamivir 75 mg po bid for 5 days or zanamivir two 5 mg inhalations twice a day for 5 days.		No known efficacious drugs for adenovirus, coronavirus, hantavirus, metapneumovirus, parainfluenza or RSV. Need travel (MERS/SARS) & exposure (Hanta) history. RSV and human metapneumovirus as serious as influenza in the elderly (NEJM 352:1749 & 1810, 2005; CID 44:1152 & 1159, 2007).
Yersinia pestis (Plague) CID 49:736, 2009; MMWR 64:918, 2015	Y. pestis if aerosolized, suspect bioterror.	Gentamicin 5 mg/kg IV q24h or Streptomycin 30 mg/kg/day in 2 div doses x 10 days	Doxy 200 mg IV x 1 day, then 100 mg po bid x 7-10 days	Cipro 500 mg po bid or 400 mg IV q12h also an option. Chloramphenicol also effective but potentially toxic. Consider if evidence of plague meningitis.

18 IV Pen G dosage: no meningitis, 2 million units IV q4h. If concomitant meningitis, 4 million units IV q4h.

*NOTE: All dosage recommendations are for adults (unless otherwise indicated) and assume normal renal function. PK, compliance, local resistance, cost...

Abbreviations on page 2.

ANATOMIC SITE/DIAGNOSIS/ MODIFYING CIRCUMSTANCES	ETIOLOGIES (usual)	SUGGESTED REGIMENS*		ADJUNCT DIAGNOSTIC OR THERAPEUTIC MEASURES AND COMMENTS
		PRIMARY	ALTERNATIVE†	
LUNG—Other Specific Infections				
Aspiration pneumonia/anaerobic lung infection/lung abscess	Transthoracic culture in 90 pts—% of total isolates: anaerobes 34%, Gm-pos. cocci 26%, S. milleri 16%, Klebsiella pneumoniae 25%, nocardia 3%	Clindamycin 300-450 mg po tid OR Ampicillin-sulbactam 3 g IV q6h OR A carbapenem (e.g., ertapenem 1 g IV q24h)	Ceftriaxone 1 gm IV q24h plus metro 500 mg IV q6h or 1 gm IV q12h	Typically anaerobic infection of the lung: aspiration pneumonitis, necrotizing pneumonia, lung abscess and empyema (REF: Anaerobe 18:235, 2012) Other treatment options: PIP-TZ 3.325 g IV q6h (for mixed infections with resistant Gram-negative aerobes) or Moxi 400 mg IV q24h (CID 41:764, 2005)
Chronic pneumonia with fever, night sweats and weight loss	M. tuberculosis, coccidioido-mycosis, histoplasmosis	See Table 11, Table 12. For risk associated with TNF inhibitors, see CID 41(Suppl 3):S187, 2005.		HIV+, foreign-born, alcoholism, contact with TB, travel into developing countries
Cystic fibrosis				Cystic Fibrosis Foundation Guidelines:
Acute exacerbation of pulmonary symptoms *BMC Medicine 9:32, 2011*	S. aureus or H. influenzae early in disease; P. aeruginosa later in disease Nontuberculous mycobacteria emerging as an important pathogen (Semin Respir Crit Care Med 34:124, 2013)	For P. aeruginosa: (Peds doses) Tobra 3.3 mg/kg q8h or 12 mg/kg IV q24h, combine tobra with PIP-TZ 4.5 gm IV q6h or ceftaz 50 mg/kg IV q8h to max of 6 gm per day. If resistant to above, CIP/Levo if P. aeruginosa susceptible. See footnote[19] & Comment	For S. aureus: (1) MSSA: oxacillin/nafcillin 2 gm IV q6h. (2) MRSA—vanco 15-20 mg/kg (actual wt) IV q8-12h (to achieve target trough concentration of 15-20 µg/mL	1. Combination therapy for P. aeruginosa infection. 2. Once-daily dosing for aminoglycosides. 3. Need more data on continuous infusion beta-lactam therapy. 4. Routine use of steroid not recommended. Inhalation options (P. aeruginosa suppression): 1) Nebulized tobra 300 mg bid x 28 days, no rx for 28 days, repeat; 2) Inhaled tobra powder-hand held; 4-28 mg bid x 28 days, no rx for 28 days, repeat; Nebulized aztreonam (Cayston): 75 mg tid after pre-dose bronchodilator. Ref Lancet 56:51, 2014.
	Burkholderia (Pseudomonas) cepacia. Mechanisms of resistance (Semin Respir Crit Care Med 34:124, 2013)	Chloro 15-20 mg per kg IV/po q6h Need culture & sens results to guide rx	TMP-SMX 5 mg per kg (TMP) IV q6h	B. cepacia has become a major pathogen. Patients develop progressive respiratory failure, 62% mortality in 1 yr. Fail to respond to aminoglycosides, anti-pseudomonal beta-lactams. Patients with B. cepacia should be isolated from other CF patients.
Empyema. IDSA Treatment Guidelines for Children, CID 53:617, 2011; exudative pleural effusion criteria (JAMA 311:2422, 2014).				
Neonatal	Staph. aureus	See Pneumonia, neonatal, page 38		Drainage indicated.
Infants/children (1 month–5 yrs)	Staph. aureus, Strep. pneumoniae, H. influenzae	See Pneumonia, age 1 month–5 years, page 38		Drainage indicated.
Child >5 yrs to ADULT—Diagnostic thoracentesis; chest tube for empyemas				
Acute, usually parapneumonic. For dosage, see Table 10B or footnote page 25	Strep. pneumoniae, Group A strep	Cefotaxime or ceftriaxone (Dosage, see footnote[11] page 25)	Vanco	Usually complication of S. aureus pneumonia &/or bacteremia.
	Staph. aureus; Check for MRSA	Nafcillin or oxacillin if MSSA	Vanco or linezolid if MRSA	
	H. influenzae	Ceftriaxone	TMP-SMX	
Subacute/chronic	Anaerobic strep, Strep. milleri, Bacteroides sp., Entero-bacteriaceae, M. tuberculosis	Clinda 450-900 mg IV q6h + ceftriaxone	Cefoxitin or IMP or PIP-TZ or AM-SB (Dosage, see footnote[11] page 25)	Pleomorphic Gm-neg. bacilli. ↑ resistance to TMP-SMX. Intrapleural tissue plasminogen activator (t-PA) 10 mg + DNase 5 mg via intrapleural chest tube twice daily for 3 days improved fluid drainage, reduced frequency of surgery, and reduced duration of the hospital stay, neither agent effective alone (N Engl J Med 365:518, 2011). Pro/con debate: Chest 145:14, 17, 20, 2014. Pleural biopsy with culture for mycobacteria and histology if TBc suspected.

Tissue Plasminogen Activator (10 mg) + DNase (5 mg) bid x 3 days via chest tube improves outcome (NEJM 365:518, 2011).

[19] Other options: (Tobra + aztreonam 50 mg per kg IV q8h); (IMP 15-25 mg per kg IV q6h + tobra); **CIP commonly used in children.**

NOTE: All dosage recommendations are for adults (unless otherwise indicated) and assume normal renal function. §Alternatives consider allergy, PK, compliance, local resistance, cost

Abbreviations on page 2.   *Abbreviations on page 2.

See footnote† & Comment

TABLE 1 (41)

ANATOMIC SITE/DIAGNOSIS/ MODIFYING CIRCUMSTANCES	ETIOLOGIES (usual)	SUGGESTED REGIMENS*		ADJUNCT DIAGNOSTIC OR THERAPEUTIC MEASURES AND COMMENTS
		PRIMARY	ALTERNATIVE[1]	
LUNG—Other Specific Infections *(continued)*				
Human immunodeficiency virus infection (HIV+): See SANFORD GUIDE TO HIV/AIDS THERAPY				
CD4 T-lymphocytes <200 per mm³ or clinical AIDS	Pneumocystis carinii most likely; also MTB, fungi, Kaposi's sarcoma, & lymphoma	Rx listed here is for **severe** pneumocystis; see Table 11A, page 132 for regimens for **mild** disease. **Prednisone 1** (See Comment), **then:**		Diagnosis (**induced sputum or bronchial wash**) for: histology or monoclonal antibody strains or PCR. Serum beta-glucan (Fungitell) levels under study (CID 46:1928 & 1930, 2008). **Prednisone 40 mg bid po times 5 days then 40 mg po times 5 days then 20 mg q24h po**
Dry cough, progressive dyspnea, & diffuse infiltrate	NOTE: AIDS pts may develop pneumonia due to DRSP or other pathogens—see box below	**TMP-SMX** [IV: 15 mg per kg per day div q8h (TMP component) or po: 2 DS tabs q8h], total of 21 days	**Clinda** 600 mg IV q8h + **primaquine** 30 mg po q24h) or (**pentamidine isethionate** 4 mg per kg per day IV) times 21 days. See Comment	**times 11 days is indicated with PCP** (pO₂ <70 mmHg), **should be given at initiation of anti-PCP rx; don't wait until pt's condition deteriorates.** If PCP studies negative, consider bacterial pneumonia, TBc, cocci, histo, crypto, Kaposi's sarcoma or lymphoma.
Prednisone first if suspect pneumocystis (See Comment)				**Pentamidine not active vs. bacterial pathogens.** NOTE: **Pneumocystis resistant to TMP-SMX,** albeit rare, does exist.
CD4 T-lymphocytes normal Acute onset, purulent sputum & pulmonary infiltrates ± pleuritic pt until **TBc excluded: Adults**	Strep. pneumoniae, H. influenzae, aerobic Gm-neg. bacilli (including P. aeruginosa), Legionella, see MTB.	Ceftriaxone 1 gm IV q24h (over age 65 1 gm IV q24h) + **azithro** Could use **Levo,** or **Moxi** IV as alternative (see Comment)		If Gram stain of sputum shows Gm-neg. bacilli, options include **P Ceph 3** AP, PIP-TZ, IMP, or MER. **FQs: Levo** 750 mg po/IV q24h. **Moxi** 400 mg q24h. Gati not available in US due to hypo- & hyperglycemic reactions.
As above: Children	Same as adult with HIV + lymphocytic interstitial pneumonia (LIP)	As for HIV + adults with pneumonia. If diagnosis is LIP, rx with steroids.		In children with AIDS, LIP responsible for 1/3 of pulmonary complications, usually < 1 yr of age vs. PCP, which is seen at 1 yr of age. Clinically: clubbing, hepatosplenomegaly, salivary glands enlarged (take up gallium), lymphocytosis.
LYMPH NODES (approaches below apply to lymphadenitis without an obvious primary source)				
Lymphadenitis, acute				
Generalized	Etiologies: EBV, early HIV infection, syphilis, toxoplasma, tularemia, Lyme disease, sarcoid, lymphoma, systemic lupus erythematosus, **Kikuchi-Fujimoto** disease and others. For differential diagnosis of fever and lymphadenopathy see NEJM 369:2333, 2013.			
By Region:				
Cervical—see cat-scratch disease (CSD), below	CSD (B. henselae), Grp A strep, Staph. aureus, anaerobes, History & physical exam directs evaluation. If nodes fluctuant, aspirate and base rx on Gram & acid-fast MTB (scrofula), M. avium, M. scrofulaceum.			stains. **Kikuchi-Fujimoto** disease causes fever and benign self-limited adenopathy.
	M. malmoense, toxo, tularemia			is unknown (CID 39:138, 2004).
Inguinal				
Sexually transmitted	HSV, chancroid, syphilis, LGV.			
Not sexually transmitted	GAS, SA, tularemia, CSD, Y. pestis (plague).			Consider bubonic plague & glandular tularemia.
Axillary	GAS, SA, CSD, tularemia, Y. pestis, sporotrichosis.			Consider bubonic plague & glandular tularemia.
Extremity, with associated nodular lymphangitis	Sporotrichosis, leishmania, Nocardia brasiliensis, Mycobacterium marinum, Mycobacterium chelonae.			Treatment varies with specific etiology	A distinctive form of lymphangitis characterized by subcutaneous swellings along inflamed lymphatic channels. Primary site of skin invasion usually present; regional adenopathy variable.
Nocardia lymphadenitis & skin abscesses	N. asteroides, N. brasiliensis	**TMP-SMX** 5-10 mg/kg/day based on TMP IV/po div in 2-4 doses	Sulfisoxazole 2 gm po qid or minocycline 100-200 mg po bid	**Duration:** 3 mos. if immunocompromised, 6 mos. if immunocompetent. Effective (Ann Pharmacother 41:1694, 2007). **Linezolid** 600 mg po/IV reported effective—but compliance, local resistance, cost

*NOTE: All dosage recommendations are for adults (unless otherwise indicated) and assume normal renal function. & alternatives consider allergy, PK, compliance, local resistance, cost

TABLE 1 (47)

ANATOMIC SITE/DIAGNOSIS/ MODIFYING CIRCUMSTANCES	ETIOLOGIES (usual)	SUGGESTED REGIMENS*		ADJUNCT DIAGNOSTIC OR THERAPEUTIC MEASURES AND COMMENTS
		PRIMARY	ALTERNATIVE§	
By Pathogen:				
Cat-scratch disease— **Immunocompetent patient** Axillary/epitrochlear nodes 46%, neck 26%, inguinal 17%. Ref: *Am J Fam Pract.*	Bartonella henselae	**Azithro dosage—Adults** (>45.5 kg): 500 mg po x 1, then 250 mg/day x 4 days. **Children** (<45.5 kg): liquid azithro 10 mg/kg x 1, then 5 mg/kg per day x 4 days	Adult: Clarithro 500 mg po bid or TMP-SMX DS 1 tab po bid or CIP 500 mg po bid (duration at least 10 days)	**Dx:** Antibody titer; PCR increasingly available. Can spread: For hepatosplenic infection: (Doxy 100 mg po bid) x 10-14 days. For CNS or retinal infection: same as above, but treat for 4-6 wks.
Bubonic plague (see also, plague pneumonia) Ref: *MMWR 64:918, 2015*	Yersinia pestis	**Streptomycin** 30 mg/kg/day IV in 2 div doses or **Gentamicin** 5 mg/kg IV single dose) x 10 days	**Doxy** 200 mg IV/po bid x 1 day, then 100 mg IV/po bid x 10 days	FQs effective in animals (**Levo** 500 mg IV/po once daily or CIP 500 mg po bid (or 400 mg IV) q12h) x 10 days or Moxi 400 mg IV/po q24h x 10-14 days
MOUTH				
Aphthous stomatitis, recurrent	Etiology unknown	Topical steroids (Kenalog in Orabase) may ↓ pain and swelling; if AIDS, see SANFORD GUIDE TO HIV/AIDS THERAPY.		Note: Metro not active vs actinomyces
Actinomycosis: "Lumpy jaw" after dental or jaw trauma	Actinomyces israelii	**AMP** 50 mg/kg/d IV div q6-8h x 4-6 wks, then **Pen VK** 2-4 gm/d x 3-6 mos	(**Ceftriaxone** 2 gm IV q24h or **Clinda** 600-900 mg IV q8h) x 4-6 wks, then **Pen VK** 2-4 gm/d x 3-6 mos	
Buccal cellulitis Children < 5 yrs	H. influenzae	**Ceftriaxone** 50 mg/kg IV q24h	**AM-CL** 45-90 mg/kg po div bid or **TMP-SMX** 8-12 mg/kg bid (TMP comp) IV/po div bid	With Hib immunization, invasive H. influenzae infections have ↓ by 95%. Now occurring in infants prior to immunization.
Candida Stomatitis ("Thrush")	C. albicans	Fluconazole	Echinocandin	See Table 11, page 122.
Dental (Tooth) abscess	Aerobic & anaerobic Strep spp.	Mild: **AM-CL** 875/125 mg po bid	Severe: **PIP-TZ** 3.375 gm IV q6h	Surgical drainage / debridement. If Pen-allergic: **Clinda** 600 mg IV q6-8h
Herpetic stomatitis	Herpes simplex virus 1 & 2	See Table 14		
Submandibular space infection, bilateral (Ludwig's angina)	Oral anaerobes, facultative streptococci, S. aureus (rare)	**PIP-TZ** or (**Pen G** IV + **Metro** IV)	**Clinda** 600 mg IV q6-8h (for Pen-allergic pt)	Ensure adequate airway and early surgical debridement. Add Vanco IV if gram-positive cocci on gram stain.
Ulcerative gingivitis (Vincent's angina or Trench mouth)	Oral anaerobes + vitamin deficiency	**Pen G** 4 million units IV q4h or **Metro** 500 mg IV q8h	**Clinda** 600 mg IV q8h	Replete vitamins (A-D). Can mimic scurvy. Severe form is NOMA (Cancrum oris) (*Ln 368:147, 2006*)
MUSCLE				
"Gas gangrene" Contaminated traumatic wound. Can be spontaneous without trauma.	C. perfringens, other histotoxic Clostridium sp.	(**Clinda** 900 mg IV q8h) + (**pen G** 24 million units/day div. q4-6h IV)		Susceptibility of C. tertium to penicillins and metronidazole is variable; resistance to clindamycin and 3GCs is common, so vanco or mer (500 mg q8h) recommended. IMP or MER expected to have activity in vitro against Clostridium spp.
Pyomyositis	Staph. aureus, Group A strep, (rarely Gm-neg. bacilli), variety of anaerobic organisms	(**Nafcillin** or **oxacillin** 2 gm IV q4h) or **Cefazolin** 2 gm IV q8h if MSSA	**Vanco** 15-20 mg/kg q8-12h if MRSA	No benefit of prophylactic antibiotics in uncomplicated acute pancreatitis. Clinical deterioration in the presence of pancreatic necrosis raises concerns for infection. Empirical antibiotic therapy to suspected infected pancreatic necrosis: either IMP 0.5-1 gm IV q8h; or Moxi 400 mg IV q24h. If patient worsens, CT-guided fine-needle aspiration for culture and sensitivity testing to re-direct therapy. Candida spp may complicate necrotizing pancreatitis.

Abbreviations on page 2.   *NOTE: All dosage recommendations are for adults (unless otherwise indicated) and assume normal renal function. § Alternatives consider allergy, PK, compliance, local resistance, cost

TABLE 1 (43)

ANATOMIC SITE/DIAGNOSIS/ MODIFYING CIRCUMSTANCES	ETIOLOGIES (usual)	SUGGESTED REGIMENS* PRIMARY	ALTERNATIVE[1]	ADJUNCT DIAGNOSTIC OR THERAPEUTIC MEASURES AND COMMENTS
PANCREAS: Review: *NEJM 354:2142, 2006*				
Acute alcoholic (without necrosis) (idiopathic) pancreatitis	Not bacterial	None No necrosis on CT		1-9% become infected but prospective studies show no advantage of prophylactic antimicrobials. Observe for pancreatic abscesses or necrosis which require therapy.
Post-necrotizing pancreatitis; infected pseudocyst; pancreatic abscess	Enterobacteriaceae, enterococci, S. aureus, S. epidermidis, anaerobes, candida	Need culture of abscess/infected pseudocyst; **PIP-TZ** is reasonable empiric therapy.		Can often get specimen by fine-needle aspiration. **Moxi, MER, IMP, ERTA** are all options (*AAC 56:6434, 2012*).
Antimicrobic prophylaxis, necrotizing pancreatitis	As above	If > 30% pancreatic necrosis on CT scan (with contrast), initiate antibiotic therapy: **IMP** 0.5-1 gm IV q6h or **MER** 1 gm IV q8h. No need for empiric Fluconazole. If patient worsens CT guided aspiration for culture & sensitivity. Controversial: *Cochrane Database Sys Rev 2003: CD 002941; Gastroenterol 126:977, 2004; Ann Surg 245:674, 2007.*		
PAROTID GLAND				
"Hot" tender parotid swelling	S. aureus, S. pyogenes, oral flora, & aerobic Gm-neg. bacilli (rare); mumps, rarely enteroviruses/ influenza, parainfluenza	**Nafcillin** or **oxacillin** 2 gm IV q4h or **cefazolin** 2 gm IV q8h if MSSA, **vanco** if MRSA, **metro** or **clinda** for anaerobes		Predisposing factors, stone(s) in Stensen's duct, dehydration. Therapy depends on ID of specific etiologic organism.
"Cold" non-tender parotid swelling	Granulomatous disease (e.g., mycobacteria, fungi, sarcoidosis, Sjögren's syndrome); drugs (iodides, et al.), diabetes, Cirrhosis, tumors			History/lab results may narrow differential; may need biopsy for diagnosis
PERITONEUM/PERITONITIS: Reference—*CID 50:133, 2010*				
Primary (spontaneous bacterial peritonitis, SBP) *Hepatology 49:2087, 2009.* Dx: Pos. culture & ≥ 250 neutrophils/μL of ascitic fluid	Enterobacteriaceae 63%, S. pneumo 15%, enterococci 6-10%, anaerobes <1%. Extended β-lactamase (ESBL) positive Klebsiella species.	**Cefotaxime** 2 gm IV (if life-threatening, q4h) OR **PIP-TZ** OR **ceftriaxone** 2 gm IV q24h or **ERTA** 1 gm IV q24h	If resistant E. coli/Klebsiella species **(ESBL+)**, then: (**DORI, ERTA, IMP** or **MER**) or (**FQ: CIP, Levo, Moxi**). Check in vitro susceptibility *(Dosage in footnote²)*.	One-year **risk of SBP** in pts with ascites and cirrhosis as high as 29% (*Gastro 104:1133, 1993*). Diagnosis of SBP: 30-40% of pts have neg. cultures of blood and ascitic fluid. % pos. cultures ↑ if 10 mL of pt's ascitic fluid added to blood culture bottles (*JAMA 299:1166, 2008*). **Duration of rx unclear.** Treat for at least 5 days, perhaps longer if pt bacteremic (*Pharm & Therapeutics 34:204, 2009*). **IV albumin** (1.5 gm/kg at dx & 1 gm/kg on day 3) may ↓ frequency of renal impairment (p 0.002) & ↓ hospital mortality (p 0.01) (*NEJM 341:403, 1999*).
			TMP-SMX-DS 1 tab po 5-7 days/wk or **CIP** 750 mg po q wk	
Prevention of SBP (*Amer J Gastro 104:993, 2009*): Cirrhosis & ascites *For prevention after UGI bleeding, see Liver, page 36*			**TMP-SMX-DS** 1 tab po q wk	**TMP-SMX,** ↓ peritonitis or spontaneous bacteremia from 27% to 3% (*AnIM 122:595, 1995*). Ref. for CIP: *Hepatology 22:1171, 1995*

²⁰ Parenteral **IV therapy** for peritonitis: **PIP-TZ** 3.375 gm q6h or 4.5 gm q8h or 4-hr infusion of 3.375 gm q8h *(See Table 10)*, **Dori** 500 mg IV q8h (1-hr infusion), **IMP** 0.5-1 gm q6h, **MER** 1 gm q8h, **FQ [CIP** 400 mg q12h, **Oflox** 400 mg q12h, **Levo** 750 mg q24h, **Moxi** 400 mg q24h], **AMP** 1 gm q6h, **aminoglycoside** (see *Table 10D, page 118*), **cefotetan** 2 gm q12h, **cefoxitin** 2 gm q6h, **P Ceph 3** [**cefotaxime** 2 gm q4-8h, **ceftriaxone** 1-2 gm q24h, **ceftizoxime** 1-2 gm q8h], **P Ceph 4** [**CFP** 2 gm q12h], **cefepime**^NUS 2 gm q8h, (**Ceftolozane-tazobactam** 2 gm 2.5 gm IV over 2 hrs q8h + **Metro**) **clinda** 600-900 mg q8h, **Metronidazole** 1 gm (15 mg/kg) loading dose IV, then 1 gm IV q12h or 500 mg IV q6h (Some data supports once-daily dosing, see *Table 10A, page 112*), **AP Pen aztreonam** 2 gm q8h)

Abbreviations on page 2

* *NOTE: All dosage recommendations are for adults (unless otherwise indicated) and assume normal renal function. # alternatives consider allergy, PK, compliance, local resistance...*

TABLE 1 (44)

ANATOMIC SITE/DIAGNOSIS/ MODIFYING CIRCUMSTANCES	ETIOLOGIES (usual)	SUGGESTED REGIMENS*		ADJUNCT DIAGNOSTIC OR THERAPEUTIC MEASURES AND COMMENTS
		PRIMARY	ALTERNATIVE¹	
PERITONEUM/PERITONITIS (continued)				
Secondary (bowel perforation, ruptured appendix, ruptured diverticulum) Ref: CID 50:133, 2010 (IDSA Guidelines) **Antifungal rx?** No need if successful uncomplicated 1st surgery for viscus perforation. Treat for candida if: pure culture from abdomen or blood, in controlled study, no benefit from preemptive rx to prevent invasive candidiasis (CID 61:1671, 2015).	Enterobacteriaceae, Bacteroides sp., enterococci, P. aeruginosa (3-15%) C. albicans (see Comment) If VRE documented, dapto may work (Int J Antimicrob Agents 32:369, 2008).	**Mild-moderate disease—Inpatient—parenteral rx:** (e.g. local periappendiceal peritonitis, peridiverticular abscess): **Usually require surgery for source control.** PIP-TZ 3.375 gm IV q6h or 4.5 gm IV q8h or 4-hr infusion of 3.375 gm IV q8h **OR ERTA** 1 gm IV q24h **OR MOXI** 400 mg IV q24h	[CIP 400 mg IV q12h or Levo 750 mg IV q24h] or [metro 1 gm IV q12h)] or (CFP 2 gm q12h + metro) Note: avoid tigecycline unless no other alternative due to increased mortality risk (FDA warning).	Must "cover" both Gm-neg. aerobic & Gm-neg. anaerobic bacteria. Empiric coverage of MRSA, enterococcus and candida not necessary unless culture indicates infection. Cover enterococcus if valvular heart disease. **Drugs active only vs. anaerobic Gm-neg. bacilli:** metro. **Drugs active only vs. aerobic Gm-neg. bacilli:** aminoglycosides, P Ceph 2/3/4, aztreonam, AP Pen, CIP, Levo. **Drugs active vs. both aerobic/anaerobic Gm-neg. bacteria:** TC-CL, PIP-TZ, DORI, IMP, MER. Increasing resistance (R) of Bacteroides species (Anaerobe 17:147, 2013; AAC 56:1247, 2012) to:
				%R: **metro** -, **PIP-TZ, TC-CL** -; **Clindamycin** 19-35
				Cefotetan 17-87, **Cefoxitin** 5-30
		Severe life-threatening disease—ICU patient: Surgery for source control is important. IMP 500 mg IV q6h or MER 1 gm IV q8h or DORI 500 mg IV q8h (1-hr infusion) or (Ceftolozane-tazobactam 1.5 gm IV q8h + Metro 500 mg q6h) or (Ceftazidime-avibactam 2.5 gm IV over 2 hrs q8h + Metro 500 mg q8h) Concomitant surgical management important.	[AMP + metro + (CIP 400 mg IV q8h or Levo 750 mg IV q24h)] OR [AMP 2 gm IV q6h + metro 500 mg IV q6h + aminoglycoside] (see Table 10D, page 118)	Essentially no resistance of Bacteroides to: **metro, PIP-TZ, TC-CL.** **Carbapenems.** Case report of B. fragilis resistant to all drugs except minocycline, tigecycline & linezolid (MMWR 62:694, 2013). **Ertapenem** not active vs. P. aeruginosa/Acinetobacter species. If absence of ongoing fecal contamination, **aerobic/anaerobic culture** of peritoneal exudate/abscess may be of help in guiding specific therapy. Less need for aminoglycosides. **With severe allergy, can "cover"** Gm-neg. aerobes with **CIP or aztreonam. Remember DORI/IMP/MER are β-lactams.** MIC to Moxi increased to Moxi increasing. Resistance increased to 1 gm q6h if suspect P. aeruginosa and pt. is critically ill. See CID 59:698, 2014 (suscept. of anaerobic bacteria). Recent data suggest that short course antibiotic Rx (approx. 4 days) may be sufficient where there is adequate source control of complicated intra-abdominal infections (NEJM 372:21, 2015).
Abdominal actinomycosis	A. Israelii and rarely others	AMP 50 mg/kg/day IV div in 3-4 doses x 4-6 wks, then Pen VK 2-4 gm/day po x 3-6 mos.	Doxy or ceftriaxone or clinda	Presents as mass +/- fistula tract after abdominal surgery, e.g. for ruptured appendix. Can use IV Pen G instead of AMP: 10-20 million units/day IV x 4-6 wks.
Associated with chronic ambulatory peritoneal dialysis (Abdominal pain, cloudy dialysate, dialysate WBC >100/μL with >50% neutrophils; normal = <8 cells/μL. Ref: Perit Dial Int 30:393, 2010)	Gm+ 45%, Gm- 15%, Multiple 1%, Fungi 2%, MTB 0.1% (Perit Dial Int 24:424, 2004)	**Empiric therapy:** Need activity vs. MRSA (Vanco) & aerobic gram-negative bacilli (Ceftaz, CFP, Carbapenem, CIP, Aztreonam, Gent). Add Fluconazole if gram stain shows yeast. Use intraperitoneal dosing, unless bacteremia (rare). For dosing detail, see Table 19, page 231.	**For diagnosis:** concentrate several hundred mL of removed dialysis fluid by centrifugation. Gram stain and culture pellet. Resuspend in 3 mL of saline and then inject into aerobic/anaerobic blood culture bottles. A positive Gram stain will guide initial therapy. If culture shows Staph. epidermidis and no pus, good chance of "saving" dialysis catheter: **If multiple Gm-neg. bacilli cultured, consider catheter-induced bowel perforation and need for catheter removal.** Other indications for catheter removal: relapsing/refractory peritonitis, fungal peritonitis, catheter tunnel infection. See Perit Dialysis Int 29:5, 2009.

Abbreviations on page 2   *NOTE: All dosage recommendations are for adults (unless otherwise indicated) and assume normal renal function. § Alternatives consider allergy, PK, compliance, local resistance, cost

TABLE 1 (45)

ANATOMIC SITE/DIAGNOSIS/ MODIFYING CIRCUMSTANCES	ETIOLOGIES (usual)	SUGGESTED REGIMENS*		ADJUNCT DIAGNOSTIC OR THERAPEUTIC MEASURES AND COMMENTS
		PRIMARY	ALTERNATIVE†	
PHARYNX				
Pharyngitis/Tonsillitis: "Strept throat" Exudative or Diffuse Erythema				
Associated cough, rhinorrhea, hoarseness and/or oral ulcers suggest viral etiology. IDSA Guidelines on Group A Strep: CID 55:1279, 2012; CID 55:e86, 2012. F. necrophorum not yet commercially available (12/2015)	[Group A, C, G Strep.; Fusobacterium, EBV; (in research studies); Primary HIV, N. gonorrhea; Respiratory viruses. Student health clinic pts: Group A Strep in 20%, F. necrophorum in 10% (AnIM 162:241; 311 & 876, 2015)	**For Strep pharyngitis:** (Pen V or Benzathine Pen) or **Cefdinir** or **Cefpodoxime**. If suspect F. necrophorum: **AM-CL** or **Clinda** Doses in footnote 21	**For Strep pharyngitis:** **Clinda** or **Azithro** or If suspect F. necrophorum: Doses in footnote 21. Resistant to macrolides: Doses in footnote 21.	**Do not use: sulfonamides (TMP-SMX), tetracyclines or FQs due to resistance, clinical failures.** Do not use if penicillin test neg., do culture (CID 59:643, 2014). No need for post-treatment test of cure rapid strep test or culture. **Complications of Strep pharyngitis:** 1) Acute rheumatic fever 48 – follows Grp A S. pyogenes infection, rare after Grp C/G infection. See footnote*. For prevention, start treatment within 9 days of onset of symptoms. 2) Children age < 7 yrs at risk for post-streptococcal glomerulonephritis. 3) Pediatric autoimmune neuropsychiatric disorder associated with Grp A Strep (PANDAS) infection. 4) Peritonsillar abscess; Suppurative phlebitis are potential complications. Not effective for pharyngeal GC: spectinomycin, cefixime, cefpodoxime and cefuroxime. Ref. MMWR 61:590, 2012. **See MMWR 64(RR-3):1, 2015** for most recent CDC STD guidelines.
Gonococcal pharyngitis		**Ceftriaxone** 250 mg IM x 1 dose + **Azithro** 1 gm po x 1 dose	FQs not recommended due to resistance	Doses in footnote 21.
Proven S. pyogenes recurrence or documented relapse: Grp A infections: 6 in 1 yr; 4 in 2 consecutive yrs		**Cefdinir** or **Cefpodoxime** Tonsillectomy may be reasonable	**AM-CL** or **Clinda**	Hard to distinguish true Grp A Strep infection from chronic Grp A Strep carriage and/or repeat viral infections.
Peritonsillar abscess – Sometimes a serious complication of exudative pharyngitis ("Quinsy") (JAC 68:1941, 2013)	F. necrophorum (44%) Grp A Strep (33%) Grp C/G Strep (9%) Strep anginosus grp	**Surgical drainage plus PIP-TZ** 3.375 gm IV q6h or (**Metro** 500 mg IV/po q6-8h) + **Ceftriaxone** 2 gm IV q24h)	Pen allergic: **Clinda** 600-900 mg IV q6-8h	**Avoid macrolides: Fusobacterium is resistant.** Reports of beta-lactamase production by oral anaerobes (Anaerobe 9:105, 2003). See jugular vein suppurative phlebitis, page 49. See JAC 68:1941, 2013. Etiologies ref: CID 49:1467, 2009
Other complications		See parapharyngeal space infection and jugular vein suppurative phlebitis (see next page)		

21 **Treatment of Group A, C & G strep: Treatment durations are from approved package inserts. Subsequent studies indicate efficacy of shorter treatment courses.** All po unless otherwise indicated. PEDIATRIC DOSAGE: Benzathine penicillin 25,000 units/kg x 10 days; **Pen V** 25-50 mg per kg per day div. q6h x 10 days; **amox** 1000 mg po once daily x 10 days. **AM-CL** 45 mg per kg per day div. q12h x 10 days; **cephalexin** 20 mg/kg/dose (max 500 mg/dose) bid x 10 days; **cefdinir** 7 mg per kg q12h x 5-10 days or 14 mg per kg q24h x 10 days; **cefprozil** 15 mg per kg q12h x 10 days; **cefuroxime axetil** 20 mg per kg per day div. bid x 10 days; **cefpodoxime proxetil** 10 mg per kg div. bid x 10 days; **clarithro** 15 mg per kg per day div. bid or clarithro 7 mg per kg q12h x 5-10 days; **cefadroxil** 30 mg/kg once daily x 10 days. ADULT DOSAGE: **Benzathine** penicillin 1.2 million units x 1; **Pen V** 500 mg po bid or 250 mg qid x 10 days; **azithro** 12 mg per kg per day div. q6h x 10 days; **cefpodoxime proxetil** 100 mg bid x 5 days; **cefdinir** 300 mg q12h x 5-10 days or 600 mg q24h; **cefprozil** 500 mg bid; **cefuroxime axetil** 250 mg bid x 4 days; **cefpodoxime proxetil** 100 mg bid x 5 days; **clarithro** 250 mg bid or **clarithro** 500 mg q24h x 4 days or **clarithro** 250 mg q12h x 10 days. **azithro** 500 mg x 1 and then 250 mg q24h x 4 days or 500 mg q24h x 3 days. **Benzathine penicillin G** has been shown in clinical trials to ↓ rate of ARF from 2.8 to 0.2%.
22 Primary rationale for therapy is eradication of Group A strep (GAS) and prevention of acute rheumatic fever (ARF). Treatment decreases duration of symptoms. This was associated with clearance of GAS on pharyngeal cultures (CID 19:1110, 1994). Subsequent studies have been based on cultures, not actual prevention of ARF.

Abbreviations on page 2.   *NOTE: All dosage recommendations are for adults (unless otherwise indicated) and assume normal renal function. § Alternatives consider allergy, PK, compliance, local resistance, cost

TABLE 1 (46)

ANATOMIC SITE/DIAGNOSIS/ MODIFYING CIRCUMSTANCES	ETIOLOGIES (usual)	SUGGESTED REGIMENS*		ADJUNCT DIAGNOSTIC OR THERAPEUTIC MEASURES AND COMMENTS
		PRIMARY	ALTERNATIVE†	
PHARYNX/Pharyngitis/Tonsillitis/Exudative or Diffuse Erythema (continued)				
Membranous pharyngitis: due to **Diphtheria** Respiratory isolation, nasal & pharyngeal cultures (special media), obtain antitoxin. **Place pt. in respiratory droplet isolation.**	*C. diphtheriae* (human to human), C. ulcerans and C. pseudotuberculosis (animal to human) (rare)	**Treatment: antibiotics + antitoxin.** **Antibiotic therapy:** Erythro 500 mg IV qid OR Pen G 50,000 units/kg (max 1.2 million units) IV q12h. Can switch to Pen VK 250 mg po qid when able. Treat for 14 days	**Diphtheria antitoxin:** Horse serum. Obtain from CDC, +1 404-639-2889. Do scratch test before IV therapy. Dose depends on stage of illness: < 48hrs: 20,000-40,000 units; If NP membranes: 40,000; tonsils: 20,000-40,000 units. > 3 days & bull neck: 80,000-120,000 units	**Ensure adequate airway.** EKG & cardiac enzymes. F/U cultures 2 wks post-treatment to document cure. Then, diphtheria toxoid immunization. Culture contacts; treat contacts with either single dose of **Pen G IM**: 600,000 units if age < 6 yrs, 1.2 million units if age ≥ 6 yrs. If Pen-allergic, **Erythro** 500 mg po qid x 7-10 days. Assess immunization status of close contacts; toxoid vaccine as indicated. In vitro, C. diphtheriae suscept. to clarithro, azithro, clinda, FQs, TMP/SMX.
Vesicular, ulcerative pharyngitis (viral)	Coxsackie A9, B1-5, ECHO (multiple types), Enterovirus 71, Herpes simplex 1,2	Antibacterial agents not indicated. For HSV-1, 2: **acyclovir** 400 mg po tid x 10 days	HIV: Famciclovir 250 mg po tid x 7-10 days or Valacyclovir 1000 mg po bid x 7-10 days	Small vesicles posterior pharynx suggests enterovirus. Viruses are most common etiology of acute pharyngitis. **Suspect viral if concurrent conjunctivitis, coryza, cough, skin rash, hoarseness.**
Epiglottitis (Supraglottis): Concern in life-threatening obstruction of the airway				
Children	H. influenzae (rare), S. pyogenes, S. pneumoniae, S. aureus (includes MRSA), viruses	**Peds dosage:** **Cefotaxime** 50 mg per kg IV q8h or **ceftriaxone** 50 mg per kg IV q24h) + **Vanco**	**Peds dosage: Levo** 10 mg/kg IV q24h + **Clinda** 7.5 mg/kg IV q6h	Have tracheostomy set "at bedside." **Levo** use in children is justified as emergency empiric therapy in pts with severe beta-lactam allergy. Use of steroids is controversial; do not recommend. *Ref: Ped Clin No Amer 53:215, 2006.*
Adults	Group A strep, H. influenzae (rare) & many others	Same regimens as for children. See footnote[23]	**Adult dosage:**	
Parapharyngeal space infection [Spaces include: sublingual, submandibular (Ludwig's angina), (see page 45) lateral pharyngeal, retropharyngeal, pretracheal]				
Poor dental hygiene, dental extractions, foreign bodies (e.g. toothpicks, fish bones) *Ref: CID 49:1467, 2009*	Polymicrobic: Strep sp., anaerobes, Eikenella corrodens. Anaerobes outnumber aerobes 10:1.	[(**Clinda** 600-900 mg IV q8h) or (**pen G** 24 million units/day by cont. infusion in div. q4-6h IV)+ **metro** 1 gm load and then 0.5 gm IV q6h]	PIP-TZ 3.375 gm IV q6h or **AM-SB** 3 gm IV q6h	Close observation. MRI or CT to identify abscess; **surgical drainage.** Metro may be given 1 gm IV q12h. Complications: infection of carotid artery & jugular vein phlebitis.
Jugular vein suppurative phlebitis (Lemierre's syndrome) [†] *LnID 12:808, 2012.*	Fusobacterium necrophorum in vast majority	PIP-TZ 4.5 gm IV q6h or IMP 500 mg IV q6h or (**Metro** 500 mg po/IV q8h + **ceftriaxone** 2 gm IV once daily)	**Clinda** 600-900 mg IV q8h. **Avoid macrolides:** **fusobacterium are resistant**	Emboli: pulmonary and systemic common. Erosion into carotid artery can occur. Lemierre described F. necrophorum in 1936, other anaerobes & Gm-positive cocci are less common etiologies of suppurative phlebitis post-pharyngitis.
Laryngitis (hoarseness)	Viral (90%)	Not indicated		

[23] Parapharyngeal space infection: **Ceftriaxone** 2 gm IV q24h; **cefotaxime** 2 gm IV q4-8h; **PIP-TZ** 3.375 gm IV q6h or 4-hr infusion of 3.375 gm q8h; **TMP-SMX** 8-10 mg per kg per day (based on TMP component) div q6h, q8h, or q12h; **Clinda** 600-900 mg IV q6-8h; **Levo** 750 mg IV q24h; **vanco** 15 mg/kg IV q12h.

*NOTE: All dosage recommendations are for adults (unless otherwise indicated) and assume normal renal function. § Alternatives consider allergy, PK, compliance, local resistance, cost

Abbreviations on page 2. *   *NOTE: All dosage recommendations on page 2.

TABLE 1 (47)

ANATOMIC SITE/DIAGNOSIS/ MODIFYING CIRCUMSTANCES	ETIOLOGIES (usual)	SUGGESTED REGIMENS*		ADJUNCT DIAGNOSTIC OR THERAPEUTIC MEASURES AND COMMENTS
		PRIMARY	ALTERNATIVE§	
SINUSES, PARANASAL				
Sinusitis, acute (Ref: CID 54:e72, 2012); Guidelines: Pediatrics 132:e262 & 284, 2013 (American Academy of Pediatrics)				
Treatment goals: • Speed resolution from virus or allergy. • Prevent bacterial complications (see Comment) • Prevent chronic sinusitis • Avoid unnecessary use of antibiotics	S. pneumonia 33% H. influenza 32% M. catarrhalis 9% Anaerobes 6% Grp A strep 2% Viruses 15–18% S. aureus 10% (see Comment)	Most common: obstruction of sinus ostia by inflammation from virus or allergy. Treatment: Saline irrigation **Antibiotics for bacterial sinusitis if:** 1) fever, pain, purulent nasal discharge; 2) still symptomatic after 10 days with no antibiotic; 3) clinical worsening after 5–6 days despite antibiotic therapy. **No clinical allergy:** **Peds:** Amox 90 mg/kg/day divided q12h or **Amox-Clav** suspension 90 mg/kg/day (Amox comp) divided q12h. Treat for 10–14 days **Adult: Amox-Clav** 1000/62.5-2 tabs po bid x 5–7 days	**Peds (if anaphylaxis): Clinda** 30–40 mg/kg/day divided po or qid x 10–14 days (see Comment) **Peds (no anaphylaxis): Cefpodoxime** 10 mg/kg/day po div q12h **Adult (if anaphylaxis): Levo** or doxy **Adult (no anaphylaxis):** Cefpodoxime 200 mg po bid	**Treatment:** • Clinda: Haemophilus & Moraxella sp. are resistant; may need 2nd drug • Duration of rx: 5–7 days (IDSA Guidelines); 10–14 days (Amer Acad Ped Guidelines) • Adjunctive rx: 1) do not use topical decongestant for > 3 days; 2) no definite benefit from nasal steroids & antihistamines; 3) saline irrigation may help. • Avoid macrolides and TMP-SMx due to resistance • Empiric rx does not target S. aureus: incidence same in pts & controls (CID 45:e121, 2007) Potential complications: transient hyposmia, orbital infection, epidural abscess, brain abscess, meningitis, cavernous sinus thrombosis. For other adult drugs and doses, see footnote[24]
Clinical failure after 3 days	As above; consider diagnostic tap/aspirate	**Mild/Mod. Disease: AM-CL-ER** (cefpodoxime), cefprozil, or cefdinir Treat 5–10 days. Adult doses in footnote[24] See Table 11, pages 121 & 131.	**Severe Disease:** Gati[NUS], Gemi, Levo, Moxi	
Diabetes mellitus with acute ketoacidosis; neutropenia; deferoxamine rx: Mucormycosis	Rhizopus sp. (mucor), aspergillus			
Hospitalized + nasotracheal or nasogastric intubation	Gm-neg. bacilli 47% (pseudomonas, acinetobacter, E coli common), Gm+ (S. aureus) 35%, yeasts 18%. Polymicrobial in 80%	Remove nasotracheal tube; recommend sinus aspiration (fluid in sinuses) for C/S & S. aureus PCR prior to empiric therapy **IMP** 0.5 gm IV q6h or **MER** 1 gm IV q8h. Add vanco for MRSA if Gram stain suggestive	After 7 days of nasotracheal or nasogastric tubes, 95% have x-ray "sinusitis" (fluid in sinuses), but on transnasal puncture only 38% culture + (AJRCCM 150:776, 1994). For pts requiring mechanical ventilation with nasotracheal tube for ≥1 wk, bacterial sinusitis occurs in < 10% (CID 27:851, 1998). May feel fluconazole if yeast on Gram stain of sinus aspirate. [Ceftaz 2 gm IV q8h + vanco] or [CFP 2 gm IV q12h + vanco]
Sinusitis, chronic Adults **Defined:** (drainage, blockage, facial pain, ↓ sense of smell) + (Polyps, purulence or abnormal endoscopy or sinus CT scan: JAMA 314:926, 2015)	Multifactorial inflammation of upper airways	Standard maintenance therapy: Saline irrigation + topical corticosteroids	Intermittent/Rescue therapy: For symptomatic nasal polyp: oral steroid x 1–3 wks. For polyps + purulence: Doxy 200 mg po x 1 dose, then 100 mg po once daily x 20 days	Leukotriene antagonists considered only for pts with nasal polyps. No antihistamines unless clearly allergic sinusitis. Some suggest > 12 wks of macrolide rx; data only somewhat supportive: worry about AEs.

[24] **Adult doses for sinusitis (all oral): AM-CL-ER** 2000/125 **mg** bid, **amox high-dose (HD)** 1 gm tid, **clarithro** 500 mg bid or **clarithro ext. release** 1 gm q24h, **doxy** 100 mg bid, **respiratory FQs** (Gati 400 mg q24h[NUS] due to hypo/hyperglycemia), **Gemi** 320 mg q24h (not FDA indication but should work), **Levo** 750 mg q24h x 5 days, **Moxi** 400 mg q24h); **O Ceph** (**cefdinir** 300 mg q12h or 600 mg q24h, **cefpodoxime** 200 mg q12h, **cefprozil** 250–500 mg bid, **cefuroxime** 250 mg q12h. **TMP-SMX** 1 double-strength (TMP 160 mg) bid (results after 3- and 10-day rx similar).

Abbreviations on page 2.

NOTE: All dosage recommendations are for adults (unless otherwise indicated) and assume normal renal function. § Alternatives consider allergy, PK, compliance, local resistance, cost

TABLE 1 (48)

ANATOMIC SITE/DIAGNOSIS/ MODIFYING CIRCUMSTANCES	ETIOLOGIES (usual)	SUGGESTED REGIMENS*		ADJUNCT DIAGNOSTIC OR THERAPEUTIC MEASURES AND COMMENTS
		PRIMARY	ALTERNATIVE§	
SKIN See IDSA Guideline: *CID 59:147, 2014.*				
Acne vulgaris (*Med Lett Treatment Guidelines 11 (Issue 125): 1, 2013*).				
Comedonal acne, "blackheads", "whiteheads"; earliest form, no inflammation	Excessive seburm production & gland obstruction. No Propionibacterium acnes	Once-q24h: Topical **tretinoin** 0.025 or 0.05%) or (gel 0.01 or 0.025%)	All once-q24h: Topical **adapalene** 0.1% gel OR **azelaic acid** 20% cream or **tazarotene** 0.1% gel	Goal is prevention, ↓ number of new comedones and create an environment unfavorable to P. acnes. Adapalene causes less irritation than tretinoin. Azelaic acid less potent but less irritating than retinoids. **Tazarotene: Do not use in pregnancy.**
Mild inflammatory acne: small papules or pustules	Proliferation of P. acnes + abnormal desquamation of follicular cells	Topical **erytho 3% + benzoyl peroxide 5%**, bid	Can substitute **clinda** 1% gel for erythro	In random. controlled trial, topical benzoyl peroxide + erytho of equal efficacy to oral minocycline & tetracycline and not affected by antibiotic resistance of propionibacteria (*Ln 364:2188, 2004*)
Inflammatory acne: comedones, papules & pustules. Less common: nodules (cysts). Isotretinoin ref: *JAMA 317: 2121, 2133, 2014.*	Progression of above events, e.g., obstruction, P. acnes proliferation, inflammation. Also, drug induced, e.g., corticosteroids, phenytoin, lithium, INH & others.	(Topical **erytho 3% + benzoyl peroxide 5% bid**) + (topical [**clinda**]) See Comment for mild acne	Oral drugs: (**doxy** 50-100 mg bid) or (**minocycline** 50 mg bid). Others: **tetracycline, erytho, TMP-SMX, clinda.** Expensive extended release once-daily minocycline (Solodyn) 1 mg/kg/d	Systemic **isotretinoin** reserved for pts with severe widespread nodular cystic lesions that fail oral antibiotic rx: 4-5 mos. course of 0.1-1 mg per kg per day. **Teratogenic (Preg category X).** Aggressive/violent behavior reported. **Doxy** can cause photosensitivity. **Minocycline** side-effects: urticaria, vertigo, pigment deposition in skin or oral mucosa. Rare induced autoimmunity in children: fever; polyarthralgia, positive ANCA (*J Peds 153:314, 2008*)
Acne rosacea Ref: *NEJM 352:793, 2005.*	Skin mite: Demodex folliculorum (*Arch Derm 146:896, 2010*)	Facial erythema: Brimonidine gel (Mirvaso) applied to affected area bid (*J Drugs Dermatol 12:650, 2013*)	Papulopustular rosacea: **Azelaic acid** gel bid, topical or **Metro** topical cream once daily or q24h.	Avoid activities that provoke flushing, e.g., alcohol, spicy food, sunlight.
Anthrax, cutaneous To report bioterrorism event: 770-488-7100; For info: www.bt.cdc.gov Treat as inhalation anthrax (if systemic illness). Ref: *AJRCCM 184:1333, 2011* (Review). *CID 59:147, 2014* (Clinical Prac Guideline). *Pediatrics 133:e1411, 2014.*	**B. anthracis** Spores are introduced into/under the skin by contact with infected animals/animal products. See *Lung, page 40.*	**Adults: CIP** 500 mg po q12h or **Doxy** 10 mg po q12h. **Children: CIP** 15 mg/kg (max dose 500 mg) po q12h or for pen-susceptible strain **Amox** 25 mg/kg (max dose 1 gm) po q8h. For bioterrorism exposure, 3-dose series of Biothrax Anthrax Vaccine Adsorbed is indicated.	**Children: Doxy** 10 mg po q12h.	1. Duration of therapy 60 days for bioterrorism event because of potential inhalational exposure and 7-10 days for naturally acquired disease. 2. Consider alternative to Doxy for pregnancy. 3. Alternatives for adults: Levo 750 mg q24h or Moxi 400 mg q24h or Clinda 600 mg q8h or (for pen-susceptible strains Amox 1 gm q8h or Pen VK 500 mg q6h. Alternatives for children: Doxy 2.2 mg/kg (max dose 100 mg) q12h (tooth staining likely with 60-day regimen age < 8 years) or Clindamycin 10 mg/kg (max dose 600 mg) q8h or Levo 8 mg/kg q12h (max dose 250 mg) if < 50 kg and 500 mg q24h if > 50 kg.
Bacillary angiomatosis: For other Bartonella infections, see *Cat-scratch disease lymphadenitis, page 45, and Bartonella systemic infections, page 57* In immunocompromised (HIV-1, bone marrow transplant) patients Also see SANFORD GUIDE TO HIV/AIDS THERAPY	Bartonella henselae and quintana	**Clarithro** 500 mg po qid or azithro 250 mg po q24h or extended release **Erythro** 500 mg po q24h or (see Comment)	**Erythro** 500 mg po qid or doxy 100 mg po bid or (**Doxy** 100 mg po bid + **RIF** 300 mg po bid)	For AIDS pts, continue suppressive therapy until HIV treated and CD4 > 200 cells/μL for 6 mos.

*NOTE: All dosage recommendations are for adults (unless otherwise indicated) and assume normal renal function. §Alternatives consider allergy, PK, compliance, local resistance, cost

TABLE 1 (49)

ANATOMIC SITE/DIAGNOSIS/ MODIFYING CIRCUMSTANCES	ETIOLOGIES (usual)	SUGGESTED REGIMENS*		ADJUNCT DIAGNOSTIC OR THERAPEUTIC MEASURES AND COMMENTS
		PRIMARY	**ALTERNATIVE†**	
SKIN (continued)				
Bite: Remember tetanus prophylaxis— See Table 20B, page 233 for rabies prophylaxis. Review: CMR 24:231, 2011. **Avoid primary wound closure.**				
Alligator (Alligator mississipiensis)	Gram negatives including Aeromonas hydrophilia, Clostridia sp.	Severe wound: Surgical debridement + (**CIP** 400–750 mg po bid or **Levo** 750 mg/d)	Severe wound: **TMP-SMX** 8–10 mg/kg/d IV div q6h or q8h or **Cefepime** 2 gm IV q8h + **Doxy** 100 mg po bid	Oral flora of American alligator isolated: anaerobes, including Aeromonas hydrophila and Clostridia sp. (S Med J 82:262, 1989).
Bat, raccoon, skunk	Strep & staph from skin; rabies			In Americas, **anti-rabies rx indicated:** rabies immune globulin + vaccine. (See Table 20B, page 233)
Camel	S. aureus, P. aeruginosa, Other Gm-neg bacilli	**Diclox** 250–500 mg po qid + **CIP** 750 mg po bid	**Cephalexin** 500 mg po qid	See EJCMID 18:918, 1999
Cat: 80% get infected; culture & treat empirically.	**Pasteurella multocida** Streptococci, Staph. aureus, Neisseria, Moraxella	**AM-CL** 875/125 mg po bid or 500/125 mg po tid + **CIP**	**Doxy** 100 mg po bid / **Cefuroxime axetil** 0.5 gm po q12h or **doxy** 100 mg po bid. **Do not use cephalexin.** Sens to FQs in vitro.	**P. multocida resistant to dicloxacillin, cephalexin, clinda; many strains resistant to erythromycin** (most sensitive to azithro but no clinical data). P. multocida infection develops within 24 hrs. Observe for osteomyelitis if culture + for only — P. multocida can switch to pen VK po. See Dog Bite. (See Table 20B, page 233)
Cat-scratch disease page 45				
Catfish sting page 45	Toxins	See Comments		Presents as immediate pain, erythema and edema. Resembles strep cellulitis.
Dog: Only 5% get infected; treat only if bite severe or bad co-morbidity (e.g. diabetes).	Pasteurella canis, S. aureus, Streptococcus, Fusobacterium sp. Capnocytophaga canimorsus	**AM-CL** 875/125 mg po bid or 1000/62.5 mg 2 tabs po bid	**Adult: Clinda** 300 mg po q6h + FQ; **Child: Clinda + TMP-SMX**	May develop secondarily infected; AM-CL is reasonable choice for prophylaxis (see Table 20B). Capnocytophaga in splenectomized pts may cause local eschar, sepsis with DIC. P. multocida, see cat. Consider prophylaxis for deep wounds adjacent to joints/bone and erythro; sensitive to ceftriaxone, cefuroxime, cefpodoxime and FQs.
Human For bacteriology, see CID 37:1481, 2003	Viridans strep 100%, Staph epidermidis 53%, corynebacterium 41%, **Staph. aureus 29%**, Eikenella 15%, bacteroides 82%, peptostrep 26%	**Early (not yet infected): AM-CL** 875/125 mg po q8h x 5 days. **Later (Signs of infection usually in 3–24 hrs): AM-SB** 1.5 gm IV q6h or **cefoxitin** 2 gm IV q8h or 4.5 gm q6h or 4-hr infusion of 3.375 gm q8h)	Pen allergy: **Clinda** + (either **CIP** or **TMP-SMX**) / **CIP** 400 mg IV q12h or 750 mg po bid	**Cleaning, irrigation and debridement most important.** fist injuries, x-rays should be obtained. Bites inflicted by hospitalized pts, consider aerobic Gm-neg. bacilli. **Eikenella resistant to clinda, nafcillin/oxacillin, metro, P Ceph 1, and erythro; susceptible to FQs and TMP-SMX.**
Leech (Medicinal) (Ln 381:1686, 2013)	Aeromonas hydrophila		**TMP-SMX DS** 1 tab po bid	Aeromonas found in GI tract of leeches. Some use prophylactic antibiotics when leeches used medicinally, but not universally accepted or necessary.
Pig (swine)	Polymicrobic: Gm+ cocci, Gm-neg. bacilli, anaerobes, Pasteurella sp.	**AM-CL** 875/125 mg po bid	**P Ceph 3** or **AM-SB** or **IMP**	Information limited but infection is common and serious (Ln 348:888, 1996).
Prairie dog	Monkeypox	See Table 14A, page 174. No rx recommended		CID 20:421, 1995
Primate, non-human	Herpesvirus simiae	**Acyclovir:** See Table 14B, page 177		
Rat	Spirillum minus & Streptobacillus moniliformis	**AM-CL** 875/125 mg po bid	**Doxy**	Anti-rabies rx not indicated. Causes rat bite fever (Streptobacillus moniliformis): Pen G or doxy, alternatively erythro or clinda.
Seal	Marine mycoplasma	Tetracycline times 4 wks		Can take weeks to appear after bite (Ln 364:448, 2004).
Snake: pit viper (Ref.: NEJM 347:347, 2002)	Pseudomonas sp., Clostridium sp.	**Primary therapy is antivenom**		Primary therapy is antivenom. Penicillin generally used but would not be effective vs organisms isolated. Ceftriaxone should be the drug if organisms isolated. Tetanus prophylaxis indicated. Ref: CID 43:1309, 2006

*NOTE: All dosage recommendations are for adults (unless otherwise indicated) and assume normal renal function. §Alternatives consider allergy, PK, compliance, local resistance, cost

TABLE 1 (50)

ANATOMIC SITE/DIAGNOSIS/MODIFYING CIRCUMSTANCES	ETIOLOGIES (usual)	SUGGESTED REGIMENS*		ADJUNCT DIAGNOSTIC OR THERAPEUTIC MEASURES AND COMMENTS
		PRIMARY	ALTERNATIVE†	
SKIN/Bite (continued)				
Spider bite: Most necrotic ulcers attributed to spiders are probably due to another cause. e.g.				
Widow (Latrodectus)	Not infectious	None		cutaneous anthrax (spider bite painful; anthrax not painful) or **MRSA infection** (Ln 364:549, 2004) or MRSA infection. May be confused with "acute abdomen". Diazepam or calcium gluconate helpful to control pain, muscle spasm. Tetanus prophylaxis.
Brown recluse (Loxosceles) NEJM 352:700, 2005	Not infectious. "Overdiagnosed". Spider distribution limited to S. Central & desert SW of US	Bite usually self-limited & self-healing. No therapy of proven efficacy	**Dapsone** 50 mg po q24h often used despite marginal supportive data	Dapsone causes hemolysis (check for G6PD deficiency). Can cause hepatitis; baseline & weekly liver panels suggested.
Boils—Furunculosis				
Active lesions See Table 6, page 82	Staph aureus, both MSSA & MRSA IDSA Guidelines: CID 59:147, 2014; CID 59:147, 2014.	**Boils and abscesses** uncomplicated patient (e.g., no immunosuppression, diabetes): **I&D** + **TMP/SMX** 1 DS (2 DS for BMI > 40) bid or **I&D** + **Clinda** 300 mg tid equally efficacious (NEJM 372:1093, 2015)		Other options: **Doxy** 100 mg po bid or **Minocycline** 100 mg po bid for 5-10 days; **Fusidic acid**^NUS 250-500 mg po q8-12h ± **RIF**; **cephalexin** 500 mg po tid-qid or dicloxacillin 500 mg po tid-qid, only in low prevalence setting for MRSA. For uncertainty or for assessing adequacy of I&D, ultrasound is helpful (NEJM 370:1039, 2014). **Note: needle aspiration is inadequate.**
		Incision and Drainage mainstay of therapy!		
To lessen number of furuncle recurrences --decolonization For surgical prophylaxis, see Table 15B, page 200.	MSSA & MRSA. IDSA Guidelines, CID 59:e10, 2014	7-day therapy. **Chlorhexidine** (2%) washes daily, **mupirocin ointment** anterior nares 2x daily + (**rifampin** 300 mg bid + **doxy** 100 mg bid).	**Mupirocin ointment** in anterior nares bid x 7 days + **chlorhexidine** (2%) washes daily x 7 days + (**TMP-SMX DS** 1 tab po bid) + **RIF** 300 mg po bid) x 7 days	Optimal regimen uncertain. Can substitute bleach baths for chlorhexidine (Inf Control Hosp Epidemiol 32:872, 2011) but only modest effect (CID 58:679, 2014). In vitro resistance of mupirocin & retapamulin roughly 10% (AAC 58:2878, 2014). One review found mupirocin resistance ranging from 1-81% (JAC 70:2681, 2015).
Hidradenitis suppurativa Not infectious disease, but bacterial superinfection occurs	Lesions secondarily infected: S. aureus, Enterobacteriaceae, pseudomonas, anaerobes	**Clinda** 1% topical cream. **Adalimumab** 40 mg once weekly beneficial (AnIM 157:846, 2012)	**Clinda** 300 mg po bid + **RIF** 300 mg po bid x 6 mos (NEJM 366:158, 2012)	Caused by keratinous plugging of apocrine glands of axillary, inguinal, perineal, perianal, infra-mammary areas. Other therapy: antiperspirants, loose clothing and anti-androgens. Dermatol Clin 28:779, 2010.
Burns. Overall management: NEJM 360:810, 2004 - step-by-step case outline				
Initial wound care Use burn unit, if available Topical rx options (NEJM 359:1037, 2006; Clin Plastic Surg 36:597, 2009)	**Not infected** Prophylaxis for potential pathogens: Gm-pos cocci Gm-neg bacilli Candida	Early excision & wound closure. Variety of skin grafts/substitutes. Shower hydrotherapy. Topical antimicrobials	**Silver sulfadiazine** cream 1% applied 1-2 x daily. Minimal pain. Transient reversible neutropenia due to margination in burn - not marrow toxicity.	Mafenide acetate cream is an alternative but painful to apply. Anti-tetanus prophylaxis indicated.
Burn wound sepsis Proposed standard est. of J Burn Care Res 28:776, 2007. Need quantitative wound cultures	Strep pyogenes, S. aureus, Enterobacter sp, S. epidermidis, E. faecalis, E. coli, P. aeruginosa. Fungi (rare). Herpesvirus (rare).	**Vanco** high dose to rapidly achieve trough concentration of 15-20 μg/mL + (**MER** 1 gm IV q8h or **cefepime** 2 gm IV q8h) + **Fluconazole** 6 mg/kg IV qd	See Comments for alternatives	Vanco allergic/intolerant: **Dapto** 6-10 mg/kg IV qd. IgE mediated allergy to beta lactams: **Aztreonam** 2 gm IV q6h. ESBL- or carbapenemase-producing MDR gm-neg bacilli: only option is **[Polymyxin B** (preferred) or **Colistin]** + (**MER** or **IMP**)

Abbreviations on page 2.

*NOTE: All dosage recommendations are for adults (unless otherwise indicated) and assume normal renal function. § Alternatives consider allergy, PK, compliance, local resistance, cost

TABLE 1 (51)

ANATOMIC SITE/DIAGNOSIS/ MODIFYING CIRCUMSTANCES	ETIOLOGIES (usual)	SUGGESTED REGIMENS*		ADJUNCT DIAGNOSTIC OR THERAPEUTIC MEASURES AND COMMENTS
		PRIMARY	**ALTERNATIVE§**	
SKIN (continued)				
Cellulitis, erysipelas: NOTE: Consider diseases that masquerade as cellulitis (Clev Clin J Med 79:547, 2012)				
Extremities, non-diabetic. For diabetes, see below. Practice guidelines: CID 59:147, 2014.	B & G Strep. Groups A, B, C & G Staph. aureus, including MRSA (bid rare) Strep sp: No purulence Staph sp: Purulence	For no purulence. **Inpatients: Elevate legs. Pen G** 1–2 million units IV q6h or **cefazolin** 1 gm IV q8h. If Pen-allergic: **Vanco** 15 mg/kg IV q12h. When afebrile: **Pen VK** 500 mg po qid & hs. Total therapy: 10 days.	**Outpatient: Elevate legs.** **Pen VK** 500 mg po qid ac & hs. If Pen-allergic: **Azithro** 500 mg po x 1, then 250 mg po qid x 4 days (total 5 days). **Linezolid** 600 mg po bid or **Tedizolid** 200 mg po q24h	• Erysipelas: elevation, IV antibiotic, treat T. pedis if present, if no purulence, no need for culture. TMP-SMX may be equivalent to clinda in clinical trial of cellulitis treatment (NEJM 372: 1093, 2015). Purulence due to presence of deep abscess, bedside ultrasound can help. If present: furunculosis (boils) • **TMP-SMX** 1 DS bid effective for uncomplicated cellulitis in non-diabetic outpatients (NEJM 372:2460, 2015) • **Oritavancin** 1500 mg IV x1 OR **Dalbavancin** 1000 mg IV x1 then 500 mg x1 a week later also effective for outpatient therapy of more severe infections in patients who might otherwise be admitted to the hospital (see NEJM 370:2180, 2014, NEJM 370:2169,2014)
Facial, adult (erysipelas)	Strep. sp. (Grp A, B, C & G), Staph. aureus (to include MRSA), S. pneumo	**Vanco** 15 mg/kg (actual wt) IV q8–12h (to achieve target trough concentration of 15–20 µg/mL) x 7-10 days	**Dapto** 4 mg/kg IV q24h or **Linezolid** 600 mg IV q12h. Treat 7-10 days if not bacteremic.	**Choice of empiric therapy must have activity vs. S. aureus.** S. aureus erysipelas of face can mimic streptococcal erysipelas of an extremity. Avoid to treat empirically for MRSA until in vitro susceptibilities available.
Diabetes mellitus and erysipelas (See Foot, "Diabetic", page 16)	Strep. sp. (Grp A, B, C & G), Staph. aureus, Enterobacteriaceae, Anaerobes	**Early mild: TMP-SMX-DS** 1-2 tabs po bid + (**Pen VK** 500 mg po qid or **cephalexin** 500 mg po qid). **For severe disease:** (**IMP or MER** 1 gm IV q6h or **ERTA** 1 gm IV q24h) or **DORI** 0.5 gm IV q8h + **vanco** 1 gm IV q12h	**Dapto** 4 mg/kg IV q24h + **linezolid** 600 mg IV (po if tolerating) q12h	Prompt surgical debridement indicated to rule out necrotizing fasciitis and to obtain cultures. If septic, consider x-ray of extremity to demonstrate gas. **Prognosis dependent on blood supply: assess arteries.** See diabetic foot, page 16. For severe disease, use regimen that targets both aerobic gram-neg bacilli & MRSA.
Erysipelas 2° to lymphedema (congenital = Milroy's disease); post-breast surgery with lymph node dissection	Streptococcus sp., Groups A, C, G	**Benzathine pen G** 1.2 million IM q4 wks or **Pen VK** 500 mg po bid or **azithro** 250 mg po qd		**Dosage,** see page 16. Diabetic foot, page 16. Benefit in controlled clinical trial if pt is having frequent episodes of cellulitis (NEJM 368:1695, 2013).
Dandruff (seborrheic dermatitis)	Malassezia species	Ketoconazole shampoo 2% or selenium sulfide 2.5% (see page 10, chronic external otitis)		Treat underlying disorder. Remove offending drug, symptomatic Rx.
Erythema multiforme	H. simplex type 1, mycoplasma, Strep. pyogenes, drugs (sulfonamides, phenytoin, penicillins)			Rx: **NSAIDs; glucocorticoids** (if refractory) Identify and treat precipitant disease if possible
Erythema nodosum	Sarcoidosis, inflammatory bowel disease, MTB, coccidioidomycosis, yersinia, sulfonamides, Whipple's disease.			
Erythrasma	Corynebacterium minutissimum	Localized infection: **Topical Clinda** 2-3 x daily	Widespread infection: **Clarithro** 500 mg po bid or **Erythro** 500 mg po bid x 14 days	Dx: Coral red fluorescence with Wood's lamp. If extensive: prophylactic bathing with anti-bacterial soap or wash with benzyl peroxide. One-time dose of Clari 1 gm po reported to be effective (Int'l J Derm 52:516, 2013; J Derm Treatm 14:70, 2013).
Folliculitis	S. aureus, candida P. aeruginosa common	Usually self-limited, no Rx needed. Could use topical mupirocin for Staph and topical antifungal for Candida		
Furunculosis	Staph. aureus	See Boils, page 53		
Hemorrhagic bullous lesions Hx of sea water-contaminated abrasion or eating raw seafood in cirrhotic pt.	Vibrio vulnificus (CID 52:788, 2011; JAC 67:488, 2012)	**Ceftriaxone** 2 gm IV q24h + (**Doxy** IV/po or **Minocycline** 100 mg IV/po bid)	**CIP** 750 mg po bid or 400 mg IV bid	Wound infection in healthy hosts, but bacteremia mostly in cirrhotics. Pathogenesis: Open wounds and eating raw oysters (seawater). Can cause necrotizing fasciitis (JAC 67:488, 2012). Surgical debridement (Am J Surg 206:32, 2013).
Herpes zoster (shingles). See Table 14				

*NOTE: All dosage recommendations are for adults (unless otherwise indicated) and assume normal renal function. § Alternatives consider allergy, PK, compliance, local resistance, cost

Abbreviations on page 2.

TABLE 1 (52)

ANATOMIC SITE/DIAGNOSIS/ MODIFYING CIRCUMSTANCES	ETIOLOGIES (usual)	SUGGESTED REGIMENS* PRIMARY	ALTERNATIVE§	ADJUNCT DIAGNOSTIC OR THERAPEUTIC MEASURES AND COMMENTS
SKIN (continued)				
Impetigo—See CID 59:147, 2014. "Honey-crust" lesions (non-bullous). Ecthyma is closely related. Causes "punched out" skin lesions.	**Group A strep impetigo** (rarely Strep. sp. Groups B, C or G). Staph. aureus can be Staph. aureus + streptococci. Staph. aureus may be secondary colonizer.	Few lesions: (Mupirocin ointment 2% or fusidic acid cream[NUS] 2%, or retapamulin[NUS] 1%) bid. Treat for 5 days	Numerous lesions: **Pen VK** 250-500 mg po q6h x 5 days or **Benzathine Pen** 600,000 units IM x 1 or TMP-SMX po x 5 days	Topical rx: OTC ointments (bacitracin, neomycin, polymyxin B not as effective as prescription ointments. For mild disease, topical rx as good as po antibiotics (Cochrane Database Syst Rev CD003261, 2012). **Ecthyma:** Infection deeper into epidermis than impetigo. May need parenteral penicillin. Military outbreaks reported: CID 48: 1213 & 1220, 2009 (good images).
Bullous (if ruptured, thin "varnish-like" crust)	**Staph. aureus.** MSSA & MRSA, strains that produce exfoliative toxin A.	For MSSA: po therapy with **dicloxacillin, oxacillin, cephalexin, AM-CL, clinda, TMP-SMX-DS,** or **mupirocin ointment** or **retapamulin ointment**	For MRSA: po therapy with, TMP-SMX-DS, minocycline, doxy, clinda. Treat for 7 days	
Infected wound, extremity—Post-trauma (for bites, see page 52; for post-operative, see page 54)				
Mild to moderate, uncomplicated. Debride wound, if necessary.	Polymicrobic: S. aureus (MSSA & MRSA), aerobic & anaerobic strep.	Clinda 300-450 mg po bid	**Minocycline** 100 mg po bid or **linezolid** 600 mg po bid	**Culture & sensitivity, check Gram stain. Tetanus toxoid if indicated. Mild infection:** check Gram stain. **If suspect Gm-neg. bacilli,** add **AM-CL-ER** 1000/62.5 two tabs po bid. If MRSA is erythro-resistant, may have inducible resistance to clinda.
Febrile with sepsis—hospitalized. Debride wound, if necessary.	Enterobacteriaceae, C. perfringens, C. tetani; if water exposure, Pseudomonas sp., Aeromonas sp. Acinetobacter in soldiers in Iraq (see CID 47:444, 2006).	[**PIP-TZ** or **DORI**[NAI] or **IMP** or **MER** or **ERTA** (Dosage, page 25)] + **vanco** 15-20 mg/kg q8-12h	(**Vanco** 15-20 mg/kg IV q8-12h or **dapto** 6 mg/kg IV q24h or **ceftaroline** 600 mg IV q12h or **telavancin** 10 mg/kg q12h (q8h if P. aeruginosa) or **Levo** 750 mg IV q24h)	**Fever—sepsis:** Another alternative is **linezolid** 600 mg IV/po q12h. If Gm-neg. bacilli & severe pen allergy, **CIP** or **Levo**
Infected wound, post-operative—Gram stain positive cocci - see below				
—Gram stain negative		For dosages, see Table 10A		
			— Gram stain negative	
Surgery not involving GI or female genital tract				
Without sepsis (mild, afebrile)	Staph. aureus, Group A, B, C or G strep sp.	**Clinda** 300-450 mg po bid	**Dapto** 6 mg per kg IV q24h or **telavancin** 10 mg/kg IV q24h	Check Gram stain of exudate. If Gm-neg. bacilli **add** β-lactam/β-lactamase inhibitor. **AM-CL-ER** po or (**ERTA** or **PIP-TZ**) IV. Dosage on page 25.
With sepsis (severe, febrile)		**Vanco** 15-20 mg/kg (actual wt) IV q8-12h to achieve target trough concentration of 15-20 μg/mL		
Surgery involving GI tract (includes oropharynx, esophagus) or female genital tract.—fever, neutrophilia	MSSA/MRSA, coliforms, bacteroides & other anaerobes	[**PIP-TZ** or (**P Ceph 3** + **metro**) or **DORI** or **ERTA** or **IMP** or **MER**] + (**vanco** 1 gm IV q12h or **dapto** 6 mg/kg IV q 24h) If severely ill: **AM-CL-ER** 1000/62.5 mg 2 tabs po bid + **TMP-SMX-DS** 1-2 tabs po bid if Gm+ cocci on Gram stain. Dosages Table 10A & footnote 26, page 56		For all treatment options, see Peritonitis, page 46. Most important: Drain wound & get cultures. Can sub **vanco for dapto** for vanco. Can sub **CIP** or **Levo** if susceptibility permits.
Meleney's synergistic gangrene	See Necrotizing fasciitis, page 63			

*NOTE: All dosage recommendations are for adults (unless otherwise indicated) and assume normal renal function. § Alternatives consider allergy, PK, compliance, local resistance, cost

TABLE 1 (53)

ANATOMIC SITE/DIAGNOSIS/MODIFYING CIRCUMSTANCES	ETIOLOGIES (usual)	SUGGESTED REGIMENS*		ADJUNCT DIAGNOSTIC OR THERAPEUTIC MEASURES AND COMMENTS
		PRIMARY	ALTERNATIVE†	
SKIN/Infected wound, post-operative—Gram stain negative *(continued)*				
Infected wound, post-op, febrile patient— Positive gram stain: **Gram-positive cocci in clusters**	S. aureus, possibly MRSA	Do culture & sensitivity; open & drain wound. **Oral:** TMP-SMX-DS 1 tab po bid or **clinda** 300-450 mg po bid (see Comment)	**IV: Vanco** 15-20 mg/kg q8-12h or **dapto** 4-6 mg/kg IV q24h or **ceftaroline** 600 mg IV q12h or **televancin** 10 mg/kg q24h	Need culture & sensitivity to verify MRSA. Other po options for CA-MRSA include minocycline 100 mg q12h or **Doxy** 100 mg po bid (inexpensive) & linezolid 600 mg po q12h (expensive). If MRSA clinda-sensitive but erythro-resistant, watch out for inducible clinda resistance. Dalbavancin and oritavancin recently FDA-approved for treatment of acute bacterial skin and skin structure infections.
Necrotizing fasciitis ("flesh-eating bacteria") See Gas Gangrene, page 45, & Toxic shock, page 65. Refs: CID 59:147, 2014; NEJM 360:281, 2009.	**5 types:** (1) Strep sp, Grp A, C, G. (2) Clostridia sp. (3) polymicrobic, aerobic + anaerobic (if S. aureus + anaerobic strep = Meleney's synergistic gangrene). (4) Community-associated MRSA (NEJM 352:1445, 2005). (5) K. pneumoniae, esp. in SE Asia (CID 55:930 & 946, 2012)	For treatment of clostridia, see Muscle, gas gangrene, page 45. Meleney's synergistic gangrene, Fournier's gangrene, necrotizing fasciitis have common pathophysiology. **All require prompt surgical debridement + antibiotics**. Dx of necrotizing fasciitis req incision & probing Subcut with fascial plane involvement (fascial plane) = necrotizing fasciitis. **Need Gram stain/culture** to determine if etiology is strep, clostridia, polymicrobial, or S. aureus. **Treatment: Pen G** if strep or clostridia. **IMP** or **MER** if polymicrobial. **vanco OR dapto** if MRSA suspected. **NOTE:** If strep necrotizing fasciitis, reasonable to treat with penicillin & clinda; if clostridia ± gas gangrene, add clinda to penicillin (see page 45). See toxic shock syndrome, streptococcal, page 65. Use of hyperbaric oxygen (HBO) for necrotizing soft tissue infection long debated, see Arch Surg 139:1339, 2004. Recent study limited to centers with on-site HBO found survival benefit for those in most extremely ill category (J Infect Dis/Jacimovic) 15:328, 2014).		
Puncture wound—nail, toothpick Through tennis shoe.	P. aeruginosa	Local debridement to remove foreign body & tetanus prophylaxis; no antibiotic therapy.		Osteomyelitis evolves in only 1-2% of plantar puncture wounds. Consider x-ray if chance of radio-opaque foreign body.
Staphylococcal scalded skin syndrome Ref: PIDJ 19:819, 2000.	Toxin-producing S. aureus	**Nafcillin** or **oxacillin** 2 gm IV (children: 150 mg/kg/day div q6h) x 5-7 days for MSSA, **vanco** 15-20 mg/kg q8-12h (children 40-60 mg/kg/day div q6h) for MRSA		Toxin causes **intradermal split** and positive Nikolsky sign. Biopsy differentiates: drugs cause epidermal/dermal split, called **toxic epidermal necrolysis**—more serious.
Ulcerated skin lesions: Differential Dx	Consider: anthrax, tularemia, P. aeruginosa (ecthyma gangrenosum), plague, blastomycosis, YAWS, arterial insufficiency, venous stasis, and others.			diphtheria, mycobacteria, mycobacteria, leishmania, mucormycosis, spider (rarely).
Ulcerated skin: venous/arterial insufficiency; pressure with secondary infection (infected decubiti) Care of non-healing, non-infected ulcers (AIM 159:ITC8, 2013).	Polymicrobic: Streptococcus sp. (Groups A, C, G), enterococci, anaerobic strep, Enterobacteriaceae, Pseudomonas sp., Bacteroides sp., Staph. aureus.	Severe local or possible bacteremia: **IMP** or **MER** or **DORI** or **PIP-TZ** or **ERTA**. If Gm-pos cocci on gram stain, add **Vanco**.	**(CIP** or **Levo) + Metro)** or **(CFP** or **Ceftaz) + Metro)**. If Gm-pos cocci on gram stain, add **Vanco**.	If ulcer clinically inflamed, rx IV with no topical rx. If not clinically inflamed, consider debridement, removal of foreign body, lessening direct pressure for weight-bearing limbs & leg elevation (if no arterial insufficiency). Topical rx to reduce bacterial counts: silver sulfadiazine 1% or combination antibiotic ointment. **Chlorhexidine & povidone iodine may harm "granulation tissue."** Avoid. If not inflamed, healing improved on air bed; protein supplement; radiant heat; electrical stimulation (AJM 159:39, 2013).
Whirlpool: (Hot Tub) folliculitis	Pseudomonas aeruginosa	Usually self-limited, treatment not indicated		Decontaminate hot tub: drain and chlorinate. Also associated with exfoliative beauty aids (loofah sponges). Ref: CID 38:38, 2004.
Whirlpool: Nail Salon, soft tissue infection	Mycobacterium (fortuitum or chelonei)	**Minocycline**, **doxy** or **CIP**		
SPLEEN. For post-splenectomy prophylaxis, see Table 15A, page 199, for Septic Shock Post-Splenectomy, see Table 1, pg 64.				
Splenic abscess	Staph. aureus, streptococci	**Nafcillin** or **oxacillin** 2 gm **Vanco** 15-20 mg/kg IV q8-IV q4h or **cefazolin** 2 gm IV 12h (to achieve target trough q8h if MSSA	concentration of [15-20 μg/mL).	Burkholderia (Pseudomonas) pseudomallei is common cause of splenic abscess in SE Asia. Presents with fever and LUQ pain. Usual treatment is antimicrobial therapy and splenectomy.
Endocarditis, bacteremia				
Contiguous from intra-abdominal site Immunocompromised	Polymicrobic Candida sp.	Treat as Peritonitis, secondary, page 46. **Amphotericin B** (Dosage, see Table 11, page 122)	**Fluconazole, caspofungin**	Vaccines: CID 58:309, 2014.

Abbreviations on page 2.   *NOTE: All dosage recommendations are for adults (unless otherwise indicated) and assume normal renal function. §Alternatives consider allergy, PK, compliance, local resistance, cost

TABLE 1 (34)

ANATOMIC SITE/DIAGNOSIS/ MODIFYING CIRCUMSTANCES	ETIOLOGIES (usual)	SUGGESTED REGIMENS*		ADJUNCT DIAGNOSTIC OR THERAPEUTIC MEASURES AND COMMENTS
		PRIMARY	ALTERNATIVE§	
SYSTEMIC SYNDROMES (FEBRILE/NON-FEBRILE) Spread by Infected TICK, FLEA, or LICE				
Babesiosis, Lyme disease, & Anaplasma (Ehrlichiosis) have same reservoir & tick vector. Epidemiologic history crucial.				**Seven diseases where pathogen visible in peripheral blood smear:** African/American trypanosomiasis; babesia; bartonellosis; filariasis; malaria; relapsing fever.
Babesiosis: see NEJM 366:2397, 2012. Do not treat if asymptomatic, young, has spleen, and immunocompetent; can be fatal in lymphoma pts.	Etiol.: B. microti et al. Vector: Usually Ixodes ticks Host: White-footed mouse & others	[[Atovaquone 750 mg po q12h) + (azithro 600 mg po day 1, then 250 mg/day times 7-10 days)] If severe infection [clinda 1.2 gm IV bid or 600 mg po times 7 days + quinine 650 mg po tid times 7 days. Ped. dosage: Clinda 20-40 mg per kg per day and quinine 25 mg per kg per day]. See Comment	Atovaquone 750 mg po q12h) + (azithro 600 mg po day 1, then 250 mg/day times 7-10 days) If severe infection [clinda 1.2 gm IV bid or 600 mg po times 7 days + quinine 650 mg po tid times 7 days. Ped. dosage: Clinda 20-40 mg per kg per day and quinine 25 mg per kg per day]. See Comment	**Dx:** Giemsa-stained blood smear; antibody test available. PCR if available. **Rx: Exchange transfusions successful adjunct if used early, in severe disease.** May need treatment for 6 or more wks if immunocompromised. Look for Lyme and/or Anaplasma co-infection.
Bartonella infections: Review EID 12:389, 2006	B. quintana, B. henselae			
Bartonella, asymptomatic	B. quintana, B. henselae	Doxy 100 mg po/IV times 15 days		Can lead to endocarditis &/or trench fever: found in homeless, alcoholics, esp. if lice/leg pain. Often missed since asymptomatic.
Cat-scratch disease	B. henselae	Azithro 500 mg po x 1 dose, then 250 mg/day po x 4 days	Azithro 250 mg po once daily x 3 months or longer	**Or** symptomatic only—see Lymphadenitis, page 45; usually lymphadenitis, hepatitis, splenitis, FUO, neuroretinitis, transverse myelitis, oculoglandular syndrome
Bacillary angiomatosis; Peliosis hepatis—pts with AIDS MMWR 58(RR-4):39, 2009; AAC 48:1921, 2004;	B. henselae, B. quintana	Erythro 500 mg po qid or Doxy 100 mg po bid x 3 months or longer. If CNS involvement: Doxy 100 mg IV/po q12h + RIF 300 mg po bid	Azithro 250 mg po once daily or longer	**Do not use:** TMP-SMX, CIP, Pen, Ceph. **Manifestations of Bartonella infections:** **Immunocompetent Patient:** Bacteremia/endocarditis/FUO encephalitis Cat scratch disease Vertebral osteo Trench fever Parinaud's oculoglandular syndrome **HIV/AIDS Patient:** Bacillary angiomatosis Bacillary peliosis Bacteremia/endocarditis/FUO
		Regardless of CD4 count, DC therapy after 3-4 mos & observe. If no relapse, no suppressive rx. If relapse, doxy, azithro or erythro x 3 mos. Stop when CD4 >200 x 6 mos.		
Endocarditis (see page 28) (Circ 111:3167, 2005; AAC 48:1921, 2004)	B. henselae, B. quintana	If suspect endocarditis: Ceftriaxone 2 gm IV once daily x 6 weeks + Gent 1 mg/kg IV q8h x 14 days + Doxy 100 mg IV/po bid x 6 wks	If proven endocarditis: Doxy 100 mg IV/po bid x 6 wks + Gent 1 mg/kg IV q8h x 11 days	**Gentamicin toxicity:** If Gent toxicity, substitute Rifampin 300 mg IV/po bid x 14 days. Role of valve removal surgery to cure unclear. Presents as SBE. Diagnosis: ECHO, serology, & PCR of resected heart valve.
	B. henselae, B. quintana	Surgical removal of infected valve		
Oroya fever (acute) & Verruga peruana (chronic) (AAC 48:1921, 2004)	B. bacilliformis	Oroya fever: CiP 500 mg po bid or Doxy 100 mg po bid x 14 d. Alternative: Chloro 500 mg IV or po q6h x 14 days or Azithro 500 mg po q24h	Verruga peruana: RIF 10 mg/kg po once daily x 14 d or Streptomycin 15-20 mg/Kg IM/IV once daily x 10 days	Oroya fever transmitted by sand-fly bite in Andes Mtns. Related Bartonella (B. rochalimae) caused bacteremia, fever and splenomegaly (NEJM 356:2346 & 2381, 2007). **CIP and Chloro preferred due to prevention of secondary Salmonella infections.**
		Oroya fever: CiP 500 mg po bid or Doxy 100 mg po bid x 14 days		
Trench fever (FUO) (AAC 48:1921, 2004)	B. quintana	No endocarditis: Doxy 100 mg po bid x 4 wks + Gentamicin 3 mg/kg once daily for 1st 2 wks of therapy (AAC 48:1921, 2004).		Vector is body louse. Do not use: TMP-SMX, FQs, cefazolin or Pen. If endocarditis, need longer rx. See Emerg ID 2:217, 2006).

Abbreviations on page 2.   *NOTE: All dosage recommendations are for adults (unless otherwise indicated) and assume normal renal function. § Alternatives consider allergy, PK, compliance, local resistance, cost

TABLE 1 (55)

ANATOMIC SITE/DIAGNOSIS/ MODIFYING CIRCUMSTANCES	ETIOLOGIES (usual)	SUGGESTED REGIMENS*		ADJUNCT DIAGNOSTIC OR THERAPEUTIC MEASURES AND COMMENTS
		PRIMARY	ALTERNATIVE†	
SYSTEMIC SYNDROMES (FEBRILE/NON-FEBRILE)/Spread by infected TICK, FLEA, or LICE *(continued)*				
Ehrlichiosis[25] CDC def. of (1) 4x↑ IFA antibody, (2) detection of Ehrlichia DNA in blood or CSF by PCR, (3) visible morulae in WBC and IFA ≥1:64. New species in WI. *MN MN 365:422, 2011).*				
Human monocytic ehrlichiosis (HME) (*Ehrlichia chaffeensis* (Lone Star tick is vector) *(MMWR 55(RR-4), 2006; CID 43:1089, 2006)*	*Ehrlichia chaffeensis*	**Doxy** 100 mg po/IV bid times 7-10 days	**Tetracycline** 500 mg po qid x 7-10 days. No current rec. for children or pregnancy	30 states: mostly SE of line from NJ to III to Missouri to Oklahoma to Texas. History of outdoor activity and tick exposure. April-Sept. Fever, rash (36%), leukopenia and thrombocytopenia. Blood smears no help. PCR for early dx.
Human Anaplasmosis (formerly known as **Human granulocytic ehrlichiosis**)	Anaplasma (Ehrlichia) phagocytophilum (Ixodes sp. ticks are vector). Dog variant is Ehrlichia ewingii (*NEJM 341:148 & 195, 1999*)	**Doxy** 100 mg bid po or IV times 7-14 days	**Tetracycline** 500 mg po qid times 7-14 days. Not in children or pregnancy *See Comment*	Upper Midwest, NE, West Coast & Europe. H/O tick exposure. April-Sept. Febrile flu-like illness after outdoor activity. No rash. Leukopenia/ thrombocytopenia common. **Dx:** PCR best; blood smear insensitive (*Am J Trop Med Hyg 93:66, 2015).* **Rx:** RIF active in vitro (*IDCNA 22:433, 2008)* but worry about resistance developing. Minocycline should work if doxy not available.
Lyme Disease NOTE: Think about concomitant tick-borne disease—e.g., babesiosis and ehrlichiosis. **Guidelines:** *CID 51:1, 2010; NEJM 370:1724, 2014.*	Bite by ixodes-infected tick in an endemic area — *Borrelia burgdorferi*			
Postexposure prophylaxis	**IDSA guidelines:** *CID 43:1089, 2006; CID 51:1, 2010*	**If endemic area**, if nymphal partially engorged deer tick: **doxy** 200 mg po times 1 dose with food.	**If not endemic area**, not engorged not deer tick: No treatment	Prophylaxis study in endemic area: erythema migrans developed in 3% of the control group and 0.4% doxy group (*NEJM 345:79 & 133, 2001).* Can substitute **Minocycline** for Doxy, if Doxy is unavailable.
Early (erythema migrans) *See Comment*	**IgM**—Need 2 of 3 positive of kilodaltons (KD): 23, 39, 41	**Doxy** 100 mg po bid, or **amoxicillin** 500 mg po tid. All regimens to 14-21 days. (10 days as good as 20) *AnM 138:697, 2003)*	**Cefuroxime axetil** 500 mg po bid times 14-21 days; or **erythro** 250 mg po qid. See Comment for peds doses	High rate of clinical failure with azithro & erythro (*Drugs 57:157, 1999).* **Amox** 50 mg per kg per day in 3 div. doses or **cefuroxime axetil** 30 mg per kg per day in 2 div. doses or **erythro** 30 mg per kg per day in 3 div. doses. Lesions usually homogeneous—not target-like (*AnIM 136:423, 2002)*
Carditis *See Comment*	**IgG**—Need 5 of 3 positive of KD: 18, 21, 28, 30, 39, 41, 45, 58, 66, 93	(**Ceftriaxone** 2 gm IV q24h) or (**cefotaxime** 2 gm IV q8h) or **Pen G** 3 million units IV q4h) times 14-21 days	**Doxy** (see Comments) 100 mg po bid times 14-21 days or **amoxicillin** 500 mg po tid times 14-21 days.	First degree AV block. Oral regimen. Generally self-limited. High degree AV block (PR >0.3 sec.): IV therapy—permanent pacemaker not necessary, but temporary pacing in 39% (*CID 59:996, 2014).*
Facial nerve paralysis (isolated finding, early)	Interest in 2 tier diagnostic approach: 1 standard Lyme ELISA & if positive: 2) C6 peptide ELISA. Better sensitivity/specificity. Applicable to European cases (*CID 57:333 & 341, 2013).*	(**Doxy** 100 mg po bid or **amoxicillin** 500 mg po tid) times 14-21 days.	**Ceftriaxone** 2 gm IV q24h times 14-21 days	LP suggested excluding central neurologic disease. If LP neg., oral regimen OK. If abnormal or not done, suggest parenteral Ceftriaxone.
Meningitis, encephalitis For encephalopathy, *see Comment*	Western blot diagnostic criteria.	**Ceftriaxone** 2 gm IV q24h times 14-28 days	(**Pen G** 20 million units IV q24h in div. dose) or (**cefotaxime** 2 gm IV q8h) times 14-28 days	Encephalopathy: memory difficulty, depression, somnolence, or headache. CSF abnormalities 89% had objective CSF abnormalities. 18/18 pts improved with ceftriaxone 2 gm per day times 30 days (*JID 180:377, 1999).* No compelling evidence that prolonged treatment has any benefit in chronic Lyme syndrome (*Neurology 69:91, 2007).*
Arthritis		**Doxy** 100 mg po bid or **amoxicillin** 500 mg po tid, both times 30-60 days	(**Ceftriaxone** 2 gm IV q24h) or (**pen G** 20-24 million units per day IV) times 14-28 days	Start with 1 mo. of therapy. If only partial response, treat for a second mo.
Pregnancy		**Amoxicillin** 500 mg po tid times 21 days	If **pen. allergic: azithro** 500 mg po qid times 7-10 days or (**erythro** 500 mg po times 14-21 days)	
Post-Lyme Disease Syndromes		None indicated	Choice depends on clinical picture	No benefit from tx (*AJM 128:865, 2013; CID 51:1, 2010; AAC 58:6701, 2014; NEJM 345:85, 2001).*

[25] In endemic area (New York), high % of both adult ticks and nymphs were jointly infected with both Anaplasma (HGE) and B. burgdorferi (*NEJM 337:49, 1997).*

Abbreviations on page 2   * *NOTE: All dosage recommendations are for adults (unless otherwise indicated) and assume normal renal function. & Alternatives consider allergy, PK, compliance, local resistance, cost*

TABLE 1 (56)

SYSTEMIC SYNDROMES (FEBRILE/NON-FEBRILE)/Spread by infected TICK, FLEA, or LICE (continued)

ANATOMIC SITE/DIAGNOSIS/ MODIFYING CIRCUMSTANCES	ETIOLOGIES (usual)	SUGGESTED REGIMENS*		ADJUNCT DIAGNOSTIC OR THERAPEUTIC MEASURES AND COMMENTS
		PRIMARY	ALTERNATIVE§	
Plague, bacteremic (see also Bubonic plague and plague pneumonia)	Yersinia pestis	(**Streptomycin** 30 mg/kg/day IV in 2 div doses or **Gentamicin** 5 mg/kg/day IV single dose) x 10 days	**Doxy** 200 mg IV/po bid x 1 day, then 100 mg IV/po bid x 7-10 days	FQs effective in animals: [**Levo** 500 mg IV/po once daily or **CIP** 500 mg po (or 400 mg IV) q12h] x 10 days or **Moxi** 400 mg IV/po q24h x 10-14 days
Relapsing fever Louse-borne (LBRF)	Borrelia recurrentis Reservoir: human Vector: Louse pediculus humanus	**Tetracycline** 500 mg IV/po x 1 dose	**Erythro** 500 mg IV/po x 1 dose	Jarisch-Herxheimer (fever, ↑ pulse, ↑ resp., ↓ blood pressure) in most patients (occurs in ~2 hrs). Not prevented by prior steroids. **Dx: Examine peripheral blood smear during fever for spirochetes.** Can relapse up to 10 times. Postexposure **doxy** pre-emptive therapy highly effective (NEJM 355:148, 2006). B. miyamoto: Dx by ref lab serum PCR. Fever, headache, thrombocytopenia & tick exposure (NE USA). Seems to respond to Doxy, Amox, Ceftriaxone (AnIM 163:91 & 141, 2015; NEJM 373:468, 2015).
Tick-borne (TBRF)	No Amer: B. hermsii, B. turicata, Africa: B. hispanica, B. crocidurae, B. duttonii; Russia: B. miyamoto (see Comment)	**Doxy** 100 mg po bid x 7-10 days	**Erythro** 500 mg po qid x 7-10 days	

Abbreviations on page 2.   *NOTE: All dosage recommendations are for adults (unless otherwise indicated) and assume normal renal function. § Alternatives consider allergy, PK, compliance, local resistance, cost

TABLE 1 (57)

ANATOMIC SITE/DIAGNOSIS/ MODIFYING CIRCUMSTANCES	ETIOLOGIES (usual)	SUGGESTED REGIMENS*		ADJUNCT DIAGNOSTIC OR THERAPEUTIC MEASURES AND COMMENTS
		PRIMARY	ALTERNATIVE†	
SYSTEMIC SYNDROMES (FEBRILE/NON-FEBRILE)/Spread by Infected TICK, FLEA, or LICE (continued)				
Rickettsial diseases. Review—Disease in travelers (CID 39:1493, 2004)				
Spotted fevers—Disease in travelers (CID 39:1493, 2004)				
Rocky Mountain spotted fever (RMSF)	R. rickettsii [Dermacentor tick vector]	**Doxy** 100 mg po/IV bid times 7 days or for 2 days after temp. normal. Do not use in pregnancy. Some suggest loading dose: 200 mg IV/po q 12h x 3 days, then 100 mg po bid	**Pregnancy: Chloro** 50 mg/kg/day in 4 div doses. If cannot obtain Chloro, no choice but Doxy despite risks (fetal bone & teeth malformation, maternal toxicity).	Fever, rash (88%), petechiae 40-50%. **Rash spreads from distal extremities to trunk.** Rash in <50% pts in 1st 72 hrs. Dx: Immunohistology on skin biopsy; confirmation with antibody titers. Highest incidence in SE and South Central states; also seen in Oklahoma, S. Dakota, Montana. Cases reported from 42 U.S. states. **NOTE: Only 3-18% of pts present with fever, rash, and hx of tick exposure; many early deaths in children & empiric doxy reasonable** (MMWR 49: 885, 2000).
Ref: LnID 8:143, 2008 and MMWR 55 (RR-4), 2007				
NOTE: Can mimic ehrlichiosis. Pattern of rash important—see Comment				
Other spotted fevers, e.g., Rickettsial pox, African tick bite fever	At least 8 species on 6 continents (CID 45 (Suppl 1) S39, 2007).	**Doxy** 100 mg po bid times 7 days	**Chloro** 500 mg po/IV po times 7 days Children <8 y.o.: **azithro** or **clarithro** (if mild disease)	Clinical diagnosis suggested by: 1) fever, intense myalgia, headache; 2) exposure to mites or ticks; 3) localized eschar (tache noire) or rash. Definitive Dx: PCR of blood, skin biopsy or sequential antibody tests.
Typhus group—Consider in returning travelers with fever				
Louse-borne: epidemic typhus Ref: LnID 8:417, 2008.	R. prowazekii [vector is body or head louse]	**Doxy** 100 mg po/IV po bid times 7 days; single 200 mg dose 95% effective.	**Chloro** 500 mg IV/po times 5 days	**Brill-Zinsser disease** (Ln 357:1198, 2001) is a relapse of typhus acquired during WWII. Truncal rash (64%) spreads centrifugally—opposite of RMSF. Louse borne typhus is a winter disease. Diagnosis by serology. R. prowazekii found in flying squirrels in SE US. Delouse clothing of infected pt.
Murine typhus (cat flea typhus): Ref: EID 14:1019, 2008	R. typhi [rat reservoir and flea vector] CID 46:913, 2008	**Doxy** 100 mg IV/po bid times 7 days	**Chloro** 500 mg IV/po times 5 days	Rash in 20-54%, not diagnostic. Without treatment most pts recover in 2 wks. Faster recovery with treatment. Dx based on suspicion; confirmed serologically.
Scrub typhus	O. Tsutsugamushi [rodent reservoir; vector is larval stage of mites (chiggers)]	**Doxy** 100 mg po/IV bid x 7 days. In pregnancy: **Azithro** 500 mg po x one dose	**Chloro** 500 mg IV/po qid x 7 days	Asian rim of Pacific. Confirm with serology. If Doxy resistance consider, alternatives are **Doxy + RIF** 900 or 600 mg once daily (Ln 356:1057, 2000) or **Azithro** 500 mg q24h (AAC 58:1488, 2014).
Tularemia, typhoidal type Ref: **bioterrorism**, see JAMA 285:2763, 2001; ID Clin No Amer 22:489, 2008; MMWR 58:744, 2009.	Francisella tularensis. [Vector depends on geography: ticks, biting flies, mosquitoes identified]	**Moderate/severe:** [(**Gentamicin** or **tobra** 5 mg per kg per day div. q8h IV) or (**Streptomycin** 10 mg/kg IV/IM q12h)] x10 days	**Mild:** [**CIP** 400 mg IV (or 750 mg po) bid or **Doxy** 100 mg IV/po bid] x 14-21 days	Diagnosis: Culture on cysteine-enriched media & serology. Dangerous in the lab. Meningoencephalitis is a complication; treatment is **Streptomycin** + **Chloro** 50-100 mg/kg/day IV in 4 divided doses (Arch Neurol 66:523, 2009).

*NOTE: All dosage recommendations are for adults (unless otherwise indicated) and assume normal renal function. § Alternatives consider allergy, PK, compliance, local resistance, cost

Abbreviations on page 2.   *NOTE: All dosage recommendations are for adults (unless otherwise indicated) and assume normal renal function.

TABLE 1 (58)

ANATOMIC SITE/DIAGNOSIS/ MODIFYING CIRCUMSTANCES	ETIOLOGIES (usual)	SUGGESTED REGIMENS*		ADJUNCT DIAGNOSTIC OR THERAPEUTIC MEASURES AND COMMENTS
		PRIMARY	ALTERNATIVE†	
SYSTEMIC SYNDROMES (FEBRILE/NON-FEBRILE)/Spread by infected TICK, FLEA, or LICE *(continued)*				
Other Zoonotic Systemic Bacterial Febrile Illnesses (not spread by fleas, lice or ticks): Obtain careful epidemiologic history				
Brucellosis Refs: *NEJM 352:2325, 2005; CID 46:426, 2008; MMWR 57:603, 2008; BMJ 336:701, 2008; PLoS One 7:e32090, 2012.*	B. abortus-cattle B. suis-swine B. melitensis-goats B. canis-dogs	**Non focal disease:** [**Doxy** 100 mg po bid x 6 wks + **Gent** 5 mg/kg once daily for 1st 7 days] ---------- **Spondylitis, Sacroiliitis:** [**Doxy** + **Gent** (as above) + **RIF**] x min 3 mos ---------- **Neurobrucellosis:** [**Doxy** + **RIF** (as above) + **ceftriaxone** 2 gm IV q12h until CSF returned to normal (AAC 56:1523, 2012) **Endocarditis:** Surgery + [(**RIF** + **Doxy** + **TMP-SMX**) x 1-1/2 to 6 mos + **Gent** for 2-4 wks (CID 56:1407, 2013) **Pregnancy:** Not much data. **RIF** 900 mg po once daily x 6 wks	[**Doxy** 100 mg po bid x 6 wks + **RIF** 600-900 mg po once daily) x 6 wks. Less optimal: **CIP** 500 mg po bid + (**Doxy** or **RIF**)] x 6 wks ---------- [(**CIP** 750 mg po bid + **RIF** 600-900 mg po once daily) x 3 mos] ---------- RIF 900 mg po once daily + **TMP-SMX** 5 mg/kg (TMP comp) po bid x 4 wks.	Bone involvement, esp. sacroiliitis in 20-30%. **Neurobrucellosis:** Usually meningitis. 1% of all pts with brucellosis. Role of corticosteroids unclear; not recommended. **Endocarditis:** Rare but most common cause of death. Need surgery + antimicrobials. **Pregnancy:** TMP-SMX may cause kernicterus if given during last week of pregnancy.
Leptospirosis *(CID 36:1507 & 1514, 2003; LnID 3:757, 2003)*	Leptospira—in urine of domestic livestock, dogs, small rodents	Severe illness: **Pen G** 1.5 million units IV q6h or **Ceftriaxone** 2 gm q24h. Duration: 7 days	Mild illness: (**Doxy** 100 mg IV/po q12h or **Amoxicillin** 500 mg po q8h x 7 days	**Severity varies.** Varies from mild anicteric illness to severe icteric disease (Weil's disease) with renal failure and myocarditis. AST/ALT do not exceed 5x normal. **Rx:** Aztho 1 gm once, then 500 mg daily x 2 days; non-inferior to, and fewer side effects than, doxy in standard dose (AAC 51:3259, 2007). Jarisch-Henxheimer reaction can occur post-Pen therapy.
Salmonella bacteremia other than S. typhi-non-typhoidal	Salmonella enteritidis—a variety of serotypes from animal sources	If NOT acquired in Asia: (**CIP** 400 mg IV q12h or **Levo** 750 mg po once daily) x 14 days *(See Comment)*	If acquired in Asia: **Ceftriaxone** 2 gm IV q24h or **Azithro** 1 gm x 1 dose, then 500 mg po once daily x 5-7 days. Do NOT use FQs until susceptibility determined. *(See Comment)*	In vitro resistance to nalidixic acid indicates relative resistance to FQs. Bacteremia can infect any organ/tissue: look for infection of atherosclerotic aorta, osteomyelitis in sickle cell pts. Rx duration range 14 days (immunocompetent) to ≥6 wks if mycotic aneurism or endocarditis. Alternative, if susceptible: **TMP-SMX** 8-10 mg/kg/day (TMP comp) divided q6h. CLSI has established new interpretive breakpoints for susceptibility to Ciprofloxacin: susceptible strains, MIC < 0.06 μg/mL. (CID 55:1107, 2012).

Abbreviations on page 2.   *NOTE: All dosage recommendations are for adults (unless otherwise indicated) and assume normal renal function. † Alternatives consider allergy, PK, compliance, local resistance, cost*

TABLE 1 (59)

ANATOMIC SITE/DIAGNOSIS/ MODIFYING CIRCUMSTANCES	ETIOLOGIES (usual)	SUGGESTED REGIMENS*		ADJUNCT DIAGNOSTIC OR THERAPEUTIC MEASURES AND COMMENTS
		PRIMARY	ALTERNATIVE¹	
SYSTEMIC SYNDROMES (FEBRILE/NON-FEBRILE) (continued)				
Miscellaneous Systemic Febrile Syndromes				
Fever in Returning Travelers Etiology by geographic exposure & clinical syndrome (AnIM 158:456, 2013).	Dengue (Flavivirus)	Supportive care: see Table 14A, page 166		Average incubation period 4 days; serodiagnosis.
	Malaria (Plasmodia sp)	Diagnosis: peripheral blood smear		See Table 13A, page 153
	Typhoid (Salmonella sp)	See Table 1, page 61.		Average incubation 7-14 days; diarrhea in 45%.
Kawasaki syndrome 6 weeks to 12 yrs of age, peak at 1 yr of age, 85% below age 5. *Pediatrics 124:1, 2009. tongue image [NEJM 373:467, 2015]*	Self-limited vasculitis with ↑ temp., rash, conjunctivitis, strawberry tongue, cervical adenitis, red hands/feet & coronary artery aneurysms	**IVIG** 2 gm per kg over 8-12 hrs x 1 + **ASA** 20-25 mg per kg qid **THEN** **ASA** 3-5 mg per kg per day po q24h times 6-8 wks	If still febrile after 1st dose of IVIG, some give 2nd dose. In Japan: **IVIG** + **prednisolone** 2 mg/kg/day. Continue steroid until CRP normal for 15 days (Lancet 379:1571, 2012).	IV gamma globulin (2 gm per kg over 10 hrs) in pts rx before 10th day of illness ↓ coronary artery lesions. See Table 14A, page 175 for IVIG adverse effects. In children, wait 11+ months after IVIG before giving live virus vaccines.
Rheumatic Fever, acute Ref: Ln 366:155, 2005	Post-Group A strep pharyngitis (not Group B, C, or G)	(1) Symptom relief: **ASA** 80-100 mg per kg per day in children; 4-8 gm per day in adults. (2) Eradicate Group A strep: **Pen** times 10 days (see Pharyngitis, page 48). Start prophylaxis: see below		
Prophylaxis				
Primary prophylaxis: Treat S. pyogenes pharyngitis		**Benzathine pen G** 1.2 million units IM (see Pharyngitis, pg. 48)		**Penicillin** for 10 days prevents rheumatic fever even when started 7-9 days after onset of illness (see page 48). Alternative: **Penicillin V** 250 mg po bid or **sulfadiazine (sulfisoxazole)** 1 gm po q24h or **erythro** 250 mg po bid.
Secondary prophylaxis (previous documented rheumatic fever)		**Benzathine pen G** 1.2 million units IM q3-4 wks (AAC 58:6735, 2014).		**Duration?** No cardiac: 5 yrs or until age 21, whichever is longer; carditis without residual heart disease: 10 yrs since last attack; carditis with residual valvular disease: 10 yrs since last episode or until age 40 whichever is longer (PEDS 96:758, 1995).
Typhoid syndrome (typhoid fever, enteric fever) Global susceptibility results: CID 50:241, 2010. Treatment: BMJ 338 b1159 & b1865, 2009	Salmonella typhi, S. paratyphi A, B, C & S. choleraesuis. **NOTE: In vitro resistance to nalidixic acid predicts clinical failure of CIP (FQs).** Do not use empiric FQs if Asia-acquired infection. Need susceptibility data.	**If NOT acquired in Asia:** **CIP** 400 mg IV q12h or **Levo** 750 mg po/IV q24h x 7-14 days. (See Comment) In children, **azithro** 10 mg/kg once daily x 7 days (AAC 51:819, 2007)	**If acquired in Asia:** (**Ceftriaxone** 2 gm IV daily x 5 days) or (**CIP** 1 gm po x 1 dose, then 500 mg po daily x 7 days) or (**Chloro** 500 mg q6h x 14 d) (See Comment)	
Sepsis: Following suggested *empiric* therapy assumes pt is bacteremic; mimicked by viral, fungal, rickettsial infections and pancreatitis (Intensive Care Medicine 34:17, 2008; IDC No Amer 22:1, 2008).				
Neonatal—early onset <1 week old	Group B strep, E. coli, Klebsiella, enterobacter, Staph. aureus (uncommon), listeria (rare in U.S.)	**AMP** 25 mg/kg IV q8h + **cefotaxime** 50 mg/kg q12h	(**AMP** + **gent** 2.5 mg/kg IV/IM q12h or (**AMP** + **ceftriaxone** 50 mg/kg IV/IM q24h)	Dexamethasone: Use in severely ill pts: 1st dose just prior to antibiotic, 3 mg/kg IV, then 1 mg/kg q6h x 8 doses. **Complications:** perforation of terminal ileum &/or cecum, osteo, septic arthritis, **mycotic aneurysm,** meningitis, hematogenous pneumonia. FQs, including Gati, narrow best treatment if isolate susceptible (BMJ 338 b1159 & 1865, 2009; LnID 11:445, 2011). CLSI has established new interpretive breakpoints for susceptibility. Ciprofloxacin: susceptible strains, MIC < 0.06 µg/mL (CID 55:1107, 2012).
Neonatal—late onset 1-4 weeks old	As above + H. influenzae & S. epidermidis	(**AMP** 25 mg/kg IV q6h + **cefotaxime** 50 mg/kg q8h) or (**AMP** + **ceftriaxone** 75 mg/kg IV q24h)	**AMP** + **gent** 2.5 mg/kg IV or IM	If MSSA/MRSA a concern, add vanco.

*NOTE: All dosage recommendations are for adults (unless otherwise indicated) and assume normal renal function. § Alternatives consider allergy, PK, compliance, local resistance, cost

TABLE 1 (60)

ANATOMIC SITE/DIAGNOSIS/ MODIFYING CIRCUMSTANCES	ETIOLOGIES* (usual)	SUGGESTED REGIMENS*		ADJUNCT DIAGNOSTIC OR THERAPEUTIC MEASURES AND COMMENTS
		PRIMARY	ALTERNATIVE§	
SYSTEMIC SYNDROMES (FEBRILE/NON-FEBRILE)/Sepsis *(continued)*				
Child; not neutropenic	Strep, pneumoniae, meningococci, Staph. aureus (MSSA & MRSA), H. influenzae now rare	(Cefotaxime 50 mg/kg IV q8h or ceftriaxone 100 mg/kg IV q24h) + vanco 15 mg/kg IV q6h	Aztreonam 7.5 mg/kg IV q6h + linezolid	Major concerns are S. pneumoniae & community-associated MRSA. Coverage for Gm-neg. bacilli included but H. influenzae infection now rare. Meningococcemia probably remains key risk (*Ln* 356:961, 2000).
Adult; not neutropenic: NO HYPOTENSION but LIFE-THREATENING; see page 64				Systemic inflammatory response syndrome (**SIRS**): 2 or more of the following: 1. temperature >38°C or <36°C 2. Heart rate >90 beats per min. 3. Respiratory rate >20 breaths per min. 4. WBC >12,000 per mcL or > 10% bands
Source unclear—consider primary bacteremia, intra-abdominal or skin source. May be **Life-threatening**. Survival greater with quick, effective empiric antibiotic Rx (*CCM* 38:1045 & 1211, 2010).	Aerobic Gm-neg. bacilli; S. aureus; streptococci; others	(IMP or MER) + vanco] or (PIP-TZ) + vanco + PIP-TZ. ↑ESBL-associated/carbapenemase-producing GNB. Empiric options pending clarification of clinical syndrome/culture results: **Low prevalence: Vanco + PIP-TZ** **High prevalence: Colistin + (MER or IMP)** (See Table 5B, page 81)	(Dapto 6 mg/kg IV q24h) + cefepime or PIP-TZ	**Sepsis:** SIRS + a documented infection (+ culture) **Severe sepsis:** Sepsis + organ dysfunction: hypotension or hypoperfusion abnormalities (lactic acidosis, oliguria, ↓ mental status) **Septic shock:** Sepsis-induced hypotension (systolic BP <90 mmHg) not responsive to 500 mL IV fluid challenge + peripheral hypoperfusion If enterococci a concern, add ampicillin or vanco to metro regimens
		Dosages in footnote[26]		
if suspect biliary source (see Gallbladder pg. 17)	Enterococci + aerobic Gm-neg. bacilli	**For Colistin combination dosing, see Table 10A, page 112.** **PIP-TZ** or **TC-CL**	Ceftriaxone + metro or CIP or Levo) + metro[26] *Dosages—footnote[26]*	Many categories of CAP, see material beginning at page 39. Suggestions based on most severe CAP; e.g., MRSA after influenza or Klebsiella pneumonia in an alcoholic.
if community-acquired pneumonia (see page 39 and following pages)	S. pneumoniae; MRSA; Legionella, Gm-neg. bacilli, others	(Levo or moxi) + (PIP-TZ) + Vanco	Aztreonam + (Levo or moxi) + linezolid	In vitro nafcillin increased production of In vitro nafcillin increased production of toxins by CA-MRSA (*JID* 195:202, 2007). Dosages—footnote 26, page 63
if illicit use IV drugs	S. aureus			
if suspect intra-abdominal source	Mixture aerobic & anaerobic Gm-neg. bacilli	See secondary peritonitis, page 47		
if petechial rash	Meningococcemia	**Ceftriaxone 2 gm IV q12h** (until sure no meningitis), consider Rocky Mountain spotted fever—see page 60		
if suspect urinary source, e.g. pyelonephritis	Aerobic Gm-neg. bacilli	See pyelonephritis, page 34		
Neutropenic: Child or Adult (absolute PMN count <500 per mm³) in cancer and transplant patients. Guideline: *CID* 52:427, 2011 (inpatients); *J Clin Oncol* 31:794, 2013 (outpatients)				
Post-chemotherapy— impending neutropenia		In patients expected to have PMN < 100 for > 7 days consider Levo 500-750 mg po q24h. Acute leukemics undergoing intensive induction consider addition of Fluc. In patients with AML or MDS who have prolonged neutropenia, consider Posa instead at 200 mg TID (*N Engl J Med* 356:348, 2007).		
Prophylaxis: Child or Adult (absolute PMN count <500 per mm³)	Pneumocystis (PCP); Viridans strep			
Post allogeneic stem cell transplant	Aerobic Gm-neg bacilli ↑ risk pneumocystis, herpes viruses, candida infection	TMP-SMX (vs. PCP) + Acyclovir (vs. HSV/VZV) + pre-emptive monitoring for CMV (vs. mold)		In autologous HCT, not active prophylaxis nor CMV screening is recommended. Fluc OK with TMP-SMX and acyclovir.

[P Ceph 3 (**cefotaxime** 2 gm IV q4-6h, use q4h if life-threatening; **ceftizoxime** 2 gm IV q8h; **ceftriaxone** 2 gm IV q24h; **ceftazidime** 2 gm IV q8h; **cefepime** 2 gm IV q8-12h if neutropenic), **cefpirome**[NUS] 2 gm IV q12h. CIP 400 mg IV q12h.** **Aminoglycosides** (see Table 10D, page 118), **AMP** 200 mg/kg/day divided q6h, **clinda** 900 mg IV q8h, **IMP** 0.5 gm IV q6h, **MER** 1 gm IV q8h, **ERTA** 1 gm IV q24h, **DORI** 500 mg IV q8h (1-hr infusion), **Nafcillin** or **oxacillin** 2 gm IV q4h, **aztreonam** 2 gm IV q8h, **metro** 1 gm loading dose then 0.5 gm q6h or 1 gm q12h, **vanco** 1 gm loading dose 25-30 mg/kg IV, then 15-20 mg/kg IV q8-12h (dose in obese pt, see Table 17C, page 229), **Cefepime** 2 gm IV q8h.]

*NOTE: All dosage recommendations are for adults (unless otherwise indicated) and assume normal renal function. § Alternatives consider allergy, PK, compliance, local resistance, cost

Abbreviations on page 2.

TABLE 1 (61)

ANATOMIC SITE/DIAGNOSIS/ MODIFYING CIRCUMSTANCES	ETIOLOGIES (usual)	SUGGESTED REGIMENS*		ADJUNCT DIAGNOSTIC OR THERAPEUTIC MEASURES AND COMMENTS
		PRIMARY	ALTERNATIVE†	
SYSTEMIC SYNDROMES (FEBRILE/NON-FEBRILE)/Neutropenia *(continued)*				
Empiric therapy—febrile neutropenia (≥38.3°C for > 1 hr or sustained >38°C and absolute neutrophil count <500 cells/μL)				(IDSA Guidelines: *CID 52:427, 2012*); (Outpatients: *J Clin Oncol 31:794, 2013*)
Low-risk adults Anticipate < 7 days neutropenia, no co-morb., can take po meds	Aerobic Gm-neg. bacilli, Viridans strep	**CIP** 750 mg po bid + **AM-CL** 875/125 mg po bid. Treat until absolute neutrophil count ≥1000 cells/μL.	Treat as outpatients with fever if: no focal findings, no COPD, no fungal infection, no dehydration, age range 16-60 yrs. motivated and compliant pts and family: can substitute clinda 300 mg po qid for AM-CL	
High-risk adults and children (Anticipate > 7 days profound neutropenia, active co-morbidities)	**Aerobic Gm-neg. bacilli** to include **P. aeruginosa:** cephalosporin-resistant **viridans strep:** MRSA	**Empiric therapy:** **CFP, IMP, MERO, DORI,** or **PIP-TZ.** Consider addition of **Vanco** as below. ----	**Combination therapy:** If pt has severe sepsis/shock, consider add **Tobra** AND **Vanco** AND **Echinocandin**	Increasing resistance of viridans streptococci to penicillins, cephalosporins (*NEJM 341:469 & 1445, 1999*). **What if severe IgE-mediated β-lactam allergy?** Aztreonam plus Tobra. Work-up should include blood, urine. CXR with additional testing based on symptoms. Low threshold for CT scan. If cultures remain neg, but pt afebrile, treat until absolute neutrophil count ≥ 500 cells/μL.
		Include empiric vanco if: Suspected CLABSI; severe mucositis, SSTI, PNA, or hypotension		
		Dosages: *Footnote⁴ and Table 10B*		
Persistent fever and neutropenia after 5 days of empiric antibacterial therapy—see *CID 52:427, 2011.*				
	Candida species, aspergillus, VRE, resistant GNB	Add either (**caspofungin** 70 mg IV day 1 then 50 mg IV q24h or **Micafungin** 100 mg IV q24h or **Anidulafungin** 200 mg IV 1 dose, then 100 mg IV q24h) **OR voriconazole** 6 mg per kg IV q12h times 2 doses, then 4 mg per kg IV q12h		Conventional **ampho B** causes more fever & nephrotoxicity & lower efficacy than lipid-based ampho B. both **caspofungin & voriconazole** better tolerated & perhaps more efficacious than lipid-based ampho B (*NEJM 346:225, 2002 & 351:1391 & 1445, 2005*).
Shock syndromes				
Septic shock: Fever & hypotension **Bacteremic shock, endotoxin shock**	Bacteremia with aerobic Gm-neg. bacteria or Gm + cocci	Lower mortality with **sepsis-based "bundle"** (*AJRCCM 188:77, 2013*) • Blood cultures & serum lactate • Initiate effective antibiotic therapy:		• Hydrocortisone in stress dose: 100 mg IV q8h if BP still low after fluids and one vasopressor (*ARJCCM 185:135, 2012*); Benefit in pts with severe shock (*CCM 42:333, 2014*).
Goals:		○ No clear source & MDR GNB are rare: **PIP-TZ** +		• Insulin Rx: Current target is glucose level of 140-180 mg/dL. Attempts at tight control (80-110 mg/dL) resulted in excessive
1. Effective antibiotics 2. Fluid resuscitation 3. Vasoactive drugs, if needed 4. Source control		**Vanco** ○ No clear source but high prevalence of MDR GNB: [**Polymyxin B** (preferred) or **Colistin** + (**MER** or **IMP**)]		hypoglycemia (*NEJM 363:2540, 2010*). • Impact of early effective antibiotic therapy (*CCM 38:1045 & 1211, 2010*). • Bacteremia due to carbapenemase-producing K. pneumoniae: lowest mortality with combination rx: carbapenem + Polymyxin B
Refs: *Chest 145:1407, 2014; NEJM 369:840, 2013; CCM 188:77, 2013*		• IV crystalloid: 20-40 mL/kg for hypotension or elevated lactate: use lactated Ringers (*AnIM 161:347 & 372, 2014*) • If hypotensive after fluids, non-epinephrine • Attempt to identify & correct source of bacteremia • Monitor central venous O₂ sat (target ≥ 70%) • Low tidal volume (6 mL/kg) mechanical ventilation (*NEJM 369:2126, 2013*) • Transfuse if hematocrit < 30% (*NEJM 371:1381, 2014*) See Comment for continuation		(preferred over Colistin) (*AAC 58:2322, 2014*). • Number of pts needed to treat with appropriate antimicrobial rx to prevent one pt death reported as 4 (*CCM 42:2342 & 2444, 2014*). • Shock associated with leaky capillaries which results in increased volume of drug distribution. Hence, need loading dose of antibiotics, and, early in treatment, larger maintenance dose (*AAC 59:2995, 2015*).
Septic shock: post-splenectomy or functional asplenia Asplenic pt care: *NEJM 371:349, 2014*	S. pneumoniae, N. meningitidis, H. influenzae, Capnocytophaga (DF-2)	No dog bite: **Ceftriaxone** 2 gm IV q24h (1 to 2 gm q12h if meningitis). ---- Post-dog bite: [**PIP-TZ** 3.375 gm IV q6h OR **MER** 1 gm IV q8h] + **Clinda** 900 mg IV q8h	No dog bite: [**Levo** 750 mg or **Moxi** 400 mg] once IV q24h	Howell-Jolly bodies in peripheral blood smear confirm absence of functional spleen. Often results in **symmetrical peripheral gangrene of digits** due to severe DIC. For prophylaxis, see Table 15A, page 199. Vaccines: *CID 58:309, 2014.*

Abbreviations on page 2.   *NOTE: All dosage recommendations are for adults (unless otherwise indicated) and assume normal/renal function. PK compliance, local resistance cost.

† Alternatives consider allergy.

TABLE 1 (62)

ANATOMIC SITE/DIAGNOSIS/ MODIFYING CIRCUMSTANCES	ETIOLOGIES (usual)	SUGGESTED REGIMENS*		ADJUNCT DIAGNOSTIC OR THERAPEUTIC MEASURES AND COMMENTS
		PRIMARY	ALTERNATIVE[1]	
SYSTEMIC SYNDROMES (FEBRILE/NON-FEBRILE)/Shock syndromes (continued)				
Toxic shock syndrome, Clostridium sordellii Clinical picture: shock, capillary leak, hemoconcentration, leukemoid reaction, afebrile. Ref: CID 43:1436 & 1447, 2006.	Clostridium sordellii–hemorrhagic & lethal toxins	Fluids, aq. **penicillin G** 18–20 million units per day div. q4–6h + **clindamycin** 900 mg IV q8h. **Surgical debridement is key.**		Occurs in variety of settings that produce anaerobic tissue, e.g., illicit drug use, post-partum. Several deaths reported after use of abortifacient regimen of mifepristone (RU486) & misoprostol. (NEJM 363:2540, 2010). 2001–2006 standard medical abortion: mifepristone orally instead of vaginal misoprostol. Since 2006, switch to buccal, instead of vaginal misoprostol. Doxy resulted in dramatic decrease in TSS (NEJM 361:145, 2009). Mortality nearly 100% if WBC >50,000/μL.
Toxic shock syndrome, staphylococcal. Review LnID 9:281, 1009 **Colonization** by toxin-producing Staph. aureus, e.g.: vagina (tampon-assoc.), surgical/traumatic wounds, endometrium, burns	Staph. aureus (toxic shock–mediated)	(**Nafcillin** or **oxacillin** 2 gm IV q8h) or (if MRSA, **vanco** 15-20 mg/kg q8-12h) + **Clinda** 600-900 mg IV q8h + **IVIG** (Dose in Comment)	(**Cefazolin** 1–2 gm IV q8h) or (if MRSA, **vanco** 15-20 mg/kg IV q8-12h OR **dapto** 6 mg/kg IV q24h) **Clinda** 600-900 mg IV q8h+ **IVIG** (Dose in Comment)	**IVIG reasonable** (see Streptococcal TSS) — dose 1 gm per kg on day 1, then 0.5 gm per kg day 2 & 3. — antitoxin antibodies present. If suspect TSS, "turn off" toxin production with clinda; report of success with **linezolid** (JID 195:202, 2007). Exposure of MRSA to nafcillin increased toxin production in vitro: JID 195:202, 2007.
Toxic shock syndrome, streptococcal. NOTE: For necrotizing fasciitis see page 56. Ref: LnID 9:281, 2009. **Associated with invasive disease,** i.e., erysipelas, necrotizing fasciitis; secondary strep infection of varicella. Secondary household contact cases reported (NEJM 335:547 & 590, 1996; CID 27:150, 1998)	Group A, B, C, & G Strep. pyogenes, Group B strep ref: EID 75:223, 2009.	(**Pen G** 24 million units per day IV in div. doses) + (**clinda** 900 mg IV q8h)	**Ceftriaxone** 2 gm IV q24h + **clinda** 900 mg q8h	**Definition:** Isolation of Group A strep, hypotension and ≥2 of: renal impairment, coagulopathy, liver involvement, ARDS, generalized rash, soft-tissue necrosis, i.e., necrotizing fasciitis, myositis, or gangrene. **Surgery usually required.** Mortality with fasciitis 30–50%, even with early rx (CID 14:2, 1992). Clinda ↓ toxin production. Use of NSAID may predispose to TSS. For reasons Pen G may fail in fulminant S. pyogenes infections (see JID 167:1401, 1993).
		For Necrotizing fasciitis without toxic shock, see page 56. Ref: LnID 9:281, 2009		
		Prospective observational study (CID 59:358, 366 & 851, 2014) indicates: • Clinda decreases mortality • IVIG perhaps on days 2, 3 • High incidence of secondary cases in household contacts		
Toxin-Mediated Syndromes—no fever unless complicated				
Botulism (CID 41:1167, 2005. As **biologic weapon:** JAMA 285:1059, 2001: www.bt.cdc.gov)	Clostridium botulinum	For all: Follow vital capacity, other supportive care. If no ileus, purge GI tract		**Equine antitoxin:** Heptavalent currently only antitoxin available (U.S) for non-infant botulism. CDC (+1 404-639-2206 M-F OR +1 404-639-2888 evenings/weekends). For infants, use Baby BIG (human botulism immune globulin): California Infant Botulism Treat & Prevent Program
Food-borne Dyspnea at presentation bad sign (CID 43:1247, 2006)		Hexavalent equine serum antitoxin—CDC (see Comment)		**Antimicrobials:** May make adult botulism worse. Untested in wound botulism. When used (1 to 20 million units per day as usual dose. If complications (pneumonia, UTI) occur, avoid antimicrobials with assoc. neuromuscular blockade, i.e., aminoglycosides, tetracycline, polymyxins, clindamycin.
Infant (Adult intestinal botulism is rare variant: EIN 18:1, 2012)		Human botulinum immunoglobulin (BIG) IV, single dose. Do not use equine antitoxin.	**No antibiotics:** may lyse C. botulinum in gut and ↑ load of toxin	
Wound		Debridement & anaerobic cultures. No proven value of local antitoxin untested	Trivalent equine antitoxin (see Comment)	**Differential dx:** Guillain-Barré, myasthenia gravis, tick paralysis, organo-phosphate toxicity, West Nile virus. Wound botulism can result from spore contamination of tar heroin. Ref: CID 31:1018, 2000. Mouse bioassay failed to detect toxin in 1/3 of patients (CID 48:1669, 2009).

Abbreviations on page 2.

*NOTE: All dosage recommendations are for adults (unless otherwise indicated) and assume normal renal function. § Alternatives consider allergy; PK, compliance, local resistance, cost

TABLE 1 (63)

ANATOMIC SITE/DIAGNOSIS/ MODIFYING CIRCUMSTANCES	ETIOLOGIES (usual)	SUGGESTED REGIMENS*		ADJUNCT DIAGNOSTIC OR THERAPEUTIC MEASURES AND COMMENTS
		PRIMARY	ALTERNATIVE†	
SYSTEMIC SYNDROMES/Toxin-Mediated Syndromes *(continued)*				
Tetanus: Trismus, generalized muscle rigidity, muscle spasm. Ref: *Ann IntMed* 154:329, 2011.	C. tetani–production of tetanospasmin toxin	**Six treatment steps:** 1—Urgent endotracheal intubation to protect the airway. Laryngeal spasm is common. Early tracheostomy. 2—Eliminate reflex spasms with diazepam, 20 mg/kg/day IV or midazolam. Reports of benefit combining diazepam with magnesium sulfate (*LD 368:1436, 2006*). Worst cases need neuromuscular blockade with vecuronium. 3—Neutralize toxin. Human hyperimmune globulin IM; start tetanus immunization—no immunity from clinical tetanus. 4—Surgically debride infected source tissue. Start antibiotic. (**Pen G** 3 million units IV q4h or **Doxy** 100 mg IV q12h) x7-10 days. 5—Avoid light as may precipitate muscle spasms. 6—Use beta blockers, e.g., short acting esmolol, to control sympathetic hyperactivity.		
VASCULAR				
IV line Infection *(See IDSA Guidelines CID 49:1, 2009.)* Heparin lock, plastic venous catheter, **non-tunneled** central venous catheter (subclavian, internal jugular); peripherally inserted central catheter (PICC). 2008 study found ↑ infection risk if femoral vein used, esp. if BMI >28.4 (*JAMA 299:2413, 2008*). **See Comment**	Staph. epidermidis, Staph. aureus (MSSA/MRSA). **Diagnosis:** Fever & either + blood cult from line & peripheral site **OR** >15 colonies on semi-quantitative culture of removed line **OR** culture from catheter positive 2 hrs earlier than peripheral vein culture.	**Vanco** 15-20 mg/kg q8-12h. **See Comment**	Other rx and duration: **(1)** If **S. aureus**, remove catheter. Can use TEE result to determine if 2 or 4 wks of therapy (*JAC 57:1172, 2006*). **(2)** If **S. epidermidis**, can try to "save" catheter. 80% cure after 7-10 days of therapy with systemic antibiotics; high rate of recurrence (*CID 49:1187, 2009*). If **leuconostoc** or **lactobacillus**, which are **Vanco** resistant, need **Pen G, Amp** or **Clinda.**	For documented MSSA **nafcillin** or **oxacillin** 2 gm IV q4h or **cefazolin** 2 gm IV q8h, if no response to, or intolerant of, **vanco** switch to **daptomycin** 6 mg per kg IV q24h. Culture removed catheter. With "roll" method, >15 colonies suggests infection. Cultures not require "routine" changing when not infected. When infected, do not insert new catheter over a wire. Antimicrobial-impregnated catheters may ↓ infection risk; the debate is likely (*CID 37:65, 2003 & 38:1287, 2004 & 39:1829, 2004*). Are femoral lines more prone to infection than subclavian or internal jugular lines? Meta-analysis: no difference (*CCM 40:2479, 2012*). In random trial, subclavian site had lowest risk of infection & thrombosis (*NEJM 373:1220, 2015*).
Tunnel type indwelling venous catheters and ports (Broviac, Hickman, Groshong, Quinton), dual lumen hemodialysis catheters (Permacath). For prevention, see below.	Staph. epidermidis, Staph. Aureus, (Candida sp.) Rarely leuconostoc or lacto-bacillus—both resistant to vanco (see Table 2, page 69) (Dx, see above).			If subcutaneous tunnel infected, very low cure rates; need to remove catheter. Beware of silent infection in clotted hemodialysis catheters. Indium scans detect (*Am J Kid Dis 40:832, 2002*).
Impaired host (burn, neutropenic)	As above + Pseudomonas sp., Enterobacteriaceae, Corynebacterium jeikeium, aspergillus, rhizopus	[**Vanco + (Cefepime** or **Ceftaz** or **(Vanco + PIP-TZ)** or **IMP + (Cefepime** or **Ceftaz** or **Aminoglycoside)**] *(Dosage in footnotes⁶,⁸, pages 46 and 63.)*		Usually have associated septic thrombophlebitis: biopsy of vein to rule out fungi. If fungal, surgical excision + amphotericin B. Surgical drainage, ligation or removal often indicated.
Hyperalimentation	With tunnel, Candida sp. common (*see Table 11,* resistant Candida species)	If candida, **voriconazole** or an **echinocandin (anidulafungin, micafungin, caspofungin)** if clinically stable. Dosage: see Table 11B, page 134.		Remove venous catheter and discontinue antimicrobial agents if possible. Ophthalmologic consultation recommended. **Rx all patients with + blood cultures.** See Table 11A, Candidiasis, page 122
Intravenous lipid emulsion	Staph. epidermidis Malassezia furfur	**Vanco** 1 gm IV q12h **Fluconazole** 400 mg IV q24h		Discontinue intralipid

NOTE: All dosage recommendations are for adults (unless otherwise indicated) and assume normal renal function. § *Alternatives consider allergy, PK compliance, local resistance, cost*

† *Alternatives consider allergy, PK compliance, local resistance, cost*

TABLE 1 (64)

ANATOMIC SITE/DIAGNOSIS/ MODIFYING CIRCUMSTANCES	ETIOLOGIES (usual)	SUGGESTED REGIMENS* PRIMARY	SUGGESTED REGIMENS* ALTERNATIVE[§]	ADJUNCT DIAGNOSTIC OR THERAPEUTIC MEASURES AND COMMENTS
VASCULAR/IV line infection *(continued)*				
Prevention of Infection of Long-Term IV Lines *CID 52:1087, 2011*	To minimize risk of infection: **Hand washing and** 1. Maximal sterile barrier precautions during catheter insertion 2. Use >0.5% chlorhexidine prep with alcohol for skin antisepsis 3. If infection rate high despite # 1 & 2, use either chlorhexidine/silver sulfadiazine or minocycline/rifampin-impregnated catheters or "lock" solutions (see *Comment*) 4. If possible, use subclavian vein, avoid femoral vessels. Lower infection risk in jugular vs femoral vein if BMI >28.4 *(JAMA 299:2413, 2008)*			**IV line "lock" solutions under study. No FDA-approved product.** Reports of the combination of TMP, EDTA & ethanol *(AAC 55:4430, 2011)*. Trials to begin in Europe. Another report: lock soln of sodium citrate, methylene blue, methylparabens *(CCM 39:613, 2011)*. Recent meeting abstracts support 70% ethanol.
Mycotic aneurysm	S. aureus (28–71%). S. epidermidis, Salmonella sp. (15–24%), M.Tbc, S. pneumonia, many others	**Vanco** (dose sufficient to achieve trough level of 15-20 µg/mL) + **(ceftriaxone** 2 gm IV q12h) or **PIP-TZ** or **CIP**. Treatment is combination of antibiotic + surgical resection with revascularization.	**Dapto** could be substituted for Vanco. For GNB: **cefepime** or **carbapenems** For MDR-GNB, **[Polymyxin B** (preferred) or **Colistin]** + **MER**	No data for ceftaroline or telavancin. Best diagnostic imaging: CT angiogram. Blood cultures positive in 50–85%. **De-escalate to specific therapy once culture results known.** Treatment duration varies but usually 6 wks from date of definitive surgery.
Suppurative (Septic) Thrombophlebitis				
Cranial dural sinus: **Cavernous Sinus**	S. aureus (70%) Streptococcus sp. Anaerobes Mucormycosis (diabetes)	**Vanco** (dose for trough conc of 15-20 mcg/mL) + **Ceftriaxone** 2 gm IV q12h, add **Metro** 500 mg IV q8h if dental/sinus source	**[Dapto** 8-12 mg/kg IV q24h OR **Linezolid** 600 mg IV q12h), add **Metro** 500 mg IV q8h if dental/sinus source	• Diagnosis: CT or MRI • Treatment: 1) obtain specimen for culture; 2) empiric antibiotics; 3) may need adjunctive surgery; 4) heparin until afebrile, then coumadin for several weeks
Lateral Sinus: Complication of otitis media/mastoiditis	Polymicrobial (often) Aerobes S. aureus P. aeruginosa B. fragilis Other GNB	**Cefepime** 2 gm IV q8h + **Metro** 500 mg IV q8h + **Vanco** (dose for trough conc of 15-20 mcg/mL)	**Meropenem** 1-2 gm IV q8h + **Linezolid** 600 mg IV q12h	• Diagnosis: CT or MRI • Treatment: 1) consider radical mastoidectomy; 2) obtain cultures; 3) antibiotics; 4) anticoagulation controversial • Prognosis: favorable
Superior Sagittal Sinus: Complication of bacterial meningitis or bacterial frontal sinusitis	S. pneumoniae N. meningitides H. influenzae (rare) S. aureus (very rare)	As for meningitis: **Ceftriaxone** 2 gm IV q12h + **Vanco** (dose for trough conc of 15-20 mcg/mL) + **dexamethasone**	As for meningitis: **Meropenem** 1-2 gm IV q8h + **Vanco** (dose for trough conc of 15-20 mcg/mL) + **dexamethasone**	• Diagnosis: MRI • Prognosis: bad; causes cortical vein thrombosis, hemorrhagic infarcts and brainstem herniation. • Anticoagulants not recommended

*NOTE: All dosage recommendations are for adults (unless otherwise indicated) and assume normal renal function. § Alternatives consider allergy, PK, compliance, local resistance, cost

TABLE 1 (65)

ANATOMIC SITE/DIAGNOSIS/ MODIFYING CIRCUMSTANCES	ETIOLOGIES (usual)	SUGGESTED REGIMENS*		ADJUNCT DIAGNOSTIC OR THERAPEUTIC MEASURES AND COMMENTS
		PRIMARY	ALTERNATIVE†	
VASCULAR/Suppurative (Septic) Thrombophlebitis *(continued)*				
Jugular Vein, Lemierre's Syndrome: Complication of pharyngitis, tonsillitis, dental infection, EBV. Ref: *NEJM* 371:2018, 2015.	Fusobacterium necrophorum (anaerobe) Less often: Other Fusobacterium S. pyogenes Bacteroides sp.	(**PIP-TZ** 3.375 gm IV q6h OR **Amp-Sulb** 3 gm IV q6h) x 4 weeks	[**Imipenem** 500 mg IV q6h OR (**Metro** 500 mg IV q8h + **Ceftriaxone** 2 gm IV once daily)] x 4 weeks. Another option: **Clinda** 600-900 mg IV q8h	• Diagnosis: Preceding pharyngitis and antibiotics therapy, persistent fever and pulmonary emboli • Imaging: Hi-res CT scan • Role of anticoagulants unclear
Pelvic Vein: Includes ovarian vein and deep pelvic vein phlebitis	Aerobic gram-neg bacilli Streptococcus sp. Anaerobes	Antibiotics + anticoagulation (heparin, then coumadin) *Low prevalence of MDR GNB:* **PIP-TZ** 3.375 gm IV q6h or 4.5 gm IV q8h OR (**Ceftriaxone** 2 gm IV once daily + **Metro** 500 mg IV q8h)	*High prevalence of MDR GNB:* **Meropenem** 1 gm IV q8h. If severe beta-lactam allergy: (**CIP** 400 mg IV q12h + **Metro** 500 mg IV q8h)	• Diagnosis: ovarian vein infection presents 1 week post-partum with fever & local pain; deep pelvic vein presents 3-5 days post-delivery with fever but no local pain. CT or MRI may help. • Treat until afebrile for 48 hrs & WBC normal • Coumadin for 6 weeks
Portal Vein (Pylephlebitis): Complication of diverticulitis, appendicitis and (rarely) other intra-abdominal infection	Aerobic gram-neg bacilli: E. coli, Klebsiella & Proteus most common Other: aerobic/anaerobic streptococci, B. fragilis, Clostridia	*Low prevalence of MDR GNB (<20%):* **PIP-TZ** 4.5 gm IV q8h OR (**CIP** 400 mg IV q12h + **Metro** 500 mg IV q8h)	*High prevalence of MDR GNB (≥20%):* If ESBL producer: **Meropenem** 1 gm IV q8h. If carbapenemase producer: [**Polymyxin B** (preferred) or **Colistin**] + **MER**	• Diagnosis: Pain, fever, neutrophilia in pt with intra-abdominal infection. • Abdominal CT scan • Pyogenic liver abscess is a complication • No anticoagulants unless hypercoaguable disease (neoplasm) • Surgery on vein not indicated

Abbreviations on page 2. *NOTE: All dosage recommendations are for adults (unless otherwise indicated) and assume normal renal function. § Alternatives consider allergy, PK, compliance, local resistance, cost.

TABLE 2 – RECOMMENDED ANTIMICROBIAL AGENTS AGAINST SELECTED BACTERIA

BACTERIAL SPECIES	ANTIMICROBIAL AGENT (See page 2 for abbreviations)		
	RECOMMENDED	ALTERNATIVE	ALSO EFFECTIVE[1] (COMMENTS)
Achromobacter xylosoxidans spp xylosoxidans (formerly Alcaligenes)	IMP, MER, DORI (no DORI for pneumonia)	TMP-SMX. Some strains susc. to ceftaz, PIP-TZ	Resistant to aminoglycosides, most cephalosporins & FQs.
Acinetobacter calcoaceticus— baumannii complex	If suscept: IMP or MER or DORI. For MDR strains: (Polymyxin B + Colistin) + (IMP or MER)	AM-SB used for activity of sulbactam (CID 51:79, 2010). Perhaps Minocycline IV	Resistant to aminoglycosides, FQs. Minocycline, effective against many strains (CID 51:79, 2010) (See Table 5A, pg 81)
Actinomyces israelii	AMP or Pen G	Doxy, ceftriaxone	Clindamycin, erythro
Aeromonas hydrophila & other sp.	CIP or Levo	TMP-SMX or (P Ceph 3, 4)	See AAC 56:1110, 2012.
Arcanobacterium (C.) haemolyticum	Erythro; azithro	Benzathine Pen G, Clinda	Sensitive to most drugs, resistant to TMP-SMX (AAC 38:142, 1994)
Bacillus anthracis (anthrax): inhalation	See Table 1, page 40		
Bacillus cereus, B. subtilis	Vancomycin, clinda	FQ, IMP	
Bacteroides sp., B. fragilis & others	Metronidazole or PIP-TZ	DORI, ERTA, IMP, MER, AM-CL	Increasing resistance to: clinda, cefoxitin, cefotetan, moxi. Ref: CID 59:698, 2014.
Bartonella henselae, quintana See Table 1, pages 30, 45, 51, 57	Varies with disease entity & immune status. Active: Azithro, clarithro, erythro, doxy in combination: RIF, gent, ceftriaxone. Not active: CIP, TMP-SMX, Pen, most cephalosporins, aztreonam		
Bordetella pertussis	Azithro or clarithro	TMP-SMX	See PIDJ 31:78, 2012.
Borrelia burgdorferi, B. afzelii, B. garinii (Lyme & relapsing fever)	See specific disease entity		
Brucella sp.	Drugs & duration vary with localization or non-localization. See specific disease entities. PLoS One 7:e32090, 2012.		
Burkholderia (Pseudomonas) cepacia	TMP-SMX or MER or CIP	Minocycline or chloramphenicol	Multiple mechanisms of resistance. Need C/S to guide therapy (Sem Resp Crit Care Med 36:99, 2015)
Burkholderia (Pseudomonas) pseudomallei Curr Opin Infect Dis 23:554, 2010; CID 41:1105, 2005	Initially, IV ceftaz or IMP or MER, then po (TMP-SMX + Doxy x 3 mos) ± Chloro (AAC 49:4010, 2005)		(Thai, 12–80% strains resist to TMP-SMX). FQ active in vitro. MER also effective (AAC 48: 1763, 2004)
Campylobacter jejuni	Azithro	Erythro or CIP	TMP-SMX, Pen & cephalosporins not active.
Campylobacter fetus	Gentamicin	IMP or ceftriaxone	AMP, chloramphenicol
Capnocytophaga ochracea (DF-1)	Dog bite: Clinda or AM-CL	Septic shock, post-splenectomy: PIP-TZ, Clinda, IMP, DORI, MER	FQ activity variable; aminoglycosides, TMP-SMX & Polymyxins have limited activity. LN ID 9:439, 2009.
Capnocytophaga canimorsus (DF-2)	Dog bite: AM-CL		
Chlamydophila pneumoniae	Doxy	Erythro, FQ	Azithro, clarithro
Chlamydia trachomatis	Doxy or azithro	Erythro	
Citrobacter diversus (koseri), C. freundii	Life threatening illness: IMP, MER, DORI	Non-life threatening illness: CIP or Gent	Emergence of resistance: AAC 52:995, 2007.
Clostridium difficile	Mild illness: Metronidazole	Moderate/severe illness: Vancomycin (po) or Fidaxomicin (CID 51:1306, 2010).	See also Table 1, page 18 re severity of disease.
Clostridium perfringens	Pen G ± clindamycin	Doxy	Erythro, chloramphenicol, cefazolin, cefoxitin, PIP-TZ, carbapenems
Clostridium tetani	Metronidazole	Doxy	Role of antibiotics unclear.
Corynebacterium diphtheriae	Erythro + antitoxin	Pen G + antitoxin	RIF reported effective (CID 27:845, 1998)
Corynebacterium jeikeium	Vancomycin + aminoglycoside	Pen G + aminoglycoside	Many strains resistant to Pen (EJCMID 25:349, 2006).
Corynebacterium minutissimum	Clinda 1% lotion	Clarithro or Erythro	Causes erythrasma
Coxiella burnetii (Q fever) acute disease (CID 52:1431, 2011).	Doxy, FQ (see Table 1, page 31)	Erythro, Azithro, Clarithro	Endocarditis: doxy + hydroxychloroquine (JID 188:1322, 2003; LnID 3:709, 2003; LnID 10:527, 2010).
chronic disease, e.g., endocarditis	Doxy + hydroxy chloroquine	TMP-SMX, Chloro	

TABLE 2 (2)

BACTERIAL SPECIES	ANTIMICROBIAL AGENT (See page 2 for abbreviations)		
	RECOMMENDED	ALTERNATIVE	ALSO EFFECTIVE[1] (COMMENTS)
Ehrlichia chaffeensis, Ehrlichia ewubguum Anaplasma (Ehrlichia) phagocytophillium	Doxy	RIF (CID 27:213, 1998), Levo (AAC 47:413, 2003).	CIP, ofloxa, chloramphenicol also active in vitro. Resist to clinda, TMP-SMX, IMP, AMP, erytho, & azithro (AAC 41:76, 1997).
Eikenella corrodens	AM-CL, IV Pen G	TMP-SMX, FQ	Resistant to clinda, cephalexin, erytho, metro, diclox
Elizabethkingae meningosepticum (formerly Chryseobacterium)	Levo or TMP-SMX	CIP, Minocycline	Resistant to Pen, cephalosporins, carbapenems, aminoglycosides, vancomycin (JCM 44:1181, 2006)
Enterobacter species	Recommended agents vary with clinical setting and degree & mechanism of resistance.		
Enterococcus faecalis	Highly resistant. See Table 5A, page 81		
Enterococcus faecium	Highly resistant. See Table 5A, page 81		
Erysipelothrix rhusiopathiae	Penicillin G or amox	P Ceph 3, FQ	IMP, PIP-TZ (vancomycin, APAG, TMP-SMX resistant)
Escherichia coli	Highly resistant. Treatment varies with degree & mechanism of resistance, see TABLE 5B.		
Francisella tularensis (tularemia) See Table 1, page 42	Gentamicin, tobramycin, or streptomycin	Mild infection: Doxy or CIP	Chloramphenicol, RIF. Doxy/chloro bacteriostatic → relapses CID 53:e133, 2011.
Gardnerella vaginalis (bacterial vaginosis)	Metronidazole or Tinidazole	Clindamycin	See Table 1, page 26 for dosage
Helicobacter pylori	See Table 1, pg 21		Drugs effective in vitro often fail in vivo.
Haemophilus aphrophilus (Aggregatibacter aphrophilus)	[(Penicillin or AMP) + gentamicin] or [AM- SB ± gentamicin]	(Ceftriaxone + Gent) or CIP or Levo	Resistant to vancomycin, clindamycin, methicillin
Haemophilus ducreyi (chancroid)	Azithro or ceftriaxone	Erytho, CIP	Most strains resistant to tetracycline, amox, TMP-SMX
Haemophilus influenzae Meningitis, epiglottitis & other life-threatening illness	Cefotaxime, ceftriaxone	AMP if susceptible and ß-lactamase neg, FQs	Chloramphenicol (downgrade from 1st choice due to hematotoxicity).
non-life threatening illness	AM-CL, O Ceph 2/3		Azithro, clarithro, telithro
Klebsiella ozaenae/ rhinoscleromatis	CIP	Levo	Acta Otolaryngol 131:440, 2010.
Klebsiella species	Treatment varies with degree & mechanism of resistance, see Table 5B.		
Lactobacillus species	Pen G or AMP	Clindamycin	**May be resistant to vancomycin**
Legionella sp.	Levo or Moxi	Azithro	Telithro active in vitro.
Leptospira interrogans	Mild: Doxy or amox	Severe: Pen G or ceftriaxone	
Leuconostoc	Pen G or AMP	Clinda	**NOTE: Resistant to vancomycin**
Listeria monocytogenes	AMP + Gent for synergy	TMP-SMX	Erythro, penicillin G (high dose), APAG may be synergistic with ß-lactams. Meropenem active in vitro. **Cephalosporin-resistant!**
Moraxella (Branhamella) catarrhalis	AM-CL or O Ceph 2/3, TMP-SMX	Azithro, clarithro, dirithromycin, telithro	Erythro, doxy, FQs
Mycoplasma pneumoniae	Doxy	Azithro, Minocycline	Clindamycin & ß lactams NOT effective. Increasing macrolide resistance (JAC 68:506, 2013; JAC 58:1034, 2014).
Neisseria gonorrhoeae (gonococcus)	Ceftriaxone,	Azithro (high dose)	FQs and oral cephalosporins no longer recommended: high levels of resistance.
Neisseria meningitidis (meningococcus)	Ceftriaxone	Chloro, MER	(Chloro less effective than other alternatives: see JAC 70:979, 2015)
Nocardia asteroides or **Nocardia brasiliensis**	TMP-SMX + IMP	Linezolid	Amikacin + (IMP or ceftriaxone or cefotaxime) (AAC 58:795, 2014).
Pasteurella multocida	Pen G, AMP, amox, cefuroxime, cefpodoxime	Doxy, Levo, Moxi, TMP-SMX	Resistant to cephalexin, oxacillin, clindamycin, erythro, vanco.
Plesiomonas shigelloides	CIP	TMP-SMX	AM-CL, Ceftriaxone & Chloro active. Resistant to: Amp, Tetra, aminoglycosides
Propionibacterium acnes (not acne)	Penicillin, Ceftriaxone	Vanco, Dapto, Linezolid	May be resistant to Metro.
Proteus sp, **Providencia sp**, Morganella sp. (Need in vitro susceptibility)	CIP, PIP-TZ; avoid cephalosporins	May need carbapenem if critically ill	Note: Proteus sp. & Providencia sp. have intrinsic resistance to Polymyxins.
Pseudomonas aeruginosa (ID Clin No Amer 23:277, 2009). Combination therapy? See Clin Micro Rev 25: 450, 2012.	No in vitro resistance: PIP-TZ, AP Ceph 3, DORI, IMP, MER, tobramycin, CIP, aztreonam. For serious inf., use AP ß-lactam + (tobramycin or CIP)	For UTI, if no in vitro resistance, single drugs effective: PIP-TZ, AP Ceph 3, cefepime, IMP, MER, aminoglycoside, CIP, aztreonam	If resistant to all beta lactams, FQs, aminoglycosides: Colistin + MER or IMP. Do not use DORI for pneumonia.

TABLE 2 (3)

BACTERIAL SPECIES	ANTIMICROBIAL AGENT (See page 2 for abbreviations)		
	RECOMMENDED	ALTERNATIVE	ALSO EFFECTIVE[1] (COMMENTS)
Rhodococcus (C. equi)	Two drugs: Azithro, Levo or RIF	(Vanco or IMP) + (Azithro, Levo or RIF)	Vancomycin active in vitro; intracellular location may impair efficacy (CID 34:1379, 2002). Avoid Pen, cephalosporins, clinda, tetra, TMP-SMX.
Rickettsia species (includes spotted fevers)	Doxy	Chloramphenicol (in pregnancy), azithro (age < 8 yrs)	See specific infections (Table 1).
Salmonella typhi (CID 50:241, 2010; AAC 54:5201, 2010; BMC ID 51:37, 2005)	If FQ & nalidixic acid susceptible: CIP	Ceftriaxone, cefixime, azithro, chloro	Concomitant steroids in severely ill. Watch for relapse (1-6%) & ileal perforation. FQ resistance reported with treatment failures (AAC 52:1278, 2008). Chloro less effective than other alternatives: see JAC 70:979, 2015).
Serratia marcescens	If no in vitro resistance: PIP-TZ, CIP, LEVO, Gent	If in vitro resistance: Carbapenem	Avoid extended spectrum Ceph if possible Table 5A.
Shigella sp.	FQ or azithro	Ceftriaxone is alternative; TMP-SMX depends on susceptibility.	
Staph. aureus, methicillin-susceptible	Oxacillin/nafcillin	P Ceph 1, vanco, teicoplanin[NUS] clinda ceftriaxone	ERTA, IMP, MER, BL/BLI, FQ, PIP-TZ, linezolid, dapto, televancin.
Staph. aureus, methicillin-resistant (health-care associated) IDSA Guidelines: CID 52 (Feb 1):1, 2011.	Vancomycin	Teicoplanin[NUS], TMP-SMX (some strains resistant), linezolid, daptomycin, telavancin, ceftaroline	Fusidic acid[NUS] >60% CIP-resistant in U.S. (Fosfomycin + RIF). Partially vancomycin-resistant strains (GISA, VISA) & highly resistant strains now described—see Table 6, pg 82.
Staph. aureus, methicillin-resistant [community- associated (CA-MRSA)]			CA-MRSA usually not multiply-resistant. Oft resist. to erythro & variably to FQ. Vanco, teico[NUS], telavancin, daptomycin, ceftaroline can be used in pts requiring hospitalization (see Table 6, pg 82). Also, ceftaroline.
Mild-moderate infection	(TMP-SMX or doxy or mino)	Clinda (if D-test neg— see Table 5A & 6).	
Severe infection	Vanco or teico[NUS]	Linezolid or daptomycin	
Staph. epidermidis	Vancomycin ± RIF	RIF + (TMP-SMX or FQ), daptomycin (AAC 51:3420, 2007)	Cephalothin or nafcillin/oxacillin if sensitive to nafcillin/oxacillin but 75% are resistant. FQs. (See Table 5A).
Staph. haemolyticus	TMP-SMX, FQ, nitrofurantoin	Oral cephalosporin	Recommendations apply to UTI only.
Staph. lugdunensis	Oxacillin/nafcillin or penicillin G (if β-lactamase neg.)	P Ceph 1 or vancomycin or teico[NUS]	Approx. 75% are penicillin-susceptible.
Staph. saprophyticus (UTI)	Oral cephalosporin or AM-CL	FQ	Almost always methicillin-susceptible.
Stenotrophomonas (Xanthomonas, Pseudomonas) maltophilia	TMP-SMX	FQ (AAC 58:176, 2014) if suscept in vitro	JAC 62:889, 2008
Streptobacillus moniliformis	Penicillin G	Doxy	Maybe erythro, clinda, ceftriaxone
Streptococcus, anaerobic (Peptostreptococcus)	Penicillin G	Clindamycin	Doxy, vancomycin, linezolid, ERTA (AAC 51:2205, 2007).
Streptococcus anginosus group	Penicillin	Vanco or Ceftriaxone	Avoid FQs; macrolide resistance emerging
Streptococcus pneumoniae penicillin-susceptible	Penicillin G, Amox	Multiple agents effective, e.g., Ceph 2/3, Clinda	If meningitis, higher dose, see Table 1, page 9.
penicillin-resistant (MIC ≥2.0)	Vancomycin, Levo, ceftriaxone, Amox (HD), Linezolid		
Streptococcus pyogenes, (Grp A), **Streptococcus sp** (Grp B, C, G). Erysipelas, bacteremia, TSS	Penicillin G + Clinda	Pen (alone) or Clinda (alone- low incidence of resistance)	JCM 49:439, 2011. Pockets of macrolide resistance. Do not use: FQs, TMP-SMX or tetracyclines
Tropheryma whipplei	Doxy + Hydroxychloroquine	None	Clinical failures with TMP-SMX
Vibrio cholerae	Doxy, FQ	Azithro, erythro	Maybe CIP or Levo; some resistance.
Vibrio parahaemolyticus	Doxy	Azithro, CIP	If bacteremic, treat as for V. vulnificus
Vibrio vulnificus, damsela alginolyticus,	Doxy + ceftriaxone	Levo	CID 52:788, 2011
Yersinia enterocolitica	CIP or ceftriaxone	TMP-SMX; CIP (if bacteremic)	CIP resistance (JAC 53:1068, 2004), also resistant to Pen, AMP, erythro.
Yersinia pestis (plague)	Streptomycin or Gent	Doxy or CIP	Levo, Moxi

[1] Agents are more variable in effectiveness than "Recommended" or "Alternative". Selection of "Alternative" or "Also Effective" based on in vitro susceptibility testing, pharmacokinetics, host factors such as auditory, renal, hepatic function, & cost.

TABLE 3 – SUGGESTED DURATION OF ANTIBIOTIC THERAPY IN IMMUNOCOMPETENT PATIENTS[1,2]

	CLINICAL SITUATION	DURATION OF THERAPY
SITE	**CLINICAL DIAGNOSIS**	**(Days)**
Bacteremia	Bacteremia with removable focus (no endocarditis)	10–14 (See Table 1)
Bone	Osteomyelitis; adult; acute	42 (Ln 385:875, 2015)
	adult; chronic	Until ESR normal (often > 3 months)
	child; acute; staph. and enterobacteriaceae[3]	21
	child; acute; strep, meningococci, haemophilus[3]	14
Ear	Otitis media with effusion	<2 yrs: 10; ≥2 yrs: 5–7
Endo-cardium	Infective endocarditis, native valve	
	Viridans strep	14 or 28 (See Table 1, page 28)
	Enterococci	28 or 42 (See Table 1, page 29)
	Staph. aureus	14 (R-sided only) or 28 (See Table 1, page 29)
GI *Also see Table 1*	Bacillary dysentery (shigellosis)/traveler's diarrhea	3
	Typhoid fever (S. typhi): Azithro	7 (children/adolescents)
	Ceftriaxone	7–14 [Short course † effective (AAC 44:450, 2000)]
	FQ	5–7
	Chloramphenicol	14
	Helicobacter pylori	10–14. For triple-drug regimens, 7 days.
	Pseudomembranous enterocolitis (C. difficile)	10
Genital	Non-gonococcal urethritis or mucopurulent cervicitis	7 days doxy or single dose azithro
	Pelvic inflammatory disease	14
Heart	Pericarditis (purulent)	28
Joint	Septic arthritis (non-gonococcal) Adult	14–28
	Infant/child	Rx as osteomyelitis above.
		10-14 days of therapy sufficient (CID 48:1201, 2009), but not complete agreement on this (CID 48:1211, 2009).
	Gonococcal arthritis/disseminated GC infection	7 (See Table 1, page 23)
Kidney	Cystitis (bladder bacteriuria)	3 (Single dose extended-release cipro also effective) (AAC 49:4137, 2005)
	Pyelonephritis (Ln 380:484, 2012)	7 (7 days if CIP used; 5 days if levo 750 mg)
Lung *(Curr Op ID 28:177, 2015)*	Pneumonia, pneumococcal	Until afebrile 3–5 days (minimum 5 days)
	Community-acquired pneumonia	Minimum 5 days and afebrile for 2-3 days (Peds ref: PIDJ 33:136, 2014).
	Pneumonia, enterobacteriaceae or pseudomonal	21, often up to 42
	Pneumonia, staphylococcal	21–28
	Pneumocystis pneumonia (PCP) in AIDS;	21
	other immunocompromised	14
	Legionella, mycoplasma, chlamydia	7–14
	Lung abscess	Usually 28–42[4]
Meninges[5]	N. meningitidis	7
	H. influenzae	7
	S. pneumoniae	10–14
	Listeria meningoencephalitis, gp B strep, coliforms	21 (longer in immunocompromised)
Multiple systems	Brucellosis (See Table 1, page 61)	42 (add SM or gent for 1ˢᵗ 7–14 days) (PLoS One 7:e32090, 2012)
	Tularemia (See Table 1, pages 44, 60)	7–14 (MMWR 58:744, 2009)
Muscle	Gas gangrene (clostridial)	10
Pharynx	Group A strep pharyngitis	10 O Ceph 2/3, azithromycin effective at 5 days
	Also see Pharyngitis, Table 1, page 48	(CID 55:1279, 2012)
	Diphtheria (membranous)	7–14
	Carrier	7
Prostate	Chronic prostatitis (TMP-SMX)	30–90
	(FQ)	28–42
Sinuses	Acute sinusitis	5–14[6]
Skin	Cellulitis	Until 3 days after acute inflamm disappears
Systemic	Lyme disease	See Table 1, page 58
	Rocky Mountain spotted fever (See Table 1, page 60)	Until afebrile 2 days

---

[1] Early change from IV to po regimens (about 72 hrs) is cost-effective with many infections, i.e., intra-abdominal. There is emerging evidence that dc of antibiotic rx concomitant with normalization of serum procalcitonin level shortens treatment duration for pneumonia and peritonitis (JAMA 309:717, 2013).

[2] The recommended duration is a minimum or average time and should not be construed as absolute.

[3] These times are with proviso: sx & signs resolve within 7 days and ESR is normalized.

[4] After patient afebrile 4-5 days, change to oral therapy.

[5] In children relapses seldom occur until 3 days or more after termination of rx. For meningitis in children, see Table 1, page 8.

[6] Duration of therapy dependent upon agent used and severity of infection. Longer duration (10-14 days) optimal for beta-lactams and patients with severe disease. For sinusitis of mild-moderate severity shorter courses of therapy (5-7 days) effective with "respiratory FQs" (including gemifloxacin, levofloxacin 750 mg), azithromycin. Courses as short as 3 days reported effective for TMP-SMX and azithro and one study reports effectiveness of single dose extended-release azithro. Authors feel such "super-short" courses should be restricted to patients with mild-mod disease (Otolaryngol-Head Neck Surg 134:10, 2006).

TABLE 4A – ANTIBACTERIAL ACTIVITY SPECTRA

The data provided are intended to serve as a general guide to antibacterial usefulness based on treatment guidelines and recommendations, in vitro activity, predominant patterns of susceptibility or resistance and/or demonstrated clinical effectiveness. Variability in resistance patterns due to regional differences or as a consequence of clinical setting (e.g., community-onset vs. ICU-acquired infection) should be taken into account when using this table because activities of certain agents can differ significantly from what is shown in the table, which are by necessity based on aggregate information. We have revised and expanded the color / symbol key to provide a more descriptive categorization of the table data.

++ = Recommended: Agent is a first line therapy; reliably active in vitro, clinically effective, guideline recommended, recommended as a first-line agent or acceptable alternative agent in the Sanford Guide

+ = Active: Agent is a potential alternative agent (active in vitro, possesses class activity comparable to known effective agents or a therapeutically interchangeable agents and hence likely to be clinically effective, but second line due to overly broad spectrum, toxicity, limited clinical experience, or paucity of direct evidence of effectiveness)

± = Variable: Variable activity such that the agent, although clinically effective in some settings or types of infections is not reliably effective in others, or should be used in combination with another agent, and/or its efficacy is limited by resistance which has been associated with treatment failure

0 = Not recommended: Agent is a poor alternative to other agents because resistance is likely to be present or occur, due to poor drug penetration to site of infection or an unfavorable toxicity profile, or limited or anecdotal clinical data to support effectiveness

? = Insufficient Data to recommend use

NA = No activity: Agent has no activity against this pathogen

	Penicillin G	Penicillin VK	Nafcillin	Oxacillin	Cloxacillin	Flucloxacillin	Dicloxacillin	Ampicillin	Amoxicillin	Amox-Clav	Amp-Sulb	Pip-Tazo	Doripenem	Ertapenem	Imipenem	Meropenem	Aztreonam	Ciprofloxacin	Ofloxacin	Levofloxacin	Moxifloxacin	Gemifloxacin	Gatifloxacin	Cefazolin	Cefotetan	Cefoxitin	Cefuroxime	Cefotaxime	Ceftizoxime	Ceftriaxone	Ceftazidime	Cefepime	Ceftaz-Avibac	Ceftaroline	Ceftol-Tazo
Aerobic gram-pos cocci																																			
E. faecalis	++	++	0	0	0	0	0	++	++	+	+	+	±	±	+	±	0	±	±	+	+	±	+	0	0	0	0	0	0	±	0	0	0	+	0
E. faecium	±	±	0	0	0	0	0	±	±	±	±	0	0	0	0	0	0	0	0	0	0	0	0	0	0	0	0	0	0	0	0	0	0	?	0
VRE faecalis	±	±	0	0	0	0	0	±	±	0	0	0	0	0	0	0	0	0	0	0	0	0	0	0	0	0	0	0	0	0	0	0	0	0	0
VRE faecium	±	±	0	0	0	0	0	±	±	0	0	0	0	0	0	0	0	0	0	0	0	0	0	0	0	0	0	0	0	0	0	0	0	0	0
S. aureus MSSA	±	±	++	++	++	++	++	±	±	++	++	+	+	+	+	+	0	±	±	+	±	+	+	++	+	+	++	+	+	+	±	+	+	++	+
S. aureus HA-MRSA	0	0	0	0	0	0	0	0	0	0	0	0	0	0	0	0	0	0	0	±	±	±	±	0	0	0	0	0	0	0	0	0	0	++	0
S. aureus CA-MRSA	0	0	0	0	0	0	0	0	0	0	0	0	0	0	0	0	0	±	±	±	±	±	±	0	0	0	0	0	0	0	0	0	0	++	0
Staph coag-neg (S)	±	±	++	++	++	++	++	±	±	++	++	+	+	+	+	+	0	±	±	+	+	+	+	++	+	+	+	+	+	+	±	+	+	+	+
Staph coag-neg (R)	0	0	0	0	0	0	0	0	0	0	0	0	0	0	0	0	0	±	±	±	±	±	±	0	0	0	0	0	0	0	0	0	0	+	0
S. lugdunensis	±	±	++	++	++	++	++	±	±	++	++	+	+	+	+	+	0	±	±	+	+	+	+	++	+	+	+	+	+	+	±	+	+	+	+
S. saprophyticus	±	±	+	+	+	+	+	+	+	++	++	+	+	+	+	+	0	+	+	+	+	+	+	+	+	+	+	+	+	+	±	+	+	+	+
Strep. anginosus gp	++	++	+	+	+	+	+	++	++	++	++	++	+	+	+	+	0	±	±	+	+	+	+	+	±	±	+	+	+	+	±	+	+	+	+
Strep. gp. A,B,C,F,G	++	++	+	+	+	+	+	++	++	++	++	++	+	+	+	+	0	±	±	+	+	+	+	+	+	+	+	+	+	+	±	+	+	+	+
Strep. pneumoniae	±	±	0	0	0	0	0	±	±	+	+	+	+	+	+	+	0	±	±	+	+	+	+	±	±	±	±	+	+	+	±	+	+	++	+
Viridans Strep.	+	+	0	0	0	0	0	+	+	+	+	+	+	+	+	+	0	±	±	+	+	+	+	±	±	±	±	+	+	+	±	+	+	+	+
Aerobic gram-pos bacilli																																			
Arcanobacter sp	+	+	?	?	?	?	?	+	+	+	+	?	?	?	?	?	0	?	?	+	?	?	?	?	?	?	?	?	?	?	0	?	?	?	0
C. diphtheriae	++	++	0	0	0	0	0	+	+	+	+	+	?	?	+	+	0	+	+	+	+	?	+	?	?	?	?	+	?	+	0	?	?	?	0
C. jeikeium	0	0	0	0	0	0	0	0	0	0	0	0	?	?	?	?	0	0	0	±	±	?	±	0	0	0	0	0	0	0	0	0	0	0	0
L. monocytogenes	+	+	0	0	0	0	0	++	++	+	+	+	+	?	+	+	0	0	0	±	+	?	±	0	0	0	0	0	0	0	0	0	0	0	0
Nocardia sp.	0	0	0	0	0	0	0	0	0	0	0	0	?	?	+	?	0	±	±	+	+	?	+	0	0	0	0	±	?	±	0	0	0	0	0

TABLE 4A (2)

Aerobic gram-neg bacilli - Enterobacteriaceae

Drug	Aeromonas sp.	C. jejuni	Citrobacter sp.	Enterobacter sp.	E. coli	E. coli, Klebs ESBL	E. coli, Klebs KPC	Klebsiella sp.	Morganella sp.	P. mirabilis	P. vulgaris	Providencia sp.	Salmonella sp.	Serratia sp.	Shigella sp.	Y. enterocolitica
Penicillins																
Penicillin G	o	o	o	o	o	o	o	o	o	o	o	o	o	o	o	o
Penicillin VK	o	o	o	o	o	o	o	o	o	o	o	o	o	o	o	o
Nafcillin	o	o	o	o	o	o	o	o	o	o	o	o	o	o	o	o
Oxacillin	o	o	o	o	o	o	o	o	o	o	o	o	o	o	o	o
Cloxacillin	o	o	o	o	o	o	o	o	o	o	o	o	o	o	o	o
Flucloxacillin	o	o	o	o	o	o	o	o	o	o	o	o	o	o	o	o
Dicloxacillin	o	o	o	o	o	o	o	o	o	o	o	o	o	o	o	o
Ampicillin	o	o	o	o	+l	o	o	o	o	+	o	o	o	o	+l	o
Amoxicillin	o	o	o	o	+l	o	o	o	o	+l	o	o	o	o	o	o
Amox-Clav	+l	o	o	o	+	o	o	+	o	+	o	+	o	o	+	+l
Amp-Sulb	+l	o	o	o	+	o	o	+	o	+	o	+	o	o	+	+l
Pip-Tazo	+	o	+l	+l	+	o	o	+	+	+	+	+	+	+	+	+
Carbapenems																
Doripenem	+	+	+	+	+	+	o	+	+	+	+	+	+	+	+	+
Ertapenem	+	+	+	+	+	+	o	+	+	+	+	+	+	+	+	~
Imipenem	+	+	+	+	+	+	o	+	+l	+	+	+	+	+	+	+
Meropenem	+	+	+	+	+	+	o	+	+	+	+	+	+	+	+	+
Aztreonam	+	~	+l	+l	+	o	o	+	+	+	+	+	+	+	+	+
Fluoroquinolone																
Ciprofloxacin	+	+	+	+	+	+l	o	+	+	+	+	+	+	+	+	+l
Ofloxacin	+	+	+	+	+	+l	o	+	+	+	+	+	+	+	+	+l
Levofloxacin	+	+	+	+	+	+l	o	+	+	+	+	+	+	+	+	+l
Moxifloxacin	+	+	+	+	+	+l	o	~	+	+	~	+	+	+	+	~
Gemifloxacin	+	+	+	+	+	+l	o	~	+	+	~	+	+	+	+	~
Gatifloxacin	+	+	+	+	+	+l	o	~	+	+	~	+	+	+	+	~
Parenteral Cephalosporins																
Cefazolin	o	o	o	o	+	o	o	+	o	+	o	o	o	o	o	+l
Cefotetan	o	o	o	o	+	+l	o	+	+	+	+	~	o	+	~	+l
Cefoxitin	o	o	o	o	+	+l	o	+	+	+	+	~	o	+	~	+l
Cefuroxime	~	o	o	o	+	o	o	+	o	+	+	o	~	o	~	~
Cefotaxime	+	o	+	+l	+	o	o	+	+	+	+	+	+	+	+	+l
Ceftizoxime	+	o	+	+l	+	o	o	+	+	+	+	+	o	+	+	+l
Ceftriaxone	+	o	+	+l	+	o	o	+	+	+	+	+	+	+	+	+l
Ceftazidime	+	o	+	+l	+	o	o	+	+	+	+	+	+	+	+	+l
Cefepime	+	o	+	+	+	o	o	+	+	+	+	+	~	+	+	+
Ceftaz-Avibac	+	o	+	+	+	+	+	+	+	+	+	+	o	+	o	+
Ceftaroline	~	~	+	o	+	o	o	+	~	~	~	~	~	~	+	~
Ceftol-Tazo	~	~	+	+	+	+	o	+	+	+	~	+	+	+	~	~

Aerobic gram-neg bacilli - Miscellaneous

Drug	Bartonella sp.	B. pertussis	B. burgdorferi	Brucella sp.	Capnocytophagia	C. burnetii	Ehrlichia, Anaplas	Eikenella sp	F. tularensis	H. ducreyi	H. influenzae	Kingella sp.	K. granulomatis	Legionella sp.	Leptospira sp.	M. catarrhalis	N. gonorrhoeae
Penicillins																	
Penicillin G	o	o	+	o	+l	o	o	+	o	o	o	+	o	o	+l	o	o
Penicillin VK	o	o	+l	o	+l	o	o	+	o	o	o	+l	o	o	o	o	o
Nafcillin	o	o	o	o	o	o	o	o	o	o	o	o	o	o	o	o	o
Oxacillin	o	o	o	o	o	o	o	o	o	o	o	o	o	o	o	o	o
Cloxacillin	o	o	o	o	o	o	o	o	o	o	o	o	o	o	o	o	o
Flucloxacillin	o	o	o	o	o	o	o	o	o	o	o	o	o	o	o	o	o
Dicloxacillin	o	o	o	o	o	o	o	o	o	o	o	o	o	o	o	o	o
Ampicillin	o	o	+l	o	+	o	o	+l	o	o	+l	+l	o	o	+l	o	o
Amoxicillin	o	o	+	o	+	o	o	+l	o	o	+l	+l	o	o	o	o	o
Amox-Clav	o	o	+	o	+	o	o	+	o	+	+	+	o	o	+l	+	o
Amp-Sulb	o	o	+	o	+	o	o	+	o	+	+	+	o	o	o	+	+l
Pip-Tazo	o	o	o	o	+	o	o	+	o	+l	+	+	o	o	o	+	o
Carbapenems																	
Doripenem	o	o	o	o	+	o	o	+	o	+	+	+	o	o	o	+	+
Ertapenem	o	o	o	o	+	o	o	+	o	+	+	+	o	o	o	+	+
Imipenem	o	o	o	+l	+	o	o	+	+l	+	+	+	o	~	o	+	+
Meropenem	o	o	o	o	+	o	o	+	+l	+	+	+	o	+	o	+	+
Aztreonam	o	o	o	o	o	o	o	~	o	~	+	~	o	o	o	+	+
Fluoroquinolone																	
Ciprofloxacin	o	~	o	+	~	+	+l	+	+	+	+	+	~	+	+	+	+l
Ofloxacin	o	~	o	+	~	+	+l	+	+	+	+	+	~	+	+	+	+l
Levofloxacin	o	+	o	+	+	+	+l	+	+	+	+	+	+	+	+	+	+l
Moxifloxacin	~	+	o	+	+	+	+l	+	+	+	+	+	+	+	+	+	+
Gemifloxacin	~	+	o	+	~	+	+l	+	+	+	+	+	+	+	+	+	+
Gatifloxacin	~	+	o	+	~	+	+l	+	~	+	+	+	~	+	+	+	+
Parenteral Cephalosporins																	
Cefazolin	o	o	o	o	+l	o	o	o	o	o	o	~	o	o	o	+	+l
Cefotetan	o	o	o	o	o	o	o	~	o	+	+	~	o	o	o	+	+l
Cefoxitin	o	o	o	o	o	o	o	~	o	+	+	~	o	o	o	+	+l
Cefuroxime	o	o	+	o	+	o	o	+	o	+l	+	~	o	o	o	+	o
Cefotaxime	o	o	+	o	+	o	o	+	o	+	+	+	o	o	+l	+	+
Ceftizoxime	o	o	+	o	+	o	o	+	o	+	+	+	o	o	+l	+	+
Ceftriaxone	o	o	+	o	+	o	o	+	o	+	+	+	o	o	+l	+	+
Ceftazidime	o	o	+	o	+	o	o	+	o	+	+	+	o	+l	o	+	+
Cefepime	o	o	+	o	+	o	o	+	o	+	+	+	o	o	o	+	+
Ceftaz-Avibac	o	o	+	o	o	o	o	+	o	o	+	+	o	o	o	+	+l
Ceftaroline	o	o	o	o	o	o	o	+	o	o	+	+	o	o	o	+	~
Ceftol-Tazo	o	o	o	o	o	o	o	+	o	o	+	~	o	o	o	+	~

TABLE 4A (3)

	Penicillins												Carbapenems					Fluoroquinolones						Parenteral Cephalosporins											
	Penicillin G	Penicillin VK	Nafcillin	Oxacillin	Cloxacillin	Flucloxacillin	Dicloxacillin	Ampicillin	Amoxicillin	Amox-Clav	Amp-Sulb	Pip-Tazo	Doripenem	Ertapenem	Imipenem	Meropenem	Aztreonam	Ciprofloxacin	Ofloxacin	Levofloxacin	Moxifloxacin	Gemifloxacin	Gatifloxacin	Cefazolin	Cefotetan	Cefoxitin	Cefuroxime	Cefotaxime	Ceftizoxime	Ceftriaxone	Ceftazidime	Cefepime	Ceftaz-Avibac	Ceftaroline	Ceftol-Tazo
Aerobic gram-neg bacilli - Miscellaneous *(continued)*																																			
N meningitidis	+	+	0	0	0	0	0	+	+	0	0	+	+	+	+	+	0	?	?	+	+	+	+	0	0	0	+	+	+	++	+	+	+	?	?
P. multocida	++	+	0	0	0	0	0	++	++	+	+	+	+	+	+	+	0	+	+	+	+	+	+	0	0	0	?	+	+	+	?	+	?	?	?
R. rickettsii	0	0	0	0	0	0	0	0	0	0	0	0	0	0	0	0	0	+	+	+	+	?	?	0	0	0	0	0	0	0	0	0	0	0	0
T. pallidum	++	+	0	0	0	0	0	0	0	0	0	0	0	0	0	0	0	0	0	0	0	0	0	0	0	0	0	+	+	++	0	0	0	0	0
U. urealyticum	0	0	0	0	0	0	0	0	0	0	0	0	0	0	0	0	0	±	±	±	+	?	?	0	0	0	0	0	0	0	0	0	0	0	0
V. cholerae	0	0	0	0	0	0	0	0	0	0	0	0	?	?	?	?	?	+	+	+	?	?	?	0	0	0	0	+	+	+	?	+	?	?	?
V. parahaemolyticus	0	0	0	0	0	0	0	0	0	0	0	+	?	?	?	?	?	+	+	+	+	?	?	0	0	0	?	+	+	+	?	+	?	?	?
V. vulnificus	0	0	0	0	0	0	0	0	0	0	0	+	?	?	?	?	?	+	+	+	+	?	?	0	0	0	0	+	+	+	?	+	?	?	?
Y. pestis	0	0	0	0	0	0	0	0	0	0	0	0	0	0	0	0	0	+	+	+	+	+	+	0	0	0	0	+	+	++	0	+	0	0	0
Aerobic gram-neg bacilli - Selected non-fermentative GNB (NF-GNB)																																			
Acinetobacter sp.	0	0	0	0	0	0	0	0	0	0	±	+	+	0	+	+	0	+	+	+	?	?	?	0	0	0	0	0	0	0	?	?	0	0	0
B. cepacia	0	0	0	0	0	0	0	0	0	0	0	+	±	0	0	+	0	+	+	+	+	?	?	0	0	0	0	0	0	0	?	?	?	0	0
P. aeruginosa	0	0	0	0	0	0	0	0	0	0	0	+	+	0	+	+	+	+	+	+	0	0	?	0	0	0	0	0	0	0	+	+	+	0	+
S. maltophilia	0	0	0	0	0	0	0	0	0	0	0	0	0	0	0	0	0	+	0	+	±	?	?	0	0	0	0	0	0	0	0	0	0	0	0
Aerobic cell wall-deficient bacteria																																			
C. trachomatis	0	0	0	0	0	0	0	0	0	+	0	0	0	0	0	0	0	+	+	++	+	+	+	0	0	0	0	0	0	0	0	0	0	0	0
Chlamydophila sp.	0	0	0	0	0	0	0	0	0	0	0	0	0	0	0	0	0	+	+	++	+	+	+	0	0	0	0	0	0	0	0	0	0	0	0
M. genitalium	0	0	0	0	0	0	0	0	0	0	0	0	0	0	0	0	0	+	+	++	+	+	+	0	0	0	0	0	0	0	0	0	0	0	0
M. pneumoniae	0	0	0	0	0	0	0	0	0	0	0	0	0	0	0	0	0	+	+	++	+	+	+	0	0	0	0	0	0	0	0	0	0	0	0
Anaerobic gram-negative bacteria																																			
B. fragilis	0	0	0	0	0	0	0	0	0	++	++	++	++	+	++	++	0	0	0	0	+	0	0	0	+	+	0	0	0	0	0	0	+	0	+
F. necrophorum	±	±	0	0	0	0	0	±	±	+	+	+	+	0	+	+	0	0	0	0	+	0	0	0	+	+	0	+	+	+	?	?	?	+	+
P. melaninogenica	±	±	0	0	0	0	0	±	±	+	+	+	+	0	+	+	0	0	0	0	+	0	0	0	+	+	+	+	+	+	?	?	+	+	+
Anaerobic gram-positive bacteria																																			
Actinomyces sp.	++	++	0	0	0	0	0	++	++	++	+	+	+	+	++	+	0	0	0	0	+	0	0	+	+	+	+	+	+	+	?	?	?	?	+
C. difficile	0	0	0	0	0	0	0	0	0	0	0	0	0	0	0	0	0	0	0	0	0	0	0	0	0	0	0	0	0	0	0	0	0	0	0
Clostridium sp.	++	+	0	0	0	0	0	+	+	++	+	+	+	+	++	+	0	0	0	0	+	0	0	+	+	+	+	+	+	+	?	?	?	+	+
P. acnes	++	+	0	0	0	0	0	++	++	+	+	+	+	+	+	+	0	0	0	0	+	0	0	+	+	+	+	+	+	+	?	?	?	+	+
Peptostreptococci	++	++	0	0	0	0	0	++	++	++	+	+	+	+	++	+	0	0	0	0	+	+	+	+	+	+	+	+	+	+	?	?	?	+	+

TABLE 4A (4)

	Oral Cephalosporins										Aminoglyco					Macrolides				Tetracycline				Glyco/Lipo					Ox-lid											
	Cefadroxil	Cephalexin	Cefaclor	Cefprozil	Cefurox-Axe	Cefixime	Ceftibuten	Cefpodoxime	Cefdinir	Cefditoren	Gentamicin	Tobramycin	Amikacin	Chloramphen	Clindamycin	Erythromycin	Azithromycin	Clarithromycin	Telithromycin	Doxycycline	Minocycline	Tigecycline	Daptomycin	Vancomycin	Teicoplanin	Telavancin	Oritavancin	Dalbavancin	Linezolid	Tedizolid	Fusidic Acid	Rif (comb)	TMP-SMX	Nitrofurantoin	Fosfomycin	Metronidazole	Quinu-Dalfo	Polymyxin B	Colistin
Aerobic gram-pos cocci																																							
E. faecalis	0	0	0	0	0	0	0	0	0	0	±	0	0	±	0	0	0	0	0	±	±	+	+	+	+	+	+	+	+	+	±	±	0	+	+	0	0	0	0
E. faecium	0	0	0	0	0	0	0	0	0	0	±	0	0	±	0	0	0	0	0	±	±	+	+	+	±	+	+	+	+	+	±	±	0	+	+	0	+	0	0
VRE faecalis	0	0	0	0	0	0	0	0	0	0	±	0	NA	±	0	0	0	0	0	±	±	+	±	0	0	0	±	±	+	+	±	±	0	+	+	0	+	0	0
VRE faecium	0	0	0	0	0	0	0	0	0	0	±	0	?	±	0	0	0	0	0	±	±	+	±	0	0	0	±	±	+	+	±	±	0	+	+	0	+	0	0
S. aureus MSSA	+	+	+	+	+	0	0	+	+	+	+	+	?	+	+	±	±	±	+	+	+	+	+	+	+	+	+	+	+	+	+	±	+	+	+	0	+	0	0
S. aureus HA-MRSA	0	0	0	0	0	0	0	0	0	0	?	?	?	+	±	0	0	0	±	+	+	+	+	+	+	+	+	+	+	+	+	±	+	+	+	0	+	0	0
S. aureus CA-MRSA	0	0	0	0	+	0	0	+	0	+	?	?	?	+	±	±	0	±	±	+	+	+	+	+	+	+	+	+	+	+	+	±	+	+	+	0	+	0	0
Staph coag-neg (S)	+	+	+	+	+	0	0	+	+	+	±	±	?	+	+	±	±	±	+	+	+	+	+	+	+	+	+	+	+	+	+	±	+	+	+	0	+	0	0
Staph coag-neg (R)	0	0	0	0	0	0	0	0	0	0	?	?	?	+	±	0	0	0	±	+	+	+	+	+	±	+	+	+	±	+	+	±	+	+	+	0	+	0	0
S. lugdunensis	+	+	+	+	+	+	0	+	+	+	±	±	?	+	+	±	±	±	+	+	+	+	+	+	+	+	+	+	+	+	+	±	+	+	+	0	+	0	0
S. saprophyticus	+	+	+	+	+	+	0	+	+	+	±	±	?	+	+	+	+	+	+	+	+	+	+	+	+	+	+	+	+	+	±	±	+	+	+	0	+	0	0
Strep. anginosus gp	±	+	+	+	+	±	±	+	+	+	0	0	0	+	+	±	±	±	+	+	+	+	+	+	+	+	+	+	+	+	+	±	±	0	+	0	+	0	0
Strep. gp A,B,C,G	+	+	+	+	+	±	±	+	+	+	0	0	0	+	+	±	±	±	+	±	±	+	+	+	+	+	+	+	+	+	+	±	±	0	+	0	+	0	0
Strep. pneumoniae	±	±	±	+	+	±	0	+	+	+	0	0	0	±	+	±	±	±	+	±	±	+	+	+	+	+	+	+	+	+	±	±	±	0	+	0	+	0	0
Viridans Strep	+	+	+	+	+	±	0	+	+	+	0	0	0	+	+	±	±	±	+	±	±	+	+	+	+	+	+	+	+	+	?	?	±	0	+	0	+	0	0
Aerobic gram-pos bacilli																																							
Arcanobacter. sp	?	?	?	?	?	?	?	?	?	?	+	+	+	+	+	+	+	+	+	+	+	+	?	+	+	?	?	?	+	?	?	?	0	?	?	0	+	0	0
C. diphtheriae	+	+	+	+	+	?	?	+	+	+	+	+	+	+	±	+	+	+	+	+	+	+	?	+	+	?	?	?	+	?	+	+	0	?	?	0	+	0	0
C. jeikeium	0	0	0	0	0	0	0	0	0	0	?	?	?	±	±	0	0	0	?	+	+	+	?	+	+	?	?	?	+	?	+	+	0	?	?	0	+	0	0
L. monocytogenes	+	+	±	+	+	0	0	0	0	0	±	0	0	+	0	+	+	+	+	+	+	+	?	0	0	?	?	?	+	?	0	+	+	?	?	0	0	0	0
Nocardia sp.	0	0	0	0	0	0	0	0	0	0	+	+	±	0	0	0	0	0	0	+	+	+	0	0	0	0	0	0	+	0	0	0	+	0	0	0	0	0	0
Aerobic gram-neg bacilli - Enterobacteriaceae																																							
Aeromonas sp.	?	?	?	?	?	+	+	+	+	+	+	+	+	+	0	0	0	0	0	+	+	+	0	0	0	0	0	0	0	0	0	0	+	?	±	0	?	+	+
C. jejuni	?	?	?	?	?	?	0	0	0	0	+	+	+	+	0	+	+	+	+	±	±	+	0	0	0	0	0	0	0	0	0	0	±	?	?	0	?	±	±
Citrobacter sp.	0	0	0	0	0	±	+	+	+	+	+	+	+	+	0	0	0	0	0	±	±	+	0	0	0	0	0	0	0	0	0	0	+	±	+	0	?	+	+
Enterobacter sp.	0	0	0	0	0	±	+	+	+	+	+	+	+	+	0	0	0	0	0	±	±	+	0	0	0	0	0	0	0	0	0	0	+	±	+	0	?	+	+
E. coli	0	±	±	±	±	+	+	+	+	+	+	+	+	+	0	0	0	0	0	±	±	+	0	0	0	0	0	0	0	0	0	0	+	+	+	0	?	+	+
E. coli, Klebs ESBL	0	0	0	0	0	0	0	0	0	0	±	±	±	±	0	0	0	0	0	±	±	+	0	0	0	0	0	0	0	0	0	0	±	+	+	0	?	+	+
E. coli, Klebs KPC	0	0	0	0	0	0	0	0	0	0	±	±	±	±	0	0	0	0	0	±	±	+	0	0	0	0	0	0	0	0	0	0	±	±	+	0	?	+	+
Klebsiella sp.	0	±	±	±	±	+	+	+	+	+	+	+	+	+	0	0	0	0	0	±	±	+	0	0	0	0	0	0	0	0	0	0	+	±	+	0	?	+	+
Morganella sp.	0	0	0	0	0	+	+	+	+	+	+	+	+	+	0	0	0	0	0	0	0	±	0	0	0	0	0	0	0	0	0	0	+	0	±	0	?	0	0
P. mirabilis	0	+	+	+	+	+	+	+	+	+	+	+	+	+	0	0	0	0	0	0	0	0	0	0	0	0	0	0	0	0	0	0	+	0	+	0	?	0	0
P. vulgaris	0	0	0	0	0	+	+	+	+	+	+	+	+	+	0	0	0	0	0	0	0	±	0	0	0	0	0	0	0	0	0	0	+	0	±	0	?	0	0
Providencia sp.	0	0	0	0	0	+	+	+	+	+	+	+	+	+	0	0	0	0	0	0	0	?	0	0	0	0	0	0	0	0	0	0	+	0	?	0	?	0	0
Salmonella sp.	0	0	0	0	0	+	+	+	+	+	+	+	+	+	0	0	+	0	0	±	±	+	0	0	0	0	0	0	0	0	0	0	+	?	+	0	?	+	+
Serratia sp.	0	0	0	0	±	+	+	+	+	+	+	+	+	+	0	0	0	0	0	±	±	+	0	0	0	0	0	0	0	0	0	0	+	0	±	0	?	0	0

TABLE 4A (5)

	Oral Cephalosporins										Aminoglyco					Macrolides				Tetracycline			Glyco/Lipo						Ox-lid		Other								
	Cefadroxil	Cephalexin	Cefaclor	Cefprozil	Cefurox-Axe	Cefixime	Ceftibuten	Cefpodoxime	Cefdinir	Cefditoren	Gentamicin	Tobramycin	Amikacin	Chloramphen	Clindamycin	Erythromycin	Azithromycin	Clarithromycin	Telithromycin	Doxycycline	Minocycline	Tigecycline	Daptomycin	Vancomycin	Teicoplanin	Telavancin	Oritavancin	Dalbavancin	Linezolid	Tedizolid	Fusidic Acid	Rif (comb)	TMP-SMX	Nitrofurantoin	Fosfomycin	Metronidazole	Quinu-Dalfo	Polymyxin B	Colistin
Aerobic gram-neg bacilli - Enterobacteriaceae (continued)																																							
Shigella sp.	0	0	0	0	0	+	+	+	+	?	+	+	+	+	0	0	+	0	0	+l	+l	+	0	0	0	0	0	0	0	0	0	0	+l	0	0	0	0	0	0
Y. enterocolitica	0	0	0	0	0	+	+	?	+	?	+	+	+	+	0	0	+	0	0	+	?	?	0	0	0	0	0	0	0	0	0	0	+	0	0	0	0	0	0
Aerobic gram-neg bacilli - Miscellaneous																																							
Bartonella sp.	0	0	0	0	0	0	0	0	0	0	‡	0	0	+	0	+	++	++	?	++	+	?	0	0	0	0	0	0	0	0	0	+l	o	0	0	0	0	0	0
B. pertussis	0	0	0	0	0	0	0	0	0	0	0	0	0	+	0	+	++	++	?	+	?	?	0	0	0	0	0	0	0	0	0	+	+	0	0	0	0	0	0
B. burgdorferi	0	0	‡	0	+	0	0	+	0	0	0	0	0	+	0	+	++	+	0	++	+	?	0	0	0	0	0	0	0	0	0	0	o	0	0	0	0	0	0
Brucella sp.	0	0	0	0	0	0	0	0	0	0	+	0	?	+	0	o	?	o	?	++	++	?	0	0	0	0	0	0	0	0	0	+l	+	0	0	0	0	0	0
Capnocytophagia	0	0	0	0	0	0	0	0	0	0	0	0	0	+	++	+	+	+	?	+	+	?	0	0	0	0	0	0	0	0	0	o	+l	0	0	0	0	0	0
C. burnetii	0	0	0	0	0	0	0	0	0	0	0	0	0	+l	0	o	o	o	0	++	?	?	0	0	0	0	0	0	0	0	0	+l	+	0	0	0	0	0	0
Ehrlichia, Anaplas	0	0	0	0	0	0	0	0	0	0	0	0	0	0	0	0	?	0	0	++	?	?	0	0	0	0	0	0	0	0	0	+l	o	0	0	0	0	0	0
Eikenella sp	0	0	0	0	0	+	+	+	0	0	0	0	0	+	+	++	++	?	+	++	+	+	0	0	0	0	0	0	0	0	0	o	+	0	0	0	0	0	0
F. tularensis	0	0	0	0	0	0	0	0	0	0	+l	0	0	+	0	+	+	+	+	+	+	?	0	0	0	0	0	0	0	0	0	o	++	0	0	0	0	0	0
H. ducreyi	0	0	0	0	+	+	+	+	+	+	‡	0	0	0	0	+	++	++	0	+l	+l	+	0	0	0	0	0	0	0	0	0	o	+	0	0	0	0	0	0
H. influenzae	0	0	0	+	+	+	+	+	+	+	‡	0	0	+	0	+l	+	?	+	+	+	0	0	0	0	0	0	0	0	0	0	o	+	0	0	0	0	?	0
Kingella sp.	0	0	0	0	0	+	+	+	0	0	0	0	0	+	0	0	++	0	0	+	+	?	0	0	0	0	0	0	0	0	0	0	?	0	0	0	0	0	0
K. granulomatis	0	0	0	0	0	0	0	0	0	0	0	0	0	0	0	++	++	?	0	O	O	?	0	0	0	0	0	0	0	0	0	+l	+	0	0	0	0	0	0
Legionella sp.	0	0	0	0	0	0	0	0	0	0	0	0	0	+	0	+	++	++	+	+	+	?	0	0	0	0	0	0	0	0	0	+l	+	0	0	0	0	0	0
Leptospira sp.	0	0	?	0	?	+	+	+	+	?	0	0	0	0	0	+	++	?	?	+l	?	?	0	0	0	0	0	0	0	0	0	0	o	0	0	0	0	0	0
M. catarrhalis	0	0	0	+	+	+	+	+	+	+	0	0	0	+	0	+	+	+	+	+	+	O	0	0	0	0	0	0	0	0	0	+l	+	0	0	0	0	0	0
N. gonorrhoeae	0	0	0	0	0	+	+	+	+	+	0	0	0	0	0	0	++	0	0	++	++	+	0	0	0	0	0	0	0	0	0	0	o	0	0	0	0	0	0
N. meningitidis	0	0	0	0	0	+	+	+	0	0	0	0	0	+	0	0	+	0	0	+l	+l	?	0	0	0	0	0	0	0	0	0	+l	o	0	0	0	0	0	0
P. multocida	0	0	?	0	0	+	+	+	0	+	+l	0	0	+	0	?	+	++	O	++	++	?	0	0	0	0	0	0	0	0	0	0	+	0	0	0	0	0	0
R. rickettsii	0	0	0	0	0	0	0	0	0	0	0	0	0	0	0	0	+	0	0	++	?	?	0	0	0	0	0	0	0	0	0	+l	o	0	0	0	0	0	0
T. pallidum	0	0	0	0	0	0	0	0	0	0	0	0	0	0	0	++	++	?	0	+	?	?	0	0	0	0	0	0	0	0	0	0	o	0	0	0	0	0	0
U. urealyticum	0	0	0	0	0	0	0	0	0	0	0	0	0	0	0	++	++	+	0	+	+	?	0	0	0	0	0	0	0	0	0	0	o	0	0	0	0	0	0
V. cholera	0	0	0	0	0	0	0	0	0	0	?	0	0	+	0	+	+	?	?	+	+	?	0	0	0	0	0	0	0	0	0	0	o	0	0	0	0	0	0
V. parahemolyticus	0	0	0	0	0	+	+	+	0	0	?	0	0	+	0	+l	+l	?	0	++	?	?	0	0	0	0	0	0	0	0	0	0	?	0	0	0	0	0	0
V. vulnificus	0	0	0	0	0	+	+	+	0	0	?	0	0	+	0	+	+	?	0	+	+	?	0	0	0	0	0	0	0	0	0	0	?	0	0	0	0	0	0
Y. pestis	0	0	0	0	0	+	+	+	0	+	+	?	?	+	0	+	+	?	0	+	+	?	0	0	0	0	0	0	0	0	0	0	+	0	0	0	0	0	0

TABLE 4A (6)

Drug Class	Drug	Acinetobacter sp.	B. cepacia	P. aeruginosa	S. maltophilia	C. trachomatis	Chlamydophila sp.	M. genitalium	M. pneumoniae	B. fragilis	F. necrophorum	P. melaninogenica	Actinomyces sp.	C. difficile	Clostridium sp.	P. acnes	Peptostreptococci
Other	Colistin	+	o	+	+					o	o	o	o	o	o	o	o
	Polymyxin B	+	o	+	+					o	o	o	o	o	o	o	o
	Quinu-Dalfo	o	o	o	o					o	o	o	o	+	o	+	?
	Metronidazole	o	o	o	o					+	+	+	o	±	+	o	±
	Fosfomycin	o	o	±	o					o	o	o	o	o	o	o	o
	Nitrofurantoin	o	o	o	o					o	o	o	o	o	o	o	o
	TMP-SMX	±	±	o	+					o	o	o	o	o	o	±	o
	Rif (comb)	o	o	o	o		o	±	o	o	o	o	o	o	o	o	o
	Fusidic Acid	o	o	o	o					o	o	o	o	o	o	o	o
Ox-lid	Tedizolid	o	o	o	o					o	o	o	?	o	o	o	?
	Linezolid	o	o	o	o					o	o	o	o	o	+	o	+
Glyco/Lipo	Dalbavancin	o	o	o	o					o	o	o	o	o	+	+	+
	Oritavancin	o	o	o	o					o	o	o	o	+	+	+	+
	Telavancin	o	o	o	o					o	o	o	?	o	+	+	+
	Teicoplanin	o	o	o	o					o	o	o	o	o	+	+	+
	Vancomycin	o	o	o	o					o	o	o	?	±	+	+	+
	Daptomycin	o	o	o	o					o	o	o	?	±	+	+	+
Tetracycline	Tigecycline	+	o	o	+		o	+	+	+	+	+	?	+	+	+	+
	Minocycline	±	±	o	+		+	+	±	±	+	+	+	o	+	+	+
	Doxycycline	o	o	o	+		±	±	±	±	+	+	+	o	+	+	+
Macrolides	Telithromycin	o	o	o	o		?	+	?	±	o	o	o	?	o	?	?
	Clarithromycin	o	o	o	o		+	+	?	±	o	o	±	+	o	+	±
	Azithromycin	o	o	o	o		+	+	±	±	o	o	±	+	o	±	±
	Erythromycin	o	o	o	o		+	+	?	±	o	o	±	+	o	±	±
	Clindamycin	o	o	o	o					±	+	+	+	+	o	+	+
	Chloramphen	o	±	o	+					+	+	+	+	o	+	+	+
Aminoglyco	Amikacin	±	o	+	o					o	o	o	o	o	o	o	o
	Tobramycin	o	o	+	o					o	o	o	o	o	o	?	o
	Gentamicin	o	o	+	o					o	o	o	o	o	?	o	o
Oral Cephalosporins	Cefditoren	o	o	o	o					?	?	?	?	?	?	?	?
	Cefdinir	o	o	o	o					?	?	?	?	?	?	?	?
	Cefpodoxime	o	o	o	o					?	o	?	?	o	?	+	+
	Ceftibuten	o	±	o	o					?	o	?	?	o	?	+	+
	Cefixime	o	o	o	o					?	o	?	?	o	?	+	+
	Cefurox-Axe	o	o	o	o					?	o	?	?	o	+	+	+
	Cefprozil	o	o	o	o					?	o	?	?	o	+	+	+
	Cefaclor	o	o	o	o					?	o	?	?	o	+	+	+
	Cephalexin	o	o	o	o					?	?	?	?	o	+	+	+
	Cefadroxil	o	o	o	o					?	?	?	?	+	+	+	+

Aerobic gram-neg bacilli - Selected non-fermentative GNB (NF-GNB): Acinetobacter sp., B. cepacia, P. aeruginosa, S. maltophilia
Aerobic cell wall-deficient bacteria: C. trachomatis, Chlamydophila sp., M. genitalium, M. pneumoniae
Anaerobic gram-negative bacteria: B. fragilis, F. necrophorum, P. melaninogenica
Anaerobic gram-positive bacteria: Actinomyces sp., C. difficile, Clostridium sp., P. acnes, Peptostreptococci

TABLE 4B – ANTIFUNGAL ACTIVITY SPECTRA

	Antifungal Drugs								
	Fluconazole	Itraconazole	Voriconazole	Posaconazole	Isavuconazole	Anidulafungin	Caspofungin	Micafungin	Amphotericin B
Fungi									
Aspergillus fumigatus	0	±	++	+	++	±	±	±	+
Aspergillus terreus	0	±	++	+	++	±	±	±	0
Aspergillus flavus	0	±	++	+	++	±	±	±	+
Candida albicans	++	+	+	+	+	++	++	++	+
Candida dubliniensis	++	+	+	+	+	++	++	++	++
Candida glabrata	±	±	±	±	±	++	++	++	++
Candida guilliermondii	++	++	++	++	+	++	++	++	++
Candida krusei	0	0	+	+	+	++	++	++	++
Candida lusitaniae	++	+	+	+	+	++	++	++	±
Candida parapsilosis	++	+	+	+	+	+	+	+	++
Candida tropicalis	++	+	+	+	+	++	++	++	++
Cryptococcus sp.	++	+	+	+	+	0	0	0	++
Dematiaceous molds	0	++	++	+	+	±	±	±	+
Fusarium sp.	0	±	±	±	+	0	0	0	±
Mucormycosis	0	0	0	+	+	0	0	0	++
Scedo apiospermum	0	0	+	±	±	0	0	0	0
Scedo prolificans	0	0	0	0	0	0	0	0	0
Trichosporon spp.	±	+	+	+	?	0	0	0	+
Dimorphic Fungi									
Blastomyces	±	++	+	+	?	0	0	0	++
Coccidioides	++	++	+	+	?	0	0	0	++
Histoplasma	±	++	+	+	?	0	0	0	++
Sporothrix	±	++	+	+	?	0	0	0	++

TABLE 4C – ANTIVIRAL ACTIVITY SPECTRA

	Viruses											
	Adenovirus	BK Virus	Cytomegalovirus	Hepatitis B	Hepatitis C	Herpes simplex	HPV	Influenza A	Influenza B	JC Virus / PML	RSV	Varicella-zoster
Hepatitis B												
Adefovir	NA	NA	NA	++	NA	NA	NA	NA	NA	NA	NA	NA
Emtricitabine	NA	NA	NA	±	NA	NA	NA	NA	NA	NA	NA	NA
Entecavir	NA	NA	NA	++	NA	NA	NA	NA	NA	NA	NA	NA
Lamivudine	NA	NA	NA	±	NA	NA	NA	NA	NA	NA	NA	NA
Telbivudine	NA	NA	NA	±	NA	NA	NA	NA	NA	NA	NA	NA
Tenofovir	NA	NA	NA	++	NA	±	NA	NA	NA	NA	NA	NA
Hepatitis C												
Daclatasvir	NA	NA	NA	NA	++	NA	NA	NA	NA	NA	NA	NA
Dasabuvir	NA	NA	NA	NA	++	NA	NA	NA	NA	NA	NA	NA
Interferon alfa, peg	NA	NA	NA	++	+	NA	NA	NA	NA	NA	NA	NA
Ledipasvir	NA	NA	NA	NA	++	NA	NA	NA	NA	NA	NA	NA
Ombitasvir	NA	NA	NA	NA	++	NA	NA	NA	NA	NA	NA	NA
Paritaprevir	NA	NA	NA	NA	++	NA	NA	NA	NA	NA	NA	NA
Ribavirin	±	NA	NA	0	+	NA	NA	NA	NA	NA	±	NA
Simeprevir	NA	NA	NA	NA	+	NA	NA	NA	NA	NA	NA	NA
Sofosbuvir	NA	NA	NA	NA	++	NA	NA	NA	NA	NA	NA	NA

TABLE 4C (2)

	Viruses											
	Adenovirus	BK Virus	Cytomegalovirus	Hepatitis B	Hepatitis C	Herpes simplex	HPV	Influenza A	Influenza B	JC Virus / PML	RSV	Varicella-zoster
Influenza												
Amantadine	NA	NA	NA	NA	NA	NA	NA	±	±	NA	NA	NA
Oseltamivir	NA	NA	NA	NA	NA	NA	NA	++	+	NA	NA	NA
Peramivir	NA	NA	NA	NA	NA	NA	NA	+	+	NA	NA	NA
Rimantadine	NA	NA	NA	NA	NA	NA	NA	±	±	NA	NA	NA
Zanamivir	NA	NA	NA	NA	NA	NA	NA	++	+	NA	NA	NA
Herpes, CMV, VZV, misc.												
Acyclovir	NA	NA	0	NA	NA	++	NA	NA	NA	NA	NA	+
Cidofovir	+	+	++	NA	NA	+	NA	NA	NA	+	NA	+
Famciclovir	NA	NA	0	NA	NA	++	NA	NA	NA	NA	NA	+
Foscarnet	NA	NA	++	NA	NA	+	NA	NA	NA	NA	NA	+
Ganciclovir	±	NA	++	NA	NA	+	NA	NA	NA	NA	NA	+
Valacyclovir	NA	NA	0	NA	NA	++	NA	NA	NA	NA	NA	++
Valganciclovir	±	NA	++	NA	NA	+	NA	NA	NA	NA	NA	+
Topical Agents												
Imiquimod	NA	NA	NA	NA	NA	NA	++	NA	NA	NA	NA	NA
Penciclovir	NA	NA	0	NA	NA	+	NA	NA	NA	NA	NA	0
Podofilox	NA	NA	NA	NA	NA	NA	++	NA	NA	NA	NA	NA
Sinecatechins	NA	NA	NA	NA	NA	NA	+	NA	NA	NA	NA	NA
Trifluridine	NA	NA	NA	NA	NA	+	NA	NA	NA	NA	NA	NA

TABLE 5A – TREATMENT OPTIONS FOR SYSTEMIC INFECTION DUE TO MULTI-DRUG RESISTANT GRAM-POSITIVE BACTERIA

ORGANISM	RESISTANT TO	PRIMARY TREATMENT OPTIONS	ALTERNATIVE TREATMENT OPTIONS	COMMENTS
Enterococcus faecium; (VRTE) **Enterococcus faecalis** (Consultation suggested)	Vancomycin Ampicillin, Penicillin G, Gentamicin (high level resistance)	**E. faecium: Dapto** 8-12 mg/kg IV q24h + **AMP** 2 gm IV q4h OR **Ceftaroline** 600 mg IV q8h). Less desirable alternatives: [**Linezolid** 600 mg po/IV q12h OR **Penicillin G** (if Pen-susceptible) 7.5 mg/kg IV q4h] **Quinu-dalfo** 7.5 mg/kg IV (central line) + **AMP** 2 gm IV q4h	**E. faecalis:** Resistance to AMP or Pen rare. If no resistance: **AMP** 2 gm IV q4h + **Ceftriaxone** 2 gm IV q12h. If Pen-resistant due to beta-lactamase: **Dapto** 8-12 mg/kg IV q12h + **AM-SB** 3 gm IV q6h	Addition of a beta lactam reverses Dapto resistance & impedes development of resistance. E. faecalis rarely resistance to penicillins. Enterococcal endocarditis ref: *Curr Infect Dis Rep 16: 431, 2014.*
Staphylococcus aureus (See also Table 6 for more details)	Vancomycin (VISA or VRSA) and all other beta lactams (except Ceftaroline)	**Daptomycin** 6-12 mg/kg IV q24h or (**Daptomycin** 6-12 mg/kg IV q24h + **Ceftaroline** 600 mg IV q8h)	**Telavancin** 10 mg/kg IV q24h or **Linezolid** 600 mg IV/po q12h	Confirm dapto susceptibility as VISA strains may be non-susceptible. If prior vanco therapy (or persistent infection on vanco) there is significant chance of developing resistance to dapto (*JAC 66: 1696, 2011*). Addition of an anti-staphylococcal beta-lactam (nafcillin or oxacillin) may restore susceptibility against Dapto-resistant MRSA (*AAC 54:3161, 2010*). Combination of Dapto + oxacillin has been successful in clearing refractory MRSA bacteremia (*CID 53:158, 2011*). Dapto + ceftaroline may also be effective.
Streptococcus pneumoniae	Penicillin G (MIC ≥ 4 µg/mL)	If no meningitis **Ceftriaxone** 2 gm IV once daily OR **Ceftaroline** 600 mg IV q12h OR **Linezolid** 600 mg IV/po q12h	Meningitis **Vancomycin** 15 mg/kg IV q8h OR **Meropenem** 2 gm IV q8h	Ceftriaxone 2 gm IV q12h should also work for meningitis.

TABLE 5B: TREATMENT OPTIONS FOR SYSTEMIC INFECTION DUE TO SELECTED MULTI-DRUG RESISTANT GRAM-NEGATIVE BACILLI

The suggested treatment options in this Table are usually not FDA-approved. Suggestions are variably based on in vitro data, animal studies, and/or limited clinical experience.

ORGANISM	RESISTANT TO	PRIMARY TREATMENT OPTIONS	ALTERNATIVE TREATMENT OPTIONS	COMMENTS
Acinetobacter baumannii	All Penicillins, All Cephalosporins, Aztreonam, Carbapenems, Aminoglycosides and Fluoroquinolones	Combination therapy. **Polymyxin E (Colistin)** + **(Imipenem or Meropenem)** See *Table 10A, page 112,* for guidance on Colistin dosing.	**Minocycline** (*IDCP 20:184, 2012*) (in vitro synergy between minocycline and imipenem)	Refs: *Int J Antimicrob Agts 37:244, 2011; BMC Int Dis 11:109, 2011.* Detergent effect of colistin reconstitutes antibiotic activity of carbapenems and other drugs. Do not use colistin as monotherapy. Colistin → Rifampin failed to influence infection-related mortality (*CID 57:349, 2013*).
Extended spectrum beta lactamase (ESBL) producing E. coli, Klebsiella pneumoniae, or other Enterobacteriaceae	All Cephalosporins, Fluoroquinolones, Aminoglycosides	**Imipenem** 500 mg IV q6h OR **Meropenem** 1 gm IV q8h OR **Doripenem** 500 mg IV q8h (*CID 39:31, 2004*) (Note: **DORI** is **not** FDA approved for treatment of pneumonia)	Perhaps high dose **Cefepime** 2 gm IV q8h (See Comment) **Polymyxin E (Colistin)** + **(MER or IMP)**. For dosing, see *Table 10A, page 112.*	For UTI: Fosfomycin, nitrofurantoin (*AAC 53:1278, 2009*) Avoid PIP-TZ even if susceptible (*AAC 57:3402, 2013*). Ceftolozane-tazobactam (see *Lancet 385:1949, 2015* and *CID 60:1462, 2015*) and ceftazidime-avibactam (see *Med Lett Drugs Ther 57:79, 2015*) recently approved for treatment of complicated UTI and intra-abdominal infections caused by ESBL+ enterics.
Carbapenemase producing aerobic gram-negative bacilli or P. aeruginosa	All Penicillins, Cephalosporins, Aztreonam, Carbapenems, Aminoglycosides, Fluoroquinolones	Combination therapy. **Polymyxin E (Colistin)** + **(MER or IMP)**. Ceftazidime-avibactam (*Med Lett Drugs Ther. 57:79, 2015*) active against some carbapenemase producing Gram-negatives (not those producing a metallo-beta-lactamase).	Pneumonia. Inhaled **Colistin^MA** 50-75 mg IV q12h + saline via nebulizer + **Colistin** + **(MER or IMP)**	See *Table 10A, page 112* for guidance on **Colistin** dosing for inhalation dosing, see *Table 10F.* Anecdotal reports of successful dual carbapenem rx. (MER + ERTA) for KPCs (*JAC 69:1718, 2014*). **Ceftazidime-avibactam** active in vitro against some carbapenemase-producing (but not metallo-beta-lactamases) organisms.
Stenotrophomonas maltophilia	All beta-lactams, Aminoglycosides, Fluoroquinolones	**TMP-SMX** 15 mg/kg/day IV divided q6h/q8h/q12h (based on TMP component)	**FQ** if suscept in vitro	Ref: *Sem Resp & CCM 36:99, 2015.*

TABLE 6 – SUGGESTED MANAGEMENT OF SUSPECTED OR CULTURE-POSITIVE COMMUNITY-ASSOCIATED METHICILLIN-RESISTANT S. AUREUS INFECTIONS
(See footnote[1] for doses)

IDSA Guidelines: CID 52 (Feb 1):1, 2011. With the magnitude of the clinical problem and a number of new drugs, it is likely new data will require frequent revisions of the regimens suggested. (See page 2 for abbreviations).
NOTE: Distinction between community and hospital strains of MRSA blurring.

CLINICAL ILLNESS	ABSCESS, NO IMMUNOSUPPRESSION, OUT-PATIENT CARE	PNEUMONIA	BACTEREMIA OR POSSIBLE ENDOCARDITIS OR BACTEREMIC SHOCK	TREATMENT FAILURE (See footnote[2])
Management Drug doses in footnote.	TMP/SMX 1 DS (2 DS if BMI > 40) po bid OR Clinda 300 mg (450 mg for BMI > 40) po tid (NEJM 372:1093, 2015). For larger abscesses, multiple lesions or systemic inflammatory response: **I&D + (Oritavancin** 1500 mg x1 or **Dalbavancin** 1000 mg x1 than 500 mg x1 a wk later)** an option for outpatient management of sicker patients with more extensive infection who might otherwise be admitted (see NEJM 370:2180, 2014, NEJM 370:2169, 2014).	**Vanco** IV or **linezolid**	**Vanco** 15-20 mg/kg IV q8-12h. Confirm adequate vanco troughs of 15-20 µg/mL Switch to alternative regimen if **vanco MIC > 2 µg/mL** If patient has slow response to vancomycin and isolate has MIC = 2, consider alternative therapy. **Dapto** 6 mg/kg IV q24h (FDA-approved dose but some authorities recommend 8-12 mg/kg for MRSA bacteremia)	**Dapto** 8-12 mg IV q24h; confirm in vitro susceptibility as prior vanco therapy may select for daptomycin non-susceptibility (MIC > 1 µg/mL) & some VISA strains are daptomycin non-susceptible. Use combination therapy for bacteremia or endocarditis: dapto + beta-lactam combination therapy (dapto 8-12 mg/kg IV q24h + (Nafcillin 2 gm IV q4h OR Oxacillin 2 gm IV q4h + Ceftaroline 600 mg IV q8h) appears effective against MRSA strains as salvage therapy even if non-susceptible to dapto (Int J Antimicrob Agents 42:450, 2013; AAC 54:3161, 2010; AAC 56:6192, 2013). **Ceftaroline** 600 mg IV q8h (J Antimicrob Chemother 67:1267, 2012; 3 Infect Chemother 19:42, 2013; Int J Antimicrob Agents 42:450, 2013; AAC 58:2541, 2014. **Linezolid** 600 mg IV/PO q12h (Linezolid is bacteriostatic and should not be used as a single agent in suspected endovascular infection). **Telavancin** 10 mg/kg IV q24h (CID 52:31, 2011; AAC 58:2030, 2014).
Comments	**Fusidic acid** 500 mg tid (not available in the US) + **rifampin** also an option; do not use rifampin alone as resistance rapidly emerges.	Patients not responding after 2-3 days should be evaluated for complicated infection and switched to **vancomycin**. Prospective study of **Linezolid** vs **Vanco** showed slightly higher cure rate with Linezolid, no difference in mortality (CID 54:621, 2012).	TMP-SMX NOT recommended in bacteremic pts: inferior to Vanco (BMJ 350:2219, 2015)	

[1] **Clindamycin:** 300 mg po tid. **Daptomycin:** 6 mg/kg IV q24h is the standard, FDA-approved dose for bacteremia and endocarditis bud 8:12 mg/kg q24h is recommended by some and for treatment failures. **Doxycycline or minocycline:** 100 mg po/IV bid. **Linezolid:** 600 mg po/IV bid **Quinupristin-dalfopristin (Q-D):** 7.5 mg per /kg IV q8h via central line. **Rifampin:** Long serum half-life justifies dosing 600 mg po q24h; however, frequency of nausea less with 300 mg po bid. **TMP-SMX-DS:** Standard dose 8–10 mg per kg per day. For 70 kg person = 700 mg TMP component po bid. 1 DS tablet contains 1 160 mg TMP and 800 mg SMX. The dose for treatment of CA-MRSA skin and soft tissue infections (SSTI) is 1 DS tablet twice daily. **Vancomycin:** 1 gm IV q12h; up to 45-60 mg/kg/day in divided doses may be required to achieve target trough concentrations of 15-20 mcg/ml; recommended for serious infections.

[2] The median duration of bacteremia in endocarditis is 7-9 days in patients treated with vancomycin (AnM 115:674, 1991). Longer duration of bacteremia, greater likelihood of endocarditis (JID 190:1140, 2004). Definition of failure unclear. **Unsatisfactory clinical response especially if blood cultures remain positive >4 days.**

TABLE 7 – ANTIBIOTIC HYPERSENSITIVITY REACTIONS & DRUG DESENSITIZATION METHODS

Penicillin. Oral route (Pen VK) preferred. 1/3 pts develop transient reaction, usually mild. **Perform in ICU setting. Discontinue β-blockers. Have IV line, epinephrine, ECG, spirometer available.** Desensitization works as long as pt is receiving Pen, allergy returns after discontinuance. History of Steven-Johnson, exfoliative dermatitis, erythroderma are contraindications. Skin testing for evaluation of Pen allergy. Testing with major determinant (benzyl Pen polylysine) and minor determinants has negative predictive value (97-99%). Risk of systemic reaction to skin testing <1% (Ann Allergy Asth Immunol 106:1, 2011). General refs. CID 58:1140, 2014.

- **Method:** Prepare dilutions using **Pen-VK** oral soln, 250 mg/5mL. Administer each dose @ 15 min intervals in 30 mL water/flavored Bev. After Step 14 observe pt for 30 min, then give full therapeutic dose by route of choice. Ref. Allergy, Prin & Prac. Mosby, 1993, pg. 1726

Step	Dilution (mg/mL)	mL Administered	Dose/Step mg	Dose/Step units	Cumulative Dose Given mg	Cumulative Dose Given units
1	0.5	0.1	0.05	80	0.05	80
2	0.5	0.2	0.1	160	0.15	240
3	0.5	0.4	0.2	320	0.35	560
4	0.5	0.8	0.4	640	0.75	1,200
5	0.5	1.6	0.8	1,280	1.55	2,480
6	0.5	3.2	1.6	2,560	3.15	5,040
7	0.5	6.4	3.2	5,120	6.35	10,160
8	5	1.2	6	9,600	12.35	19,760
9	5	2.4	12	19,200	24.35	38,960
10	5	4.8	24	38,400	48.35	77,360
11	50	1	50	80,000	98.35	157,360
12	50	2	100	160,000	198.35	317,360
13	50	4	200	320,000	398.35	637,360
14	50	8	400	640,000	798.35	1,277,360

Penicillin. Parenteral (Pen G) route. Follow procedures/notes under Oral (Pen-VK) route. Ref. Allergy, Prin & Prac. Mosby, 1993, pg. 1726.

- **Method:** Administer **Pen G** IM, IV or sc as follows:

Step	Dilution (units/mL)	mL Administered	Dose/Step (units)	Cumulative Dose Given (units)
1	100	0.2	20	20
2		0.4	40	60
3		0.8	80	140
4	1,000	0.2	200	340
5		0.4	400	740
6		0.8	800	1,540
7	10,000	0.2	2,000	3,540
8		0.4	4,000	7,540
9		0.8	8,000	15,540
10	100,000	0.2	20,000	35,540
11		0.4	40,000	75,540
12		0.8	80,000	155,540
13	1,000,000	0.2	200,000	355,540
14		0.4	400,000	755,540
15		0.8	800,000	1,555,540

Ceftriaxone. Ref. Allergol Immunopathol (Madr) 37:105, 2009.

- **Method:** Infuse **Ceftriaxone IV** @ 20 min intervals as follows:

Day	Dose (mg)
1	0.001, then 0.01 then 0.1, then 1
2	1, then 5, then 10, then 50
3	100, then 250, then 500
4	1000

TMP-SMX. Perform in hospital/clinic. Refs CID 20:849, 1995, AIDS 5:311, 1991.

- **Method:** Use **TMP-SMX** oral susp. (40 mg TMP/200 mg SMX)/5 mL. Take with 6 oz water after each dose. Corticosteroids, antihistamins NOT used.

Hour	Dose (TMP/SMX) (mg)
0	0.004/0.02
1	0.04/0.2
2	0.4/2
3	4/20
4	40/200
5	160/800

Desensitization Methods for Other Drugs (References)
- **Imipenem-Cilastatin.** Ann Pharmacother 37:513, 2003
- **Meropenem.** Ann Pharmacother 37:1424, 2003.
- **Metronidazole.** Allergy Rhinol 5:1, 2014
- **Daptomycin.** Ann All Asthma Immun 100:87, 2008.
- **Ceftazidime.** Curr Opin All Clin Immunol 6(6): 476, 2006
- **Vancomycin.** Intern Med 45:317, 2006
- General review, including desensitization protocols for Amp, CFP, CIP, Clarithro, Clinda, Dapto, Linezold, Tobra (CID 58:1140, 2014).

TABLE 7 (2)

Ceftaroline. 12-step IV desensitization protocol. Ref. Open Forum Infect Dis 2:1. 2015.
- Method: Cumulative drug infused: 600 mg. Total time required for all 12 steps: 318 minutes.

Step	Conc (mg/mL)	Vol Infused (mL)	Infusion duration (min)	Drug infused this step (mg)	Cumulative drug infused (mg)
1	0.0002	5	15	0.001	0.001
2	0.0002	15	15	0.003	0.004
3	0.002	5	15	0.01	0.014
4	0.002	15	15	0.03	0.04
5	0.02	5	15	0.1	0.14
6	0.02	15	15	0.3	0.4
7	0.2	5	15	1	1.4
8	0.2	15	15	3	4.4
9	2	5	15	10	14.4
10	2	15	15	30	44.4
11	2	25	15	50	94.4
12	2	255	153	510	604.4

Valganciclovir. 12-step oral desensitization protocol. Ref. Transplantation 98:e50. 2014.
- Method: Administer doses at 15-minute intervals; entire protocol takes 165 minutes. Cumulative dose administered: 453.6 mg

Step	Drug administered this step (mg)	Cumulative drug administered (mg)
1	0.1	0.1
2	0.2	0.3
3	0.4	0.7
4	0.8	1.5
5	1.6	3.1
6	3.5	6.6
7	7	13.6
8	14	27.6
9	28	55.6
10	58	113.6
11	115	228.6
12	225	453.6

TABLE 8 – PREGNANCY RISK AND SAFETY IN LACTATION

Drug	Risk Category (Old)	Use during Lactation
Antibacterials		
Amikacin	D	Probably safe, monitor infant for GI toxicity
Azithromycin	B	Safe, monitor infant for GI toxicity
Aztreonam	B	Safe, monitor infant for GI toxicity
Cephalosporins	B	Safe, monitor infant for GI toxicity
Chloramphenicol	C	Avoid use
Ciprofloxacin	C	Avoid breastfeeding for 3-4 hrs after a dose, monitor infant for GI toxicity
Clarithromycin	C	Safe, monitor for GI toxicity
Clindamycin	B	Avoid use if possible, otherwise monitor infant for GI toxicity
Colistin (polymyxin E)	C	Probably safe, but data limited
Dalbavancin	C	Probably safe with monitoring, but no data available
Daptomycin	B	Probably safe with monitoring, but data limited
Doripenem	B	Probably safe with monitoring, but no data available
Doxycycline	D	Short-term use safe, monitor infant for GI toxicity
Ertapenem	B	Safe
Erythromycin	B	Safe
Fidaxomicin	B	Probably safe
Fosfomycin	B	Probably safe with monitoring
Fusidic acid	-	Safety not established
Gatifloxacin	C	Short-term use safe
Gemifloxacin	C	Short-term use safe
Gentamicin	D	Probably safe
Imipenem	C	Safe, monitor infant for GI toxicity
Isepamicin	D	Safety not established, avoid use
Levofloxacin	C	Avoid breastfeeding for 4-6 hrs after a dose, monitor infant for GI toxicity
Linezolid	C	Probably safe with monitoring, but no data available; avoid if possible
Meropenem	B	Probably safe with monitoring, but no data available
Metronidazole	B	Data and opinions conflict; best to avoid
Minocycline	D	Short-term use safe, monitor infant for GI toxicity
Moxifloxacin	C	Short-term use safe, monitor infant for GI toxicity; avoid if possible
Netilmicin	D	Safety not established
Nitrofurantoin	B	Avoid if infant <8 days of age
Ofloxacin	C	Avoid breastfeeding for 4-6 hrs after a dose, monitor infant for GI toxicity
Oritavancin	C	Probably safe with monitoring, but no data available; avoid if possible
Penicillins	B	Safe, monitor infant for GI toxicity
Polymyxin B	C	Topical administration safe (no data with systemic use)
Quinupristin-Dalfopristin	B	Probably safe with monitoring, but no data available; avoid if possible
Rifaximin	C	Probably safe with monitoring, but no data available; avoid if possible
Streptomycin	D	Probably safe, monitor infant for GI toxicity
Tedizolid	C	Probably safe with monitoring, but no data available; avoid if possible
Telavancin	C	Probably safe with monitoring, but no data available; avoid if possible
Telithromycin	C	Probably safe with monitoring, but no data available; avoid if possible
Tetracycline	D	Short-term use safe, monitor infant for GI toxicity
Tigecycline	D	Safety not established, avoid use
TMP-SMX	C	Risk of kernicterus in premature infants; avoid if infant G6PD-deficient
Tobramycin	D	Probably safe, monitor infant for GI toxicity
Vancomycin	C	Safe with monitoring
Antifungals		
Amphotericin B (all products)	B	Probably safe, but no data available
Anidulafungin	B	Safety not established, avoid use
Caspofungin	C	Probably safe with monitoring, but no data available; avoid if possible
Fluconazole (other regimens)	D	Safe with monitoring
Fluconazole (single dose)	C	Safe with monitoring
Flucytosine	C	Safety not established, avoid use
Griseofulvin	C	Safety not established, avoid use
Isavuconazole	C	Avoid use
Itraconazole	C	Little data available, avoid if possible
Ketoconazole	C	Little data available, avoid if possible
Micafungin	C	Safety not established, avoid use

TABLE 8 (2)

Drug	Risk Category (Old)	Use during Lactation
Antifungals *(continued)*		
Posaconazole	C	Safety not established, avoid use
Terbinafine	B	Little data available, avoid if possible
Voriconazole	D	Safety not established, avoid use
Antimycobacterials		
Amikacin	D	Probably safe, monitor infant for GI toxicity
Bedaquiline	B	Safety not established, avoid use
Capreomycin	C	Probably safe, monitor infant for GI toxicity
Clofazimine	C	May color breast milk pink; probably safe but avoid if possible
Cycloserine	C	Probably safe
Dapsone	C	Safe
Ethambutol	"safe"	Probably safe
Ethionamide	C	Probably safe with monitoring
Isoniazid	C	Safe
Para-aminosalicylic acid	C	Probably safe
Pyrazinamide	C	Probably safe
Rifabutin	B	Probably safe
Rifampin	C	Probably safe
Rifapentine	C	Probably safe
Streptomycin	D	Probably safe
Thalidomide	X	Safety not established
Antiparasitics		
Albendazole	C	Data limited; one-time dose considered safe by WHO
Artemether/Lumefantrine	C	Data limited; probably safe, particularly if infant weighs at least 5 kg
Atovaquone	C	Data limited; probably safe, particularly if infant weighs at least 5 kg
Atovaquone/Proguanil	C	Data limited; probably safe, particularly if infant weighs at least 5 kg
Benznidazole	avoid	Safe with monitoring
Chloroquine	C	Probably safe with monitoring, but data limited; avoid if possible
Dapsone	C	Safe, but avoid if infant G6PD-deficient
Eflornithine	C	Probably safe, monitor infant for toxicity
Ivermectin	C	Probably safe, monitor infant for toxicity
Mebendazole	C	Probably safe, monitor infant for toxicity
Mefloquine	B	Probably safe, monitor infant for toxicity
Miltefosine	D	Safety not established, avoid use
Nitazoxanide	B	Probably safe with monitoring, but data limited; avoid if possible
Pentamidine	C	Safety not established, avoid use
Praziquantel	B	Probably safe, monitor infant for toxicity
Pyrimethamine	C	Safe with monitoring
Quinidine	C	Probably safe, monitor infant for toxicity
Quinine	X	Probably safe, but avoid if infant G6PD-deficient
Sulfadoxine/Pyrimethamine	C	Little data available, avoid use if possible
Tinidazole	C	Safety not established, avoid use
Antivirals		
Acyclovir	B	Safe with monitoring
Adefovir	C	Safety not established, avoid use if possible
Amantadine	C	Avoid use
Cidofovir	C	Avoid use
Daclatasvir	No human data	Safety not established, avoid use if possible
Entecavir	C	Safety not established, avoid use if possible
Famciclovir	B	Safety not established, avoid use
Foscarnet	C	Safety not established, avoid use
Ganciclovir	C	Safety not established, avoid use
Interferons	C	Probably safe, monitor infant for toxicity
Oseltamivir	C	Probably safe, monitor infant for toxicity
Peramivir	C	Safety not established, avoid use if possible
Ribavirin	X	No data, but probably safe with monitoring
Rimantadine	C	Avoid use
Simeprevir	C (X w/ribavirin)	Safety not established, avoid use if possible
Sofosbuvir	B (X w/ribavirin)	Safety not established, avoid use if possible
Telbivudine	B	Safety not established, avoid use if possible

TABLE 8 (3)

Drug	Risk Category (Old)	Use during Lactation
Antivirals (continued)		
Valacyclovir	B	Safe with monitoring
Valganciclovir	C	Safety not established, avoid use
Zanamivir	C	Probably safe, but no data
Antivirals (hep C combinations)		
Harvoni	B	Safety not established
Technivie	B	Safety not established
Viekira Pak	B	Safety not established
Antiretrovirals		
Abacavir	C	See general statement about antiretrovirals below
Atazanavir	B	See general statement about antiretrovirals below
Darunavir	C	See general statement about antiretrovirals below
Delavirdine	C	See general statement about antiretrovirals below
Didanosine	B	See general statement about antiretrovirals below
Dolutegravir	B	See general statement about antiretrovirals below
Efavirenz	D	See general statement about antiretrovirals below
Elvitegravir	B	See general statement about antiretrovirals below
Emtricitabine	B	See general statement about antiretrovirals below
Enfuvirtide	B	See general statement about antiretrovirals below
Etravirine	B	See general statement about antiretrovirals below
Fosamprenavir	C	See general statement about antiretrovirals below
Indinavir	C	See general statement about antiretrovirals below
Lamivudine	C	See general statement about antiretrovirals below
Lopinavir/r	C	See general statement about antiretrovirals below
Maraviroc	B	See general statement about antiretrovirals below
Nelfinavir	B	See general statement about antiretrovirals below
Nevirapine	B	See general statement about antiretrovirals below
Raltegravir	C	See general statement about antiretrovirals below
Rilpivirine	B	See general statement about antiretrovirals below
Ritonavir	B	See general statement about antiretrovirals below
Saquinavir	B	See general statement about antiretrovirals below
Stavudine	C	See general statement about antiretrovirals below
Tenofovir	B	See general statement about antiretrovirals below
Tipranavir	C	See general statement about antiretrovirals below
Zalcitabine	C	See general statement about antiretrovirals below
Zidovudine	C	See general statement about antiretrovirals below

GENERAL STATEMENT ABOUT ANTIRETROVIRALS
1) HIV-infected mothers are generally discouraged from breastfeeding their infants
2) In settings where breastfeeding is required, country-specific recommendations should be followed.

TABLE 9A – SELECTED PHARMACOLOGIC FEATURES OF ANTIMICROBIAL AGENTS

For pharmacodynamics, see Table 9B; for Cytochrome P450 interactions, see Table 9C. Table terminology key at bottom of each page. Additional footnotes at end of Table 9A, page 98.

DRUG	REFERENCE DOSE (SINGLE OR MULTIPLE)	PREG RISK	FOOD REC (PO DRUGS)[1]	ORAL ABS (%)	PEAK SERUM CONC[2] (µg/mL)	PROTEIN BINDING (%)	VOLUME OF DISTRIBUTION (Vd)[3]	AVG SERUM T½ (hr)[4]	BILE PEN (%)[5]	CSF/BLOOD (%)	CSF PENETRATION[6]	AUC[a] (µg·hr/mL)	Tmax (hr)
ANTIBACTERIALS													
Aminoglycosides													
Amik, Gent, Kana, Tobra	See Table 10D	D			See Table 10D	0-10	0.26 L/kg	2-3	10-60	0-30	No	ND	
Neomycin	po	D	Tab/soln ± food	<3	0	ND	ND	ND	ND	ND	ND	ND	ND
Carbapenems													
Doripenem	500 mg IV	B			23 (SD)	8.1	16.8 L Vss	1	117 (0-611)	ND	ND	36.3	
Ertapenem	1 gm IV	B			154 (SD)	95	0.12 L/kg Vss	4	10	ND	ND	572.1	
Imipenem	500 mg IV	C			40 (SD)	15-25	0.27 L/kg	1	minimal	8.5	Possibly[g]	42.2	
Meropenem	1 gm IV	B			49 (SD)	2	0.29 L/kg	1	3-300	≈ 2	Possibly[g]	72.5	
Cephalosporins (IV)													
Cefazolin	1 gm IV	B			188 (SD)	73-87	0.19 L/kg	1.9	29-300	1-4	No	236	
Cefotetan	1 gm IV	B			158 (SD)	78-91	10.3 L	4.2	2-21			504	
Cefoxitin	1 gm IV	B			110 (SD)	65-79	16.1 L Vss	0.8	280	3	No		
Cefuroxime	1.5 gm IV	B			100 (SD)	33-50	0.19 L/kg Vss	1.5	35-80	17-88	Marginal	150	
Cefotaxime	1 gm IV	B			100 (SD)	30-51	0.28 L/kg	1.5	15-75	10	Yes	70	
Ceftizoxime	1 gm IV	B			60 (SD)	30	0.34 L/kg	1.7	34-82			85	
Ceftriaxone	1 gm IV	B			150 (SD)	85-95	5.6-13.5 L	8	200-500	8-16	Yes	1006	
Cefepime	2 gm IV	B			164 (SD)	20	18 L Vss	2	10-20	10	Yes	284.8	
Ceftazidime	2 gm IV	B			69 (SD)	<10	0.24 L/kg Vss	1.9	13-54	20-40	Yes	127	
Ceftazidime /avibactam	2.5 gm IV q8h	B			Ceftaz 90.4, Avi 14.6 (SS)	Ceftaz <10, Avi 5.7-8.2	Ceftaz 17 L, Avi 22.2 L (Vss)	Ceftaz 2.8, Avi 2.7	ND	ND	ND	Ceftaz 291, Avi 38.2 (8 hr)	
Ceftolozane /tazobactam	1.5 gm IV q8h	B			Ceftolo 74.4, Tazo 18 (SS)	Ceftolo 16-21, Tazo 30	Ceftolo 13.5 L, Tazo 18.2 L (Vss)	Ceftolo 3.1, Tazo 1.0	ND	ND	ND	Ceftolo 182, Tazo 25 (8 hr)	
Ceftaroline	600 mg IV q12h	B			21.3 (SS)	20	20.3 L Vss	2.7	ND	ND	ND	56.3 (12 hr)	
Ceftobiprole[*US]	500 mg IV	B			33-34.2 (SD)	16	18 L Vss	2.9-3.3	ND	ND	ND	116	

Preg Risk: FDA risk categories: **A** = no risk in adequate human studies. **B** = animal studies suggest no fetal risk, but no adequate studies in humans; potential benefit may warrant use despite potential risk. **C** = evidence of fetal risk, but potential benefit may warrant use despite potential risk. **D** = evidence of human risk, but potential benefit may warrant use despite potential risk. **X** = evidence of human risk that clearly exceeds potential benefits. **Food Effect (PO dosing):** **+ food** = take with food. **no food** = take without food. **± food** = take with or without food. **Oral % AB** = % absorbed. **Peak Serum Level: SD** = after single dose. **SS** = steady state after multiple doses. **Volume of Distribution (Vd): V/F** = Vd/oral bioavailability. **Vss** = Vd at steady state/oral bioavailability. **Vss/F** = Vd at steady state/oral bioavailability. **AUC** = area under drug concentration curve; **24hr** = AUC 0-24; **Tmax** = time to max plasma concentration. **CSF Penetration:** therapeutic efficacy comment based on dose, usual susceptibility of target organism & penetration into CSF.

TABLE 9A (2) (Footnotes at the end of table)

DRUG	REFERENCE DOSE (SINGLE OR MULTIPLE)	PREG RISK	FOOD REC (PO DRUGS)[1]	ORAL ABS (%)	PEAK SERUM CONC[2] (µg/mL)	PROTEIN BINDING (%)	VOLUME OF DISTRIBUTION (Vd)[3]	AVG SERUM T½ (hr)[4]	BILE PEN (%)[5]	CSF/BLOOD[6] (%)	CSF PENETRATION[7]	AUC[8] (µg*hr/mL)	Tmax (hr)
Cephalosporins (po)													
Cefadroxil	500 mg po	B	Cap/susp/tab ± food	90	16 (SD)	20	0.31 L/kg V/F	1.5	22			47.4	ND
Cephalexin	500 mg po	B	Cap/tab/susp ± food	90	18 (SD)	5-15	0.38 L/kg V/F	1	216			29	1
Cefaclor	500 mg po	B	Cap/susp ± food	93	13 (SD)	22-25	0.33 L/kg V/F	0.8	≥ 60			20.5	0.5-1.0
Cefaclor ER	500 mg po	B	Tab + food		8.4 (SD)	22-25	0.23 L/kg Vss/F	0.8	≥ 60			18.1	2.5
Cefprozil	500 mg po	B	Tab/susp ± food	95	10.5 (SD)	36	0.66 L/kg V/F	1.5				25.7	1.5
Cefuroxime axetil	250 mg tab po	B	Susp + food, tab ± food	52	4.1 (SD)	50	0.35 L/kg V/F	1.5				12.9	2.5
Cefdinir	300 mg po	B	Cap/susp ± food	25	1.6 (SD)	60-70		1.7				7.1	2.9
Cefditoren pivoxil	400 mg po	B	Tab + food	16	4 (SD)	88	9.3 L Vss/F	1.6				20	1.5-3.0
Cefixime	400 mg po	B	Tab/susp ± food	50	3-5 (SD)	65	0.93 L/kg V/F	3.1	800			25.8	4
Cefpodoxime proxetil	200 mg po	B	Tab + food, Susp ± food	46	2.3 (SD)	40	0.7 L/kg V/F	2.3	115			14.5	2-3
Ceftibuten	400 mg po	B	Cap/susp no food	80	15 (SD)	65	0.21 L/kg V/F	2.4				73.7	2.6
Monobactams													
Aztreonam	1 gm IV	B			90 (SD)	56	12.6 L Vss	2	115-405	3-52	ND	271	
Penicillins													
Benzathine Penicillin G	1.2 million units IM	B			0.15 (SD)								
Penicillin G	2 million units IV	B			20 (SD)	65	0.35 L/kg	0.5	500	5-10	Yes: Pen-sens S pneumo		
Penicillin V	500 mg po	B	Tab/soln ± food	60-73	5-6 (SD)	65		0.5					ND
Amoxicillin	500 mg po	B	Cap/tab/susp ± food	80	5.5-7.5 (SD)	17	0.36 L/kg	1.2	100-3000	13-14	Yes (IV only)	22	1-2
Amoxicillin ER	775 mg po	B	Tab + food		6.6 (SD)	20		1.2-1.5				29.8	3.1
Amox/Clav	875/125 mg po	B	Cap/tab/susp ± food	80/30-98	11.6/2.2 (SD)	18/25	0.36/0.21 (both L/kg)	1.4/1.0	amox 100-3000	ND	ND	26.8/5.1 (0-∞)	ND

Preg Risk: FDA risk categories: A = no risk, B = No risk - human studies, C = toxicity in animals - inadequate human studies, D = human risk, but benefit may outweigh risk, X = fetal abnormalities - risk > benefit; Food Effect (PO dosing): + food = take with food, no food = take without food, ± food = take with or without food; Oral % = % absorbed; SD = after single dose; SS = steady state after multiple doses; Volume of Distribution (Vd): V/F = Vd/oral bioavailability, Vss = Vd at steady state, Vss/F = Vd/oral bioavailability; CSF Penetration: therapeutic efficacy comment based on dose, usual susceptibility of target organism & penetration into CSF; 24hr = AUC 0-24; Tmax = time to max plasma concentration.

TABLE 9A (3) *(Footnotes at the end of table)*

DRUG	REFERENCE DOSE (SINGLE OR MULTIPLE)	PREG RISK	FOOD REC (PO DRUGS)[1]	ORAL ABS (%)	PEAK SERUM CONC[2] (µg/mL)	PROTEIN BINDING (%)[3]	VOLUME OF DISTRIBUTION (Vd)[3]	AVG SERUM T½ (hr)[4]	BILE PEN (%)[5]	CSF/ BLOOD[6] (%)	CSF PENETRATION[7]	AUC[8] (µg·hr/mL)	Tmax (hr)
Penicillins *(continued)*													
Amox/Clav ER	2 tabs [total 2000/125 mg]	B	Tab + food	ND	17/2.1 (SD)	18/25	0.36/0.21 (both L/kg)	1.4/1.0	amox 100-3000	ND	ND	71.6/5.3 (0-∞)	1.5/1.03
Ampicillin	2 gm IV	B			100 (SD)	18-22	0.29 L/kg	1.2	100-3000	13-14	Yes	120/71 (0-∞)	
Amp/Sulb	3 gm IV	B			109-150/ 48-88 (SD)	28/38	0.29/0.3 (both L/kg)	1.4/1.7	amp 100-3000	ND	ND		
Cloxacillin[NUS]	500 mg po	B	Cap no food	50	7.5-14 (SD)	95	0.1 L/kg	0.5	5-8	ND	ND	ND	1-1.5
Dicloxacillin	500 mg po	B	Cap no food	37	10-17 (SD)	98	0.1 L/kg	0.7	>100	ND	ND	18.1 (0-∞)	1-1.5
Nafcillin	500 mg IV	B			30 (SD)	90-94	27.1 L Vss	0.5-1	25	9-20	Yes w/high doses	ND	
Oxacillin	500 mg IV	B	Cap no food	50	43 (SD)	90-94	0.4 L/kg	0.5-0.7	>100	10-15	Yes		
Pip/Tazo	3.375 gm IV	B			242/24 (SD)	16/48	0.24/0.4 (both L/kg)	1/1	>100	ND	ND	242/25	
Fluoroquinolones[10]													
Ciprofloxacin	750 mg po q12h	C	Tab/susp ± food	70	3.6 (SS)	20-40	2.4 L/kg	4	2800-4500		Inadequate for Strep	31.6 (24 hr)	1-2
Ciprofloxacin	400 mg IV q12h	C			4.6 (SS)	20-40	2.4 L/kg	4	2800-4500	26		25.4 (24 hr)	
Ciprofloxacin	500 mg ER po q24h	C	Tab ± food		1.6 (SS)	20-40	2.4 L/kg	6.6				8 (24 hr)	1-4
Gemifloxacin	320 mg po q24h	C	Tab ± food	71	1.6 (SS)	55-73	2-12 L/kg Vss/F	7				9.9 (24 hr)	0.5-2.0
Levofloxacin	750 mg po/IV q24h	C	Tab ± food, soln no food	99	po 8.6, IV 12.1 (SS)	24-38	244 L Vss	7				po 90.7, IV 108 (24 hr)	po 1.6
Moxifloxacin	400 mg po/IV q24h	C	Tab ± food	89	4.2-4.6 (SS)	30-50	2.2 L/kg	10-14		>50	Yes (CID 49:1080, 2009)	po 48, IV 38 (24 hr)	po 1-3
Norfloxacin	400 mg po q12h	C	Tab no food	30-40	1.5 (400 mg SD)	10-15	1.7 L/kg	3-4	700	ND	No	6.4 (400 mg)	1
Ofloxacin	400 mg po q12h	C	Tab ± food	98	4.6-6.2 (SS)	32	1-2.5 L/kg	7		ND		82.4 (24 hr)	1-2
Prulifloxacin[NUS]	600 mg po	ND	Tab ± food	ND	1.6 (SD)	45	1231 L	10.6-12.1		negligible		7.3	1

Preg Risk: FDA risk categories: **A** = no risk, **B** = No risk – human studies, **C** = toxicity in animals – inadequate human studies, **D** = human risk, but benefit may outweigh risk, **X** = fetal abnormalities – risk > benefit; **Food Effect (PO dosing):** ± food = take with or without food, + food = take with food, no food = take without food; **SS** = steady state after multiple doses; **Volume of Distribution (Vd):** V/F = Vd/oral bioavailability, **Vss** = Vd at steady state, **Vss/F** = Vd at steady state/oral bioavailability, **SD** = after single dose; **Peak Serum Level:** SD = after single dose; **CSF Penetration:** therapeutic efficacy comment based on dose, usual susceptibility or target organism & penetration into CSF; **AUC** = area under drug concentration curve; **24hr** = AUC 0-24; **Tmax** = time to max plasma concentration

TABLE 9A (4) *(Footnotes at the end of table)*

DRUG	REFERENCE DOSE (SINGLE OR MULTIPLE)	PREG RISK	FOOD REC (PO DRUGS)[1]	ORAL ABS (%)	PEAK SERUM CONC[2] (μg/mL)	PROTEIN BINDING (%)	VOLUME OF DISTRIBUTION (Vd)[3]	AVG SERUM T½ (hr)[4]	BILE PEN (%)[5]	CSF/ BLOOD[6] (%)	CSF PENETRATION[7]	AUC[8] (μg·hr/mL)	Tmax (hr)
GLYCOPEPTIDES, LIPOGLYCOPEPTIDES, LIPOPEPTIDES													
Dalbavancin	1 gm IV	C			280-300 (SD)	93-98	0.11 L/kg	147-258	ND	ND	ND	23.443	
Daptomycin	4-6 mg/kg IV q24h	B			58-99 (SS)	92	0.1 /kg Vss	8-9	ND	0-8	ND	494-632 (24 hr)	
Oritavancin	1200 mg IV	C			138 (SD)	85	87.6 L	245 (terminal)	ND	ND	ND	2800 (0-∞)	-
Telavancin	6 mg/kg IV	C			40-50 (SD)	90-95	0.9-1.6 L/kg Vss	70-100	ND	negligible	No	500-600 (0-∞)	-
Teicoplanin	10 mg/kg IV q24h	C			108 (SS)	90	0.13 L/kg	8.1	Low			780 (24 hr)	
Vancomycin	1 gm IV q12h	C			20-50 (SS)	<10-55	0.7 L/kg	4-6		7-14	Need high doses	500-600 if trough 20 (24 hr)	
MACROLIDES, AZALIDES, LINCOSAMIDES, KETOLIDES													
Azithromycin	500 mg po	B	Tab/susp ± food	37	0.4 (SD)	7-51	31.1 L/kg	68	High			4.3	2.5
Azithromycin	500 mg IV	B			3.6 (SD)	7-51	33.3 L/kg	68	High			9.6 (24 hr, pre SS)	
Azithromycin ER	2 gm po	B	Susp no food	≈ 30	0.8 (SD)	7-51	31.1 L/kg	59	High			20	5
Clarithromycin	500 mg po q12h	C	Tab/susp ± food	50	3-4 (SS)	65-70	4 L/kg	5-7	7000			20 (24 hr)	2.0-2.5
Clarithromycin ER	1 gm ER po q24h	C	Tab ± food	≈ 50	2-3 (SS)	65-70							5-8
Clindamycin	150 mg po	B	Cap ± food	90	2.5 (SD)	85-94	1.1 L/kg	2.4	250-300		No	ND	0.75
Clindamycin	900 mg IV q8h	B			14.1 (SS)	85-94	1.1 L/kg	2.4	250-300		No	ND	
Erythromycin base, esters	500 mg po	B	Tab/susp no food, DR caps ± food	18-45	0.1-2 (SD)	70-74	0.6 L/kg	2.4		2-13	No		delay rel. 3
Erythromycin lactobionate	500 mg IV	B			3-4 (SS)	70-74	0.6 L/kg	2.4					
Telithromycin	800 mg po q24h	C	Tab ± food	57	2.3 (SS)	60-70	2.9 L/kg	10	7			12.5 (24 hr)	1
MISCELLANEOUS ANTIBACTERIALS													
Chloramphenicol	1 gm po q6h	C	Cap ± food	High	18 (SS)	25-50	0.8 L/kg	4.1		45-89	Yes		
Fosfomycin	3 gm po	C	Sachet ± food	<10	26 (SD)	<10	136 L Vss/F	5.7		ND		150	2
Fusidic acid[AUS]	500 mg po	-	Tab ± food	91	30 (SD)	95-99	0.3 L/kg	15	100-200	ND	ND	442 (0-∞)	2-4

Preg. Risk: FDA risk categories: A = no risk. **B** = No risk in humans. **C** = toxicity in animals - inadequate human studies. **D** = human risk, but benefit may outweigh risk. **X** = fetal abnormalities - risk > benefit. **Food Effect (PO dosing): ± food** = take with or without food. **± food** = take with food. **no food** = take without food. **Oral %** = % absorbed. **Peak Serum Level: SD** = after single dose, **SS** = steady state after multiple doses. **Volume of Distribution (Vd): V/F** = Vd/oral bioavailability. **Vss** = Vd at steady state. **Vss/F** = Vd at steady state/oral bioavailability. **CSF Penetration:** therapeutic efficacy comment based on dose, usual susceptibility or target organism & penetration into CSF. **AUC** = area under drug concentration curve. **24hr** = AUC 0-24; **Tmax** = time to max plasma concentration.

TABLE 9A (5) (Footnotes at the end of table)

DRUG	REFERENCE DOSE (SINGLE OR MULTIPLE)	PREG RISK	FOOD REC (PO DRUGS)[1]	ORAL ABS (%)	PEAK SERUM CONC[2] (µg/mL)	PROTEIN BINDING (%)	VOLUME OF DISTRIBUTION (Vd)[3]	AVG SERUM T½ (hr)[4]	BILE PEN (%)[5]	CSF/BLOOD[6] (%)	CSF PENETRATION[7]	AUC[8] (µg*hr/mL)	Tmax (hr)
MISCELLANEOUS ANTIBACTERIALS (continued)													
Metronidazole	500 mg IV/po q6h	B	ER tab no food, tab/cap ± food	100	20-25 (SS)	20	0.6-0.85 L/kg	6-14	100	45-89		560 (24 hr)	ER 6.8, regular 1.6
Quinupristin-dalfopristin	7.5 mg/kg IV q8h	B			Q 3.2/D 8 (SS)	ND	Q 0.45/D 0.24 (L/kg)	Q 0.85/ 0.7	ND	ND	ND	Q 7.2/D 10.6 (24 hr)	
Rifampin	600 mg po	C	Cap no food	70-90	7 (SD)	80	0.65 L/kg Vss	1.5-5	10.000	7-56	Yes	40-60 (24 hr)	1.5-2
Rifaximin	200 mg po	C	Tab ± food	<0.4	0.0007-0.002 (SS)	67.5	ND	2-5				0.008	1
Trimethoprim	100 mg po	C	Tab ± food	80	1 (SD)	44	100-120 L V/F	8-15			No		1-4
TMP/SMX	160/800 mg po q12h	C	Tab/susp ± food	85	1-2/40-60 (SS)	44/70	100-120 L/ 12-18 L	11/9	100-200	50/40		ND	1-4
TMP/SMX	160/800 mg IV q8h	C			9/105 (SS)	44/70	100-120 L/ 12-18 L	11/9	40-70			ND	
OXAZOLIDINONES													
Linezolid	600 mg po/IV q12h	C	Tab/susp ± food	100	15-20 (SS)	31	40-50 L Vss	5	ND	60-70	Yes (AAC 50:3971, 2006)	po 276, IV 179 (24 hr)	po 1.3
Tedizolid	200 mg po/IV q24h	C	Tab ± food	91	po 2.2, IV 3.0 (SS)	70-90	67-80 L Vss	12	ND	ND	ND	po 25.6, IV 29.2 (24 hr)	po 3, IV 1.1
POLYMYXINS													
Colistin (polymyxin E)	150 mg IV	C			5-7.5 (SD)	≈ 50	0.34 L/kg	colistimethate 1.5-2, colistin >4	0	ND	No		
Polymyxin B	1.5 mg/kg IV q12h	C			2.8 (avg conc at SS)	60	ND	4.5-6 (old data)	ND	ND		66.9 (24 hr)	
TETRACYCLINES, GLYCYLCYCLINES													
Doxycycline	100 mg po	D	Tab/cap/susp + food		1.5-2.1 (SD)	93	53-134 L Vss	18	200-3200	26	No	31.7 (0-∞)	2
Minocycline	200 mg po	D	Cap/tab ± food	ND	2.0-3.5 (SD)	76	80-114 L Vss	16	200-3200	ND	ND	48.3 (0-∞)	2.1
Tetracycline	250 mg po	D	Cap no food	ND	1.5-2.2 (SD)	20-65	1.3 L/kg	6-12	200-3200	Poor	No	30 (0-∞)	2-4
Tigecycline	50 mg IV q12h				0.63 (SD)	71-89	7-9 L/kg	42	138	5.9-10.6	No	4.7 (24 hr)	

Preg Risk: FDA risk categories: **A** = no risk; **B** = No risk - human studies; **C** = toxicity in animals - inadequate human studies - risk > benefit; **D** = human risk, but benefit may outweigh risk; **X** = fetal abnormalities - risk > benefit. **Food Effect (PO dosing):** + **food** = take with food, **no food** = take without food, ± **food** = take with or without food; **Oral % AB** = % absorbed; **Peak Serum Level:** **SD** = after single dose, **SS** = steady state after multiple doses; **Volume of Distribution (Vd):** **V/F** = Vd/oral bioavailability; **Vss** = Vd at steady state. **Vss/F** = Vd at steady state/oral bioavailability; **CSF Penetration:** therapeutic efficacy comment based on dose, usual susceptibility of target organism & penetration into CSF; **24hr** = AUC 0-24; **Tmax** = time to max plasma concentration.

TABLE 9A (6) *(Footnotes at the end of table)*

DRUG	REFERENCE DOSE (SINGLE OR MULTIPLE)	PREG RISK	FOOD REC (PO DRUGS)[1]	ORAL ABS (%)	PEAK SERUM CONC[2] (µg/mL)	PROTEIN BINDING (%)	VOLUME OF DISTRIBUTION (Vd)[3]	AVG SERUM T½ (hr)[4]	BILE PEN (%)[5]	CSF/BLOOD[6] (%)	CSF PENETRATION[7]	AUC[9] (µg*hr/mL)	Tmax (hr)
ANTIFUNGALS													
Polyenes													
Ampho B deoxycholate	0.4-0.7 mg/kg IV q24h	B			0.5-3.5 (SS)		4 L/kg	24		0		17 (24 hr)	
Ampho B lipid complex (ABLC)	5 mg/kg IV q24h	B			1-2.5 (SS)		131 L/kg	173				14 (24 hr)	
Ampho B liposomal	5 mg/kg IV q24h	B			83 (SS)		0.1-0.4 L/kg Vss	6.8				555 (24 hr)	
Antimetabolites													
Flucytosine	2.5 gm po	C	Cap ± food	78-90	30-40 (SD)	ND	0.6 L/kg	3-5		60-100	Yes	ND	2
Azoles													
Fluconazole	400-800 mg po/IV	D	Tab/susp ± food	90	6.7-14 (SD)	10	50 L/F	20-50		50-94	Yes	140 (8 hr) after 3 mg/kg SD	po: 1-2
Isavuconazole	200 mg po/IV q24h (maint)	C	Cap ± food	98	7.5 (SS)	99	450 L Vss	130	ND	ND	ND	121.4 (24 hr)	2-3
Itraconazole	200 mg oral soln po q24h	C	Cap/tab + food, soln no food	55+	Itra 2.0, OH-Itra 2.0 (SS)	99.8	796 L	35	ND	0	ND	Itra 29.3, OH-Itra 45 (24 hr)	Itra 2.5, OH-Itra 5.3
Ketoconazole	200 mg po	C	Tab ± food	variable	3.5 (SD)	99	1.2 L/kg	8	ND	<10	No	12	1-2
Posaconazole oral susp	400 mg po bid	C	Susp + food	ND	0.2-1.0 (200 mg SD)	98-99	226-295 L	20-66	ND	ND	Yes (JAC 56:745, 2005)	9.1 (12 hr)	3-5
Posaconazole tab	300 mg tab po q24h	C	Tab + food	54	2.1-2.9 (SS)	98-99	226-295 L	20-66	ND	ND	Yes (JAC 56:745, 2005)	37.9 (24 hr)	3-5
Posaconazole injection	300 mg IV q24h	C	-	-	3.3 (SS)	98-99	226-295 L	20-66	ND	ND	Yes (JAC 56:745, 2005)	36.1 (24 hr)	1.5
Voriconazole	200 mg IV q12h	D	Tab/susp no food	96	3 (SS)	58	4.6 L/kg Vss	variable	ND	22-100	Yes (CID 37:728, 2003)	39.8 (24 hr)	1-2
Echinocandins													
Anidulafungin	100 mg IV q24h	B			7.2 (SS)	>99	30-50 L	26.5			No	112 (24 hr)	
Caspofungin	50 mg IV q24h	C			8.7 (SS)	97	9.7 L Vss	13	ND		No	87.3 (24 hr)	
Micafungin	100 mg IV q24h	C			10.1 (SS)	>99	0.39 L/kg	15-17			No	97 (24 hr)	

Preg. Risk: FDA risk categories: **A** = no risk, **B** = No risk - human studies, **C** = toxicity in animals - inadequate human studies, **D** = human risk, but benefit may outweigh risk, **X** = fetal abnormalities - risk > benefit; **Food Effect (PO dosing): + food** = take with food, **no food** = take without food, **± food** = take with or without food, **Oral % absorbed**; **SS** = steady state after multiple doses; **Volume of Distribution (Vd): V/F** = Vd/oral bioavailability, **Vss** = Vd at steady state, **Vss/F** = Vd at steady state/oral bioavailability; **Peak Serum Level: SD** = after single dose, **Peak Serum Level; CSF Penetration:** therapeutic efficacy comment based on dose, usual susceptibility of target organism & penetration into CSF; **AUC** = area under drug concentration curve; **24h** = AUC 0-24; **Tmax** = time to max plasma concentration.

TABLE 9A (7) *(Footnotes at the end of table)*

DRUG	REFERENCE DOSE (SINGLE OR MULTIPLE)	PREG RISK	FOOD REC (PO DRUGS)[1]	ORAL ABS (%)	PEAK SERUM CONC[2] (µg/mL)	PROTEIN BINDING (%)	VOLUME OF DISTRIBUTION (Vd)[3]	AVG SERUM T½ (hr)[4]	BILE PEN (%)[5]	CSF/BLOOD[6] (%)	CSF[7] PENETRATION[6]	AUC[4] (µg*hr/mL)	Tmax (hr)
ANTIMYCOBACTERIALS													
First line, tuberculosis													
Ethambutol	25 mg/kg po	C	Tab + food	80	2-6 (SD)	10-30	6 L/kg Vss/F	4		10-50	No	29.6	2-4
Isoniazid (INH)	300 mg po	C	Tab/syrup no food	100	3-5 (SD)	<10	0.6-1.2 L/kg	0.7-4		up to 90	Yes	20.1	1-2
Pyrazinamide	20-25 mg/kg po	C	Tab + food	95	30-50 (SD)	5-10		10-16		100	Yes	500	2
Rifabutin	300 mg po	B	Cap - food	20	0.2-0.6 (SD)	85	9.3 L/kg Vss	32-67	300-500	30-70	ND	4.0 (24 hr)	2.5-4.0
Rifampin	600 mg po	C	Cap no food	70-90	7 (SD)	80	0.65 L/kg Vss	1.5-5	10,000	7-56	Yes	40-60 (24 hr)	1.5-2
Rifapentine	600 mg po q72h	C	Tab + food	ND	15 (SS)	98	70 L	13-14	ND	0-30	ND	320 (72 hr)	4,8
Streptomycin	15 mg/kg IM	D			25-50 (SD)	0-10	0.26 L/kg	2.5	10-60	0-30	No	ND	
Second line, tuberculosis													
Amikacin	15 mg/kg IM	D			25-50 (SD)	0-10	0.26 L/kg	2.5	10-60	0-30	No	ND	
Bedaquiline	400 mg po qd	B	Tab + food	ND	3.3 (week 2)	>99	≈ 60 x total body water Vss	24-30 (terminal 4-5 mo)	ND	ND	ND	22 (24 hr) after 8 wk	5
Capreomycin	1 gm IM	C			30 (SD)	ND	0.4 L/kg	2-5	ND	<10	No	ND	1-2
Cycloserine	250 mg po	C	Cap no food	70-90	4-8 (SD)	<20	0.47 L/kg	10	ND	54-79	Yes	110	1-2
Ethionamide	500 mg po	C	Tab ± food	90	2.2 (SD)	10-30	80 L	1.9	ND	≈100	Yes	10.3	1.5
Kanamycin	15 mg/kg IM	D			25-50 (SD)	0-10	0.26 L/kg	2.5	10-60	0-30	No	ND	
Para-aminosalicylic acid (PAS)	4 g (granules) po	C	Granules + food	ND	9-35 (SD)	50-60	0.9-1.4 L/kg V/F	0.75-1.0	ND	10-50	Marginal	1.08 (4 gm SD, 0-∞)	8
ANTIPARASITICS													
Antimalarials													
Artemether/ lumefantrine	4 tabs (80 mg/480 mg)	C	Tab + food	ND	Art 0.06-0.08, DHA 0.09-0.1, Lum 7.4-9.8 (SD)	Art 95.4, DHA 47-76, Lum 99.7	ND	Art 1.6-2.2, DHA 1.6-2.2, Lum 101-119	ND	ND	ND	Art 0.15-0.26, DHA 0.29, Lum 158-243	Art 1.5-2, Lum 6-8
Artesunate (AS)	120 mg IV	?	-	-	DHA 2.4 (SD)	AS 62-75, DHA 66-82	AS 0.1-0.3, DHA 0.5-1 L/kg	AS 2.4 min, DHA 0.5-1 hr	ND	ND	ND	DHA 2.1 (SD, 0-∞)	25 min (to DHA)

Preg Risk: FDA risk categories: **A** = no risk. **B** = No risk – human studies. **C** = toxicity in animals – inadequate human studies. **D** = human risk, but benefit may outweigh risk – risk > benefit. **Food Effect (PO dosing):** **+ food** = take with food. **no food** = take without food. **± food** = take with or without food. **Oral % AB** = % absorbed. **Peak Serum Level: SD** = after single dose. **SS** = steady state after multiple doses; **Volume of Distribution (Vd): V/F** = Vd/oral bioavailability. **Vss** = Vd at steady state. **Vss/F** = Vd at steady state/oral bioavailability. **CSF Penetration:** therapeutic efficacy comment based on dose, usual susceptibility of target organism & penetration into CSF. **AUC** = area under drug concentration curve; **24hr** = AUC 0-24; **Tmax** = time to max plasma concentration.

TABLE 9A (B) (Footnotes at the end of table)

DRUG	REFERENCE DOSE (SINGLE OR MULTIPLE)	PREG RISK	FOOD REC (PO DRUGS)[1]	ORAL ABS (%)	PEAK SERUM CONC[2] (μg/mL)	PROTEIN BINDING (%)	VOLUME OF DISTRIBUTION (Vd)[3]	AVG SERUM T½ (hr)[3]	BILE PEN (%)[4]	CSF/ BLOOD[5] (%)	CSF PENETRATION[7]	AUC[6] (μg·hr/mL)	Tmax (hr)
ANTIPARASITICS, Antimalarials *(continued)*													
Atovaquone	750 po bid	C	Susp + food	47	24 (SS)	99.9	0.6 L/kg Vss	67	ND	<1	No	801 (750 mg x1)	ND
Chloroquine phosphate	300 mg base	C	Tab + food	90	0.06-0.09 (SD)	55	100-1000 L/kg	45-55 days (terminal)	ND	ND	ND	ND	1-6
Mefloquine	1.25 gm po	B	Tab + food		0.5-1.2 (SD)	98	20 L/kg	13-24 days	ND	ND	ND	ND	17
Proguanil[11]	100 mg po	C	Tab + food	ND	ND	75	1600-2600 L V/f	12-21	ND	ND	ND	ND	ND
Quinine sulfate	648 mg po	C	Cap + food	76-88	3.2 (SD)	69-92	2.5-7.1 L/kg V/f	9.7-12.5	ND	2-7	No	28 (12 hr)	2.8
ANTIPARASITICS, Other													
Albendazole	400 mg po	C	Tab + food		0.5-1.6 (sulfoxide)	70	ND	8-12	ND	ND	ND	ND	2-5 (sulfoxide)
Benznidazole	100 mg po	avoid	Tab + food	92	2.2-2.8	44	89.6 L V/f (newer data) 1.5 L/kg	12-15	ND	ND	ND	ND	3-4
Dapsone	100 mg po q24h	C	Tab ± food	70-100	1.1 (SS)	70	182 L V/F	10-50	ND	ND	No	52.6 (24 hr)	2-6
Diethylcarbamazine	6 mg/kg po	avoid	Tab ± food	80-85	1.93 (SD)	ND	3-3.5 L/kg	9	ND	ND	ND	23.8 (0-∞)	1-2
Ivermectin	12 mg po	C	Tab no food	60	0.05-0.08 (SD)	93	ND	20	ND	No	No		4
Miltefosine	50 mg po tid	D	Cap + food	ND	76 (diff at 23 days)	95	ND	7-31 days	ND	ND	ND	486	2.8
Nitazoxanide	500 mg po	B	Tab/susp + food	Susp 70% of tab	Tizox 9-11, gluc 7.3-10.5 (SD)	Tizox 99	ND	Tizox 1.3-1.8	ND	ND	ND	Tizox 40, gluc 46.5-63.0	Tizox, gluc: 1-4
Praziquantel	20 mg/kg po	B	Tab + food	80	0.2-2.0 (SD)	87	8000 L V/f	0.8-1.5	ND	ND	ND	1.51	1-3
Pyrimethamine	25 mg po	C	Tab ± food	High	0.1-0.3 (SD)	87	3 L/kg	96	ND	ND	ND	ND	2-6
Tinidazole	2 gm po	C	Tab/soln ± food	48	48 (SD)	12	50 L	13	ND	ND	ND	902	1.6
ANTIVIRALS (non-HIV)													
Hepatitis B													
Adefovir	10 mg po	C	Tab ± food	59	0.02 (SD)	≤4	0.37 L/kg Vss	7.5	ND	ND	ND	0.22 (24 hr)	1.75
Entecavir	0.5 mg po q24h	C	Tab/soln no food	100	4.2 ng/mL (SS)	13	>0.6 L/kg V/F	128-149 (terminal)	ND	ND	ND	0.014 (24 hr)	0.5-1.5
Telbivudine	600 mg po q24h	B	Tab/soln ± food		3.7 (SS)	3.3	>0.6 L/kg V/F	40-49	ND	ND	ND	26.1 (24 hr)	2

Preg Risk: FDA risk categories: **A** = no risk, **B** = No risk - human studies, **C** = toxicity in animals - inadequate human studies, **D** = human risk, but benefit may outweigh risk, **X** = fetal abnormalities – risk > benefit. **Food Effect (PO dosing):** ± **food** = take with food, **no food** = take without food, ± **food** = take with or without food. **Oral % AB** = % absorbed. **Peak Serum Level: SD** = after single dose. **SS** = steady state after multiple doses; **Volume of Distribution (Vd): V/F** = Vd/oral bioavailability. **Vss** = Vd at steady state. **Vss/F** = Vd/oral bioavailability. **CSF Penetration:** therapeutic efficacy comment based on dose, usual susceptibility of target organism & penetration into CSF. **AUC** = area under drug concentration curve; **24H** = AUC 0-24, **Tmax** = time to max plasma concentration.

TABLE 9A (9) *(Footnotes at the end of table)*

DRUG	REFERENCE DOSE (SINGLE OR MULTIPLE)	PREG RISK	FOOD REC (PO DRUGS)[1]	ORAL ABS (%)	PEAK SERUM CONC[2] (μg/mL)	PROTEIN BINDING (%)[3]	VOLUME OF DISTRIBUTION (Vd)[3]	AVG SERUM T½ (hr)[3]	BILE PEN (%)[4]	CSF/ BLOOD (%)[5]	CSF PENETRATION[7]	AUC[6] (μg*hr/mL)	Tmax (hr)
Hepatitis C													
Daclatasvir	60 mg po q24h		Tab ± food	67	0.18 (Cmin, SS)	99	47 Vss	12-15	ND	ND	ND	11 (24 hr)	2
Dasabuvir	250 mg po q12h	B	Tab + food	ND	0.03-3.1 (10-1200 mg SD)	ND	ND	5-8	ND	ND	ND	ND	3
Ledipasvir + Sofosbuvir	(90 mg + 400 mg) po q24h	B	Tab ± food	ND	Ledip: 0.3 (SS)	Ledip: >99.8	ND	Ledip:47	ND	ND	ND	Ledip: 7.3 (24hr)	Ledip: 4-4.5
Ombitasvir + Paritaprevir (RTV)	25 mg po q24h	B	Tab + food	77	0.56 (SS)	ND	ND	28-34	ND	ND	ND	0.53 (24 hr)	4-5
Paritaprevir/RTV (with Ombitasvir)	150 mg (+ RTV 100 mg) po q24h	B	Tab + food		ND	ND	ND	5.8	ND	ND	ND	ND	4,3
Ribavirin	600 mg po	X	Tab/cap/soln + food	64	3.7 (SS)	minimal	2825 L V/F	44 (terminal 298)	ND	ND	ND	228 (12 hr)	2
Simeprevir	150 mg po	C	Cap + food	ND	ND	>99.9	ND	41	ND	ND	ND	57.5 (24 hr)	4-6
Sofosbuvir	400 mg po q24h	B	Tab ± food	ND	Sofos: 0.6 (SS)	Sofos: 61-65	ND	Sofos: 0.5-0.75	ND	ND	ND	Sofos: 0.9 (24 hr)	0.5-2
Herpesvirus													
Acyclovir	400 mg po bid	B	Tab/susp ± food	10-20	1.21 (SS)	9-33	0.7/kg	2.5-3.5	ND	ND	ND	7.4 (24 hr)	1.5-2
Cidofovir (w/probenecid)	5 mg/kg IV	C	Probenecid: ± food	ND	19.6 (SD)	<6	0.41 L/kg Vss	2.6 (diphosphate: 17-65)	ND	0	No	40.8	1,1
Famciclovir	500 mg po	B	Tab ± food	77	3-4 (SD)	<20	1.1 L/kg (Penciclovir)	2-3 (Penciclovir)	ND	ND	ND	8.9 (Penciclovir)	0.9 (Penciclovir)
Foscarnet	60 mg/kg IV	C			155 (SD)	4	0.46 L/kg	3 (terminal 18-88)	No	ND	ND	2195 μM*hr	
Ganciclovir	5 mg/kg IV	C			8.3 (SD)	1-2	0.7 L/kg Vss	3	ND	ND	ND	24.5	
Valacyclovir	1 grm po	B	Tab ± food	55	5.6 (SD)	13-18	0.7 L/kg	3	ND	ND	ND	19.5 (Acyclovir)	
Valganciclovir	900 mg po q24h	C	Tab/soln + food	59	5.6 (SS)	1-2	0.7 L/kg	4	ND	ND	ND	29.1 (Ganciclo)	1-3 (Ganciclo)
Influenza													
Oseltamivir	75 mg po bid	C	Cap/susp ± food	75	carboxylate 0.35 (SS)	3	carboxylate 23-26 L	carboxylate 6-10	ND	ND	ND	carboxylate 5.4 (24 hr)	
Peramivir	600 mg IV	C			46.8 (SD)	<30	12.56 L	25		ND	ND	102.7 (0-∞)	
Rimantadine	100 mg po q12h	C	Tab ± food	75-93	0.4-0.5 (SS)	40	17-19/kg	25	ND		ND	3.5	6

Preg Risk: FDA risk categories: A = no risk. **B** = No risk in animals. **C** = toxicity in animals. **D** = human risk, but benefit may outweigh risk. **X** = fetal abnormalities – risk > benefit. **Food Effect (PO dosing): + food** = take with food. **no food** = take without food. **± food** = take with or without food. **Oral Abs % = AB** = % absorbed. **Peak Serum Level: SD** = after single dose. **SS** = steady state after multiple doses. **Volume of Distribution (Vd): V/F** = Vd/oral bioavailability. **Vss** = Vd at steady state. **CSF Penetration:** therapeutic efficacy comment based on dose, usual susceptibility or target organism & penetration into CSF. **AUC** = area under drug concentration curve. **24hr** = AUC 0-24. **Tmax** = time to max plasma concentration.

DRUG	REFERENCE DOSE (SINGLE OR MULTIPLE)	PREG RISK	FOOD REC (PO DRUGS)	ORAL ABS (%)	PEAK SERUM CONC (μg/mL)	PROTEIN BINDING (%)	VOLUME OF DISTRIBUTION (Vd)	AVG SERUM T½ (hr)	INTRACEL L T½ (HR)	CPE¹²	CSF/BLOOD (%)	AUC (μg*hr/mL)	Tmax (hr)
ANTIRETROVIRALS													
NRTIs													
Abacavir (ABC)	600 mg po q24h	C	Tab/soln ± food	83	4.3 (SS)	50	0.86 L/kg	1.5	20.6	3	36	12 (24 hr)	1,3
Didanosine enteric coated (ddI)	400 mg EC po q24h (pt ≥60 kg)	B	Cap/soln no food	30-40	ND	<5	308-363 L	1.6	25-40	3	ND	2.6(24 hr)	2
Emtricitabine (FTC)	200 mg po q24h	B	Cap/soln ± food	cap 93, soln 75	1.8 (SS)	<4	ND	10	39	3	ND	10 (24 hr)	1-2
Lamivudine (3TC)	300 mg po q24h	C	Tab/soln ± food	86	2.6 (SS)	<36	1.3 L/kg	5-7	18	2	ND	11 (300 mg x1)	ND
Stavudine (d4T)	30 mg po bid (pt ≥60 kg)	C	Cap/soln ± food	86	0.54 (SS)	<5	46 L	1.2-1.6	3.5	2	20	2.6 (24 hr)	1
Tenofovir (TDF)	300 mg po q24h	B	Tab ± food	39 w/food	0.3 (300 mg x1)	<7	1.2-1.3 L/kg Vss	17	>60	1	ND	2.3 (300 mg x1)	1
Zidovudine (ZDV)	300 mg po bid	C	Tab/cap/syrup ± food	60	1-2 (300 mg x1)	<38	1.6 L/kg	0.5-3	11	4	2	2.1 (300 mg x1)	0.5-1.5
NNRTIs													
Delavirdine (DLV)	400 mg po tid	C	Tab ± food	85	19 (SS)	98	ND	5.8	ND	3	ND	180 μM*hr (24 hr)	1
Efavirenz (EFV)	600 mg po q24h	D	Cap/tab no food	42	4.1 (SS)	99	252 L/F	40-55	ND	3	ND	184 μM*hr (24 hr)	3-5
Etravirine (ETR)	200 mg po bid	B	Tab + food	>90	0.3 (SS)	99.9	ND	41	ND	4	ND	9 (24 hr)	2.5-4.0
Nevirapine (NVP)	200 mg po bid	B	Tab/susp ± food	>90	2 (200 mg x1)	60	1.21 L/kg Vss	25-30	ND	4	63	110 (24 hr)	2.5-4.0
Rilpivirine (RPV)	25 mg po qd	B	Tab + food	ND	0.1-0.2 (25 mg x1)	99.7	152 L	45-50	ND	ND	ND	2.4 (24 hr)	4-5
PIs													
Atazanavir (ATV)	400 mg po q24h	B	Cap/powder + food	Good	2.3 (SS)	86	88.3 L/F	7	ND	2	ND	22.3 (24 hr)	2.5
Cobicistat	150 mg po q24h	B	Take with food	ND	0.99 (SS)	97-98	ND	4-Mar	ND	ND	ND	7.6 (24 hr)	3.5
Darunavir (DRV)	600 mg (+ RTV 100 mg) po bid	C	Tab/susp + food	82	3.5 (SS)	95	2 L/kg	15	ND	3	ND	116.8 (24 hr)	2.5-4.0
Fosamprenavir (FPV)	700 mg (+RTV 100 mg) po bid	C	Tab ± food, susp adult no. peds ±	ND	6 (SS)	90	ND	7.7	ND	3	ND	79.2 (24 hr)	2.5
Indinavir (IDV)	800 mg (+ RTV 100 mg) po bid	C	Boosted cap + food	65	20.2 μM (SS)	60	ND	1.2-2.0	ND	4	11	249 μM*hr (24 hr)	0.8 (fasting)
Lopinavir/RTV	400 mg/100 mg po bid	C	Tab ± food, soln + food	ND	9.6 (SS)	98-99	ND	LPV 5-6	ND	3	ND	LPV 186 (24 hr)	LPV 4

Preg Risk: FDA risk categories: A = no risk. **B** = No risk - human studies, **C** = toxicity in animals - inadequate human studies, **D** = human risk, but benefit may outweigh risk - risk > benefit. **Food Effect for PO Drugs:** + food = take with food. **no food** = take without food. ± food = take with or without food. **Oral % AB** = % absorbed. **Peak Serum Level: SD** = after single dose. **SS** = steady state. **Volume of Distribution (Vd): V/F** = Vd/oral bioavailability. **Vss** = Vd at steady state. **CSF Penetration:** therapeutic & penetration into CSF. **AUC** = AUC 0-24; **24hr** = AUC 0-24. **Tmax** = time to max plasma concentration. **CPE¹²** = CNS penetration-effectiveness. efficacy comment based on dose, usual susceptibility of target organism or usual susceptibility or target organism.

TABLE 9A (11) (Footnotes at the end of table)

DRUG	REFERENCE DOSE (SINGLE OR MULTIPLE)	PREG RISK	FOOD REC (PO DRUGS)	ORAL ABS (%)	PEAK SERUM CONC (µg/mL)	PROTEIN BINDING (%)	VOLUME OF DISTRIBUTION (Vd)	AVG SERUM T½ (hr)	INTRACEL L T½ (HR)	CPE[12]	CSF/BLOOD (%)	AUC (µg*hr/mL)	Tmax (hr)
PIs (continued)													
Nelfinavir (NFV)	1250 mg po bid	B	Tab/powder + food	20-80	3-4 (SS)	98	2-7 L/kg V/F	3.5-5	ND	1	0	53 (24 hr)	ND
Ritonavir (RTV)	Boosting dose varies	B	Cap/soln + food	65	11.2 (600 mg bid SS)	98-99	0.41 L/kg V/F	3-5	ND	1	ND	121.7 (600 mg soln SD)	soln 2-4
Saquinavir (SQV)	1 gm (+RTV 100 mg) po bid	B	Tab/cap + food	4 (SQV alone)	0.37 (SS)	97	700 L Vss	1-2	ND	1	ND	29.2 (24 hr)	ND
Tipranavir (TPV)	500 mg (+RTV 200 mg) po bid	C	Cap/soln + food	Low	47-57 (SS)	99.9	7.7-10 L	5.5-6	ND	1	ND	1600 µM*hr (24 hr)	3
INSTIs													
Dolutegravir (DTG)	50 mg po q24h	B	Tab ± food	ND	3.67 (SS)	>99	17.4 L V/F	14	ND	4	ND	53.6 (24 hr)	2-3
Elvitegravir (EVG)	85-150 mg po q24h	B	Tab + food	ND	1.2-1.5 (SS)	98-99	ND	8.7 (w/RTV)	ND	ND	ND	18 (24 hr)	4
Raltegravir (RAL)	400 mg po bid	C	Tab/susp ± food	ND	11.2 µM (SS)	83	287 L Vss/F	9	ND	3	1-53.5	28.7 µM*hr (12 hr)	3
Fusion, Entry Inhibitors													
Enfuvirtide (ENF, T20)	90 mg sc bid	B		84 (sc % ab)	5 (SS)	92	5.5 L Vss	3.8	ND	1	ND	97.4 (24 hr)	4-8
Maraviroc (MVC)	300 mg po bid	B	Tab ± food	33	0.3-0.9 (SS)	76	194 L	14-18	ND	3	ND	3 (24 hr)	0.5-4.0

Preg Risk: FDA risk categories: A = no risk. **B** = No risk - human studies, **C** = toxicity in animals - inadequate human studies, **D** = human risk, but benefit may outweigh risk, **X** = fetal abnormalities - risk > benefit; **Food Effect (PO dosing): + food** = take with food, **no food** = take without food, **± food** = take with or without food; **Oral % AB** = % absorbed; **Peak Serum Level; SD** = after single dose, **SS** = steady state after multiple doses, **Volume of Distribution (Vd): V/F** = Vd/oral bioavailability, **Vss** = Vd at steady state, **Vss/F** = Vd at steady state/oral bioavailability; **CSF Penetration:** therapeutic efficacy comment based on dose, usual susceptibility, or target exposure & penetration into CSF; **AUC** = area under the curve.

1 Refers to adult oral preparations unless otherwise noted; **+ food** = take with food, **no food** = take without food, **± food** = take with or without food
2 SD = after a single dose, SS = at steady state
3 V/F = Vd/oral bioavailability, Vss = Vd at steady state, Vss/F = Vd at steady state/oral bioavailability
4 Assumes CrCl >80 mL/min
5 (Peak concentration in serum) x 100. If blank, no data.
6 CSF concentrations with inflammation.
7 CSF concentrations.
8 Judgment based on drug dose and organism susceptibility. CSF concentration ideally ≥ 10x MIC.
9 AUC = area under serum concentration vs. time curve. 12 hr = AUC 0-12, 24 hr = AUC 0-24
10 Concern over seizure potential (see Table 10B)
11 Take all FQs 2-4 hours before sucralfate or any multivalent cation (calcium, iron, zinc).
11 Given with atovaquone as Malarone for malaria prophylaxis
12 CPE (CNS Penetration Effectiveness) value: 1=low penetration, 2-3=intermediate penetration, 4=highest penetration (Letendre et al, CROI 2010, abs #430)

TABLE 9B – PHARMACODYNAMICS OF ANTIBACTERIALS*

BACTERIAL KILLING/PERSISTENT EFFECT	DRUGS	THERAPY GOAL	PK/PD MEASUREMENT
Concentration-dependent/Prolonged persistent effect	Aminoglycosides; daptomycin; ketolides, quinolones, metro	High peak serum concentration	24-hr AUC²/MIC
Time-dependent/No persistent effect	Penicillins; cephalosporins; carbapenems; monobactams	Long duration of exposure	Time above MIC
Time-dependent/Moderate to long persistent effect	Clindamycin; erythro/azithro/clarithro; linezolid; tetracyclines; vancomycin	Enhanced amount of drug	24-hr AUC²/MIC

* Adapted from Craig, WA. IDC No. Amer 17:479, 2003 & Drusano, G.L. CID 44:79, 2007

TABLE 9C– ENZYME -AND TRANSPORTER- MEDIATED INTERACTIONS OF ANTIMICROBIALS

DRUG	ISOZYME/TRANSPORTER THAT DRUG IS A SUBSTRATE OF	INHIBITED BY DRUG	INDUCED BY DRUG	IMPACT ON SERUM DRUG CONCENTRATIONS*
Antibacterials				
Azithromycin	PGP	PGP (weak)		mild ↑
Chloramphenicol		2C19, 3A4		↑
Ciprofloxacin		1A2; 3A4 (minor)		↑
Clarithromycin	3A4	3A4, PGP, OAT		↑
Erythromycin	3A4, PGP	3A4, PGP, OAT		↑
Levofloxacin		OCT		↑
Metronidazole		2C9		↑
Nafcillin			2C9 (?), 3A4	
Norfloxacin		1A2 (weak)		mild ↑
Oritavancin		2C9 (weak), 2C19 (weak)	2D6 (weak), 3A4 (weak)	mild ↑ or ↓
Quinupristin–Dalfopristin		3A4		↓
Rifampin	PGP	OAT	1A2; 2B6; 2C8, 2C9, 2C19, 2D6 (weak); 3A4, PGP	↓
Telithromycin		3A4, PGP (?)		↑
TMP/SMX	SMX: 2C9 (major), 3A4	TMP: 2C8; SMX: 2C9		↑
Trimethoprim		2C8		↑
Antifungals				
Fluconazole		2C9, 2C19, 3A4		↑
Isavuconazole	3A4	3A4, PGP, OCT2		↑
Itraconazole	3A4	3A4, PGP		↑
Ketoconazole	3A4	3A4, PGP		↑
Posaconazole	PGP	3A4, PGP		↑
Terbinafine		2D6		↑
Voriconazole	2C9, 2C19, 3A4	2C9, 2C19, 3A4		↑

TABLE 9C (2)

DRUG	Substrate	Inhibits	Induces	Impact
Antimycobacterials (Rifampin listed above)				
Bedaquiline	3A4			
Isoniazid (INH)	2E1	2C19, 3A4		↑
Rifabutin	3A4		3A4	↑
Rifapentine			2C9, 3A4	↑
Thalidomide	2C19			
Antiparasitics				
Artemether/Lumefantrine	3A4 (Art, Lum)	2D6 (Lum)	3A4 (Art)	↑ or ↓
Chloroquine	2C8, 2D6	2D6		↑
Dapsone	3A4			
Halofantrine	3A4	2D6		↑
Mefloquine	3A4, PGP	PGP		↑
Praziquantel	3A4			
Proguanil	2C19 (→cycloguanil)			
Quinine sulfate	main 3A4; also 1A2, 2C9, 2D6	2D6		
Tinidazole	3A4			
Antivirals (hepatitis C)				
Daclatasvir	3A4, PGP			-
Dasabuvir	3A4, PGP, OATP1B1	2C8, UGT1A1, OATP1B1, OATP1B3		↑
Ledipasvir	PGP, BCRP	PGP, BCRP		↑
Ombitasvir	3A4, PGP	2C8, UGT1A1		↑
Paritaprevir	2C8, 2D6, 3A4, PGP	UGT1A1, OATP1B1		
Simeprevir	3A4, PGP, OAT	1A2 (weak), 3A4, PGP, OAT		↑
Sofosbuvir	PGP, BCRP			
Antivirals (herpesvirus)				
Cidofovir	OAT1, OAT3			

TABLE 3C (5)

DRUG	Substrate	Inhibits	Induces	Impact
Antiretrovirals				
Atazanavir	3A4	1A2, 2C8, 3A4, UGT1A1		↑
Cobicistat (part of Stribild)	2D6, 3A4	2D6, 3A4, PGP, BCRP, OATP1B1, OATP1B3		↑
Darunavir	3A4	3A4		↑
Delavirdine	2D6, 3A4	2C9, 2C19, 3A4		↑
Dolutegravir	3A4, UGT1A1			
Efavirenz	2B6, 3A4	2B6, 2C9, 2C19	2C19, 3A4	↑ or ↓
Elvitegravir (part of Stribild)	CYP3A4, UGT1A1/3	PGP (weak)	2C9 (weak)	mild ↑ or ↓
Etravirine	2C9, 2C19, 3A4	2C9, 2C19 (weak)	3A4	↑ or ↓
Fosamprenavir	3A4	3A4, PGP		↑
Indinavir	3A4, PGP	3A4		↑
Lopinavir	3A4	3A4		↑
Maraviroc	3A4, PGP	2D6		↓
Nelfinavir	2C9, 2C19, 3A4, PGP	3A4, PGP	3A4	↑ or ↓
Nevirapine	2B6, 3A4		3A4	↓
Raltegravir	UGT			
Rilpivirine	3A4			
Ritonavir	3A4, PGP	2D6, 3A4, PGP	long term (?): 1A2, 2B6, 2C9, 3A4, PGP	↑ or ↓
Saquinavir	3A4, PGP	3A4, PGP		↑
Tipranavir	3A4, PGP	1A2, 2C9, 2C19, 2D6	3A4, PGP (weak)	↑ or ↓

*Refers to serum concentrations of companion drugs that may be affected by the listed antimicrobial. ↑=increase, ↓=decrease, blank=no drugs should be affected

TERMINOLOGY:

BCRP = breast cancer resistance protein
CYP450 nomenclature, e.g. 3A4: 3 = family, A = subfamily, 4 = gene
OAT = organic anion transporter
OATP = organic anion transporter polypeptide
OCT = organic cation transporter
PGP = P-glycoprotein
UGT = uridine diphosphate glucuronosyltransferase

REFERENCES:

Hansten PD, Horn JR. The Top 100 Drug Interactions: A Guide to Patient Management. Freeland (WA): H&H Publications, 2014; primary literature; package inserts.

TABLE 10A – ANTIBIOTIC DOSAGE* AND SIDE-EFFECTS

CLASS, AGENT GENERIC NAME (TRADE NAME)	USUAL ADULT DOSAGE*	ADVERSE REACTIONS, COMMENTS (See Table 10B for Summary)
NATURAL PENICILLINS		**Allergic reactions a major issue.** 10% of all hospital admissions give history of pen allergy; but only 10% have allergic reaction if given penicillin. Why? Possible reasons: inaccurate history, waning immunity with age, aberrant response during viral illness. If given, **Bicillin C-R IM (procaine Pen + benzathine Pen)** could be reaction to procaine. **Most serious reaction is anaphylaxis:** incidence only 0.05% but 5-10% fatal. Other IgE-mediated reactions: urticaria, angioedema, laryngeal edema, bronchospasm, abdominal pain with emesis, or chain. **Morbilliform rash after 72 hrs is not IgE-mediated and not serious.**
Benzathine penicillin G (Bicillin L-A)	600,000–1.2 million units IM q2-4 wks	
Penicillin G	Low: 600,000-1.2 million units IM per day High: ≥20 million units IV q24h (=12 gm) div q4h	
Penicillin V (250 & 500 mg caps)	0.25–0.5 gm po bid, tid, qid before meals & at bedtime. Pen V preferred over Pen G for oral therapy due to greater acid stability.	**Serious late allergic reactions:** Coombs-positive hemolytic anemia, neutropenia, thrombocytopenia, serum sickness, interstitial nephritis, hepatitis, eosinophilia, drug fever. **Cross-allergy to cephalosporins and carbapenems** varies from 0-11%. One factor is similarity, or lack of similarity, of side chains. **For pen desensitization,** see Table 7. For skin testing, suggest referral to allergist. **High CSF** concentrations cause seizures. Reduce dosage with renal impairment, see Table 17A. Allergy refs: AJM 121:572, 2008; CID 59:1113, 2014; NEJM 354-601, 2006; CID 39:20-43, 2014.
PENICILLINASE-RESISTANT PENICILLINS		
Dicloxacillin (Dynapen) (250 & 500 mg caps)	0.125–0.5 gm po q6h before meals	Blood levels ~2 times greater than cloxacillin so preferred for po therapy. Acute hemorrhagic cystitis reported. Acute abdominal pain with GI bleeding without antibiotic-associated colitis also reported.
Flucloxacillin[3] (Floxapen, Lutropin, Staphcil)	0.25–0.5 gm po q6h 1-2 gm IV q4h	Cholestatic hepatitis occurs in 1:15,000 exposures: more frequently in age > 55 yrs, females and therapy > 2 wks duration. Can appear up to several wks after end of therapy and take wks to resolve (JAC 66:1431, 2011). **Recommendation: use only in severe infection.**
Nafcillin (Unipen, Nafcil)	1-2 gm IV/IM q4h. Due to > 90% protein binding, need 12 gm/day for bacteremia.	Extravasation can result in tissue necrosis. With dosages ≥ 200-300 mg/kg/day hypokalemia may occur. **Reversible neutropenia** (over 10% with ≥21-day rx, occasionally WBC <1000 per mm³).
Oxacillin (Prostaphlin)	1-2 gm IV/IM q4h. Due to > 90% protein binding, need 12 gm/day for bacteremia.	**Hepatic dysfunction** (with ≥12 gm per day. LFTs usually 1 2-24 days after start rx, reversible. In children, more rash and liver toxicity with oxacillin as compared to nafcillin (CID 34:50, 2002)
AMINOPENICILLINS		
Amoxicillin (Amoxil, Polymox)	250 mg–1 gm po tid	IV available in UK & Europe. IV amoxicillin rapidly converted to ampicillin. Rash with infectious mono– see Ampicillin. Increased risk of cross-allergenicity with oral cephalosporins with identical side-chains; cefadroxil, cefprozil. Allergic reactions, C. difficile associated diarrhea, false positive test for urine glucose with clinitest.
Amoxicillin extended release (Moxatag)	One 775 mg tab po once daily	
Amoxicillin-clavulanate (Augmentin) AM-CL extra-strength peds suspension (ES-600) AM-CL-ER—extended release adult tabs	See Comment for adult products. Peds Extra-Strength susp: 600/42.9 per 5 mL Dose: 90/6.4 mg/kg div bid. For adult formulations, see Comments IV amox-clav available in Europe	With bid regimen, less diarrhea & less GI upset. In pts with immediate allergic reaction to AM-CL, ⅔ due to Clav component. (Allergy Immunol 125:502, 2011). Positive blood tests for 1,3-beta D-glucan (with IV AM-CL (NEJM 354:2834, 2006). Hepatotoxicity linked to clavulanic acid. AM-CL causes 13-23% of drug-induced liver injury. Onset delayed. Usually mild; rare liver failure (JAC 66:1431, 2011). **Comparison adult Augmentin dosage regimens:** Augmentin 500/125 1 tab po tid Augmentin 875/125 1 tab po bid Augmentin-XR 1000/62.5 2 tabs po bid A maculopapular rash occurs (not urticaria), **not true penicillin allergy,** in 65-100% pts with infectious mono, 90% with chronic lymphocytic leukemia, and 15-20% in pts taking allopurinol. EBV-associated rash does not indicate permanent allergy; post-EBV no rash when challenged. Increased risk of true cross-allergenicity with oral cephalosporins with identical side chains; cephalexin, cefaclor
Ampicillin (Principen) (250 & 500 mg caps)	0.25–0.5 gm po q6h. 50–200 mg/kg IV/day.	

*NOTE: all dosage recommendations are for adults (unless otherwise indicated) & assume normal renal function. (See page 2 for abbreviations)

TABLE 10A (4)

CLASS, AGENT, GENERIC NAME (TRADE NAME)	USUAL ADULT DOSAGE*	ADVERSE REACTIONS, COMMENTS (See Table 10B for Summary)
AMINOPENICILLINS (continued)		
Ampicillin-sulbactam (Unasyn)	**1.5–3 gm IV q6h; for Acinetobacter: 3 gm (Amp 2 gm/Sulb 1 gm) IV q4h**	Supplied in vials: ampicillin 1 gm, sulbactam 0.5 gm or amp 2 gm, sulbactam 1 gm. AM-SB is not active vs pseudomonas. Total daily dose evaluated ≤4 gm. Increasing resistance of aerobic gram-negative bacilli. Subactam doses up to 9–12 gm/day evaluated (J Infect 56:432, 2008). See also CID 50:133, 2010.
ANTIPSEUDOMONAL PENICILLINS		
Piperacillin-tazobactam (PIP-TZ) (Zosyn) Prolonged infusion dosing, see Comment and Table 10E. Obesity dosing, see Table 17C.	**Formulations:** PIP/TZ: 2/0.25 gm (2.25 gm) PIP/TZ: 3/0.375 gm (3.375 gm) PIP/TZ: 4/0.5 gm (4.5 gm) **Standard Dose (no P. aeruginosa):** 3.375 gm IV q6h or 4.5 gm IV q8h **Standard Dose for P. aeruginosa:** 3.375 gm IV q4h or 4.5 gm IV q6h	Based on PK/PD studies, there is emerging evidence in support of **prolonged infusion** of PIP-TZ: Initial "loading" dose of 4.5 gm over 30 min, then, 4 hrs later, start 3.375 gm IV over 4 hrs q 8h (CrCl≥ 20) or 3.375 gm IV over 4 hrs q12h (CrCl<20) (CID 44:357, 2007; AAC 54:460, 2010). • Cystic fibrosis + P. aeruginosa infection: 350-450 mg/kg/day div q4-6h • P. aeruginosa pneumonia: PIP-TZ or CIP or Tobra. If dosed correctly, no need for dual therapy. Misc: Assoc false-pos galactomannan test for aspergillus, thrombocytopenia 2.79 mEq Na+ per gram of PIP. For obesity dosing adjustment see Table 17C., page 229. In critically ill pts, may contribute to thrombocytopenia (PLoS One 8(11):e81477).
Temocillin[AUS]	2 gm IV q12h.	Semi-synthetic penicillin stable in presence of classical & ESBLs plus AmpC beta-lactamases. Source: www.eumedica.be
CARBAPENEMS. Review: AAC 55:4943, 2011. NOTE: Cross allergenicity: **In studies of pts with history of Pen-allergy but no confirmatory skin testing, 0–11% had allergic reactions with cephalosporin therapy** (JAC 54:1155, 2004). In better studies, pts with positive skin tests for Pen allergy were given Carbapenem: **no reaction in 99%** (J Allergy Clin Immunol 124:167, 2009). Of 12 pts with IgE-mediated reaction to ceph. 2 suffered rash & 1 an IgE reaction when given a carbapenem (CID 53:1113, 2014). Incidence of carbapenem-resistant GNB highest in Georgia, Maryland & New York (JAMA 314:1455 & 1479, 2015).		
Doripenem (Doribax) Ref: CID 49:291, 2009. For prolonged infusion dosing, see Table 10E	Intra-abdominal & complicated UTI: **500 mg IV q8h (1-hr infusion).** For prolonged infusion, see Table 10E, page 119. Do not use for pneumonia	Most common adverse reactions (≥5%): Headache, nausea, diarrhea, rash & phlebitis. Seizure reported in post-marketing surveillance. Can lower serum valproic acid levels. Adjust dose in renal impairment. Somewhat more stable in solution than IMP or MER (AAC 65:1023, 2010; CID 49:291, 2009). FDA safety announcement (01/05/12): Trial of DORI for the treatment of VAP stopped early due to safety concerns. Compared to IMP, patients treated with DORI were observed to have excess mortality and poorer cure rate. **NOTE: DORI is not approved to treat any type of pneumonia; DORI is not approved for doses greater than 500 mg q8h.**
Ertapenem (Invanz)	1 gm IV/IM q24h.	**Lidocaine** diluent for IM use; ask about lidocaine allergy. Standard dosage may be inadequate in obesity (BMI 240). Reports of DRESS (drug rash eosinophilia systemic symptoms) Syndrome. Visual hallucinations reported (NZ Med J 122:76, 2009). No predictable activity vs. P. aeruginosa.
Imipenem + cilastatin (Primaxin) Ref: JAC 58:916, 2006	**0.5 gm IV q6h;** for P. aeruginosa: 1 gm q6-8h (see Comment)	Seizures: In meta-analysis, risk of seizure low but greatest with carbapenems among beta-lactams. No diff between IMP and MER (JAC 69:2043, 2014). For infection with P. aeruginosa, increase dosage to 3 or 4 gm per day div. q6h or q8h. Continuous infusion of carbapenems may be more efficacious & safer (AAC 49:1881, 2005). Comments: Does not require a dehydropeptidase inhibitor (cilastatin). Activity vs aerobic gm-neg. slightly ↓ vs IMP. activity vs staph & strep slightly ↓; anaerobes: B. ovatus, B. distasonis more resistant vs meropenem. Cilastatin blocks enzymatic degradation of Imipenem in lumen of renal proximal tubule & also prevents tubular toxicity.
Meropenem (Merrem)	**0.5-1 gm IV q8h. Up to 2 gm IV q8h for meningitis. Prolonged infusion** in critically ill: If CrCl ≥ 50: 2 gm (over 3 hr) q8h If CrCl 30-49: 1 gm (over 3 hr) q8h If CrCl 10-29: 1 gm (over 3 hr) q12h (Inten Care Med 37:632, 2011)	Seizures: In meta-analysis, risk of seizure low but shared with carbapenems among beta-lactams. No diff between IMP and MER (JAC 69:2043, 2014). Comments: Does not require a dehydropeptidase inhibitor (cilastatin). Activity vs aerobic gm-neg. slightly ↑ vs IMP activity vs staph & strep slightly ↓; anaerobes: B. ovatus, B. distasonis more resistant to meropenem.

(See page 2 for abbreviations)   *NOTE: all dosage recommendations are for adults (unless otherwise indicated) & assume normal renal function.

TABLE 10A (3)

CLASS, AGENT, GENERIC NAME (TRADE NAME)	USUAL ADULT DOSAGE*	ADVERSE REACTIONS, COMMENTS (See Table 10B for Summary)
MONOBACTAMS		
Aztreonam (Azactam)	1 gm q8h–2 gm IV q6h.	Can be used in pts with allergy to penicillins/cephalosporins. Animal data and a letter raise concern about cross-reactivity with ceftazidime as **side-chains of aztreonam and ceftazidime are identical.**
Aztreonam for inhalation (Cayston)	75 mg bronchodilator before each inhalation.	Improves respiratory symptoms in CF pts colonized with *P. aeruginosa*. Alternative to inhaled Tobra. AEs: bronchospasm, cough, wheezing. So far, no emergence of other resistant pathogens. Ref: *Chest 135:1223, 2009*.
CEPHALOSPORINS (1st parenteral, then oral drugs). NOTE: Prospective data demonstrate correlation between use of cephalosporins (esp. 3ʳᵈ generation) and ↑ risk of *C. difficile* toxin-induced diarrhea. May also ↑ risk of colonization with vancomycin-resistant enterococci. See Oral Cephalosporins, page 106, for **important note on cross-allergenicity.**		
1ˢᵗ Generation, Parenteral		
Cefazolin (Ancef, Kefzol)	1–1.5 gm IV/IM q8h, occasionally 2 gm IV q8h for serious infections, e.g., MSSA bacteremia (max. 12 gm/day)	Do not give into lateral ventricles—**seizures!** No activity vs. MRSA.
2ⁿᵈ Generation, Parenteral (Cephamycins): May be active in vitro vs. ESBL-producing aerobic gram-negative bacilli. **Do not use as there are no clinical data for efficacy.**		
Cefotetan (Cefotan)	1–3 gm IV/IM q12h. (max. dose not >6 gm q24h).	Increasing resistance of B. fragilis, Prevotella bivia, Prevotella disiens (most common in pelvic infections); do not use for intra-abdominal infections. Methylthiotetrazole (MTT) side chain can inhibit vitamin K activation. Avoid alcohol-disulfiram reaction.
Cefoxitin (Mefoxin)	1 gm q8h–2 gm IV/IM q6-8h.	Increasing resistance of B. fragilis isolates.
Cefuroxime (Kefurox, Ceftin, Zinacef)	0.75–1.5 gm IV/IM q8h.	Improved activity against H. influenzae compared with 1st generation cephalosporins. See *Cefuroxime axetil* for oral preparation.
3ʳᵈ Generation, Parenteral—Use correlates with ↑ incidence of C. difficile toxin diarrhea: most are inactivated by ESBLs and amp C cephalosporinase from aerobic gram-negative bacilli		
Cefoperazone-sulbactam^NUS (Sulperazon)	Usual dose (Cefoperazone comp) 1–2 gm IV q12h; if larger doses, do not exceed 4 gm/day of sulbactam.	Increasing resistance of B. fragilis. Prevotella bivia, Prevotella disiens (most common in pelvic infections); do not use for intra-abdominal, biliary, & gyn. infections. Other uses due to broad spectrum of activity. Possible clotting problem due to side-chain.
Cefotaxime (Claforan)	1 gm q8h–2 gm IV q4h.	Maximum daily dose: 12 gm; give as 4 gm IV q8h. Similar to ceftriaxone but, unlike ceftriaxone, but requires multiple daily doses.
Ceftazidime (Fortaz, Tazicef)	**Usual dose: 1–2 gm IV/IM q8-12h.** **Prolonged infusion dosing:** initial dose: 15 mg/kg over 30 min, then immediately begin: If CrCl > 50: 6 gm (over 24 hr) daily If CrCl 31-50: 4 gm (over 24 hr) daily If CrCl 10-30: 2 gm (over 24 hr) daily (AAC 49:3550, 2005; Infect 37:418, 2009)	Often used in healthcare-associated infections, where P. aeruginosa is a consideration. Use may result in ↑ incidence of C. difficile-assoc. diarrhea and/or selection of vancomycin-resistant E. faecium (same side chain).
Ceftazidime-avibactam] (Avycaz)	2.5 gm (2 gm ceftazidime/0.5 gm avibactam) IV q8h for gram-negative complicated UTI & complicated intra-abdominal infection (add metronidazole 500 mg IV q8h).	Infuse over 2 hrs. Active against many isolates with several ESBLs and AmpC beta-lactamases. *Cross-reaction in beta-lactam allergic pts. Decreased efficacy w/ CrCl 30-50 mL/min.
Ceftizoxime (Cefizox)	From 1–2 gm IV q8-12h up to 2 gm IV q4h.	Maximum daily dose: 12 gm; can give as 4 gm IV q8h.
Ceftriaxone (Rocephin)	**1–2 gm IV once daily.** P. aeruginosa infection 2 gm IV q12h. Can give **IM in 1% lidocaine.**	"**Pseudocholelithiasis**" 2° to sludge in gallbladder by ultrasound (50%), symptomatic (9%) (NEJM 322:1821, 1990). More likely with ≥2 gm per day, with pt on total parenteral nutrition and not eating (AnIM 115:712, 1991). Clinical significance still unclear but use caution. Increased risk of cholecystectomy (JID 17:356, 1995) and gallstone pancreatitis (Ln 17:662, 1998). In pilot study 2 gm once daily by continuous infusion superior to 2 gm bolus once daily (AAC 59:285, 2007). For Ceftriaxone Desensitization, see *Table 7, page 83*.

*NOTE: all dosage recommendations are for adults (unless otherwise indicated) & assume normal renal function.

(See page 2 for abbreviations)

TABLE 10A (4)

CEPHALOSPORINS (1st parenteral, then oral drugs) (continued)

Other Generation, Parenteral: All are substrates for ESBLs & amp C cephalosporinase for aerobic gram-negative bacilli. Cefepime penetrates to target faster than other cephalosporins. (See Table 10B for Summary)

CLASS, AGENT, GENERIC NAME (TRADE NAME)	USUAL ADULT DOSAGE*	ADVERSE REACTIONS, COMMENTS (See Table 10B for Summary)
Cefepime (Maxipime) Obesity dosing, see Table 17C	**Usual dose: 1–2 gm IV q8–12h.** **Prolonged infusion dosing:** Initial dose: 15 mg/kg over 30 min, then immediately begin: If CrCl > 60: 6 gm (over 24 hr) daily If CrCl 30–60: 4 gm (over 24 hr) daily If CrCl 11–29: 2 gm (over 24 hr) daily	Active vs P. aeruginosa and many strains of Enterobacter, Serratia, C. freundii resistant to ceftazidime, cefotaxime, aztreonam. More active vs MSSA than 3rd generation cephalosporins. Neutropenia after 14 days rx. (Scand J Infect Dis 42:156, 2010). **FDA Safety warning (June 2012):** risk of non-convulsive status epilepticus, especially in pts with renal insufficiency when doses not adjusted. Seizure activity resolved after drug discontinuation and/or hemodialysis in the majority of pts. Postulated mechanism: binding to GABA receptors (Scand J Infect Dis 46:272, 2014; Crit Care 17:R264, 2013).
CefpiromeNUS (HR 810)	**1–2 gm IV q12h**	Similar to cefepime: ↑ activity vs enterobacteriaceae, P. aeruginosa, Gm + organisms. Anaerobes: less active than cefoxitin, more active than cefotax or ceftaz.
Ceftaroline fosamil (Teflaro)	**600 mg IV q12h (5–60 min infusion)** Pneumonia/bacteremia 600 mg q8h[NAI]. *See Comment*	**Avid binding to PBP 2a; active vs. MRSA.** Inactivated by Amp C & ESBL enzymes. Approved for MRSA skin and skin structure infections and used for MRSA pneumonia and bacteremia, but not approved indications (J Infect Chemother 19:42, 2013). Active in vitro vs. VISA, VRSA. Refs: CID 52:1156, 2011; Med Lett 53:5, 2011. Used successfully for bacteremia and bone/joint infections, but NAI (AAC 58:2541, 2014).
Ceftazidime-avibactam (Avycaz)	**2.5 gm (2 gm ceftazidime/0.5 gm avibactam) IV over 2 hrs q8h for gram-negative complicated UTI & add metronidazole 500 mg IV q8h for complicated intra-abdominal infection**	Active against ESBL- & KPC-producing aerobic gm-neg bacilli. No activity vs. GNB-producing metallo-carbapenemases. Decreased efficacy in pts with w/ CrCl 30-50 mL/min (in clinical trials).
CeftobiproleNUS	**0.5 gm IV q8h for mixed gm- neg & gm-pos infections. 0.5 gm IV q12h for gm-pos infections**	Infuse over 2 hrs for q8h dosing, over 1 hr for q12h dosing. Associated with caramel-like taste disturbance. Ref.: Clin Microbiol Infections 13(Suppl 2):17 & 25, 2007. MRSA.
Ceftolozane-tazobactam (Zerbaxa)	**1.5 gm (1/0.5 gm) IV q8h for gm-neg complicated UTI & complicated intra-abdominal infection (add Metro 500 mg IV q8h)**	Infuse over 1 hr. Active vs. P. aeruginosa and many gm-neg bacteria producing beta-lactamases. Cross-reaction in beta-lactam allergic pts. Decreased efficacy w/ CrCl 30-50 mL/min.

(See page 2 for abbreviations)   *NOTE: all dosage recommendations are for adults (unless otherwise indicated) & assume normal renal function.

TABLE 10A (5)

CLASS, AGENT, GENERIC NAME (TRADE NAME)	USUAL ADULT DOSAGE*	ADVERSE REACTIONS, COMMENTS (See Table 10B for Summary)
CEPHALOSPORINS (1st parenteral, then oral drugs) (continued)		
Oral Cephalosporins		Cross-Allergenicity: **Patients with a history of IgE-mediated allergic reactions to penicillin (e.g., bronchospasm anaphylaxis, angioneurotic edema, immediate urticaria) should not receive a cephalosporin.** If the history is a "measles-like" rash to penicillin, available data suggest a 5–10% risk of rash
1st Generation, Oral		with a cephalosporin. In the absence of an advanced risk of anaphylaxis:
Cefadroxil (Duricef)	0.5–1 gm po q12h.	• In pts with history of Pen "reaction," 3.4–8.4% react to a cephalosporin (Aller Asthma Proc 26:135, 2006). If positive Pen G skin test, only 2% given a cephalosporin will react. Can predict with cephalosporin skin testing,
(500 mg caps, 1 gm tabs)		but not available (An M 141:16, 2004; AJM 125:572, 2008)
Cephalexin (Keflex)	0.25–1 gm po q6h (max 4 gm/day).	• IgE antibodies against either ring structure or side chains; 80% pts IgE over 10 yrs post-reaction (J Aller Clin
(250 & 500 mg tabs)		Immunol 103:918, 1999). Amox, Cefadroxil, Cefprozil have similar side chains; Amp, Cefaclor, Cephalexin, Cephedrine
2nd Generation, Oral		Cefprozil (Cefzil) share side chains.
Cefaclor (Ceclor, Raniclor)	0.25–0.5 gm po q8h.	• If Pen/Ceph skin test not available or clinically no time, proceed with cephalosporin if history does not suggest
(250 & 500 mg caps)		IgE-mediated reaction, prior reaction more than 10 yrs ago or cephalosporin side chain differs from implicated Pen.
Cefprozil (Cefzil)	0.25–0.5 gm po q12h.	Any of the cephalosporins can result in **C. difficile toxin**-mediated diarrhea/enterocolitis.
		The reported frequency of nausea/vomiting and non-C. difficile toxin diarrhea is summarized in Table 10B.
Cefuroxime axetil po (Ceftin)	0.125–0.5 gm po q12h.	There are **few drug-specific adverse effects, e.g.:**
3rd Generation, Oral		**Cefaclor:** Serum sickness-like reaction 0.1–0.5%—arthralgia, rash, erythema multiforme but no adenopathy, proteinuria
Cefdinir (Omnicef)	300 mg po q12h or 600 mg q24h.	or liver disease. Cause unknown, not immune complexes.
(300 mg cap)		**Cefdinir:** Drug-iron complex causes red stools; frequency 1% of pts.
Cefditoren pivoxil (Spectracef)	400 mg po bid.	**Cefditoren pivoxil:** Hydrolysis yields pivalate. Pivalate absorbed (70%) & becomes pivaloylcarnitine which is renally
(400 mg tab)		excreted; 39–63% ↓ in serum carnitine concentrations. Carnitine involved in fatty acid (FA) metabolism & FA
Cefixime (Suprax)	0.4 gm po q12–24h.	transport into mitochondria. Effect transient & reversible. Contraindicated in patients with carnitine deficiency or those
(400 mg cap)		with inborn errors of metabolism might result in clinically significant carnitine deficiency. Also contains caseinate
Cefpodoxime proxetil (Vantin)	0.1–0.2 gm po q12h.	**(milk protein); avoid in milk allergy** (not same as lactose intolerance). Need gastric acid for optimal absorption.
Ceftibuten (Cedax)	0.4 gm po q24h.	**Cefpodoxime:** There are reports of acute liver injury, bloody diarrhea, pulmonary infiltrates with eosinophilia.
(400 mg tab)		**Cephalexin:** Can cause false-neg urine dipstick test for leukocytes.
AMINOGLYCOSIDES AND RELATED ANTIBIOTICS—See Table 10D, page 118, and Table 17A, page 215		
GLYCOPEPTIDES, LIPOGLYCOPEPTIDES, LIPOPEPTIDES		
Dalbavancin (Dalvance)	1000 mg IV over 30 min; one week later, 500 mg IV over 30 min. Avoid use with saline, drug may precipitate out of solution.	If CrCl<30: 750 mg IV initial dose, then one week later 375 mg IV. **Hemodialysis:** Dose as for normal renal function. No adjustment for mild/moderate renal impairment. Red man syndrome can occur with rapid infusion. Potential cross-reaction in those with hypersensitivity to other glycopeptides.
Daptomycin (Cubicin) (Ref on resistance: CID 50:S10, 2010). Case series success in treating right- & left-sided endocarditis with higher dose of 8–10 mg/kg/day (JAC 68:936 & 2921, 2013).	**Skin/soft tissue:** 4 mg per kg IV over 2 or 30 minutes q24h. **Bacteremia/right-sided endocarditis:** 6 mg per kg IV over 2 or 30 minutes q24h; up to 12 mg/kg IV q24h under study. Morbid obesity: base dose on total body weight (AAC 51:2741 & Table 10C, p. 117, page 229, recommendations, see Table 10C, page 116). Dapto + ceftaroline may work as salvage therapy in pts with refractory MRSA bacteremia (AAC 57:66, 2012; AAC 56:5296, 2012).	**Pneumonia:** Dapto should not be used for pneumonia unless hematogenous in origin and is FDA approved for right-sided endocarditis caused by S. aureus. **Dapto Resistance:** Can occur de novo, after or during Vanco therapy, or after or during Dapto therapy (CID 50:Suppl 1):S10, 2010). As Dapto MIC increases, MRSA more susceptible to TMP-SMX; nafcillin, oxacillin (AAC 54:5187, 2010; CID 53:158, 2011). **Dapto muscle toxicity:** 0.14 mg per kg per day. ↑ CPK in 2.8% dapto pts & 1.8% comparator-treated pts. Risk increases if min conc exceeds 24.3 mg/L. Package insert: monitor CPK weekly. Check for myopathy; if CPK exceeds 10x normal level or if symptoms of myopathy and CPK >1,000. **NOTE:** Statins may ↑ risk; stop dapto x 24-48 hrs. Dapto interferes with prothrombin reagents & artificially prolongs the PT. (Blood Coag & Fibrinolysis 19:32, 2008) **NOTE:** Dapto well-tolerated in healthy volunteers at doses up to 12 mg/kg q24h x 14d (AAC 50:3245, 2006) and in pts given 4-8 mg/kg/day (CID 49:177, 2009). **Immune thrombocytopenia** reported (CID 52:e63, 2010). **Eosinophilic pneumonia**—chronic steroid-dep pneumonia reported (CID 50:737, 2010; CID 56:1239, 2012).
Oritavancin (Orbactiv) Review: CID 61:627, 2015	1200 mg IV over 3 hr x 1 dose. Dilute in D5W; do not use saline	Artificially increases PT & INR x 24h and aPTT x 48 hr. **Drug-drug interactions with warfarin:** ↑ warfarin serum levels. Acute urticarial has occurred. No dose adjustment for renal or hepatic insuff. Not removed by hemodialysis. In vitro activity vs. VRE (AAC 56:1639, 2012).

*NOTE: all dosage recommendations are for adults (unless otherwise indicated) & assume normal renal function.

(See page 2 for abbreviations)

TABLE 10A (6)

CLASS, AGENT, GENERIC NAME (TRADE NAME)	USUAL ADULT DOSAGE*	ADVERSE REACTIONS, COMMENTS (See Table 10B for Summary)
GLYCOPEPTIDES, LIPOPEPTIDES, LIPOGLYCOPEPTIDES (Continued)		
Teicoplanin[NUS] (Targocid)	**For septic arthritis—maintenance dose 12 mg/kg per day; S. aureus endocarditis—trough serum levels >20 mg/mL required (12 mg/kg q12h times 3 loading doses, then 12 mg/kg/q24h)**	Hypersensitivity, fever (at 3 mg/kg 2.2%, at 24 mg per kg 8.2%), skin reactions 2.4%. Marked ↓ platelets (high dose ≥15 mg per kg per day). Red neck syndrome less common than with vancomycin.
Telavancin[NUS] (Vibativ) Lipopeptide Ref: CID 80:787, 2015; CID 61(Suppl 2), 2015	10 mg/kg IV q24h if CrCl >50 mL/min. Infuse each dose over 1 hr.	**Avoid during pregnancy: teratogenic in animals.** Do pregnancy test before therapy. Adverse events: **dysgeusia (taste) 33%**; nausea 27%; vomiting 14%; headache 14%; ↑ creatinine (3.1%), foamy urine (13%); flushing if infused rapidly. In clin trials, **evidence of renal injury** in 3% telavancin vs. 1% vanco; in practice, renal injury reported in 1/3 of 21 complicated pts (JAC 67:723, 2012). Interferes with PT, aPTT & INR for 18 hrs post-infusion.
Vancomycin (Vancocin) Guidelines Ref: CID 49:325, 2009. See Comments for p.o. dose. Continuous infusion dosing, see Table 10E	**initial doses based on actual wt, including for obese pts.** Subsequent doses adjusted based on measured serum levels. **For critically ill pts, give loading dose of 25-30 mg/kg IV then 15-20 mg/kg IV q8-12h.** Target trough level is 15-20 µg/mL. For individual doses over 1 gm, infuse over 1.5-2 hrs. **Dosing for morbid obesity (BMI ≥40 kg/m²): If CrCl ≥50 mL/min & pt not critically ill:** 30 mg/kg/day divided q8-12h—no dose over 2 gm. Infuse doses of 1 gm or more over 1.5-2 hrs. Check trough levels. **Morbid obesity & critically ill:** Loading dose of 25-30 mg/kg (actual wt), then 15-20 mg/kg (actual wt) IV q8-12h. Infuse over 1.5-2 hrs. Limit maximal single dose to 2 gm. Oral tabs for C. difficile: 125 mg po q6h Generic drug now available	Treatment failure of MRSA bacteremia associated with Vanco trough concentration <15 µg/mL & MIC > 1 µg/mL (CID 52:975, 2011). IDSA Guideline supports target trough of 15-20 µg/mL (CID 52:e18, 2011). Pertinent issues: • Max Vanco effect vs. MRSA when ratio of AUC/MIC > 400 (CID 52:975, 2011). • MIC values vary with method used, so hard to be sure/compare (JCM 49:269, 2011). • With MRSA Vanco MIC = 1 & Vanco dose >3 gm/day IV, AUC/MIC > 400 in 80% with est. risk of nephrotoxicity of 25%. With MIC = 2 & 4 gm/day IV, AUC/MIC > 400 in only 57% (nephrotoxicity risk 35%) (CID 52:969, 2011). • Higher Vanco doses assoc with nephrotoxicity; causal relation unproven: other factors: renal disease, other nephrotoxic drugs, shock/vasopressors, radiographic contrast (AAC 52:1330, 2008; AAC 55:3278, 2011; AJM 123:182e1, 2010). • If pt clinically failing Vanco (regardless of MIC or AUC/MIC), consider other drugs active vs. MRSA: ceftaroline, daptomycin, linezolid, telavancin. (see Table 5A for MDR options) **PO vanco for C. difficile colitis: 125 mg po q6h.** Commercial po formulation very expensive. Can compound po vanco from IV formulation: 5 g, IV vanco powder + 47.5 mL sterile 0.05 gm saccharin, 0.05 gm stevia powder, 40 mL glycerin and then enough cherry syrup to yield 100 mL = 50 mg vanco/mL. Oral dose = 2.5 mL q6h po. **Intrathecal dose:** 5-10 mg/day (children & adults) to target CSF concentration of 10-20 µg/mL. **Nephrotoxicity:** Risk increases with dose and duration, reversible (AAC 57:734, 2013). **Red Neck Syndrome:** consequence of rapid infusion with non-specific histamine release. **Other adverse effects:** rash, immune thrombocytopenia (NEJM 356:904, 2007); fever, neutropenia, initial report of dose-dependent decrease in platelet count (AAC 67:727, 2012). **IgA bullous dermatitis** (CID 38:442, 2004). **Obesity dosing:** Frequent under dosing (AJM 121:515, 2008). For obesity dosing adjustments, see Table 17C, page 229. For CrCl calculation for morbidly obese patient see Table 10D or Am J Health Sys Pharm 66:642, 2009.

(See page 2 for abbreviations)

*NOTE: all dosage recommendations are for adults (unless otherwise indicated) & assume normal renal function.

TABLE 10A (7)

CLASS, AGENT GENERIC NAME (TRADE NAME)	USUAL ADULT DOSAGE*	ADVERSE REACTIONS, COMMENTS (See Table 10B for Summary)
CHLORAMPHENICOL, CLINDAMYCIN(S), ERYTHROMYCIN GROUP, KETOLIDES, OXAZOLIDINONES, QUINUPRISTIN-DALFOPRISTIN		
Chloramphenicol (Chloromycetin)	50-100 mg/kg/day po/IV div q6h (max. 4 gm/day)	No oral drug distrib in U.S. Hematologic: C RBC -- 1/3 pts, aplastic anemia 1:21,600 courses). Gray baby syndrome in premature infants, anaphylactoid reactions, optic atrophy or neuropathy (very rare), digital paresthesias, minor disulfiram-like reactions. Recent review suggests Chloro is probably less effective than current alternatives for serious infection: respiratory tract, enteric, meningitis (JAC 70:979, 2015).
Clindamycin (Cleocin)	0.15-0.45 gm po q6h. 600-900 mg IV/IM q8h.	Based on number of exposed pts, these drugs are the most frequent cause of **C. difficile toxin-mediated diarrhea**. In most severe form can cause pseudomembranous colitis/toxic megacolon. Available as caps, IV soln, topical (for acne) & intravaginal suppositories & cream. **Used to inhibit synthesis of toxic shock syndrome toxins**.
Lincomycin (Lincocin)	0.6 gm IV/IM q8h.	Risk of C. difficile colitis. Rarely used.
Erythromycin Group (Review drug interactions before use)		**Motilin:** activates duodenal/jejunal receptors that initiate peristalsis. Erytho (E) and E esters activate motilin receptors and cause uncoordinated peristalsis with resultant anorexia, nausea or vomiting. Less binding and GI distress with azithromycin/clarithromycin. No peristalsis benefit (JAC 58:347, 2007).
Azithromycin (Zithromax) Azithromycin ER (Zmax)	po preps: Tabs 250 & 600 mg. Peds suspension: 100 & 200 mg per 5 mL. Adult ER suspension: 2 gm. Dose varies with indication, see Table 1. Acute otitis media (page 11), acute exac. chronic bronchitis (pages 39-40) & sinusitis (page 50). IV: 0.5 gm q24h.	Systemic erytho in 1st 2 wks of life associated with **infantile hypertrophic pyloric stenosis** (J Ped 139:380, 2001). **Frequent drug-drug interactions:** see Table 22, page 235. Major concern is prolonged QTc. **Prolonged QTc:** Erytho, clarithro & azithro all increase risk of ventricular tachycardia via increase in QTc interval. Can be congenital or acquired (NEJM 358:169, 2008). Caution if positive family history of sudden cardiac death, electrolyte abnormalities (low K+/Mg++) or drugs that prolong QTc.
Erythromycin Base and esters (Erythrocin) IV name: E. lactobionate	0.25 gm q6h--0.5 gm q12h po /IV q6h; 15-20mg/kg up to 4 gm q24h. Infuse over 30+ min.	↑ risk QTc ≥ 500 msec] Risk amplified by other drugs [macrolides, antiarrhythmics, & drug-drug interactions (see FQs page 110 for list)]. www.qtdrugs.org & www.torsades.org. Ref. Arrh J Med 128:1362, 2015. Cholestatic hepatitis in approx. 1:1000 adults (not children) given E. estolate.
Clarithromycin (Biaxin) or clarithro extended release (Biaxin XL)	0.5 gm po q12h Extended release: Two 0.5 gm tabs po per day.	**Drug-drug interactions of note:** Erytho or clarithro with statins: high statin levels, rhabdomyolysis (Ann Int Med 158:869, 2013); concomitant clarithro & colchicine (gout) can cause fatal colchicine toxicity (pancytopenia, renal failure) (CID 41:291, 2005). Concomitant clarithro & Ca++ channel blockers increase risk of hypotension, kidney injury (JAMA 310:2544, 2013). Hypoglycemia with concomitant sulfonylureas (JAMA Int Med 174:1605, 2014). **Transient reversible tinnitus or deafness** with 24 gm per day of erytho IV in pts with renal or hepatic impairment. Reversible sensorineural hearing loss with Azithro (JID 170:2267, 2007).
Fidaxomicin (Dificid) (200 mg tab)	One 200 mg tab po bid x 10 days with or without food	Dosages of oral erythro preparations expressed as base equivalents. Variable amounts of erythro esters required to achieve same free erythro serum level. **Azithromycin** reported to exacerbate symptoms of myasthenia gravis. Approved for C. difficile toxin-mediated diarrhea, including hypervirulent NAP1/B1/027 strains. Minimal GI absorption. In trial vs. po Vanco, lower relapse rate vs. non-NAP1 strains than Vanco (NEJM 364:422, 2011). Despite absence of GI absorption, 12 pts developed allergic reactions; known macrolide allergy in 3 of 12 (CID 58:537, 2014).
Ketolide:		Drug warnings: acute liver failure & serious liver injury post treatment. (Am J Med 144:415, 447, 2006) **Uncommon:** blurred vision or visual accommodation; may cause exacerbation of **myasthenia gravis (Black Box Warning: Contraindicated in this setting).** Liver, eye and myasthenia complications may be due to inhibition of nicotinic acetylcholine receptor at neuromuscular junction. (AAC 49:2035, 2010) Prolonged QTc prolongation.
Telithromycin (Ketek) (Med Lett 46:66, 2004; Drug Safety 31:561, 2008)	Two 400 mg tabs po q24h. 300 mg tabs available.	Several **drug-drug interactions** (Table 22, page 237) (NEJM 355:2260, 2006)

*NOTE: all dosage recommendations are for adults (unless otherwise indicated) & assume normal renal function.

(See page 2 for abbreviations)   *See page 2 for abbreviations)

TABLE 10A (8)

CLASS, AGENT, GENERIC NAME (TRADE NAME)	USUAL ADULT DOSAGE*	ADVERSE REACTIONS, COMMENTS (See Table 10B for Summary)
CHLORAMPHENICOL, CLINDAMYCIN(S), ERYTHROMYCIN GROUP, KETOLIDES, OXAZOLIDINONES, QUINUPRISTIN-DALFOPRISTIN (continued)		
Tedizolid phosphate (Sivextro) Ref: CID 58(Suppl 1):S57, 2014; CID 61:1315, 2015.	200 mg IV/po once daily. Infuse IV over 1 hr.	IV dose reconstituted in 250 mL of normal saline; incompatible with lactated ringers ca due to absence of solubility in presence of divalent cations. SST clinical trial result (LnID 14:696, 2014; JAMA 309:559 & 609, 2013). Excreted by liver. No adjustment for renal insufficiency. Weak inhibitor of monoamine oxidase; low risk of serotonin syndrome, but low risk based on in vitro, animal & human study (AAC 57:3060, 2013).
Linezolid (Zyvox) (600 mg tab) Review: JAC 66(Suppl 4):3, 2011	PO or IV dose: 600 mg q12h. Available as 600 mg tabs, oral suspension (100 mg per 5 mL), & IV solution. Special populations Refs: Renal insufficiency (J Infect Chemother 17:70, 2011); Liver transplant (CID 42:434, 2006); Cystic fibrosis (AAC 48:281, 2004); Burns (J Burn Care Res 31:207, 2010). Obesity: clinical failure with standard dose in 265 kg patient (Ann Pharmacother 47:e25, 2013).	Reversible myelosuppression: thrombocytopenia, anemia, myelopenia reported. Most often after >2 wks of therapy. Increased risk on hemodialysis or peritoneal dialysis (Int J Antimicrob Ag 36:179, 2010; JAC doi:10.1093/jac/dkv184) Inhibitor of monoamine oxidase; risk of severe hypertension if taken with foods rich in tyramine. Avoid concomitant pseudoephedrine, phenylpropanolamine, and caution with SSRIs.† Serotonin syndrome (fever, agitation, mental status changes, tremors). Risk with concomitant SSRIs: (CID 42:1578 and 43:180, 2006). Actual incidence seems low (AAC 57:5901, 2013). Other adverse effects: black hairy tongue and acute interstitial nephritis (IDCP 17:61, 2009). Rhabdomyolysis: case probably related to linezolid in a patient receiving linezolid as a component of multi-drug therapy for XDR tuberculosis (CID 54:1624, 2012) Resistance: Linezolid resistant S. epidermidis and MRSA due to mutation of the 23S rRNA binding site (JAC 68:4, 2013).
Quinupristin + dalfopristin (Synercid) (CID 36:473, 2003)	7.5 mg per kg IV q12h for skin/skin structure infections, infused over 1 hour. [For previous indication of VRE infection, dose used was 7.5 mg per kg IV q8h.] Give by central line.	Venous irritation (5%); use with central venous line. Asymptomatic † in unconjugated bilirubin. Arthralgia 2%–50% (CID 36:476, 2003). Note: E. faecium susceptible; E. faecalis resistant. Drug-drug interactions: Cyclosporine, nifedipine, midazolam, many more—see Table 22.
TETRACYCLINES		
Doxycycline (Vibramycin, Doryx, Monodox, Adoxa, Periostat) (20, 50, 75, 100 mg tab)	0.1 gm po/IV q12h	Similar to other tetracyclines. † nausea on empty stomach. Erosive esophagitis, esp. if taken at bedtime: take with lots of water. Phototoxicity & photo-onycholysis occur but less than with tetracycline. Deposition in teeth less. Can be used in patients with renal failure. Comments: Effective in treatment and prophylaxis for malaria, leptospirosis, typhus fevers.
Minocycline (Minocin, Dynacin) (50, 75, 100 mg cap, 45, 90, 135 mg ext rel tab; IV prep)	200 mg po/IV loading dose, then 100 mg po/IV q12h IV minocycline available.	Vestibular symptoms (30–90% in some groups, none in others): vertigo 33%, ataxia 43%, nausea 50%, vomiting 3%, women more frequently than men. Hyperpigmentation of skin and other tissues with long-term use. Can cause slate-grey pigment of skin. ~34 cases reported (BMJ 310:1520, 1995) Comments: More effective than other tetracyclines vs staph and in prophylaxis of meningococcal disease. P. acnes: many resistant to other tetracyclines, not to minocycline. Induced autoimmunity reported in children treated for acne (J Ped 153:314, 2008). Active vs Nocardia asteroides, Mycobacterium marinum and many acinetobacter isolates. GI (oxy 19%, tetra 4), anaphylactoid reaction (rare), deposition in teeth, negative N balance, hepatotoxicity, enamel ageneis, pseudotumor cerebri/encephalopathy. Outdated drug: Fanconi syndrome. See drug-drug interactions, Table 22.
Tetracycline, Oxytetracycline (Sumycin) (250, 500 mg cap) (CID 36:462, 2003)	0.25–0.5 gm po q6h, 0.5–1 gm IV q12h	Contraindicated in pregnancy, hepatotoxicity in mother, transplacental to fetus. Comments: Pregnancy: IV dosage over 2 gm per day may be associated with fatal hepatotoxicity (Ref: JAC 66:1431, 2011).

† SSRI = selective serotonin reuptake inhibitors, e.g. fluoxetine (Prozac).

(See page 2 for abbreviations)   *NOTE: all dosage recommendations are for adults (unless otherwise indicated) & assume normal renal function.

TABLE 10A (9)

CLASS, AGENT GENERIC NAME (TRADE NAME)	USUAL ADULT DOSAGE*	ADVERSE REACTIONS, COMMENTS (See Table 10B for Summary)
TETRACYCLINES (Continued)		
Tigecycline (Tygacil) Meta-analysis & editorial: Ln ID 11:804 & 834, 2011. Also CID 54:1699 & 1710, 2012.	100 mg IV initially, then 50 mg IV q12h with po food, if possible to decrease risk of nausea. **If severe liver dis. (Child Pugh C):** 100 mg IV initially, then 25 mg IV q12h	Derivative of tetracycline. High incidence of nausea (25%) & vomiting (20%) but only 1% of pts discontinued therapy. Pregnancy Category D. Do not use in children under age 18. Like other tetracyclines, may cause photosensitivity, pseudotumor cerebri, pancreatitis, a catabolic state (elevated BUN) and maybe hyperpigmentation (CID 45:136, 2007). Decreases serum fibrinogen (AAC 59:1650, 2015). **Tetracycline, minocycline & tigecycline** associated with acute pancreatitis (Int J Antimicrob Agents, 34:486, 2009). **Black Box Warning:** In meta-analysis of clinical trials, all cause mortality higher in pts treated with tigecycline (2.5%) vs. 1.8% in comparators. Cause of mortality risk difference of 0.6% (95% CI 0.1, 1.2) not established. Tigecycline should be reserved for use in situations when alternative treatments are not suitable (FDA MedWatch Sep 27, 2013). Poor result due to low serum levels (AAC 56:1065 & 1466, 2012); high doses superior to low doses for HAP (AAC 57:1756, 2013).

FLUOROQUINOLONES (FQs): All can cause false-positive urine drug screen for opiates (Pharmacother 26:435, 2006). Toxicity review: Drugs Aging 27:193, 2010.

CLASS, AGENT GENERIC NAME (TRADE NAME)	USUAL ADULT DOSAGE*	ADVERSE REACTIONS, COMMENTS (See Table 10B for Summary)
Ciprofloxacin (Cipro) and Ciprofloxacin-extended release (Cipro XR, Proquin XR) (100, 250, 500, 750 mg tab; 500 mg ext rel tab)	Usual Parenteral Dose: **400 mg IV q12h** For P. aeruginosa: **400 mg IV q8h** Uncomplicated Urethritis/cystitis (Oral) Dose: **250 mg po bid or CIP XR 500 mg po once daily** Other Indications (Oral): **500-750 mg po bid**	FQs are a common precipitant of **C. difficile toxin-mediated diarrhea.** **Children:** No FQ approved for use under age 16 based on joint cartilage injury in immature animals. Articular SEs in children est at 2-3% (LnID 3:537, 2003). The exception is anthrax. Pathogenesis believed to involve FQ chelation of Mg++ and damaging chondrites (AAC 51:1022, 2007; Int J Antimicrob Agents 33:194, 2009). No evidence of cartilage damage with Levo in children (Pediatrics 134:e146, 2014). **CNS toxicity:** Poorly understood. Varies: lightheadedness, confusion, seizures. May be aggravated by NSAIDs. Peripheral neuropathy occurs: rapid onset, potentially permanent injury. **Gemi skin rash:** Macular rash after 8-10 days of rx. Incidence of rash with ≤5 days of therapy only 1.5%. Frequency highest females, < age 40, treated 14 days (22.6%). In men, < age 40, frequency 7.7%. Mechanism unclear, indication to DC therapy. Ref: Diag Micro Infect Dis 68:140, 2010. **Hypoglycemia/hyperglycemia (Dysglycemia):** increased risk, esp. of hypoglycemia in diabetic pts from any of the marketed FQs (CID 57:971, 2013).
Gatifloxacin (Tequin)^NUS See comments	**200-400 mg IV/po q24h.** (See comment) Ophthalmic solution (Zymar)	**Thrombocytopenia** in critically ill (PLoS One 8(11):e81477). **Opiate screen false-positives:** FQs can cause false-positive urine assay for opiates CID 57:917, 2013).
Gemifloxacin (Factive) (320 mg tab)	**320 mg po q24h.**	**Photosensitivity:** See Table 10C, page 117. **QT, (corrected QT) interval prolongation:** ↑ QT. (>500 msec or >80 msec from baseline) is considered possible with any FQ. ↑ QT. can lead to torsades de pointes and ventricular fibrillation. Overall risk is 4.7/10,000 person yrs (CID 55:1457, 2012). Risk low with current marketed drugs. Risk ↑ in women, ↓ K. ↓ Mg++; bradycardia. (Refs.: CID 43:1603, 2006). Major problem is ↑ risk with concomitant drugs.

(See page 2 for abbreviations)   *NOTE: all dosage recommendations are for adults (unless otherwise indicated) & assume normal renal function.

TABLE 10A (10)

CLASS, AGENT, GENERIC NAME (TRADE NAME)	USUAL ADULT DOSAGE*	ADVERSE REACTIONS, COMMENTS (See Table 10B for Summary)		
FLUOROQUINOLONES (FQs) (continued)		**Avoid concomitant drugs with potential to prolong QTc such as** (see www.qtdrugs.org; www.torsades.org):		
Levofloxacin (Levaquin) (250, 500, 750 mg tab)	**250–750 mg po/IV q24h.** For most indications, 750 mg is preferred dose. PO therapy, avoid concomitant dairy products, multivitamins, iron, antacids due to chelation by multivalent cations & interference with absorption. No dose adjustment for morbid obesity.	**Antiarrhythmics:** Amiodarone Disopyramide Dofetilide Flecainide Ibutilide Procainamide Quinidine, quinine Sotalol	**Anti-Infectives:** Azoles (not Posa) Clarithro/erythro FQs (not CiP) Halofantrine NNRTIs Pentamidine Protease Inhibitors Telavancin Telithromycin **Anti-Hypertensives:** Bepridil Isradipine Nicardipine Moexipril	**CNS Drugs:** Fluoxetine Haloperidol Phenothiazines Pimozide Quetiapine Risperidone Sertraline Tricyclics Venlafaxine Ziprasidone **Misc:** Dolasetron Droperidol Fosphenytoin Indapamide Methadone Naratriptan Salmeterol Sumatriptan Tamoxifen Tizanidine
		Tendinopathy: Over age 60, approx. 2–6% of all Achilles tendon ruptures attributable to use of FQ (AVM 163:1801, 2003). ↑ risk with concomitant steroid, renal disease or post-transplant (heart, lung, kidney) (CID 36:1404, 2003). **Chelation:** Risk of chelation of oral FQs by multivalent cations (Ca++, Mg++, Fe++, Zn++). Avoid dairy products, multivitamins (Clin Pharmacokinet 40 [Suppl 1]:33,2001). **Allergic/Immunologic:** Rash, anaphylaxis—IgE-mediated: urticaria, anaphylaxis. 3 pts with Moxi had immediate reactions but tolerated CiP (Ann Pharmacother 44:740, 2010). **Myasthenia gravis:** Any of the FQs may exacerbate muscle weakness in pts. with myasthenia gravis. **Retinal detachment:** Association with FQs in 2 studies (JAMA 307:1414, 2012; CID 58:197, 2014); no association found in 2 other studies (JAMA 310:2151 & 2184, 2013; JAC 69:2563, 2014).		
Moxifloxacin (Avelox)	**400 mg po/IV q24h. Note:** no need to increase dose for morbid obesity (CID 66:2330, 2011).			
	Ophthalmic solution (Vigamox)			
Ofloxacin (Floxin)	**200–400 mg po bid.** Ophthalmic solution (Ocuflox)	Not available in the U.S.		
Prulifloxacin Ref: Drugs 64:2221, 2004.	Tablets: 250 and 600 mg. Usual dose: **600 mg po once daily**			
POLYMYXINS (POLYPEPTIDES) Note: Proteus sp., Providencia sp., Serratia sp., are intrinsically resistant to polymyxins. Review: CID 59:88, 2014. B. cepacia				
Polymyxin B (Poly-Rx) 1 mg = 10,000 international units **Where available, Polymyxin B preferred over Colistin.** Avoid monotherapy, see Comment.	Doses based on actual body weight. **LOADING DOSE:** 2.5 mg/kg IV over 2 hrs. **MAINTENANCE DOSE:** 12 hrs later 1.5 mg/kg over 1 hr, then repeat q12h. Combination therapy with **carbapenem** suggested to increase efficacy and reduce risk of resistance. No dose reduction for renal insufficiency. **Intrathecal therapy for meningitis:** 5 mg/day into CSF x 3–4 days, then 5 mg every other day x 2 or more weeks.	**Adverse effects: Neurologic:** rare, but serious, is neuromuscular blockade: other, circumoral paresthesias, extremity numbness, blurred vision, drowsy, irritable, ataxia; can manifest as respiratory arrest (Chest 141:515, 2012). **Renal:** Renal injury in 42% (Polymyxin B) vs. 60% (Colistin) (CID 57:1300, 2013). PK study showed no need to reduce dose for renal insufficiency (CID 57:524, 2013). **Polymyxin B preferred over Colistin** (see Comment under Colistin for rationale). In retrospective study, lower mortality from P. aeruginosa & A. baumannii with Polymyxin B + carbapenem vs. polymyxin monotherapy (AAC 59:6575, 2015).		

(See page 2 for abbreviations)

*NOTE: all dosage recommendations are for adults (unless otherwise indicated) & assume normal renal function.

TABLE 10A (11)

CLASS, AGENT, GENERIC NAME (TRADE NAME)	USUAL ADULT DOSAGE*	ADVERSE REACTIONS, COMMENTS *(See Table 10B for Summary)*
POLYMYXINS (POLYPEPTIDES) *(continued)*		
Colistin, Polymyxin E (Colymycin) All doses are based on mg of Colistin base. Calculated doses are higher than the package insert dosing; need to avoid underdosage in the critically ill. **Do not use as monotherapy (combine with carbapenem)** Dosing formula based on PK study of 105 pts (AAC 55:3284, 2011). Loading dose (AAC 53:3430, 2009). **Recommendations are evolving; see Sanford Guide digital editions for updated information and dosing calculator.**	• **Severe Systemic Infection:** **LOADING DOSE:** 2.5 (targeted average serum steady state level) x 2 x body weight in kg (lower of ideal or actual weight) IV. This will often result in a loading dose of over 300 mg of colistin base. First maintenance dose given 12 hrs later. **MAINTENANCE DOSE:** Formula for calculating the daily maintenance dose: 2.5 x (desired serum steady state concentration) x [(1.5 x CrCl) +30] = total daily dose. Divide and give q8h or maybe q12h. The maximum suggested daily dose is 340 mg. **NOTE:** CrCln is the Creatinine Clearance (CrCl) normalized (n) to the Body Surface Area (BSA) such that the CrCln = CrCl BSA m²/1.73 m² • *Combination therapy is recommended for all pts:* **Colistin** (as above) + (**IMP** or **MER**) (based on IBW) • **intrathecal or intraventricular for meningitis:** 10 mg/day q8h • **Cystic fibrosis:** 3-8 mg/kg/day q8h • **inhalation therapy:** 50-75 mg in 3-4 mL of Saline via nebulizer 2-3x/day	• **GNB Resistance:** Some sp. are intrinsically resistant: Serratia sp, Proteus sp, Providencia sp., B. cepacia. In vitro and in animal models, gram-negative bacilli quickly become resistant. The greater the resistance of GNB to Colistin, the greater the susceptibility to beta-lactams (AM-SB, PIP-TZ, extended spectrum Ceph, maybe carbapenems). • **Caveat:** higher doses of colistin (> 5 mg/kg ideal body weight per day) are associated with increased risk of nephrotoxicity and should be reserved for critically ill patients (CID 53:879, 2011). • **Bactericidal activity concentration dependent** but no post-antibiotic effect: do not dose once daily. • **Nephrotoxic:** exact risk unknown, but increased by concomitant nephrotoxins (IV contrast), hypotension, maybe Rifampin. Rare: neuromuscular blockade with respiratory failure. • **Neurotoxicity:** Frequent: circumoral paresthesia, vertigo, abnormal vision, confusion, ataxia. Rare: neuromuscular blockade with respiratory failure. • **Caution:** Some colistimethate products are expressed in IUs. To convert IUs to mg of colistin base: 1,000,000 IUs colistimethate = 80 mg colistimethate base = 30 mg colistin base. See CID 58:139, 2014. Colistin preferred over Polymyxin B for treatment of UTIs. **Urine concentration of Polymyxin B is very low.** • Note: Polymyxin B is preferred over Colistin, except for UTIs because: 1) ease of dose calculation; 2) rapid achievement of stable serum level; 3) low inter patient variability in PK; 4) no dose adjustment for renal insufficiency (CID 59:88, 2014). • Ascorbic acid 1 gm IV q4-6h may reduce risk of nephrotoxicity (CID doi 10.1093, 2015)
MISCELLANEOUS AGENTS		
Fosfomycin (Monurol) (3 gm packet)	3 gm with water po times 1 dose. For emergency use: single patient IND for IV use. From FDA, 1-888-463-6332.	Diarrhea in 9% compared to 6% of pts given nitrofurantoin and 2.3% given TMP-SMX. Available outside U.S. IV & PO. For treatment of multi-drug resistant bacteria. For MDR-GNB 6-12 gm/day IV divided q6-8h. Ref: Int J Antimicrob Ag 37:415, 2011.
Fusidic acid[NUS] (Fucidin, Taksta)	500 mg po/IV (Denmark & Canada) US: loading dose of 1500 mg po bid x 1 day, then 600 mg po bid	Activity vs MRSA of importance. Approved outside the U.S.; currently in U.S. clinical trials. Ref for proposed US regimen: CID 52 (Suppl 7):S520, 2011.
Methenamine hippurate (Hiprex, Urex)	1 gm po bid	Nausea and vomiting, skin rash or dysuria. Overall ~3%. Methenamine requires (pH ≤ 5.5) urine to liberate formaldehyde. Useful in suppressive therapy after infecting organisms cleared; do not use for pyelonephritis. **Comment:** Do not force fluids; may dilute formaldehyde. Of no value in pts with chronic Foley. If urine pH > 5.5, co-administer ascorbic acid. Contraindicated with renal insufficiency (2 gm/600 mg tabs) after drug has been used, results ± based on long term T1/2 of 1,500 mg: rational. Do not use concomitantly with sulfonamides.
Methenamine mandelate (Mandelamine)	1 gm po qid	Contraindicated with concomitant sulfonylureas. Also: topical & vaginal gels. Can use IV such as enema for C. diff colitis. Resistant anaerobic organisms: Actinomyces, Peptostreptococci. Once-daily IV dosing of 1,500 mg: rational based on long term serum T1/2; standard in Europe; supportive retrospective studies in adults with intra-abdominal infections (AAC 19:410, 2007).
Metronidazole [Flagyl] (250, 375, 500 mg tab/cap) Ref.: Activity vs. B. fragilis Still drug of choice (CID 50 (Suppl 1):S16, 2010).	Anaerobic infections: usually Rx 7.5 mg per kg (~500 mg) (not to exceed 4 gm q24h). With long T1/2, can use IV at 15 mg per kg (1,500 mg per kg IV q24h). If life-threatening, use loading dose of IV 15 mg per kg. Oral dose: 500 mg qid; extended release tabs available 750 mg	Common AEs: nausea (12%), metallic taste, furry tongue. **Avoid alcohol during 48 hrs after last dose to avoid disulfiram reaction (N/V, flushing, tachycardia, dyspnea).** Neurologic: AEs with high dose/long Rx: peripheral autonomic and optic neuropathy, aseptic meningitis, encephalopathy, seizures & reversible cerebellar lesion reported. Risk of hypoglycemia with concomitant sulfonylureas. Also: topical & vaginal gels. Can use IV such as enema for C. diff colitis.

*NOTE: all dosage recommendations are for adults (unless otherwise indicated) & assume normal renal function.

(See page 2 for abbreviations)

CLASS, AGENT, GENERIC NAME (TRADE NAME)	USUAL ADULT DOSAGE*	ADVERSE REACTIONS, COMMENTS (See Table 10B for Summary)
MISCELLANEOUS AGENTS (continued)		
Nitazoxanide	See Table 13B, page 162	Absorption ↑ with meals. Increased activity in acid urine. Much reduced at pH 8 or over. Nausea and vomiting, **peripheral neuropathy**, pancreatitis. **Pulmonary reactions** (with chronic rx): acute ARDS type, **chronic desquamative interstitial pneumonia with fibrosis**. Intrahepatic cholestasis & **hepatitis** similar to chronic active hepatitis; Hemolytic anemia in G6PD deficiency. Drug rash, eosinophilia, systemic symptoms (DRESS) hypersensitivity syndrome reported (*Neth J Med 67:147, 2009*). Concern that efficacy may be reduced and AEs increased with CrCl under 40 mL/min. Should not be used in infants <1 month of age. Birth defects; increased risk reported (*Arch Ped Adolesc Med 163:978, 2009*).
Nitrofurantoin macrocrystals, Furadantin, Macrodantin, Furadantin) (25, 50, 100 mg caps) Systematic rev: *JAC70:2456, 2015*	Active UTI: **Furadantin/Macrodantin 50-100 mg po qid x 5-7 days OR Macrobid 100 mg po bid x 5-7 days** Dose for long-term UTI suppression: **50-100 mg at bedtime**	
Rifampin (Rifamate, Rifadin) (150, 300 mg cap)	**300 mg po/IV bid or 600 mg po/IV qd.** Rapid selection of resistant bacteria if used as monotherapy	Causes orange-brown discoloration of sweat, urine, tears, contact lens. **Many important drug-drug interactions,** see *Table 22.* Immune complex flu-like syndrome: fever, headache, myalgias, arthralgia—especially with intermittent rx. Thrombocytopenia, vasculitis reported (*C Ann Pharmacother 42: 727, 2008*). Can cause interstitial nephritis. Risk-benefit of adding RIF to standard therapies for S. aureus endocarditis (*AAC 52:2463, 2008*). See also, *Antimycobacterial Agents, Table 12B, page 148.*
Rifaximin (Xifaxan) (200, 550 mg)	Traveler's diarrhea: **200 mg po tid** times 3 days. Hepatic encephalopathy: **550 mg tab po bid.** C. diff diarrhea as "chaser": **400 mg po bid**	For traveler's diarrhea and hepatic encephalopathy (*AAC 54:3618, 2010; NEJM 362:1071, 2010*). In general, adverse events equal to or less than placebo.
Sulfonamides [e.g. sulfisoxazole (Gantrisin), sulfamethoxazole (Gantanol, Truxazole), sulfadiazine]	Dose varies with indications. See *Nocardia & Toxoplasmosis*	**CNS:** fever, headache, dizziness; **Derm:** mild rash to life threatening Stevens-Johnson syndrome, toxic epidermal necrolysis, photosensitivity; **Hem:** agranulocytosis, aplastic anemia. **Cross-allergenicity:** other sulfa drugs, sulfonylureas, diuretics, crystalluria (esp. sulfadiazine-need ≥ 1500 mL po fluid/day). **Other:** serum sickness, hemolysis if G6PD def, polyarteritis, SLE reported.
Tinidazole (Tindamax)	Tabs **250, 500 mg.** Dose for giardiasis: **2 gm** po times 1 with food.	**Adverse reactions:** metallic taste 3.7%, nausea 3.2%, anorexia/vomiting 1.5%. All higher with multi-day dosing. Avoid alcohol during & for 3 days after last dose; cause disulfiram reaction, flushing, N/V, tachycardia.
Trimethoprim (Trimpex, Proloprim, and others) (100, 200 mg tab)	**100 mg po q12h or 200 mg po q24h.**	**CNS:** drug fever, aseptic meningitis; **Derm:** rash (3-7% at 200 mg/day), phototoxicity, Stevens-Johnson syndrome (rare), toxic epidermal necrolysis (rare). **Renal:** ↑ K+, ↑ Na+, ↑ Cr; **Hem:** neutropenia, thrombocytopenia, methemoglobinemia.
Trimethoprim (TMP)-Sulfamethoxazole (SMX) (Bactrim, Septra, Sulfatrim, Cotrimoxazole) Single-strength (SS) is 80 TMP/400 SMX, double-strength (DS) 160 TMP/800 SMX	**Standard po rx: 1 DS tab bid. P. carinii:** see *Table 11A, page 132.* **IV rx** see *Table 11A, page 132.* **standard 8-10 mg per kg IV per day divided q6h, q8h, or q12h For shigellosis: 2.5 mg per kg IV q6h.**	Adverse reactions in 10%: GI: nausea, vomiting, anorexia. Skin: Rash, urticaria, photosensitivity. More serious (1-10%): TMP, ACE inhibitors & aldactone increase serum K+. Higher incidence of severity when combined. Increased risk of death (*BMJ 349:g6196, 2014*). **Stevens-Johnson syndrome & toxic epidermal necrolysis.** Skin reactions may represent toxic metabolites of SMX (rather than allergy) (*J Am Pharmacotherapy 32:381, 1998*). Daily ascorbic acid 0.5-1.0 gm on may promote detoxification (*JAIDS 36:1041, 2004*). Risk of **hypoglycemia** with concomitant sulfonylureas. **Sweet's Syndrome** can occur. Hyperkalemia. Both TMP & ACE inhibitors can block renal tubular secretions of K+ & lead to dangerous hyperkalemia (*BMJ 349:g6196, 2014*). TMP can be etiology of **aseptic meningitis**. Report of psychosis during treatment of PCP (*JAC 66:1117, 2011*). TMP-SMX contains sulfites and may trigger asthma in sulfite-sensitive pts. Frequent drug cause of thrombocytopenia. No cross allergenicity with other sulfonamide non-antibiotic drugs (*NEJM 349:1628, 2003*). **For TMP-SMX desensitization,** see *Table 7, page 83.*

*NOTE: all dosage recommendations are for adults (unless otherwise indicated) & assume normal renal function.

(See page 2 for abbreviations)

TABLE 10A (13)

CLASS, AGENT, GENERIC NAME (TRADE NAME)	USUAL ADULT DOSAGE*	ADVERSE REACTIONS, COMMENTS *(See Table 10B for Summary)*
Topical Antimicrobial Agents Active vs. S. aureus & Strep. pyogenes *(CID 49:1541, 2009)*. **Review of topical antiseptics, antibiotics** *(CID 49:1541, 2009)*		
Bacitracin (Baciguent)	20% bacitracin zinc ointment, apply 1-5 x/day.	Active vs. staph, strep & clostridium. Contact dermatitis occurs. Available without prescription.
Fusidic acid^NUS ointment	2% ointment, apply tid	Available in Canada and Europe *(Leo Laboratories)*. Active vs. S. aureus & S. pyogenes
Mupirocin (Bactroban)	**Skin cream or ointment 2%: Apply tid times 10 days. Nasal ointment 2%: apply bid times 5 days.**	Skin cream: itch, burning, stinging 1-1.5%; Nasal: headache 9%, rhinitis 6%, respiratory congestion 5%. Not active vs. enterococci or gm-neg bacteria. Summary of resistance *JAC 70:2681, 2015.* If large amounts used in azotemic pts, can accumulate polyethylene glycol *(CID 49:1541, 2009).*
Polymyxin B—Bacitracin (Polysporin)	5000 units/gm; 400 units/gm. Apply 1-4x/day	Polymyxin active vs. some gm-neg bacteria but not Proteus sp. or Serratia sp. or gm-pos bacteria. See Bacitracin comment above. Available without prescription.
Polymyxin B—Bacitracin—Neomycin (Neosporin, triple antibiotic ointment (TAO))	5000 units/gm; 400 units/gm; 3.5 mg/gm. Apply 1-3x/day.	See Bacitracin and polymyxin B comments above. Neomycin active vs. gm-neg bacteria and staphylococci; not active vs. streptococci. Contact dermatitis incidence 1%; risk of nephro- & oto-toxicity if absorbed. TAO spectrum broader than mupirocin and active mupirocin-resistant strains *(DMID 54:63, 2006)*. Available without prescription.
Retapamulin (Altabax)	1% ointment; apply bid. 5, 10 & 15 gm tubes.	Microbiologic success in 90% S. aureus infections and 97% of S. pyogenes infections *(J Am Acad Derm 55:1003, 2006).* Package insert says **for MSSA only** (not enough MRSA pts in clinical trials). Active vs. some mupirocin-resistant S. aureus strains.
Silver sulfadiazine	1% cream, apply once or twice daily.	A sulfonamide but the active ingredient is released silver ions. Activity vs. gram-pos & gram-neg bacteria (including P. aeruginosa). Often used to prevent infection in pts with 2nd/3rd degree burns. Rarely, may stain into the skin.

*NOTE: all dosage recommendations are for adults (unless otherwise indicated) & assume normal renal function

TABLE 10B – SELECTED ANTIBACTERIAL AGENTS—ADVERSE REACTIONS—OVERVIEW

Adverse reactions in individual patients represent all-or-none occurrences, even if rare. After selection of an agent, the physician should read the manufacturer's package insert [statements in the product labeling (package insert)] must be approved by the FDA.] **For unique reactions, see the individual drug** (Table 10A) For drug-drug interactions, see Table 22.
Numbers = frequency of occurrence (%); + = occurs, incidence not available; ++ = significant adverse reaction; 0 = not reported; R = rare, defined as <1%.
NOTE: Important reactions in **bold print**. A blank means no data found. Any antibacterial can precipitate C. difficile colitis.

ADVERSE REACTIONS (AR) For unique ARs, see individual drug, Table 10A	PENICILLINASE-RESISTANT ANTI-STAPH. PENICILLINS				AMINOPENICILLINS				AP PENS	CARBAPENEMS				MONOBACTAMS	AMINOGLYCOSIDES	MISC.	
	Penicillin G, V	Dicloxacillin	Nafcillin	Oxacillin	Amoxicillin	Amox-Clav	Ampicillin	Amp-Sulb	Pip-Taz	Doripenem	Ertapenem	Imipenem	Meropenem	Aztreonam	Amikacin Gentamicin Kanamycin Netilmicin^NUS Tobramycin	Linezolid	Tedizolid
Rx stopped due to AR	3					2-4.4			3.2	3.4			1.2	<1			0.5
Rash	3		R	4	**5**	3	**5**	**2**	4	1-5	+	+	+	2		**2**	
+ Coombs	3	0	R	R	0	0	0	0	+								
Neutropenia	R	0	+	R	2	+	2	2	+	R	+	2	+	R		1.1	0.5
Eosinophilia	+	+	22	22	2	+	22	22	+	8	+	+	8	+			
Thrombocytopenia	R	0	R	R	R	R	R	+	2		3	2	5	R		3	2.3
Nausea/vomiting		+	0	0	2	3	2	**2**	7	4-12	3	2	4	R		6/4	8/3
Diarrhea		R	R	R	**5**	**9**	**10**	6	**11**	6-11	6	2	5	2		8.3	10
↑ LFTs	R	+	R	+	R	3	R	+	R	+	6	6	4	R			
↑ BUN, Cr	R	0	0	0	0	0	0	0	+	+	2	2	4	0	5-25		
Seizures	R	0	0	0	0	R	0	0	R	See footnote²				+			
Ototoxicity	R	0	0	0	0	0	0	0	0	0	0			0	3-14		
Vestibular	0	0	0	0	0	0	0	0	0	0	0			0	4-6		

¹ Eosinophilia in 25% of pts; of those 30% have clinical event (rash 30%, renal injury 15%, liver injury 6%, DRESS in 0.8% (J Allergy Clin Immuno doi 10.1076/j.jaci.2015.04.005

² **All β-lactams in high concentration can cause seizures.** In rabbit, IMP 10x more neurotoxic than benzyl penicillin (JAC 22:687, 1988). In clinical trial of IMP for pediatric meningitis, trial stopped due to seizures in 7/25 IMP recipients; hard to interpret as purulent meningitis causes seizures (PIDJ 10:122, 1991). Risk with IMP↓ with careful attention to dosage (Epilepsia 42:1590, 2001).
Postulated mechanism: Drug binding to GABAₐ receptor. IMP binds with greater affinity than MER.
Package Insert, percent seizures: ERTA 0.5, IMP 0.4, MER 0.7. However, in 3 clinical trials of MER for bacterial meningitis, no drug-related seizures (Scand J Inf Dis 31:3, 1999; Drug Safety 22:191, 2000).
In meta-analysis, seizure risk low but greatest with carbapenems vs. other beta-lactams. No difference in incidence between IMP & MER (IAC 69:2043, 2014).

TABLE 10B (2)

CEPHALOSPORINS/CEPHAMYCINS

ADVERSE REACTIONS (AR) For unique ARs, see individual drug, Table 10A	Cefazolin	Cefotetan	Cefoxitin	Cefuroxime	Cefotaxime	Ceftazidime	Ceftaz-avi	Ceftizoxime	Ceftriaxone	Cefepime	Ceftaroline	Ceftobiprole^NUS	Ceftolo-tazo	Cefaclor/Cef.ER/Loracarbef^NUS	Cefadroxil	Cefdinir	Cefixime	Cefpodoxime	Cefprozil	Ceftibuten	Cefditoren pivoxil	Cefuroxime axetil	Cephalexin
Rx stopped due to AR	+			R	2	2			2	1.5	2.7	4	2	1		3	1	2.7	2	2	2	2.2	1
Rash	3	+	2	R	6	4	<5			2	3	2.7		R	+	R	1	R	1	1	R	2	1
+ Coombs	+	+	2	R	1	1	2	2	2	14	9.8		<1		+	R	R	R		R	R	R	+
Neutropenia				R	1	8	<5	+		1		+	+				R	R	2	R	R	R	+
Eosinophilia	+		3	7			<5	4	6		4/2	+	3/1	2		15	7	3		3	6/1	3	9
Thrombocytopenia	+	+			+	+	+	+	+	+	+		+			1	16	R	R	R	1.4	4	+
↑ PT/PTT	++	++		R	+	+	+	R	R	+	1	+	2	1-4			R	4	R	R	R	2	+
Nausea/vomiting				R	+	2	<5	3	R	1	5	9.1/4.8	3/1	2	+	15	7	4	4	2	6/1	3	3
Diarrhea	4	4	3	R	1	3		3	3	+	2	<2	2	1-4	+	1	16	7	3	3	1.4	4	9
↑ LFTs	+	1	4	R	6	4	1.5	+	4	+	1.7		1.7	3	+	R	R	4	2	R	R	2	+
Hepatic failure	0	0	0	0	0	0		0	0	0		R											+
↑ BUN, Cr	0	0	3	0	1	10	1.5		R	+	R	1.5		+		R	+	4		R	R	R	+
Headache	0	2	3	0	2				R	2	2	4.5		3		2	+		R	R	2	R	9

MACROLIDES / FLUOROQUINOLONES / OTHER AGENTS

ADVERSE REACTIONS (AR) For unique ARs, see individual drug, Table 10A	Erythromycin	Clarithromycin, Reg. & ER	Azithromycin, Reg. & ER	Ciprofloxacin/Cipro XR	Gatifloxacin^NUS	Gemifloxacin	Levofloxacin	Moxifloxacin	Ofloxacin	Chloramphenicol	Clindamycin	Polymyxin B & E (Colistin)	Dalbavancin	Oritavancin	Daptomycin	Metronidazole	Quinupristin-dalfopristin	Rifampin	Telavancin	Tetracycline/Doxy/Mino	Tigecycline	TMP-SMX	Vancomycin
Rx stopped due to AR	1	3	1	3.5	2.9	2.2	4.3	3.8	4				3	3.8	2.8						5		
Rash	R		+	3	R	1-2	2	R	2	+	+	+	2.7	<1.5	4		R	+	4	+		+	3
Nausea/vomiting	3	3	25	5	8/<3	2.7	7/2	7/2	4	+	+	+	6/3	9.9/4.6	6.3	12	2	+	27/14	+	30/20	+	+
Diarrhea	5	3-6	8	2	4	3.6	5	7	4		7	+	4.4	3.7	5	+		+	7	+	12	+	+
↑ LFTs	R	R	+	2	R	1.5	0.1-1		R	+	+		0.8	2.8	R			+		+	4	+	4
↑ BUN, Cr	+	4		R			2	2			0	++			R			+	3	+	2	+	2
Dizziness, light headedness				3	3	0.8	3	2	3				2.7							+	3.5	+	5
Headache	R	2		R		1.2	6	2		+	+	+	4.7	7.1	5	+		+		+		+	

a Highest frequency: females <40 years of age after 14 days of rx; with 5 days or less of Gemi; incidence of rash <1.5%.

TABLE 10C – ANTIMICROBIAL AGENTS ASSOCIATED WITH PHOTOSENSITIVITY

The following drugs (listed alphabetically) are known to cause photosensitivity in some individuals. Note that photosensitivity lasts for several days after the last dose of the drug, at least for tetracyclines. There is no intent to indicate relative frequency or severity of reactions. *Ref: Drug Saf 34:821, 2011.*

DRUG OR CLASS	COMMENT
Azole antifungals	Voriconazole, Itraconazole, Ketoconazole, but not Fluconazole
Bithionol	Old reports
Cefotaxime	Manifested as photodistributed telangiectasia
Ceftazidime	Increased susceptibility to sunburn observed
Dapsone	Confirmed by rechallenge
Doxycycline	Increased susceptibility to sunburn
Efavirenz	Three reports
Flucytosine	Two reports
Fluoroquinolones	Worst offenders have halogen atom at position 8
Griseofulvin	Not thought to be a potent photosensitizer
Isoniazid	Confirmed by rechallenge
Pyrimethamine	One report
Pyrazinamide	Confirmed by rechallenge
Quinine	May cross-react with quinidine
Saquinavir	One report
Tetracyclines	Least common with Minocycline; common with Doxycycline
Trimethoprim	Alone and in combination with Sulfamethoxazole

TABLE 10D – AMINOGLYCOSIDE ONCE-DAILY AND MULTIPLE DAILY DOSING REGIMENS

(See Table 17A, page 215, if estimated creatinine clearance <90 mL per min.)

- General Note: dosages are given as **once daily dose (OD)** and **multiple daily doses (MDD).**
- For **calculation of dosing in non-obese patients** use **Ideal Body Weight (IBW):**

  Female: 45.5 kg + 2.3 kg per inch over 60 inch height = dosing weight in kg.

  Male: 50 kg + 2.3 kg per inch over 60 inch height = dosing weight in kg.

- **Adjustment for calculation of dosing weight in obese patients** (actual body weight (ABW) is ≥ 30% above IBW): IBW + 0.4 (ABW minus IBW) = adjusted weight (Pharmacotherapy 27:1081, 2007; CID 25:112, 1997).
- If CrCl >90 mL/min, use doses in Table 17A, page 215.

- For **non-obese patients, calculate estimated creatinine clearance (CrCl) as follows:**

$$\frac{(140 \text{ minus age}) \times \text{IBW(in kg)}}{72 \times \text{serum creatinine}} = \frac{\text{CrCl in mL/min for men.}}{\text{Multiply answer by 0.85 for women (estimated)}}$$

- For **morbidly obese patients, calculate estimated creatinine clearance (CrCl)** as follows (AJM 84:1053, 1988):

$$\frac{(137 \text{ minus age}) \times [0.285 \times \text{wt in kg}) + (12.1 \times \text{ht in meters}^2)]}{51 \times \text{serum creatinine}} = \text{CrCl (obese male)}$$

$$\frac{(146 \text{ minus age}) \times [0.287 \times \text{wt in kg}) + (9.74 \times \text{ht in meters}^2)]}{60 \times \text{serum creatinine}} = \text{CrCl (obese female)}$$

DRUG	MDD AND OD IV REGIMENS/ TARGETED PEAK (P) AND TROUGH (T) SERUM LEVELS	COMMENTS For more data on once-daily dosing, see AAC 55:2528, 2011 and Table 17A, page 215
Gentamicin (Garamycin), Tobramycin (Nebcin)	MDD: 2 mg per kg load, then 1.7 mg per kg q8h ------ P 4-10 mcg/mL, T 1-2 mcg per mL ------ OD: 5.1 (7 if critically ill) mg per kg q24h ------ P 16-24 mcg per mL, T <1 mcg per mL	**All aminoglycosides have potential to cause tubular necrosis and renal failure, deafness due to cochlear toxicity, vertigo due to damage to vestibular organs, and rarely neuromuscular blockade.** Risk minimal with oral or topical application due to small % absorption unless tissues altered by disease
Kanamycin (Kantrex), Amikacin (Amikin), Streptomycin	MDD: 7.5 mg per kg q12h ------ P 15-30 mcg per mL, T 5-10 mcg per mL ------ OD: 15 mg per kg q24h ------ P 56-64 mcg per mL, T <1 mcg per mL	Risk of nephrotoxicity ↑ with concomitant administration of cyclosporine, vancomycin, ampho B, radiocontrast. Risk of nephrotoxicity ↓ by once-daily dosing method (especially if baseline renal function normal). In general, same factors influence risk of ototoxicity. **NOTE: There is no known method to eliminate risk of aminoglycoside nephro/ototoxicity. Proper rx attempts to ↓ the % risk.**
Netilmicin[NUS]	MDD: 2 mg per kg q8h ------ P 4-10 mcg per mL, T 1-2 mcg per mL ------ OD: 6.5 mg per kg q24h ------ P 22-30 mcg per mL, T <1 mcg per mL	The clinical trial data of OD aminoglycosides have been reviewed extensively by meta-analysis (CID 24:816, 1997). **Serum levels:** Collect peak serum level (PSL) exactly 1 hr after the start of the infusion of the 3rd dose. In critically ill patients, PSL after the 1st dose as volume of distribution and renal function may change rapidly.
Isepamicin[NUS]	Only OD. Severe infections 15 mg per kg q24h, less severe 8 mg per kg q24h	Other dosing methods and references. For once-daily 7 mg per kg per day of gentamicin—Hartford Hospital method (may under dose if <7 mg/kg/day dose), see AAC 39:650, 1995.
Spectinomycin (Trobicin)[NUS]	2 gm IM times 1-gonococcal infections	One in 500 patients (Europe) have mitochondrial mutation that predicts cochlear toxicity (NEJM 360:640 & 642, 2009). Aspirin supplement (3 gm/day) attenuated risk of cochlear injury from gentamicin (NEJM 354:1856, 2006). Vestibular injury usually bilateral & hence no vertigo but imbalance & oscillopsia (Med J Aust 196:701, 2012).
Neomycin—oral	Prophylaxis GI surgery: 1 gm times 3 with erythro, see Table 15B, page 200 For hepatic coma: 4-12 gm per day po	
Tobramycin—inhaled (Tobi): See Cystic fibrosis, Table 1, AB & Table 10F, page 120. Adverse effects few: transient voice alteration (13%) and transient tinnitus (3%).		
Paromomycin—oral: See Entamoeba and Cryptosporidia, Table 13A, page 151.		

TABLE 10E: PROLONGED OR CONTINUOUS INFUSION DOSING OF SELECTED BETA LACTAMS

Based on current and rapidly changing data, it appears that prolonged or continuous infusion of beta-lactams is at least as successful as intermittent dosing. Hence, this approach can be part of stewardship programs as supported by recent publications.

Antibiotic stability is a concern. Factors influencing stability include drug concentration, IV infusion diluent (e.g. NS vs. D5W), type of infusion device, and storage temperature (Ref: P&T 36:723, 2011). Portable pumps worn close to the body expose antibiotics to temperatures closer to body temperature (37°C) than to room temperature (around 25°C). Carbapenems are particularly unstable and may require wrapping of infusion pumps in cold packs or frequent changes of infusion bags or cartridges.

A meta-analysis of observational studies found reduced mortality among patients treated with extended or continuous infusion of carbapenems or piperacillin-tazobactam (pooled data) as compared to standard intermittent regimens. The results were similar for extended and continuous regimens when considered separately. There was a mortality benefit with piperacillin-tazobactam but not carbapenems (CID 56:272, 2013). The lower mortality could, at least in part, be due to closer professional supervision engendered by a study environment. On the other hand, a small prospective randomized controlled study of continuous vs. intermittent Pip-Tazo, and meropenem found a higher clinical cure rate and a trend toward lower mortality in the continuous infusion patients (CID 56:236, 2013).

DRUG/METHOD	MINIMUM STABILITY	RECOMMENDED DOSE	COMMENTS
Cefepime (Continuous)	@ 37°C: 8 hours @ 25°C: 24 hours @ 4°C: ≥24 hours	Initial dose: 15 mg/kg over 30 min, then immediately begin: • If CrCl > 60: 6 gm (over 24 hr) daily • If CrCl 30-60: 4 gm (over 24 hr) daily • If CrCl 11-29: 2 gm (over 24 hr) daily	CrCl adjustments extrapolated from prescribing information, not clinical data. Refs: JAC 57:1017, 2006; Am. J. Health Syst. Pharm. 68:319, 2011.
Ceftazidime (Continuous)	@ 37°C: 8 hours @ 25°C: 24 hours @ 4°C: ≥24 hours	Initial dose: 15 mg/kg over 30 min, then immediately begin: • If CrCl > 50: 6 gm (over 24 hr) daily • If CrCl 31-50: 4 gm (over 24 hr) daily • If CrCl 10-30: 2 gm (over 24 hr) daily	CrCl adjustments extrapolated from prescribing information, not clinical data. Refs: Br J Clin Pharmacol 50:184, 2000; IJAA 17:497, 2001; AAC 49:3550, 2005; Infect 37: 418, 2009; JAC 68:900, 2013.
Doripenem (Prolonged)	@ 37°C: 8 hours (in NS) @ 25°C: 24 hours (in NS) @ 4°C: 24 hours (in NS)	• If CrCl ≥ 50: 500 mg (over 4 hr) q8h • If CrCl 30-49: 250 mg (over 4 hr) q8h • If CrCl 10-29: 250 mg (over 4 hr) q12h	Based on a single study (Crit Care Med 36:1089, 2008).
Meropenem (Prolonged)	@ 37°C: < 4 hours @ 25°C: 4 hours @ 4°C: 24 hours	• If CrCl ≥ 50: 2 gm (over 3 hr) q8h • If CrCl 30-49: 1 gm (over 3 hr) q8h • If CrCl 10-29: 1 gm (over 3 hr) q12h	Initial 1 gm dose reasonable but not used by most investigators. Ref: Intens Care Med 37:632, 2011.
PIP-TZ (Prolonged)	@ 37°C: 24 hours @ 25°C: 24 hours @ 4°C: no data	Initial dose: 4.5 gm over 30 min, then 4 hrs later start: • If CrCl ≥ 20: 3.375 gm (over 4 hr) q8h • If CrCl < 20: 3.375 gm (over 4 hr) q12h	Reasonable to begin first infusion 4 hrs after initial dose. Refs: CID 44:357, 2007; AAC 54:460, 2010. See CID 56:236, 245 & 272, 2013. In obese patients (> 120 kg), may need higher doses 6.75 gm or even 9 gm (over 4 hrs) q8h to achieve adequate serum levels of tazobactam (Int J Antimicrob Agts 41:52, 2013).
Temocillin	@ 37°C: 24 hours @ 25°C: 24 hours These apply to Temocillin 4 gm/48 mL dilution (JAC 61:382, 2008)	Initial dose: 2 gm over 30 min, then immediately begin: • If CrCl > 50: 6 gm (over 24 hr) daily • If CrCl 31-50: 3 gm (over 24 hr) daily • If CrCl 10-30: 1.5 gm (over 24 hr) daily • If CrCl <10: 750 mg (over 24 hr) daily CVVH: 750 mg (over 24 hr) daily	Offers higher probability of reaching desired PK/PD target than conventional q8h dosing. This study not designed to assess clinical efficacy (JAC 70:891, 2015).
Vancomycin (Continuous)	@ 37°C: 48 hours @ 25°C: 48 hours @ 4°C: 58 days (at conc 10 μg/mL)	Loading dose of 15-20 mg/kg over 30-60 minutes, then 30 mg/kg by continuous infusion over 24 hours. No data on pts with renal impairment.	Adjust dose to target plateau concentration of 20-25 μg/mL. Higher plateau concentrations (30-40 μg/mL) achieved with more aggressive dosing increase the risk of nephrotoxicity (Ref: Clin Micro Inf 19:E98, 2013). Continuous infusion may reduce risk of Vanco nephrotoxicity (CCM 42:2527 & 2635, 2014).

TABLE 10F: INHALATION ANTIBIOTICS

Introductory remarks: There is interest in inhaled antimicrobials for several patient populations, such as those with cystic fibrosis or as a result of other conditions. Interest is heightened by growing incidence of infection due to multi-drug resistant Gram-negative bacilli. Isolates of *P. aeruginosa, A. baumannii*, or *Klebsiella* species susceptible only to colistin are of special concern.

There are a variety of ways to generate aerosols for inhalation: inhalation of dry powder, jet nebulizers, ultrasonic nebulizers, and most recently, vibrating mesh nebulizers. The vibrating mesh inhalers generate fine particle aerosols with enhanced delivery of drug to small airways (*Cochrane Database of Systematic Reviews 4:CD007639, 2013*).

Inhaled DRUG	DELIVERY SYSTEM	DOSE	COMMENT
Amikacin + Ceftazidime	Vibrating plate nebulizer	AMK: 25 mg/kg once daily x 3 days Ceftaz: 15 mg/kg q3h x 8 days	Radiographic and clinical cure of *P. aeruginosa* ventilator-associated pneumonia (VAP) similar to IV AMK/Ceftaz, including strains with intermediate resistance (*AJRCCM 184:106. 2011*).
Aztreonam (Cayston)	Altera vibrating mesh nebulizer	75 mg tid x 28 days (every other month)	Improves pulmonary function, reduces frequency of exacerbations, and improves symptoms in cystic fibrosis (CF) pts (*Exp Opin Pharmacother 14:2115, 2013*). Cost per treatment cycle about $6070.
Colistin	Various (see comment)	Various (see comment)	Much variability and confusion in dosing. Nebulized colistimethate (CMS) 1-2 million U (33-66 mg colistin base) effective for CF (*Exp Opin Drug Deliv 9:333, 2012*). Summary of available studies (*Expert Rev Antiinfect Ther 13:1237, 2015*). Adjunctive role for VAP still unclear (*CID 43:589, 2006; CID 51:1238, 2010*). "High-dose" nebulized CMS (400 mg q8h) via **vibrating-mesh nebulizer effective for VAP due to multidrug-resistant *P. aeruginosa* and *A. baumannii*** (*Anesth 117:1335, 2012*). Efficacy of adding inhaled colistin to IV colistin for VAP due to GNB susceptible only to colistin was studied. Colistin: 1 million IU q8h (as CMS) nebulized with either jet or ultrasonic nebulizer. Higher cure rate with combined inhaled plus IV colistin as compared to IV colistin alone (*Chest 144: 1768, 2013*).
Fosfomycin + Tobramycin (FTI) 4:1 w/wt	eFlow vibrating mesh nebulizer	FTI 160/40 or 80/20 bid x 28 days	Both doses maintained improvements in FEV₁ following a 28-day inhaled aztreonam run-in (vs. placebo) in CF patients with *P. aeruginosa*; FTI 80/20 better tolerated than 160/40 (*AJRCCM 185:171, 2012*).
Levofloxacin	eFlow vibrating mesh nebulizer	240 mg bid x 28 days	Reduced sputum density of *P. aeruginosa*, need for other antibiotics, and improved pulmonary function compared to placebo in CF pts (*AJRCCM 183:1510, 2011*).
Liposomal Amikacin	PARI LC STAR jet nebulizer	500 mg qd x 28 days (every other month)	Company reports Phase 3 study in CF pts with *P. aeruginosa* has met primary endpoint of non-inferiority compared to TOBI for FEV₁ improvement. Insmed website: *http://investor.insmed.com/releasedetail.cfm?ReleaseID=774638*. Accessed November 30, 2013.
Tobramycin (TOBI, Bethkis)	PARI LC PLUS jet nebulizer	300 mg bid x 28 days (every other month)	Cost: about $6700 for one treatment cycle (*Med Lett 56:51, 2014*)
Tobramycin (TOBI Podhaler)	28 mg dry powder caps	4 caps (112 mg) bid x 28 days (every other month)	Improvement in FEV₁, similar to Tobra inhaled solution in CF patients with chronic *P. aeruginosa* but more airway irritation with the powder. Cost of one month treatment cycle about $6700 (*Med Lett 56:51, 2014*).

TABLE 11A – TREATMENT OF FUNGAL INFECTIONS—ANTIMICROBIAL AGENTS OF CHOICE*

For Antifungal Activity Spectra, see Table 4B, page 79

TYPE OF INFECTION/ORGANISM/ SITE OF INFECTION	ANTIMICROBIAL AGENTS OF CHOICE		COMMENTS
	PRIMARY	ALTERNATIVE	
Aspergillosis (A. fumigatus most common, also A. flavus and others) (See NEJM 360:1870, 2009; Chest 146:1870, 2014).			
Allergic bronchopulmonary aspergillosis (ABPA) Clinical manifestations: wheezing, pulmonary infiltrates, bronchiectasis & fibrosis. Airway colonization assoc. with ↑ blood eosinophils, ↑ serum IgE, ↑ specific serum antibodies.	Acute asthma attacks associated with ABPA: **Corticosteroids**	Rx of ABPA: **itraconazole** oral soln 200 mg po bid times 16 wks or longer	Itra decreases number of exacerbations requiring corticosteroids with improved immunological markers, improved lung function & exercise tolerance (IDSA Guidelines updated CID 46:327, 2008).
Allergic fungal sinusitis: relapsing chronic sinusitis; nasal polyps without bony invasion; asthma, eczema or allergic rhinitis; ↑ IgE levels and isolation of Aspergillus sp. or other dematiaceous fungi. (Alternaria, Cladosporium, etc.)	**Rx controversial:** systemic corticosteroids + surgical debridement (relapse common).	For failures try **itra** 200 mg po bid times 12 mos or flucon nasal spray.	Controversial area.
Aspergilloma (fungus ball)	No therapy or surgical resection. Efficacy of antimicrobial agents not proven.		Aspergillus may complicate pulmonary sequestration.
Invasive, pulmonary (IPA) or extrapulmonary Post-transplantation and post-chemotherapy in neutropenic pts (PMN <500 per mm³) but may also present with neutrophil recovery. Common pneumonia in transplant recipients. Usually a late (≥100 days) complication in allogeneic bone marrow & other transplantation: High mortality (CID 44:531, 2007). **Typical x-ray/CT lung lesions** (halo sign, cavitation, or macronodules) (CID 44:373, 2006). An immunologic test that detects circulating **galactomannan** antigen is available for dx of invasive aspergillosis (Lancet ID 4:349, 2005). Serum galactomannan relatively insensitive; antifungal rx may decrease sensitivity (Am J Respir Crit Care Med 177:27, 2008). Improved sensitivity when performed on BAL fluid. (Am J Respir Crit Care Med 177:27, 2008). **False-pos result seen in pts receiving PIP-TZ, Amox-Clav & other beta lactams, infection with other fungi & some blood product conditioning fluid (CID 40:1762, 2007). **Better diagnostic strategy:** combination of serum galactomannan & aspergillus PCR (not routinely available) (LnID 13:519, 2013).** **Beta D-Glucan:** in fungal cell wall. Can detect with immunoassay. Many false positives + low sensitivity (JCM 51:3478, 2013).	**Primary therapy** (See CID 46:327, 2006): **Voriconazole** 6 mg/kg IV q12h on day 1; then either (4 mg/kg IV q12h) or (200 mg po q12h for body weight ≥40 kg, but 100 mg po q12h for body weight <40 kg) (use actual wt) (see table 4): 1.0–5.5 mg/L associated with improved response rates and reduced adverse effects (Clin Infect Dis 55:1080, 2012). **Alternative therapies: Liposomal ampho B** (L-AMB) 3-5 mg/kg/day IV; OR **Ampho B lipid complex** (ABLC) 5 mg/kg/d IV; OR **Caspofungin** 70 mg/day then 50 mg/day thereafter; OR **Micafungin**ᴺᴬᴵ 100 mg IV/day (JAC 64:840, 2009– based on PK/PD study): OR **Posaconazole**ᴺᴬᴵ 200 mg qid, then 400 mg bid after stabilization of disease;	For failures try **itra** 200 mg po bid times 12 mos or flucon nasal spray.	**Voriconazole** more effective than ampho B. Vori, both a substrate and an inhibitor of CYP2C19, CYP2C9, and CYP3A4, has potential for deleterious drug-drug interactions (e.g., with protease inhibitors). Review concomitant medications. Measure serum level with prolonged therapy or for patients with possible drug-drug interactions. In patients with CrCl < 50 mL/min, po may be preferred due to concerns for nephrotoxicity of IV vehicle (cyclodextrin). **Isavuconazole** (prodrug isavuconazonium sulfate): A randomized control trial of isavuconazole vs. Voriconazole for invasive aspergillosis demonstrated that isavuconazole is non-inferior to voriconazole for the treatment of invasive aspergillosis (Package insert, clinical trial not published). **L-AMB & ABLC recommended as a lipid formulation**, either L-AMB 3 mg/kg/day and 3 mg/kg doses of L-AMB are equally efficacious with greater toxicity of higher dose (CID 2007: 44:1289–97). One comparative trial found greater toxicity with ABLC than with L-AMB: 34.6% vs 25.8% adverse events and 21.2% vs 2.8% nephrotoxicity (Cancer 112:1282, 2008). Vori preferred as primary therapy. **Posaconazole:** 42% response rate in open-label trial of patients refractory/intolerant to conventional therapy (Clin Infect Dis 44:2, 2007). Caution for azole-azole resistance with azole-non-responders. Measurement of serum concentrations advisable. **Caspofungin:** ~50% response rate in IPA. Licensed for salvage therapy. **Micafungin:** Favorable responses to micafungin as a single agent in 6/12 patients in primary therapy group and 9/22 in the salvage therapy group (J Infect 53: 337, 2006). **Combination therapy:** A RCT of Voriconazole plus Anidulafungin vs. Voriconazole alone showed a trend towards reduced mortality in all patients with invasive aspergillosis in the combination therapy arm (Ann Intern Med 162:81, 2015). Subgroup of patients for whom diagnosis was established by radiographic findings and GM positivity had lower mortality with combination therapy. Combination therapy should be strongly considered although further data is needed to determine which patients would benefit the most. Some experts would recommend addition of echinocandin to amphotericin-based regimen or other azoles as well.

See page 2 for abbreviations. All dosage recommendations are for adults (unless otherwise indicated) and assume normal renal function

TABLE 11A (2)

TYPE OF INFECTION/ORGANISM/ SITE OF INFECTION	ANTIMICROBIAL AGENTS OF CHOICE		COMMENTS
	PRIMARY	ALTERNATIVE	
Aspergillosis (continued)			
Blastomycosis (CID 46: 1801, 2008) (Blastomyces dermatitidis) Cutaneous, pulmonary or extrapulmonary.	**LAB**, 3-5 mg/kg per day; OR **Ampho B**, 0.7-1 mg/kg per day, for 1-2 weeks, **then Itra** oral soln 200 mg tid for 3 days, then 200 mg bid for 6-12 months	**Itra** oral soln 200 mg tid for 3 days then once or twice per day for 6-12 months for mild to moderate disease, OR **Flu** 400-800 mg per day for those intolerant to Itra	Serum levels of **Itra** should be determined after 2 weeks to ensure adequate drug exposure. Flu less effective than Itra; role of Vori or Posa unclear but active in vitro. Can look for Blastomyces in antigen in urine as aid to diagnosis.
Blastomycosis: CNS disease (CID 50:797, 2010)	**LAB** 5 mg/kg per day for 4-6 weeks, followed by **Flu** 800 mg per day	**Itra** oral soln 200 mg bid or tid; OR **Vori** 200-400 mg q12h	Flu and Vori have excellent CNS penetration. Ampho B only slightly reduced activity compared to Itra. Treat for at least 12 months and until CSF has normalized. Monitor serum Itra levels to assure adequate drug concentrations. More favorable outcome with Voriconazole (CID 50:797, 2010).
Candidiasis: Candida is a common cause of nosocomial bloodstream infection. C. albicans & non-albicans species show ↓ susceptibility to antifungal agents (esp. fluconazole). C. albicans & non-albicans candidiasis is a major manifestation of advanced HIV, & represents common AIDS-defining diagnosis. where antifungal prophylaxis (esp. fluconazole) is widely used. Oral, esophageal, vaginal candidiasis. See CID 48:503, 2009 or updated IDSA Guidelines.			
Candidiasis: Bloodstream infection			
Bloodstream: non-neutropenic patient	**Caspofungin** 70 mg IV loading dose, then 50 mg IV daily; OR **Micafungin** 100 mg IV daily; OR **Anidulafungin** 200 mg IV loading dose then 100 mg IV daily. Note: Reduce **Caspo** dose for renal impairment.	**Fluconazole** 800 mg (12 mg/kg) loading dose, then 400 mg daily IV OR Lipid-based **ampho B** 3-5 mg/kg IV daily; OR **Ampho B** 0.7 mg/kg IV daily; OR **Voriconazole** 400 mg (6 mg/kg) IV twice daily for 2 doses then 200 mg q12h.	**Echinocandin** is recommended for empiric therapy, particularly for patients with recent azole exposure or with moderately severe or severe illness, hemodynamic instability. An echinocandin should be used for treatment of Candida glabrata unless susceptibility to fluconazole or voriconazole has been confirmed. Echinocandin preferred empiric therapy in centers with high prevalence of non-albicans candida species. Echinocandin vs. polyenes or azole associated with better survival (Clin Infect Dis 54:1110, 2012).
Remove all intravascular catheters if possible: replace catheters at a new site (not over a wire).			A double-blind randomized trial of anidulafungin (n=127) and fluconazole (n=118) showed an 88% microbiologic response rate (119/135 candida species) with anidulafungin vs a 76% (99/130 candida species) with fluconazole (p=0.02) (NEJM 356: 2472, 2007).
Higher mortality associated with delay in therapy (CID 43:25, 2006).			**Fluconazole** is not recommended for empiric therapy but could be considered for patients with mild-to-moderate illness, hemodynamically stable, with no recent azole exposure. Fluconazole not recommended for treatment of documented C. krusei: use an echinocandin or voriconazole or posaconazole (note: echinocandins have better in vitro activity than either Vori or Posa against C. glabrata).
	Funduscopic examination within first week of therapy to exclude ophthalmic involvement. Ocular disease present in ~15% of patients with candidemia, but endophthalmitis is uncommon (~2%) (CID 53:262, 2011). Intraocular injections of ampho B required for endophthalmitis as echinocandins have poor penetration into the eye. For **septic thrombophlebitis,** catheter removal and incision and drainage and resection of the vein, as needed, are recommended; duration of therapy at least 2 weeks after last positive blood culture.		Fluconazole recommended for treatment of Candida parapsilosis because of reduced susceptibility of this species to echinocandins. Transition from echinocandin to fluconazole for stable patients with Candida albicans or other azole-susceptible species. **Voriconazole** with little advantage over fluconazole (more drug-drug interactions) except for oral step-down therapy of Candida krusei or voriconazole-susceptible Candida glabrata. Recommended **duration of therapy** is 14 days after last positive blood culture. Duration of systemic therapy should be extended to 4-6 weeks for eye involvement.

See page 2 for abbreviations. All dosage recommendations are for adults (unless otherwise indicated) and assume normal renal function

TABLE 11A (3)

TYPE OF INFECTION/ORGANISM/ SITE OF INFECTION	ANTIMICROBIAL AGENTS OF CHOICE		COMMENTS
	PRIMARY	**ALTERNATIVE**	
Candidiasis: Bloodstream infection (continued)			
Bloodstream: neutropenic patient Remove intravascular catheters if possible; replace catheters at a new site (not over a wire).	**Capsofungin** 70 mg IV loading dose, then 50 mg IV daily, 35 mg for moderate hepatic insufficiency; OR **Micafungin** 100 mg IV daily; OR **Anidulafungin** 200 mg IV loading dose then 100 mg IV daily; OR **Lipid-based ampho B** 3-5 mg/kg IV daily.	**Fluconazole** 800 mg (12 mg/kg) loading dose, then 400 mg daily IV or PO; OR **Voriconazole** 400 mg (6 mg/kg) IV twice daily for 2 doses then 200 mg (3 mg/kg) IV q12h.	**Duration of therapy** in absence of metastatic complications is for 2 weeks after last positive blood culture, resolution of signs, and resolution of neutropenia. Perform funduscopic examination after recovery of white count as signs of ophthalmic involvement may not be seen during neutropenia. See comments above for recommendations concerning choice of specific agents.
Candidiasis: Bone and joint infections			
Osteomyelitis	**Fluconazole** 400 mg (6 mg/kg) daily IV or PO; OR **Lipid-based ampho B** 3-5 mg/kg daily for several weeks, then oral fluconazole	**Caspo, Mica** or **Anidula** or **ampho B** 0.5-1 mg/kg IV daily for several weeks then oral **fluconazole.**	Treat for a total of 6-12 months. **Surgical debridement** often necessary; **remove hardware** whenever possible.
Septic arthritis	**Fluconazole** 400 mg (6 mg/kg) daily IV or PO; OR **Lipid-based ampho B** 3-5 mg/kg IV daily for several weeks, then oral fluconazole.	**Caspo, Mica** or **Anidula** or **ampho B** 0.5-1 mg/kg IV daily for several weeks then oral **fluconazole.**	**Surgical debridement** in all cases; removal of prosthetic joints whenever possible. Treat for at least 6 weeks and indefinitely if retained hardware.
Candidiasis: Cardiovascular infections			
Endocarditis (See Eur J Clin Microbiol Infect Dis 27:519, 2008)	**Caspofungin** 50-150 mg/day IV; OR **Micafungin** 100-150 mg/day IV; OR **Anidulafungin** 100-200 mg/day IV; OR **Lipid-based ampho B** 3-5 mg/kg/day + **5-FC** 25 mg/kg po qid.	**Ampho B** 0.6-1 mg/kg IV daily + **5-FC** 25 mg/kg po qid	Consider use of higher doses of echinocandins for endocarditis or other endovascular infections. Can switch to **fluconazole 400-800 mg orally in stable patients** with negative blood cultures and fluconazole susceptible organism. See Med 90:237, 2011. Valve replacement strongly recommended, particularly if prosthetic valve endocarditis. Duration of therapy not well defined, but treat for at least 6 weeks after valve replacement and longer in those with complications (e.g., perivalvular or myocardial abscess, extensive disease, delayed resolution of candidemia). Long-term (life-long?) suppression with fluconazole 400-800 mg daily for native valve endocarditis and no valve replacement; life-long suppression for prosthetic valve endocarditis if no valve replacement.
Myocarditis	**Lipid-based ampho B** 3-5 mg/kg IV daily; OR **Fluconazole** 400-800 mg. (6-12 mg/kg) daily IV or PO; OR **Caspo, Mica** or **Anidula** (see endocarditis)		Can switch to **fluconazole 400-800 mg orally in stable patients** with negative blood cultures and fluconazole susceptible organism. Recommended duration of therapy is for several months.

See page 2 for abbreviations. All dosage recommendations are for adults (unless otherwise indicated) and assume normal renal function

TABLE 11A (4)

TYPE OF INFECTION/ORGANISM/ Site of Infection	ANTIMICROBIAL AGENTS OF CHOICE		COMMENTS
	PRIMARY	ALTERNATIVE	
Candidiasis: Cardiovascular infections *(continued)*			
Pericarditis	**Lipid-based ampho B** 3-5 mg/kg daily; OR **Fluconazole** 400-800 mg (6-12 mg/kg) daily IV or po; OR **An echinocandin** IV *(see endocarditis)*		**Pericardial window or pericardiectomy** also is recommended. Can switch to **fluconazole 400-800 mg orally in stable patients** with negative blood cultures and fluconazole susceptible organism. Recommended duration of therapy is for several months.
Candidiasis: Mucosal, esophageal, and oropharyngeal			
Candida esophagitis Primarily encountered in HIV-positive patients Dysphagia or odynophagia predictive of esophageal candidiasis.	**Fluconazole** 200-400 (3-6 mg/kg) mg IV/po daily; OR **echinocandin (caspofungin** 50 mg IV daily; OR **micafungin** 150 mg IV daily; OR **anidulafungin** 200 mg IV loading dose then 100 mg IV daily); OR **Ampho B** 0.5 mg/kg IV daily.	An azole (**itraconazole** solution 200 mg daily; or **posaconazole** suspension 400 mg bid for 3 days then 400 mg daily or **voriconazole** IV/po 200 mg q12h.	**Duration of therapy** 14-21 days. IV echinocandin or ampho B for patients unable to tolerate oral therapy. For fluconazole refractory disease, Itra (80% will respond), Posa, Vori, an echinocandin, or ampho B. Echinocandins associated with higher relapse rate than fluconazole. ART recommended. Suppressive therapy with fluconazole 200 mg po 3x/wk until CD4 > 200/mm³.
Oropharyngeal candidiasis			
Non-AIDS patient	**Clotrimazole troches** 10 mg 5 times daily; OR **Nystatin suspension** or pastilles po qid; OR **Fluconazole** 100-200 mg daily	**Itraconazole** solution 200 mg daily; OR **posaconazole** suspension 400 mg bid for 3 days then 400 mg daily; or **voriconazole** 200 mg q12h; OR an echinocandin (**caspofungin** 70 mg IV loading dose then 50 mg IV daily; or **micafungin** 100 mg IV daily; or **anidulafungin** 200 mg IV daily); OR **Ampho B** 0.3 mg/kg daily	**Duration of therapy** 7-14 days. Clotrimazole or nystatin recommended for mild disease; fluconazole preferred for moderate-to-severe disease. Alternative agents reserved for refractory disease.
AIDS patient	**Fluconazole** 100-200 mg po daily for 7-14 days.	Same as for non-AIDS patient for 7-14 days.	ART in HIV-positive patients. Suppressive therapy until CD4 > 200/mm³, but if required fluconazole 100 mg po thrice weekly. Oral Itra, Posa, or Vori for 28 days for fluconazole-refractory disease. IV echinocandin also an option. Dysphagia or odynophagia predictive of esophageal candidiasis.

See page 2 for abbreviations. All dosage recommendations are for adults (unless otherwise indicated) and assume normal renal function

TABLE 11A (5)

TYPE OF INFECTION/ORGANISM/ SITE OF INFECTION	ANTIMICROBIAL AGENTS OF CHOICE		COMMENTS
	PRIMARY	ALTERNATIVE	
Candidiasis: Mucosal, esophageal, and oropharyngeal *(continued)*			
Vulvovaginitis			
Non-AIDS Patient	**Topical azole therapy: Butoconazole 2% cream** (5 gm), q24h at bedtime x 3 days or 2% cream SR 5 gm x 1; OR **Clotrimazole 100 mg vaginal tabs** (2 at bedtime x 3 days) or 1% cream (5 gm) at bedtime times 7 days (14 days may ↑ cure rate) or 100 mg vaginal tab x 7 days or 500 mg vaginal tab x 1; OR **Miconazole 200 mg vaginal suppos** (1 at bedtime x 3 days) or 100 mg vaginal suppos. q24h x 7 days or 2% cream (5 gm) at bedtime x 7 days; OR **Terconazole 80 mg vaginal tab** (1 at bedtime x 3 days) or 0.4% cream (5 gm) at bedtime x 7 days or 0.8% cream 5 gm intravaginal q24h x 3 days: or tioconazole 6.5% vag. ointment 1 x 1 dose. **Oral therapy:** **Fluconazole** 150 mg po x 1; OR **itraconazole** 200 mg po bid x 1 day.	**Recurrent vulvovaginal candidiasis: fluconazole** 150 mg weekly for 6 months.	
AIDS Patient	Topical **azoles** (clotrimazole, buto, mico, tico, or tercon) x3–7d; OR Topical **nystatin** 100,000 units/day as vaginal tablet x14d; OR Oral **Flu** 150 mg x1 dose.		For recurrent disease 10-14 days of topical azole or oral **Flu** 150 mg, then **Flu** 150 mg po weekly for 6 mos.
Candidiasis: Other Infections			
CNS Infection	**Lipid-based ampho B** 3-5 mg/kg IV daily ± 5-FC 25 mg/kg po qid.	**Fluconazole** 400-800 mg (6–12 mg/kg) IV or po.	Removal of **intraventricular devices** recommended. **Flu** 400-800 mg as step-down therapy in the stable patient and in patient intolerant of ampho B. Experience too limited to recommend echinocandins at this time. **Treatment duration** for several weeks until resolution of CSF, radiographic, and clinical abnormalities.
Cutaneous *(including paronychia, Table 1, page 27)*	Apply topical ampho B, clotrimazole, econazole, ketoconazole, miconazole, or nystatin 3-4 x daily for 7–14 days or ketoconazole 400 mg once daily x 14 days. Ciclopirox olamine 1% cream/lotion; apply topically bid x 7–14 days.		
Endophthalmitis / Chorioretinitis • Occurs in 10% of candidemia, thus ophthalmological consult for all pts • Diagnosis: typical white exudates on retinal exam and/or positive vitrectomy culture • Chorioretinitis accounts for 85% of ocular disease while endophthalmitis occurs in only 15% (*Clin Infect Dis* 53:262, 2011).	Chorioretinitis or Endophthalmitis: Lipid-based **Amphotericin B** 3-5 mg/kg daily + **Flucytosine** 25 mg/kg po/IV q12 OR **Voriconazole** 6 mg/kg po/IV q12 x 2 doses and then 4 mg/kg po/IV q12. Consider intravitreal **Amphotericin B** 5–10 mcg in 0.1 mL or intravitreal **Voriconazole** 100 mcg in 0.1 mL for sight threatening disease.	Chorioretinitis or Endophthalmitis: **Fluconazole** 6-12 mg/kg IV daily (poor activity against C. glabrata and C. krusei) and consider intravitreal **Amphotericin B** 5-10 mcg in 0.1 mL. Consider vitrectomy in advanced disease. *Clin Infect Dis.* 52:648, 2011.	**Duration of therapy:** 4-6 weeks or longer, based on resolution determined by repeated examinations. Vitrectomy may be necessary for those with vitritis or endophthalmitis (*Br J Ophthalmol* 92:466, 2008; *Pharmacotherapy* 27:1711, 2007).

See page 2 for abbreviations. All dosage recommendations are for adults (unless otherwise indicated) and assume normal renal function

TABLE 11A (6)

TYPE OF INFECTION/ORGANISM/ SITE OF INFECTION	ANTIMICROBIAL AGENTS OF CHOICE		COMMENTS
	PRIMARY	ALTERNATIVE	
Candidiasis: Other infections (continued)			
Neonatal candidiasis	**Ampho B** 1 mg/kg IV daily, OR **Fluconazole** 12 mg/kg IV daily.	**Lipid-based ampho B** 3-5 mg/kg IV daily.	**Lumbar puncture** to rule out CNS disease, **dilated retinal examination,** and **intravascular catheter removal** strongly recommended. Lipid-based ampho B used only if there is no renal involvement. Echinocandins considered 3rd line therapy. **Duration of therapy is at least 3 weeks.**
Peritonitis (Chronic Ambulatory Peritoneal Dialysis) See Table 19, page 231.	**Fluconazole** 400 mg po q24h x 2-3 wks; or **caspofungin** 70 mg IV on day 1 followed by 50 mg IV q24h for 14 days; or **micafungin** 100 mg IV q24h for 14 days.	**Ampho B,** continuous intraperitoneal dosing at 1.5 mg/L of dialysis fluid times 4-6 wks.	Remove cath immediately or if no clinical improvement in 4-7 days.
Candidiasis: Urinary tract Infections			
Cystitis **Asymptomatic** See CID 52:s427, 2011; CID 52:s452, 2011.	If possible, remove catheter or stent. No therapy indicated except in patients at high risk for dissemination or undergoing a urologic procedure.		**High risk patients** (neonates and neutropenic patients) should be managed as outlined for treatment of bloodstream infection. For patients undergoing urologic procedures, Flu 200 mg (3 mg/kg) IV/po daily or ampho B 0.5 mg/kg IV daily (for flu-resistant organisms) for several days pre- and post-procedure.
Symptomatic	**Fluconazole** 200 mg (3 mg/kg) IV/po daily for 14 days.	**Ampho B** 0.5 mg/kg IV daily (for fluconazole resistant organisms) for 7-10 days.	Concentration of echinocandins is low, case reports of efficacy versus azole resistant organisms (Can J Infect Dis Med Microbiol 18:149, 2007; CID 44:e46, 2007). Persistent candiduria in immunocompromised pt warrants ultrasound or CT of kidneys to rule out fungus ball.
Pyelonephritis	**Fluconazole** 200-400 mg (3-6 mg/kg) once daily orally.	**Ampho B** 0.5 mg/kg daily IV ± 5-FC 25 mg/kg po qid.	**Treat for 2 weeks.** For suspected disseminated disease treat as if bloodstream infection is present.
Chromoblastomycosis (Clin Exp Dermatol, 34:849, 2009). (Cladophialophora, Phialophora, or Fonsecaea) Cutaneous (usually feet, legs), raised scaly lesions, most common in tropical areas	If lesions small & few, **surgical excision or cryosurgery with liquid nitrogen.** If lesions chronic, extensive, burrowing: **itraconazole.**	**Itraconazole:** 200-400 mg oral soln q24h or 400 mg pulse therapy once daily for 1 week of each month for 6-12 months (or until response) NAI.	**Terbinafine** NAI 500-1000 mg once daily alone or in combination with **itraconazole** 200-400 oral soln mg, or **posaconazole** (800 mg/d) po may be effective. Anecdotal report of efficacy of topical imiquimod 5%: 5x/wk (CID 58:1734, 2014).

See page 2 for abbreviations. All dosage recommendations are for adults (unless otherwise indicated) and assume normal renal function

TABLE 11A (7)

TYPE OF INFECTION/ORGANISM/ SITE OF INFECTION	ANTIMICROBIAL AGENTS OF CHOICE		COMMENTS
	PRIMARY	ALTERNATIVE	
Coccidioidomycosis (Coccidioides immitis) *IDSA Guidelines 2005: CID 41:1217, 2005; see also Mayo Clin Proc 83:343, 2008)* **Primary pulmonary** (San Joaquin or Valley Fever): **For pts at low risk of persistence/complication:** **Primary pulmonary in pts with ↑ risk for complications or dissemination. Rx indicated:** • Immunosuppressive disease, post-transplantation, hematological malignancies or therapies (steroids, TNF-α antagonists) • Pregnancy in 3rd trimester • Diabetes • Cf antibody >1:16 • CF antibody >1:16 • Diffuse pulmonary infiltrates • Dissemination (identification of spherules or culture of organism from ulcer, joint, effusion, pus from subcutaneous abscess or bone biopsy, etc.)	**Antifungal rx not generally indicated** for pts at low risk of persistence/complication and/or fatigue that does not resolve within 4-8 wks **Mild to moderate severity** *(EID 29:193, 2011):* Itraconazole solution 200 mg po or IV bid; OR Fluconazole 400 mg po q24h IV or po **Locally severe or disseminated disease** **Ampho B** 0.6-1 mg/kg per day x 7 days then 0.8 mg/kg every other day or **liposomal ampho** B 3-5 mg/kg/d IV or **ABLC** 5 mg/kg/d IV, until clinical improvement, usually several wks or longer in disseminated disease), followed by Itra or Flu for at least 1 year. Some use combination of Ampho B & Flu for progressive severe disease; controlled series lacking. **Consultation with specialist recommended:** surgery may be required. Suppression in HIV + patients until CD4 >250 & infection controlled. Flu 200 mg po q24h or Itra oral soln 200 mg po bid *(Mycosis 46:42, 2003).*		Uncomplicated pulmonary in normal host common in endemic areas *(Emerg Infect Dis 12:958, 2006).* Influenza-like illness of 1-2 wks duration. Antifungal rx that does not resolve within 4-8 wks. ↑ fever, wt. loss **Mild to moderate severity** *(EID 29:193, 2011):* Responses to azoles are similar; Itra may have slight advantage esp. in soft tissue infection. Relapse rates after rx 40%. Relapse rate ↑ if ↑ CF titer ≥1:256. Following CF titers after completion of rx important; rising titers warrant retreatment. **Posaconazole** reported successful in 73% of pts with refractory non-meningeal cocci *(Chest 132:952, 2007).* Not frontline therapy. Treatment of pediatric cocci to include salvage therapy with Vori & Caspo *(CID 56:1573, 1579 & 1587, 2013).* Can test for delayed hypersensitivity with skin test antigen called Spherusol; helpful if history of Valley Fever.
Meningitis: occurs in 1/3 to 1/2 of pts with disseminated coccidioidomycosis Adult *(CID 42:103, 2006)* Child (Cryptococcus neoformans, C. gattii)	**Fluconazole** 400-1,000 mg q24h indefinitely **Fluconazole** (po) (Pediatric dose not established), 6 mg per kg q24h	**Ampho B** IV as for pulmonary (above) + 0.1–0.3 mg daily intrathecal (intraventricular via reservoir device) *(CID 28:870, 2009).* OR 800 mg q24h **OR voriconazole** (see Comment)	**80% relapse rate, continue flucon indefinitely.** **Voriconazole** successful in high doses (6 mg/kg IV q12h) followed by oral suppression (200 mg po q12h)
Cryptococcosis *IDSA Guideline: CID 50:291, 2010.* **Non-meningeal (non-AIDS)** Risk 57% in organ transplant & those receiving other forms of immunosuppressive agents *(EID 13:953, 2007).*	**Fluconazole** 400 mg/day IV or po for 8 wks to 6 mos **For more severe disease:** **Ampho B** 0.5–0.8 mg/kg per day IV till response then change to **fluconazole** 400 mg po q24h for 8-10 wks course	**Itraconazole** 200-400 mg po solution q24h for 6-12 mos OR (**Ampho B** 0.3 mg/kg per day IV + **flucytosine** 37.5 mg/kg po q24h x times 6 wks use ideal body wt)	**Flucon alone 90% effective for meningeal and non-meningeal forms.** Fluconazole is effective as ampho B. Addition of **interferon-γ** (IFN-γ-Ib 50 mcg per M² subcut. 3x per wk x 9 wks) assoc. with response in pt failing antifungal rx *(CID 38: 910, 2004).* Posaconazole 400-800 mg also effective in a small series of patients *(CID 45:562, 2007; Chest 132:952, 2007)*
Meningitis (non-AIDS)	**Ampho B** 0.5-0.8 mg/kg per day IV + **flucytosine** 37.5 mg/kg (some use 25 mg/kg) po q6h until pt afebrile & cultures neg (~6 wks) *(NEJM 301:126, 1979),* then stop ampho B/flucyt, start **fluconazole** 200 mg po q24h *(AnIM 113:183, 1990)* OR **Fluconazole** 400 mg po q24h x 8-10 wks (less severely ill). Some recommend Flu for 2 yrs to reduce relapse rate *(CID 28:297, 1999).* Some recommend Ampho B plus fluconazole as induction Rx. Studies underway.		**If CSF opening pressure >25 cm H₂O, repeat LP to drain fluid to control pressure.** **C. gattii** meningitis reported in the Pacific Northwest *(EID 13:42, 2007);* severity of disease and prognosis appear to be worse than with C. neoformans; initial therapy with **ampho B + flucytosine** recommended. C. gattii susceptible to flucon than C. neoformans *(Clin Microbiol Inf 14:727, 2008).* Outcomes in non-AIDS and non-AIDS cryptococcal meningitis improved with Ampho B + 5-FC induction therapy for 14 days in those with neurological abnormalities or high organism burden *(PLoS ONE 3:e2870, 2008).*

See page 2 for abbreviations. All dosage recommendations are for adults *(unless otherwise indicated)* and assume normal renal function

TABLE 11A (8)

TYPE OF INFECTION/ORGANISM/ SITE OF INFECTION	ANTIMICROBIAL AGENTS OF CHOICE		COMMENTS
	PRIMARY	ALTERNATIVE	

Cryptococcosis (continued)

TYPE OF INFECTION/ORGANISM/ SITE OF INFECTION	PRIMARY	ALTERNATIVE	COMMENTS
HIV+/AIDS: Cryptococcemia and/or Meningitis			
Treatment See Clin Infect Dis 50:291, 2010 (IDSA Guidelines). ↓ with ARV but still common presenting OI in newly diagnosed AIDS pts. Cryptococcal infection may be manifested by positive blood culture or positive serum cryptococcal antigen (CRAG >95% sens). CRAG no help in monitoring response to therapy. With ARV, symptoms of acute meningitis may return: immune reconstitution inflammatory syndrome (IRIS), ↑ CSF pressure (> **250 mm H2O**), associated with high mortality. lower with CSF removal. If frequent LPs not possible, ventriculoperitoneal shunts are an option (Surg Neurol 63:529 & 531, 2005).	**Ampho B** 0.7 mg/kg IV q24H + **flucytosine** 25 mg/kg po q6h for at least two weeks or longer until CSF is sterilized. See Comment. **Then** **Consolidation therapy: Fluconazole** 400–800 mg po q24h to complete a 10-wks course then suppression (see below). Deferring ART for 5 wks after initiation cryptococcal meningitis therapy significantly improved survival as compared to starting ART during the first 2 wks (NEJM 370:2487, 2014).	**Amphotericin B** IV or **liposomal ampho B** IV+ **fluconazole** 400 mg po or IV daily, **OR** **Amphotericin B** 0.7 mg/kg or **liposomal ampho B** 4 mg/kg IV q24h alone, **OR Fluconazole** ≥ 800 mg/day (1200 mg preferred) (po or IV) **plus flucytosine** 25 mg/kg po q6h for 4–6 weeks.	Outcome of treatment: treatment failure associated with dissemination of infection & high serum antigen titer, indicative of high burden of organisms and lack of 5FC use during inductive Rx, abnormal neurological evaluation & underlying hematological malignancy. Mortality rates still high, particularly in those with concomitant pneumonia (PLoS Medicine 4:e47, 2007). Early Dx essential for improved outcome (PLoS Medicine 4:e47, 2007). Ampho B + 5FC treatment ↓ crypto CFUs more rapidly than ampho + Flu or ampho + 5FC + Flu. Ampho B 1 mg/kg/d alone much more rapidly fungicidal in vivo than Flu 400 mg/d (CID 45:76&81, 2007). Use of lipid-based ampho B associated with lower mortality compared to ampho B deoxycholate in solid organ transplant recipients (CID 48:1566, 2009). Higher levels & ↑ Monitor 5-FC levels: peak 70-80 mg/L, trough 30-40 mg/L. Higher levels assoc. with bone marrow toxicity. No difference in outcome if given IV or po (AAC 51:1038, 2007). Failure of Flu may rarely be due to resistant organism, especially if burden of organism high at initiation of Rx. Although 200 mg qd = 400 mg qd of Flu: median survival 76 & 82 days respectively, outcomes were observed in 14/29 (48%) subjects with cryptococcal meningitis treated with posaconazole (BMC Infect Dis 6:118, 2006). Trend toward improved outcomes with fluconazole 400-800 mg combined with ampho B versus ampho B alone in AIDS patients (CID 48:1775, 2009). Role of other azoles uncertain: successful outcomes with posaconazole (JAC 56:745, 2005). Voriconazole also may be effective. **When to initiate antiretroviral therapy (ART)?** Defer ART to allow for diagnosis of cryptococcal meningitis mortality was increased when compared to initiation of ART > 5 weeks after diagnosis (NEJM 370:2487, 2014).
Suppression (chronic maintenance therapy) Discontinuation of antifungal rx can be considered with effective antiretroviral rx. Some authorities recommend dc suppressive rx. See www.hivatis.org. Authors would only dc if CSF culture negative.	**Fluconazole** 200 mg/day po [If CD4 count rises to >100/mm³ with effective antiretroviral rx, some authorities recommend dc suppressive rx. See www.hivatis.org. Authors would only dc if CSF culture negative.]	**Itraconazole** 200 mg po q12h if Flu intolerant or failure. No data on Vori for maintenance.	Itraconazole less effective than fluconazole & not recommended because of higher relapse rate (23% vs 4%). Recurrence rate of 0.4 to 3.9 per 100 patient-years with discontinuation of suppressive therapy in 100 patients on ARV with CD4 >100 cells/mm³.
Some perform a lumbar puncture before discontinuation of maintenance rx. Reappearance of pos. serum CRAG may predict relapse >100-200/mm³ for ≥6 months.	[If CD4 count rises to >100/mm³ Some perform a lumbar puncture before discontinuation of maintenance rx. Reappearance of pos. serum CRAG may predict relapse]		

See page 2 for abbreviations. All dosage recommendations are for adults (unless otherwise indicated) and assume normal renal function

TABLE 11A (9)

TYPE OF INFECTION/ORGANISM/ SITE OF INFECTION	ANTIMICROBIAL AGENTS OF CHOICE		COMMENTS
	PRIMARY	ALTERNATIVE	
Dermatophytosis			
Onychomycosis (Tinea unguium) (primarily cosmetic) Laser rx FDA approved: modestly effective, expensive (Med Lett 55:15, 2013); (NEJM 360:2108, 2009) Ref: Am J Clin Derm 15:17, 2014; BMJ 348:g1800, 2014; Clinics Derm 31:544, 2013	**Fingernail Rx Options:** **Terbinafine**[1] 250 mg po q24h [children <20 kg: 67.5 mg/day, 20–40 kg: 125 mg/day, >40 kg: 250 mg/day] x 6 wks (79% effective) OR **Itraconazole**[1] 200 mg po q24h x 3 mos NAI OR **Fluconazole** 200 mg po bid x 1 wk/mo x 2 mos OR **Fluconazole** 150–300 mg po q wk x 3–6 mos.[AAI]		**Toenail Rx Options:** **Terbinafine**[1] 250 mg po q24h [children <20 kg: 67.5 mg/day, 20–40 kg: 125 mg/day, >40 kg: 250 mg/day] x 12 wks (76% effective) OR **Itraconazole** 200 mg po q24h x 12 wks (59% effective) OR **Efinaconazole** 10% solution applied to nail once daily for 48 wks OR **Itraconazole** 200 mg bid x 1 wk/mo x 3–4 mos (63% effective)[AAI] OR **Fluconazole** 150–300 mg po q wk x 6–12 mos (48% effective)[AAI] OR topical **Tavaborole** (Kerydin) or topical **efinaconazole** (Jublia)
Tinea capitis ("ringworm") (Trichophyton tonsurans, Microsporum canis, N. America; other sp. elsewhere) (PIDJ 18:191, 1999)	**Terbinafine**[1] 250 mg po q 24h x Itraconazole[1] 5 mg/kg per day x 2 wks (adults); 5 mg/kg/day x 4 wks (children)	**Itraconazole**[1] 5 mg/kg per day x **Fluconazole** 6 mg/kg q wk x 8–12 wks OR adults 200 mg q24h x 4 wks NAI/CA; Cap at 150 mg/day x for adults **Griseofulvin**: adults 500 mg po q24h x 4–6 wks; children 10–20 mg/kg per day until hair regrows.	Durations of therapy are for T. tonsurans; treat for approx. twice as long for M. canis. All agents with similar cure rates (60–100%) in clinical studies. Addition of topical ketoconazole or selenium sulfate shampoo reduces transmissibility (Int J Dermatol 39:261, 2000)
Tinea corporis, cruris, or pedis (Trichophyton rubrum, T. mentagrophytes, Epidermophyton floccosum) "Athlete's foot, jock itch", and ringworm	**Topical rx:** Generally applied 2x/day. Available as creams, ointments, sprays, etc. Apply 2x/day for 2–3 wks. Recommend: Lotrimin Ultra or Lamisil AT contain butenafine & terbinafine—both are fungicidal	**Terbinafine** 250 mg po q24h x 2 wks NAI OR **ketoconazole** 200 mg po q24h x 4 wks OR **fluconazole** 150 mg po 1x/wk for 2–4 wks[AAI] **Griseofulvin**: adults 500 mg po q24h times 4–6 wks, children 10–20 mg/kg per day. Duration 2–4 wks for corporis, 4–8 wks for pedis	**Keto** (po) times 1 dose was 97% effective in 1 study. Another alternative: **Selenium sulfide** (Selsun), 2.5% lotion; apply as lather, leave on 10 min then wash off, 1/day x 7 day or 3–5/wk times 2–4 wks
Tinea versicolor (Malassezia furfur or Pityrosporum orbiculare) Rule out erythrasma—see Table 1, page 54	**Ketoconazole** (400 mg po single dose) or (200 mg/day x 7 days) or (2% cream 1x q24h x 2 wks)	**Fluconazole** 400 mg po single dose OR **itraconazole** 400 mg po q24h x 3–7 days	**Keto** (po) often effective in severe recalcitrant infection. Follow for hepatotoxicity; many drug-drug interactions.
Fusariosis Third most common cause of invasive mold infections, after Aspergillus and Mucorales and related molds, in patients with hematologic malignancies (Mycoses 52:197, 2009). Pneumonia, skin infections, bone and joint infections, and disseminated disease occur in severely immunocompromised patients. In contrast to other molds, blood cultures are frequently positive. Fusarium solani, F. oxysporum, F. verticillioides and F. moniliforme account for approx. 90% of isolates (Clin Micro Rev 20: 695, 2007). Frequently fatal; outcome depends on decreasing the level of immunosuppression.	**Lipid-based ampho B** 5–10 mg/kg/d IV. OR **Ampho B** 1–1.5 mg/kg/d IV	**Posaconazole** 400 mg po with meals (if not taking meals, 200 mg qid) OR **Voriconazole** IV: 6 mg per kg q12h times 1 day, then 4 mg per kg q12h; PO: 400 mg q12h, then 200 mg q12h. See comments	**Surgical debridement** for localized disease. Fusarium spp. resistance to most antifungal agents, including echinocandins, F. solani and F. verticillioides typically are resistant to azoles. F. oxysporum and F. moniliforme may be susceptible to voriconazole and posaconazole. Role of combination therapy not well defined but case reports of response (Mycoses 50: 227, 2007). Given variability in susceptibilities can consider combination therapy with Vori and ampho B awaiting speciation. Outcome dependent on reduction or discontinuation of immuno-suppression. Duration of therapy depends on response; long-term suppressive therapy for patients remaining on immunosuppressive therapy.

[1] **Serious but rare cases of hepatic failure** have been reported in pts receiving terbinafine & should not be used in those with chronic or active liver disease (see Table 11B, page 136).

[2] Use of itraconazole has been associated with myocardial dysfunction and with onset of congestive heart failure.

See page 2 for abbreviations. All dosage recommendations are for adults (unless otherwise indicated) and assume normal renal function

TABLE 11A (10)

TYPE OF INFECTION/ORGANISM/ SITE OF INFECTION	ANTIMICROBIAL AGENTS OF CHOICE		COMMENTS
	PRIMARY	**ALTERNATIVE**	
Histoplasmosis (Histoplasma capsulatum): *See IDSA Guideline: CID 45:807, 2007.* Best diagnostic test is urinary, serum, or CSF histoplasma antigen. MiraVista Diagnostics (1-866-647-2847)			
Acute pulmonary histoplasmosis	**Mild to moderate disease, symptoms <4 wks:** No rx. If symptoms last over one month: **Itraconazole** oral soln 200 mg tid or bid for 3 days then once or twice daily for 6-12 wks.		Ampho B for patients at low risk of nephrotoxicity. Check for Itra drug interactions.
	Moderately severe or severe: Liposomal ampho B, 3-5 mg/kg/d IV or **ABLC** 5 mg/kg/d IV or ampho B 0.7-1.0 mg/kg/d for 1-2 wks, then Itra 200 mg tid for 3 days, then bid for 12 wks. **+ methylprednisolone** 0.5-1 mg/kg/d for 1-2 wks.		
Chronic cavitary pulmonary histoplasmosis	**Itra** oral soln 200 mg po tid for 3 days then once or twice daily for at least 12 mos (some prefer 18-24 mos).		Document therapeutic itraconazole blood levels at 2 wks. Relapses occur in 9-15% of patients.
Mediastinal lymphadenitis, mediastinal granuloma, pericarditis; and rheumatologic syndromes	**Mild cases:** Antifungal therapy not indicated. Nonsteroidal anti-inflammatory drug for pericarditis or rheumatologic syndromes. If no response to non-steroidals, **Prednisone** 0.5-1.0 mg/kg/d tapered over 1-2 weeks for 1) pericarditis with hemodynamic compromise, 2) lymphadenitis with obstruction or compression syndromes, or 3) severe rheumatologic syndromes.		
	Itra 200 oral soln mg po once or twice daily for 6-12 wks for moderately severe to severe cases, or if prednisone is administered.		
Progressive disseminated histoplasmosis	**Mild to moderate disease: Itra** 200 mg po tid for 3 days then bid for at least 12 mos.		Check Itra blood levels to document therapeutic concentrations. Check for Itra drug-drug interactions. **Ampho B** 0.7-1.0 mg/kg/d may be used for patients at low risk of nephrotoxicity. Confirm therapeutic Itra blood levels. Azoles are teratogenic; Itra should be avoided in pregnancy, use a lipid ampho formulation. Urinary antigen levels useful for monitoring response to therapy and relapse
	Moderately severe to severe disease: Liposomal ampho B, 3 mg/kg/d or **ABLC** 5 mg/kg/d for 1-2 weeks then **Itra** 200 mg tid for 3 days, then bid for at least 12 mos.		
CNS histoplasmosis	**Liposomal ampho B,** 5 mg/kg/d, for a total of 175 mg/kg over 4-6 wks, then **Itra** 200 mg 2-3x a day for at least 12 mos. Vori likely effective for CNS disease or Itra failures. *(Arch Neurology 57:1235, 2006).*	**Itra** 200 mg po tid for 3 days then bid *(J Antimicro Chemo 65: 666, 2008; J Antimicro Chemo 57:1235, 2006).*	Monitor CNS histo antigen; monitor Itra blood levels. PCR may be better for Dx than histo antigen. Absorption of Itra (check levels) and CNS penetration may be an issue; case reports of success with Fluconazole *(Braz J Infect Dis 12:555, 2008)* and Posaconazole *(Drugs 65:1553, 2005)* following Ampho B therapy.
Prophylaxis (immunocompromised patients)	**Itra** 200 mg po daily. Check for Itra drug-drug interactions.		Consider primary **prophylaxis in HIV-infected** patients with < 150 CD4 cells/mm³ in high prevalence areas. Secondary prophylaxis (i.e. suppressive therapy) indicated in HIV-infected patients with < 150 CD4 cells/mm³ and other immunocompromised patients in who immunosuppression cannot be reversed

See page 2 for abbreviations. All dosage recommendations are for adults (unless otherwise indicated) and assume normal renal function

TABLE 11A (11)

TYPE OF INFECTION/ORGANISM/ SITE OF INFECTION	ANTIMICROBIAL AGENTS OF CHOICE		COMMENTS
	PRIMARY	ALTERNATIVE	
Madura foot (See *Nocardia* & *Scedosporium*)			
Mucormycosis & other related species—Rhizopus, Rhizomucor, Lichtheimia. **Rhinocerebral, pulmonary due to angioinvasion with tissue necrosis.** Key to lateral rx: early dx with symptoms suggestive of sinusitis (or lateral facial pain or numbness): think mucor with palatal ulcers, &/or black eschars, onset unilateral blindness in immunocompromised or diabetic. Rapidly fatal without rx. Dx by culture of tissue or stain: wide ribbon-like, non-septate with variation in diameter & right angle branching. Diabetics are predisposed to mucormycosis due to microangiopathy & ketoacidosis. Iron overload also predisposes: iron stimulates fungal growth.	**Liposomal ampho B** 5-10 mg/kg/day, OR **Ampho B** 1-1.5 mg/kg/day.	**Posaconazole** 400 mg po bid with meals (if not taking meals, 200 mg po/iv q6h x 7 days and then 200 mg po/iv q8 x 1 day and then 200 mg daily	**Ampho B** (ABLC) monotherapy relatively ineffective with 20% success rate vs 69% for other polyenes (*CID 47:364, 2008*). Complete or partial response rates of 60-80% in **posaconazole salvage protocols** (*JAC 61, Suppl 1, i35, 2008*). **Isavuconazole:** Approved for treatment of invasive mucor infection based on historical controls (Package insert, clinical trial not published). Amphotericin B is promising given safety profile, synergy in murine models, and observational clinical data (*Clin Infect Dis 54(S1):S73, 2012*). **Combination therapy:** Adjunctive echinocandin to liposomal Amphotericin B failed to demonstrate benefit (*J Antimicrob Chemother. 67:715, 2012*). Adjunctive Deferasirox therapy to liposomal Amphotericin B failed to demonstrate benefit (*J Antimicrob Chemother. 67:715, 2012*). Resistant to **voriconazole:** prolonged use of voriconazole prophylaxis predisposes to mucormycosis infections. Total duration of therapy based on response: continue therapy until 1) resolution of clinical signs and symptoms of infection, 2) resolution or stabilization of radiographic abnormalities; and 3) resolution of underlying immunosuppression. Posaconazole for secondary prophylaxis for those on immunosuppressive therapy (*CID 48:1743, 2009*).
Paracoccidioidomycosis (South American blastomycosis) *P. braziliensis* (*Dermatol Clin 26:257, 2008; Expert Rev Anti Infect Ther 6:251, 2008*). Important cause of death from fungal infection in HIV-infected patients in Brazil (*Mem Inst Oswaldo Cruz 104:513, 2009*).	**Mild-moderate disease:** Itra 200 mg po daily for 6-9 months for mild and 12-18 months for moderate disease. **Severe disease: Ampho B** 0.7-1 mg/kg IV daily to a cumulative total of 30 mg/kg followed by Itra 200 mg po daily for at least 12 months	**Ketoconazole** 200-400 mg daily for 6-18 months; OR **Ampho B** total dose > 30 mg/kg OR **TMP/SMX** 800/160 mg bid-tid for 30 days, then 400/80 mg/day indefinitely (up to 3-5 years)	Improvement in >90% pts on Itra or Keto.ᴺᴹ **Ampho B** reserved for severe cases and those intolerant to other agents. TMP-SMX suppression life-long in HIV+. Check for Itra or Keto drug-drug interactions.
Lobomycosis (keloidal blastomycosis/ P. loboi	Surgical excision, clofazimine or itraconazole		Preliminary data suggests Vori effective: *CID 43:1060, 2006*.
Penicilliosis (Penicillium marneffei): Common disseminated fungal infection in AIDS pts in SE Asia (esp. Thailand & Vietnam).	**Ampho B** 0.5-1 mg/kg per day times 2 wks followed by **itraconazole** 400 mg/day for 10 wks followed by 200 mg/day **indefinitely for HIV-infected pts.**	For less sick patients Itra oral soln 200 mg po tid x 3 days, then 200 mg po bid x 12 wks, then 200 mg po q24hᴺᴹ (Oral soln better absorbed)	3ʳᵈ most common OI in AIDS pts in SE Asia following TBc and cryptococcal meningitis. Prolonged fever, lymphadenopathy, hepatomegaly. Skin nodules are umbilicated (mimic cryptococcal infection or molluscum contagiosum).
Phaeohyphomycosis, Black molds. Dematiaceous fungi (See *Clin Microbiol Rev 27:527, 2014*). Opportunistic infection in immunocompromised hosts (e.g., HIV/AIDS, transplants). Most often presents with skin and soft tissue infection or mycetoma that can cause disease in bone and joint, brain abscess, endocarditis, and disseminated disease. Most clinically relevant species are within the genera of *Exophiala, Cladophialophora, Coniosporium, Cyphellophora, Fonsecaea, Phialophora*, and *Rhinocladiella*.	**Surgery + itraconazole** oral soln 400 mg/day po, duration not defined, probably 6 moᴺᴹ	**Voriconazole** 6 mg/kg po bid x 1 day and then 4 mg/kg po bid or **Posaconazole** (suspension) 400 mg po bid	Both Vori and Posa have demonstrated efficacy (*Med Mycol 48:769, 2010; Med Mycol 43:91, 2005*) often in addition to surgical therapy. Consider adjunctive anti-fungal susceptibility testing.

See page 2 for abbreviations. All dosage recommendations are for adults (unless otherwise indicated) and assume normal renal function

TABLE 11A (12)

TYPE OF INFECTION/ORGANISM/ SITE OF INFECTION	ANTIMICROBIAL AGENTS OF CHOICE		COMMENTS
	PRIMARY	ALTERNATIVE	
Pneumocystis pneumonia (PCP) caused by **Pneumocystis jiroveci**. Ref. *JAMA* 301:2578, 2009			
Not acutely ill, able to take po meds. PaO₂ >70 mmHg. Diagnosis: sputum PCR. Serum Beta-D Glucan may help: reasonable sensitivity & specificity, but also many false positives (*JCM* 51:3478, 2013).	**[TMP-SMX-DS,** 2 tabs po q8h x21 days) OR **(Dapsone** 100 mg + **trimethoprim** 5mg/kg po tid x21 days)	**[Clindamycin** 300–450mg po q6h + **primaquine** 15 mg base po q24h] x21 days OR **Atovaquone** suspension 750 mg po bid with food x21 days	Mutations in gene of the enzyme target (dihydropteroate synthetase) of sulfamethoxazole identified. Unclear whether mutations result in resist to TMP-SMX or dapsone + TMP (*EID* 10:1721, 2004). Dapsone ref.: *CID* 27:191, 1998. **After 21 days, chronic suppression in AIDS pts (see below—post-treatment suppression).**
	NOTE: Concomitant use of corticosteroids usually reserved for sicker pts with PaO₂ <70 (see below)		
Acutely ill, po rx not possible. PaO2 <70 mmHg. Still unclear whether antiretroviral therapy (ART) should be started during treatment of PCP (*CID* 46: 634, 2008).	**[Prednisone**(15–30 min. before **TMP-SMX):** 40 mg po bid times 5 days, then 40 mg q24h times 5 days, then 20 mg po q24h times 11 days) + **[TMP-SMX** (15 mg of TMP component per kg per day) IV div. q6-8h times 21 days]	**Prednisone** as in primary rx. PLUS((Clinda 600 mg IV q8h) + **primaquine** 30 mg base po q24h)] times 21 days OR **Pentamidine** 4 mg per kg per day IV times 21 days. **Caspofungin** active in animal models: (*CID* 36:1445, 2003)	**After 21 days, chronic suppression in AIDS pts** (see below—post-treatment suppression). **PCP can occur in absence of HIV infection & steroids** (*CID* 25:215 & 219, 1997). Wait 4–8 days before declaring treatment failure& switching to clinda + primaquine or pentamidine (*JAIDS* 48:63, 2008), or adding caspofungin (*Transplant* 84:685, 2007).
	Can substitute IV prednisolone (reduce dose 25%) for po prednisone		
Primary prophylaxis and post-treatment suppression	**TMP-SMX-DS or -SS,** 1 tab po q24h or 1 DS 3x/wk) OR **(dapsone** 100 mg po q24h) OR DC when CD4 >200 x/3 mos (*NEJM* 344:159, 2001).	**[Pentamidine** 300 mg in 6mL sterile water by aerosol (q4wks) OR **(dapsone** 200mg po + **pyrimethamine** 75 mg po + **folinic acid** 25mg po—all once a week) or **atovaquone** 1500mg po q24h with food.	TMP-SMX-DS regimen provides cross-protection vs Toxo and other bacterial infections. Dapsone + pyrimethamine protects vs Toxo. Atovaquone suspension 1500mg once daily as effective as daily dapsone (*NEJM* 339:1889, 1998) or inhaled pentamidine (*JID* 180:369, 1999).
Scedosporium species (Scedosporium apiospermum [Pseudallescheria boydii] and Scedosporium prolificans) Infection occurs via inhalation or inoculation of skin. Normal hosts often have cutaneous disease. Immunocompromised hosts can have pulmonary colonization -> invasive disease in lung or skin -> disseminated disease.	**Scedosporium apiospermum:** Voriconazole 6 mg/kg PO/IV q12h on day 1, then 4 mg/kg PO/IV q12h. **Scedosporium prolificans:** Surgical debridement and reduction of immunosuppression, consider addition of Voriconazole as above although usually resistant	Posaconazole 400 mg po bid with meals (may be less active)	Surgical debridement should be considered in most cases. S. apiospermum is resistant Amphotericin B and Scedosporium prolificans is resistant to all antifungal agents. Synergy with Terbinafine and echinocandins have been reported in vitro although clinical data is limited (*AAC* 56:2635, 2012). S. prolificans osteomyelitis responded to miltefosine (*CID* 48:1257, 2009) in a case report. Consider susceptibility testing. Treatment guidelines/review: *Clin Microbiol Infect* 3:27, 2014. *Clin Microbiol Rev* 21:157, 2008.

See page 2 for abbreviations. All dosage recommendations are for adults (unless otherwise indicated) and assume normal renal function

TABLE 11A (13)

TYPE OF INFECTION/ORGANISM/ SITE OF INFECTION	ANTIMICROBIAL AGENTS OF CHOICE		COMMENTS
	PRIMARY	**ALTERNATIVE**	
Sporotrichosis *IDSA Guideline: CID 45:1255, 2007.*			
Cutaneous/Lymphocutaneous	**Itraconazole** oral soln po 200 mg/day for 2-4 wks after all lesions resolved, usually 3-6 mos.	If no response, **Itra** 200 mg po bid or **terbinafine** 500 mg po bid or **SSKI** 5 drops (eye drops) tid & increase to 40-50 drops tid	Fluconazole 400-800 mg daily only if no response to primary or alternative suggestions. Pregnancy or nursing: local hyperthermia (see below).
Osteoarticular	**Itra** oral soln 200 mg po bid x 12 mos.	**Liposomal ampho B** 3-5 mg/kg/d IV or **ABLC** 5 mg/kg/d IV or **ampho B deoxycholate** 0.7-1 mg/kg/d IV daily; if response, change to **Itra** oral soln 200 mg po bid x total 12 mos.	After 2 wks of therapy, document adequate serum levels of itraconazole.
Pulmonary	If severe, **lipid ampho B** 3-5 mg/kg IV or **standard ampho B** 0.7-1 mg/kg IV once daily until response, then **Itra** 200 mg po bid. Total of 12 mos.	Less severe: **Itraconazole** 200 mg po bid x 12 mos.	After 2 weeks of therapy document adequate serum levels of Itra. Surgical resection plus ampho B for localized pulmonary disease.
Meningeal or Disseminated	**Lipid ampho B** 5 mg/kg IV once daily x 4-6 wks, then—if better— **Itra** 200 mg po bid for total of 12 mos.	AIDS/Other immunosuppressed pts: chronic therapy with **Itra** oral soln 200 mg po once daily.	After 2 weeks, document adequate serum levels of Itra.
Pregnancy and children	**Pregnancy:** Cutaneous—local hyperthermia. Severe: **lipid ampho B** 3-5 mg/kg IV once daily. **Avoid itraconazole.**	**Children:** Cutaneous: **Itra** 6-10 mg/kg (max of 400 mg) daily. Alternative is **SSKI** 1 drop tid increasing to max of 1 drop/kg or 40-50 drops tid/day, whichever is lowest.	For children with disseminated sporotrichosis: Standard ampho B 0.7 mg/kg IV once daily & after response, Itra 6-10 mg/kg (max 400 mg) once daily.

See page 2 for abbreviations. All dosage recommendations are for adults (unless otherwise indicated) and assume normal renal function

TABLE 11B – ANTIFUNGAL DRUGS: DOSAGE, ADVERSE EFFECTS, COMMENTS

DRUG NAME, GENERIC (TRADE)/USUAL DOSAGE	ADVERSE EFFECTS/COMMENTS
Non-lipid amphotericin B deoxycholate (Fungizone) 0.3–1.0 mg/kg IV per day as single infusion Ampho B predictably not active vs. *Scedosporium*, *Candida lusitaniae* & *Aspergillus terreus*	**Admin:** Ampho B is a colloidal suspension that must be prepared in electrolyte-free D5W to avoid precipitation. No need to protect suspensions from light. Infusions cause chills/fever, myalgia, anorexia, nausea, rarely hemodynamic collapse/hypotension. Postulated due to proinflammatory cytokines, doesn't appear to histamine release *(Pharmaco 23:966, 2003)*. **Infusion duration usu. 4+ hrs.** No difference found in 1 vs 4 hr infus. except chills/fever occurred sooner with 1 hr infus. (reactive at 4 hrs). Rare pulmonary reactions (severe dyspnea & focal infiltrates suggest pulmonary edema) assoc with rapid infus. **Severe rigors reactions with repeat doses.** Pare 5 dose **40–50 mg**. Rx: Meperidine 25 mg IV or dantrolene, diphenhydramine. **Admin:** had no influence on rigors/fever. If cytokine postulate correct, NSAIDs or high-dose steroids may prove efficacious but their use may risk worsening infection under rx or increased risk of **nephrotoxicity** (i.e., NSAIDs). Clinical side effects ↓ with ↑ age. **Toxicity:** Major concern is nephrotoxicity. Manifest initially by kaliuresis and **hypokalemia**, then fall in serum bicarbonate (may proceed to renal tubular acidosis). ↓ in renal erythropoietin and anemia, and rising BUN/serum creatinine. Hypomagnesemia may occur. Can reduce risk of renal injury by **(a) pre- & post-infusion hydration with 500 mL saline (if clinical status allows salt load)**, **(b)** avoidance of other nephrotoxins, eg, radiocontrast, aminoglycosides, cis-platinum, **(c)** use of lipid prep of ampho B.
Lipid-based ampho B products[3]: **Amphotericin B lipid complex (ABLC)** (Abelcet); 5 mg/kg per day as single infusion	**Admin:** Consists of ampho B complexed with 2 lipid bilayer ribbons. Compared to standard ampho B, larger volume of distribution, rapid blood clearance and high tissue concentrations (liver, spleen, lung). Dosage: **5 mg/kg per day**; infuse at 2.5 mg/kg per hr: adult and ped. dose the same. Saline pre- and post-dose lessens toxicity. Do NOT use in-line filter. Do not dilute with saline or with other drugs or electrolytes.[2] **Toxicity:** Fever and chills 14–18%, nausea 9%, vomiting 8%; serum creatinine ↑ in 11%; renal failure 5%; anemia 4%; ↓ K 5%; rash 4%. A fatal fat embolism following ABLC infusion *(Exp Mol Path 177:246, 2004).* Majority of pts intolerant of liposomal ampho B can tolerate ABLC *(CID 56:701, 2013).*
Liposomal amphotericin B (LAB)[3]; 3–5 mg/kg IV per day as single infusion. Infusion rate: majority OK with lipid form *(CID 56:701, 2013).*	**Admin:** Consists of vesicular bilayer liposome with ampho B intercalated within the membrane. Dosage: **3–5 mg/kg per day** IV as single infusion over a period of approx. 120 min. If tolerated, infusion time reduced to 60 min. (See footnote[2].) Saline pre- and post-dose lessens toxicity. **Major toxicity:** Gen less than ampho B. Nephrotoxic 18.7% vs 33.7% for ampho B; chills 47% vs 75%, nausea 39.7% vs 38.7%, vomiting 31.8% vs 43.9%, rash 24% for both; ↑ Ca 18.4% vs 20.9%, ↓ K 20.4% vs 25.6%, ↓ Mg 20.4% vs 25.6%. Acute reactions common with liposomal ampho B. 20–40%. 86% occur within 5 min of infusion, incl chest pain, dyspnea, hypoxia or severe abdom, flank or leg pain; 14% clear flushing & urticaria near end of 4 hr infusion. All responded to diphenhydramine (1 mg/kg) & interruption of infusion. Reactions may be due to complement activation by liposome *(CID 36:1213, 2003).*
Caspofungin (Canicidas) 70 mg IV 1st day followed by 50 mg IV q24h (reduce to 35 mg IV q24h with moderate hepatic insufficiency)	An echinocandin which inhibits synthesis of β-(1,3)-D-glucan. Fungicidal against candida (MIC <2 mcg/mL) including those resistant to other antifungals & active against aspergillus (MIC 0.4–2.7 mcg/mL). Approved indications: empirical rx for febrile, neutropenic pts; rx of candidemia, candida intraabdominal abscesses, peritonitis, & tissue infections (see footnote[3]); esophageal candidiasis; & invasive aspergillosis in pts refractory to or intolerant of other therapies. Serum levels on rec. dosages = peak 12, trough 1.3 (24 hrs) mcg/mL. **Toxicity:** Histamine-mediated symptoms: pruritus at infusion site & headache, fever, chills, vomiting. Drug & diarrhea assoc with infusion. In 422 pts with candidemia *(LnID, Oct 12, 2005; online)*. Drug remains in liver & dosage ↓ to 35 mg in moderate to severe hepatic failure. Class C for preg (embryotoxic in rats & rabbits). See *Table 22, page 235 for drug-drug interactions*, esp cyclosporine *(hepatic toxicity)* & tacrolimus *(drug level monitoring recommended)*. Reversible thrombocytopenia reported *(Pharmacother 24:1408, 2004).* **No drug in CSF, urine or vitreous humor of the eye.**
Micafungin (Mycamine) 50 mg IV q24h for prophylaxis post-bone marrow stem cell trans; 100 mg IV q24h candidemia, 150 mg IV q24h candida esophagitis	Approved for rx of esophageal candidiasis & prophylaxis against fungal infections in HSCT[3] recipients. Active against most strains of candida sp & prophylaxis sp. incl those resist to fluconazole such as C. glabrata & C. krusei. No antagonism seen when combo with other antifungal drugs. No dosage adjust for severe renal failure or moderate hepatic impairment. Watch for drug-drug interactions with sirolimus or nifedipine. Micafungin well tolerated & common adverse events incl nausea 2.8%, vomiting 2.4%, headache 2.4%. Transient ↑ LFTs, BUN, creatinine 2.4%. **No drug in CSF or urine.** See *CID 42:1171, 2006.*

[1] Published data from patients intolerant of or refractory to conventional ampho B deoxycholate. **None of the lipid ampho B preps has shown superior efficacy compared to ampho B deoxycholate, with a single exception.**
Trials (except liposomal ampho B) was more effective vs ampho B in rx of disseminated histoplasmosis at 2 wks). Dosage equivalency has not been established *(CID 36:1500, 2003).*
[2] Comparisons between Abelcet & AmBisome suggest higher infusion-assoc. toxicity (rigors) & febrile episodes with Abelcet (70% vs 36%) but higher frequency of mild hepatic toxicity with AmBisome
(59% vs 38%, p=0.05). Mild elevations in serum creatinine were observed in 1/3 of both *(BJ Hemat 103:198, 1998; Focus on Fungal Inf #9, 1998; Bone Marrow Tx 20:39, 1997; CID 26:1383, 1998).*
[3] HSCT = hematopoietic stem cell transplant.

See page 2 for abbreviations. All dosage recommendations are for adults (unless otherwise indicated) and assume normal renal/renal function

TABLE 11B (2)

DRUG NAME, GENERIC (TRADE)/USUAL DOSAGE	ADVERSE EFFECTS/COMMENTS
Anidulafungin (Eraxis) For Candidemia: 200 mg IV on day 1 followed by 100 mg IV. Esophageal candidiasis: 100 mg IV x 1, then 50 mg IV once/d.	An echinocandin with antifungal activity (cidal) against candida sp. & aspergillus sp. including ampho B- & triazole-resistant strains. FDA approved for treatment of esophageal candidiasis (EC), candidemia, and other complicated Candida infections. Effective in 3 clinical trials of esophageal candidiasis & in 1 trial was superior to fluconazole in rx of invasive candidiasis/candidemia in 245 pts (75.6% vs 60.2%). other echinocandins, remarkably non-toxic; most common side-effects: nausea, vomiting, ↓ mg, ↓ K & headache in 11–13% of pts. No dose adjustments for renal or hepatic insufficiency. *See CID 43:215, 2006.* **No drug in CSF or urine.**
Fluconazole (Diflucan) 100 mg tabs 150 mg tabs 200 mg tabs 400 mg IV Oral suspension: 50 mg per 5 mL	IV=oral dose because of excellent bioavailability. **Pharmacology:** absorbed po, water solubility enables IV. For peak serum levels (see *Table 9A, page 93*). T½ 30hr (range 20–50 h). 12% protein bound. **CSF levels 50–90% of serum in normals,** ↑ in meningitis. No effect on mammalian steroid metabolism. **Drug-drug interactions common,** *see Table 22.* Side-effects overall 16% (more common in HIV+ pts [21%]). Nausea 3.7%, headache 1.9%, skin rash 1.8%, abdominal pain 1.7%, vomiting 1.7%, diarrhea 1.5%, ↑ SGOT 20%. Alopecia (scalp, pubic crest) in 12–20% pts on ≥400 mg po q24h after median of 3 mos (reversible in approx. 6mo). Rare: severe hepatotoxicity (*CID 41:301, 2005*). **Note: Candida krusei and Candida glabrata resistant to Flu.**
Flucytosine (Ancobon, 5-FC) 500 mg cap **Expensive:** $11,000 for 100 capsules (Sep 2015 US price)	AEs: Overall 30%. GI 6% (diarrhea, anorexia, nausea, vomiting); hematologic 22% [leukopenia, thrombocytopenia, when serum level >100 mcg/mL (esp. in azotemic pts)]; hepatotoxicity (asymptomatic ↑ SGOT, reversible); skin rash 7%, aplastic anemia (rare—2 or 3 cases). False ↑ in serum creatinine on EKTACHEM analyzer.
Griseofulvin (Fulvicin, Grifulvin, Grisactin) 500 mg tabs; susp 125 mg/mL	Photosensitivity, urticaria, GI upset, fatigue, leukopenia (rare). Interferes with warfarin drugs. Increases blood and urine porphyrins. Exacerbation of systemic lupus erythematosus.
Imidazoles, topical For vaginal and/or skin use	Not recommended in 1st trimester of pregnancy. Local reactions: 0.5–1.5%: dyspareunia, mild vaginal or vulvar erythema, burning, pruritus, urticaria, rash. Rarely similar symptoms in sexual partner.
Isavuconazole (Cresemba) PO: 186 mg caps IV: 372 mg vials	An azole antifungal agent for treatment of invasive aspergillosis and invasive mucormycosis in adults. **Contraindications:** Coadministration with strong CYP3A4 inhibitors, e.g., Ketoconazole or high-dose Ritonavir, or strong CYP3A4 inducers, e.g. Rifampin, carbamazepine, St. John's wort, or long-acting barbiturates is contraindicated. Do not use in patients with shortened QT interval. **Loading Dose:** 200 mg of Isavuconazole which equals 1 reconstituted vial of 372 mg of the prodrug Isavuconazonium sulfate, IV or po q8h x 6 doses (48 hours) and THEN **Maintenance Dose:** 200 mg of Isavuconazole which equals 1 reconstituted vial of 372 mg of the prodrug Isavuconazonium sulfate, IV or po once daily. No dosage adjustment for renal impairment. **AEs:** Most common: nausea, vomiting, diarrhea, headache, elevated liver chemistry tests, hypokalemia, constipation, dyspnea, cough, peripheral edema, and back pain. Hepatic: increased ALT, AST.
Itraconazole (Sporanox) 100 mg cap 10 mg/mL oral solution IV usual dose 200 mg bid x 4 doses followed by 200 mg q24h for a max of 14 days	**Itraconazole tablet & solution forms not interchangeable, solution preferred.** Many authorities recommend measuring drug serum concentration after 2 wks to ensure satisfactory absorption. To obtain highest plasma concentration, tablet is given with food & acidic drinks (e.g. cola) while solution is taken in fasted state. Peak plasma concentrations after IV injection (200 mg) compared to oral capsule (200 mg): **2.8 mcg/mL (do not use to treat meningitis).** Peak levels reached faster (2.2 vs 5 hrs) with solution. Peak plasma (200 mg) compared to oral capsule (200 mg) **2.8 mcg/mL** (do not use to treat meningitis). Peak levels reached faster (2.2 vs 5 hrs) with solution. Peak plasma conc. of capsule is approx. 3 mcg/mL & of solution is 4 mcg/mL. Adverse effects: dose-related nausea 10%, vomiting 6%, ↓ blood pressure 3.2%, edema 3.5%, & hepatitis 2.7% reported. Protein-binding 99.8%. concentrations in CSF (**do not use to treat meningitis**). Adverse effects: dose-related nausea 10%, for both preparations & over 99%, which explains virtual absence of penetration into CSF (**do not use to treat meningitis**). Protein-binding diarrhea 8%, vomiting 6%, & abdominal discomfort 5.7%. Allergic: rash 8.6%, ↑ bilirubin 6%, edema 3.5%, & hepatitis 2.7% reported. **Reported to produce impairment in cardiac function.** Severe liver failure req transplant in pts receiving pulse rx for onychomycosis reported (*J Neur Neurosurg Psych 81:327, 2010*). Reported in 24 cases with 11 deaths out of 50 mill people who received the drug prior to 2001. Other concern, as with fluconazole and ketoconazole, is **drug-drug interactions;** *see Table 22.* Some can be life-threatening.
Ketoconazole (Nizoral) 200 mg tab	**Gastric acid required for absorption**—cimetidine, omeprazole, antacids block absorption. In achlorhydria, dissolve tablet in 4 mL 0.2N HCl, drink with a straw. Coca-Cola ↑ absorption by 65%. CSF levels "none." **Drug-drug interactions important,** *see Table 22.* **Dose- dependent nausea and vomiting.** Liver toxicity of hepatocellular type reported in 1:10,000 exposed pts—usually after several wks to weeks of exposure. With high doses, adrenal (Addisonian) crisis reported. At doses of ≥800 mg per day serum testosterone and plasma cortisol levels fall.

See page 2 for abbreviations. All dosage recommendations are for adults (unless otherwise indicated) and assume normal renal/renal function

TABLE 11B (3)

DRUG NAME, GENERIC (TRADE)/USUAL DOSAGE	ADVERSE EFFECTS/COMMENTS
Miconazole (Monistat IV) 200 mg—*not available in U.S.*	IV miconazole indicated in patient critically ill with Scedosporium (Pseudallescheria boydii) infection. Very toxic due to vehicle needed to get drug into solution.
Nystatin (Mycostatin) 30 gm cream 500,000 units oral tab	Topical: virtually no adverse effects. Less effective than imidazoles and triazoles. PO: large doses give occasional GI distress and diarrhea.
Posaconazole (Noxafil) Suspension (40 mg/mL): 400 mg po bid with food or 200 mg po qid (with food) with meals, 200 mg qid, Delayed-release tablets (100 mg): 300 mg bid x 1 day and then 300 mg daily for prophylaxis. Intravenous formulation, 300 mg IV bid x 1 day (for prophylaxis). Takes 7-10 days to achieve steady state. No IV formulation.	**Suspension is dosed differently than delayed-release tablets (not interchangeable) – check dose carefully.** An oral triazole with activity against a wide range of fungi refractory to other antifungal rx including: aspergillosis; mucormycosis (variability by species); fusariosis; Scedosporium (Pseudallescheria), phaeohyphomycosis, histoplasmosis, refractory coccidioidomycosis, & refractory chromoblastomycosis. Clinical response in 75% of 176 AIDS pts with azole-refractory oral/esophageal candidiasis. Posaconazole has similar toxicities as other triazoles: nausea 9%, vomiting 6%, abd. pain 5%, headache 5%, diarrhea, ↑ ALT, AST, & rash (3% each). In pts rx for >6 mos., serious side-effects have included adrenal insufficiency, nephrotoxicity, & QTc interval prolongation. Significant drug-drug interactions; inhibits CYP3A4 (*see Table 22*). Consider monitoring serum concentrations (*AAC 53:24, 2009*). **100 mg delayed-release tablets:** loading dose of 300 mg (three 100 mg delayed-release tablets) twice daily on the first day, followed by a once-daily maintenance dose of 300 mg (three 100 mg delayed-release tablets) starting on the second day of therapy. Approved for prophylaxis only and not interchangeable. Intravenous formulation approved for prophylaxis at 300 mg IV daily after a loading dose of 300 mg bid x 1 day. The tablet and solution are not interchangeable. Consider therapeutic drug monitoring with a goal trough of > 0.7 for prophylaxis and > 1.0 for treatment. **Should be given with high fat meal for maximum absorption.** Approved for prophylaxis of invasive aspergillus and candidiasis. Tablets allow patients to achieve better levels than the suspension-lower dose unknown but prophylactic dose often achieves therapeutic levels. *JAC 69:1162, 2014.*
Terbinafine (Lamisil) 250 mg tab	In pts given terbinafine for onychomycosis, rare cases (8) of idiosyncratic & symptomatic hepatic injury & more rarely liver failure leading to death or liver transplant. The drug is **not recommended** for pts with **chronic or active liver disease;** hepatotoxicity may occur in pts with or without pre-existing disease. Pretreatment serum transaminases (ALT & AST) advised & alternate rx used for those with abnormal levels. Pts started on terbinafine should be monitored about symptoms suggesting liver dysfunction (persistent nausea, anorexia, fatigue, vomiting, RUQ pain, jaundice, dark urine or pale stools); if symptoms develop, drug should be discontinued & liver function immediately evaluated. In controlled trials, changes in ocular lens and retina reported—clinical significance unknown. May have drug-drug interaction is 100% ↑ rx rate of clearance by rifampin. AEs: usually mild, transient and rarely caused discontinuation of rx. % with AE, terbinafine vs placebo: nausea/diarrhea 2.6–5.6 vs 2.9; rash 5.6 vs 2.2; taste abnormality 2.8 vs 0.7. Inhibits CYP2D6 enzymes (*see Table 22*). An acute generalized exanthematous pustulosis and subacute cutaneous lupus reported.
Voriconazole (Vfend) IV: **Loading dose 6 mg per kg per kg q12h** IV x 1 day, then **4 mg per kg q12h** IV for invasive aspergillus & serious mold infections; **3 mg per kg IV q12h** for serious candida infections. Oral: **≥40 kg body weight:** 400 mg po q12h, then 200 mg po q12h, then **<40 kg body weight:** 200 mg po q12h, then 100 mg po q12h Take one dose 1 hour before or 1 hour after eating.	A triazole with activity against Aspergillus sp., **including Ampho resistant strains** of A. terreus. Active vs Candida sp. (including krusei), Fusarium sp. & various molds. Steady state serum levels reach 2.5–4 mcg per mL. Up to 20% of patients with subtherapeutic levels with oral administration; check serum drug concentrations. Treatment failure. **Toxicity** similar to other azoles/triazoles including uncommon serious hepatic toxicity (hepatitis, cholestasis & fulminant hepatic failure. Liver function tests should be monitored during rx & drug dc'd if abnormalities develop. Photosensitivity is common and can be severe. Many reports of associated skin cancers. Strongly recommend sun protective measures. *CID 58:997, 2014* & hallucinations in a 15 y/o pt with ALL reported. **Approx. 21% experience a transient visual disturbance** following IV or po administration & are attenuated with repeated doses (**do not drive at night**). Visual changes resolve within 30-60 min. after administration; altered/enhanced visual perception, blurred vision, changed color vision, or photophobia within 30-60 minutes. Visual changes resolve within 30-60 min. Hallucinations, hypoglycemia, electrolyte disturbance & pneumonitis attributed to ↑ drug concentrations. Cause unknown. In patients with ClCr <50 mL per min., the intravenous vehicle (SBECD-sulfobutylether-ß-cyclodextrin) may accumulate but clearance not obviously toxic (*AJHP Dec 1, 2012*). Oral suspension (40 mg per mL). Oral suspension dosing. Same as for oral tabs. Reduce to 50% maintenance dose for moderate hepatic insufficiency. **With prolonged use, fluoride in drug can cause a painful periostitis** (*CID 59:1237, 2014*). Potential for drug-drug interactions high—see *Table 22*. **NOTE: Not in urine in active form. No activity vs. mucormycosis.**

See page 2 for abbreviations. All dosage recommendations are for adults (unless otherwise indicated) and assume normal renal function

TABLE 12A – TREATMENT OF MYCOBACTERIAL INFECTIONS*

Tuberculin skin test (TST). Same as PPD *[Chest 136:1456, 2010].*

Criteria for positive TST after 5 tuberculin units (intermediate PPD) read at 48–72 hours:

- ≥5 mm induration: + HIV, immunosuppressed, ≥15 mg prednisone per day, recent close contact
- ≥10 mm induration: foreign-born, countries with high prevalence; IVD Users; low income; NH residents; chronic illness; silicosis
- ≥15 mm induration: otherwise healthy

Two-stage to detect sluggish positivity: If 1st PPD + but <10 mm, repeat intermediate PPD in 1 wk. Response to 2nd PPD can also happen if pt received BCG in childhood.

BCG vaccine as child: if ≥10 mm induration, & from country with TBc, should be attributed to MTB. Prior BCG may result in booster effect in 2-stage TST.

Routine energy testing not recommended.

Interferon Gamma Release Assays (IGRAs): IGRAs detect sensitivities to MTB by measuring IFN-γ release in response to MTB antigens. May be used in place of TST in all situations in which TST may be used *[MMWR 59 (RR-5), 2010].* IGRAs approved tests available in the U.S.:

- QuantiFERON-TB Gold (QFT-G) (approved 2005)
- QuantiFERON-TB Gold In-Tube Test (QFT-GIT) (approved 2007)
- T-Spot (approved 2008)

IGRAs are relatively specific for MTB and do not cross-react with BCG or most nontuberculous mycobacteria. CDC recommends IGRA over TST for persons unlikely to return for reading TST & for persons who have received BCG. TST is preferred in children age < 5 yrs (but IGRA is acceptable). IGRA or TST may be used without preference for recent contacts of TB with special utility for follow-up testing since IGRAs do not prime the immune system or cause a booster effect. May also be used without preference over TBc for occupational exposures. As with TST, testing with IGRAs in low prevalence populations will result in false-positive results *[CID 53:234, 2011].* Manufacturer's IFN-gamma cut-off ≥0.35 IU/ml for QFT-GIT may be too low for low prevalence settings, inflating positivity and conversion rates, and a higher cut-off may be more appropriate *[Am. J Respir Crit Care Med 188:1005, 2013).* For detailed discussion of IGRAs, see *MMWR 59 (RR-5), 2010 and JAMA 308:241, 2012.*

Rapid (24-hr or less) diagnostic tests for MTB: (1) the Amplified Mycobacterium tuberculosis Direct Test amplifies and detects MTB ribosomal RNA; (2) the AMPLICOR Mycobacterium tuberculosis Test amplifies and detects MTB DNA. Both tests have sensitivities & specificities >95% in sputum samples that are AFB-positive. In negative smears, specificity remains >95% but sensitivity is 40–77% *[MMWR 58:7, 2009; CID 49:46, 2009] (see: http://www.cdc.gov/tb/publications/guidelines/amplification_tests/default.htm (3) COBAS TaqMan MTB Test: real-time PCR test for detection of M. tuberculosis in respiratory specimens not available in the U.S.; with performance characteristics similar to other rapid tests (J Clin Microbiol 51:3225, 2013).*

Xpert MTB/RIF is a rapid test (2 hrs) for MTB in sputum samples which also detects RIF resistance with specificity of 99.2% and sensitivity of 72.5% in smear negative patients (*NEJM 363:1005, 2010*). Current antibody-based and ELISA-based rapid tests for TBc not recommended by WHO because they are less accurate than microscopy ± culture *(Lancet ID 11:736, 2011).*

CAUSATIVE AGENT/DISEASE	MODIFYING CIRCUMSTANCES	SUGGESTED REGIMENS	
		INITIAL THERAPY	CONTINUATION PHASE OF THERAPY
I. Mycobacterium tuberculosis exposure (baseline TST/IGRA negative (household members & other close contacts of potentially infectious cases)	Neonate: Rx essential NOTE: If fever, abnormal CXR (pleural effusion, hilar adenopathy, infiltrate) at baseline, treat for active TBc and not with INH alone.	INH (10 mg/kg/day for 8-10 wks)	Repeat tuberculin skin test (TST) in 8-12 wks: if TST neg & CXR normal & infant age at exposure > 6 mos., stop INH. If TST (≥ 5 mm) or age > 5 mos., treat with INH for total of 9 mos. If follow-up CXR abnormal, treat for active TBc
		As for neonate for 1st & 2nd mos.	If repeat TST at 8-10 wks is negative, stop. If repeat TST ≥ 5 mm, continue INH for total of 9 mos. If INH not given initially, repeat TST at 3 mos. **If + rx** with INH for 9 mos. *(see Category II below).*
	Children <5 years of age—Rx indicated		
	Older children & adults— Risk 2–4% 1st yr		Pts at high risk of progression (e.g., HIV+, immunosuppressed or on immunosuppressive therapy) and no evidence of active infection should be treated for LTBI (see below). Otherwise repeat TST/IGRA at 8-10 wks: no rx if repeat TST/IGRA neg

See page 2 for abbreviations   * Dosages are for adults (unless otherwise indicated) and assume normal renal function   † **DOT** = directly observed therapy

TABLE 12A (2)

CAUSATIVE AGENT/DISEASE	MODIFYING CIRCUMSTANCES	SUGGESTED REGIMENS	
		INITIAL THERAPY	**ALTERNATIVE**
II. Tuberculosis (LTBI, positive TST or IGRA as above, active TB ruled out) *See FIGURE 1 for treatment algorithm for pt with abnormal baseline CXR (e.g., upper lobe fibronodular disease) suspected active TBc.)* Review: *NEJM 372:2127, 2015*	Age no longer an exclusion, all persons with LTBI should be offered therapy. If pre-anti-TNF therapy, recommend at least one month of treatment for LTBI prior to start of anti-TNF therapy (*Arth Care & Res 64:625, 2012*). Overall, regimens containing a rifamycin (RIF, RFB or RFP) are most effective at preventing active tuberculosis (*AnUM 161:419 & 449, 2014*). For patients on **Isoniazid** educate and monitor clinically for signs and symptoms of hepatitis. Baseline lab testing of liver function at start of therapy not routinely indicated but is indicated for patients with HIV infection, pregnant women, and women within 3 mo of delivery, persons with a history of chronic liver disease, persons who use alcohol regularly, and persons at risk for chronic liver disease.	**INH** po once daily (adult: 5 mg/kg/day, max 300 mg/day; child: 10-15 mg/kg/day not to exceed 300 mg/day) x 9 mos. For current recommendations for monitoring hepatotoxicity on INH see *MMWR 59:227, 2010.* Supplemental pyridoxine 50 mg/day for HIV+ patients. A 12 dose once weekly DOT **INH + Rifapentine (RFP)**. **INH** po 15 mg/kg (max dose 900 mg). **RFP** po (wt-based dose): 10-14 kg: 300 mg; 14.1-25 kg: 450 mg; 25.1-32 kg: 600 mg; 32.1-49.9 kg: 750 mg; ≥50 kg: 900 mg. Not recommended for children age < 2 yrs; pts with HIV/AIDS on ART; pregnant women; or pts presumed infected with INH- or RIF-resistant MTB (*MMWR 60:1650, 2011; NEJM 365:2155, 2011*).	**INH** 300 mg once daily for 6 mo (but slightly less effective than 9 mos.; not recommended in children, HIV+ persons, or those with fibrotic lesions on chest film). **INH** 2x/wk (adult: 15 mg/kg, max 900 mg; child: 20-30 mg/kg, max dose 900 mg) x 9 mo. **RIF** once daily (adult: 10 mg/kg/day, max dose 600 mg/day; child: 10-20 mg/kg/day, max dose 600 mg/day) for 4 mos. **INH + RIF** once daily x 3 mos. Rates of flu-like symptoms, cutaneous reactions, and severe drug reactions (rare, 0.3%) higher with 3 mo INH+RFP than with 9 mo INH (*CID 61:527, 2015*), but hepatotoxicity higher with INH (1.8% vs. 0.4%) (*Int J Tuberc Lung Dis 19:1039, 2015*).
Estimating risk of active M.TBc in pts with positive TST or IGRA (www.tstt3d.com)	Lab monitoring of liver function during therapy is indicated if baseline liver function tests are abnormal, if risk factors for hepatic disease are present, or to evaluate for possible adverse effects.		
	Pregnancy	Regimens as above. Once active disease is excluded may delay initiation of therapy until after delivery unless patient is recent contact to an active case. HIV+. Supplemental pyridoxine 10-25 mg/d recommended	
LTBI, suspected INH-resistant organism		**RIF** once daily po (adult: 10 mg/kg/day, max dose 600 mg/day; child: 10-20 mg/kg/day, max dose 600 mg/day) for 4 mos.	**RFB** 300 mg once daily po may be substituted for RIF (in HIV+ patient on anti-retrovirals, dose may need to be adjusted for drug interactions).
LTBI, suspected INH and RIF resistant organism		**Moxi** 400 mg ± **EMB** 15 mg/kg once daily x 12 months	**Levo** 500 mg once daily + **EMB** 15 mg/kg or **PZA** 25 mg/kg) once daily x 12 months.

TABLE 12A (3)

CAUSATIVE AGENT/DISEASE	MODIFYING CIRCUM-STANCES	SUGGESTED REGIMENS					COMMENTS						
		INITIAL THERAPY		CONTINUATION PHASE OF THERAPY AND DIRECTLY OBSERVED THERAPY (DOT) REGIMENS (in vitro susceptibility known)			Dose in mg per kg (max. q24h dose)						
								INH	RIF	PZA	EMB	SM	RFB
		SEE COMMENTS FOR DOSAGE AND INITIAL THERAPY					Regimen* Q24h:						
		Regimen: in order of preference	Drugs	Interval/Doses (min. duration)	Regimen	Drugs	Interval/Doses (min. duration)	Range of Total Doses (min. duration)					
III. Mycobacterium tuberculosis A. Pulmonary TB General reference on rx in adults & children: MMWR 52 (RR-11):1, 2003. In pts with newly diagnosed HIV and TB, Rx for both should be started as soon as possible (NEJM 362:697, 2010).	Rate of INH resistance known to be <4% (drug-susceptible organisms)	1 (See Figure 2, page 143)	INH RIF PZA EMB	7 days per wk times 56 doses (8 wks) or 5 days per wk (DOT) times 40 doses (8 wks) If cavitary disease, treat for 9 mos. Fixed dose combination of INH, RIF, PZA & EMB currently being evaluated (JAMA 305:1415, 2011).	1a	INH/ RIF[3]	7 days per wk times 126 doses (18 wks) or 5 days per wk (DOT) times 90 doses (18 wks) If cavitary disease, treat for 9 mos.	182-130 (26 wks)	Child: 10-20 (300) Adult 5 days per wk (DOT): Child 20-40 (900) Adult 15 (900)	10-20 (600) 10-20 (600) 10-20 (600)	15-30 (2000) 50-70 (4000) 50-70 (4000)	15-25 50 50	20-40 (1000) 25-30 (1500) 25-30 (1500)	10-20 (300) 5 (300) 5 (300)
					1b	INH/ RIF	2 times per wk times 36 doses (18 wks)	92-76 (26 wks) (Not AIDS pts)	2 times per wk (DOT): Child 20-40 (900) Adult 15 (900)	10-20 (600) 10-20 (600)	50-70 (4000) 50-70 (4000)	50 50	25-30 (1500) 25-30 (1500)	10-20 (300) 5 (300)
					1c	INH/ RFP	1 time per wk times 18 doses (18 wks) (only if HIV-neg)	74-58 (26 wks)	3 times per wk (DOT): Child 20-40 (900) Adult 15 (900)	10-20 (600) 10-20 (600)	50-70 (3000) 50-70 (3000)	25-30 25-30	25-30 (1500) 25-30 (1500)	NA NA
Isolation essential! Hospitalized pts with suspected or documented active TB should be isolated in single rooms using airborne precautions until deemed non-infectious. DC isolation if 3 negative AFB smears, or 1-2 neg NAAT (Xpert MTB/RIF), (CID 59:1353 & 1361, 2014).		2 (See Figure 2, page 143)	INH RIF PZA EMB	7 days per wk times 14 doses (2 wks), then 2 times per wk times 12 doses then or 5 days per wk (DOT) times 10 doses (2 wks) then 2 times per wk times 12 doses (6 wks)	2a	INH/ RIF	2 times per wk times 36 doses (18 wks)	62-58 (26 wks) (Not AIDS pts)	Second-line anti-TB agents can be dosed as follows to facilitate DOT: Cycloserine 500-750 mg po q24h					
					2b[5]	INH/ RFP	1 time per wk times 18 doses (18 wks) (only if HIV-neg)	44-40 (26 wks)	Ethionamide 500–750 mg po q24h (5 times per wk) Kanamycin or capreomycin 15 mg per kg IM/IV q24h (3–5 times per wk) Ciprofloxacin 750 mg po q24h (5 times per wk) Ofloxacin 600–800 mg po q24h (5 times per wk) Levofloxacin 750 mg po q24h (5 times per wk)						
		3 (See Figure 2, page 143)	INH RIF PZA EMB	3 times per wk times 24 doses (8 wks)	3a	INH/ RIF	3 times per wk times 54 doses (18 wks)	78 (26 wks)						
USE DOT REGIMENS IF POSSIBLE		4 (See Figure 2, page 143)	INH RIF EMB	7 days per wk times 56 doses (8 wks) or 5 days per wk (DOT) times 40 doses (8 wks)	4a	INH/ RIF	7 days per wk times 217 doses (31 wks) or 5 days per wk (DOT) times 155 doses (31 wks)	273-195 (39 wks)	Risk factors for drug-resistant (MDR) TB: Recent immigration from Latin America or Asia or living in area of ↑ resistance (≥4%) or previous rx without RIF; exposure to known MDR TB. Incidence of primary drug resistance in US steady at 0.7%. Incidence of MDR TB is particularly high (~25%) in parts of China, Thailand, Russia, Estonia & Latvia, ~80% of US MDR cases in foreign born.					
					4b	INH/ RIF	3 times per wk times 62 doses (31 wks)	118-102 (39 wks)						

(continued on next page)

See page 2 for abbreviations

* Dosages are for adults (unless otherwise indicated) and assume normal renal function

[3] DOT = directly observed therapy

TABLE 12A (4)

CAUSATIVE AGENT/DISEASE	MODIFYING CIRCUMSTANCES	SUGGESTED REGIMEN[a]	DURATION OF TREATMENT (mos.)[a]	SPECIFIC COMMENTS[a]	COMMENTS
III. Mycobacterium tuberculosis A. Pulmonary TB (continued from previous page)	INH (± SM) resistance	RIF, PZA, EMB (a FQ may strengthen the regimen for pts with extensive disease.)	6	INH should be stopped in cases of INH resistance. Outcome similar for drug susceptible and INH-mono-resistant strains (CID 48:179, 2009).	(continued from previous page) **Alternatives for resistant strains: Moxi** and **levo** are **FQs of choice**, not CIP. FQ resistance may be seen in pts previously treated with FQ. WHO recommends using moxi (if MIC ≤ 2) if resistant to earlier generation FQs (AAC 54:4765, 2010). **Linezolid** 600 mg once daily has excellent in vitro activity, including MDR strains and effective in selected cases of MDR TB and XDR TB but watch for toxicity (NEJM 367:1508, 2012). **Clofazimine** 100 mg as one component of a multiple drug regimen may improve outcome (CID 60:1361, 2015). **Bedaquiline** recently FDA approved for treatment of MDR TB based on efficacy in Phase 2 trials (AAC 56:3271, 2012; NEJM 371:689, 723, 2014). Dose is 400 mg once daily for 2 weeks then 200 mg bw for 22 weeks administered as directly observed therapy (DOT), taken with food, and always in combination with other anti-TB meds. The investigational agent, **delamanid** (NEJM 366:2151, 2012; Eur Respir J 45:1498, 2015) at a dose of 100 mg bid, granted conditional approval for treatment of MDR-TB as one component of an optimized background regimen by the European Medicines Agency. **Consultation with an expert in MDR-TB management** strongly advised before use of this agent. For MDR-TB and XDR-TB, do drug susceptibility testing for combination FQs and other 2nd line drugs if possible (CID 59:1364, 2014).
Multidrug-Resistant Tuberculosis (MDR TB): Defined as resistant to at least 2 drugs including INH & RIF. Rx clusters with high mortality (NEJM 363:1050, 2010).	Resistance to INH & RIF (± SM)	FQ, PZA, EMB, AMK or capreomycin (SM only if confirmed susceptible). see Comment	18–24	Extended rx is needed to ↓ the risk of relapse. In cases with extensive disease, the use of an additional agent (alternative agents) may be prudent to ↓ the risk of failure & additional acquired drug resistance. Resectional surgery may be appropriate.	
	Resistance to INH, RIF & PZA	FQ, EMB or PZA (if active), AMK or capreomycin (SM only if confirmed susceptible). see Comment	24	Use the first-line agents to which there is susceptibility. Add 2 or more alternative agents in case of extensive disease. Surgery should be considered. Survival ↑ in pts receiving active active TB & surgical intervention (AJRCCM 169:1103, 2004).	
Extensively Drug-Resistant TB (XDR-TB): Defined as resistant to INH & RIF plus any FQ and at least 1 of the 3 second-line drugs: capreomycin, kanamycin or amikacin (MMWR 56:250, 2007; CID 51:379, 2010).	Resistance to RIF	INH, EMB, FQ, supplemented with PZA for the first 2 mos (an IA may be included for the first 2–3 mos. for pts with extensive disease)	12–18	Extended use of an IA may not be feasible. An all-oral regimen times 12–18 mos. should be effective but for more extensive disease &/or to shorten duration (e.g., to 12 mos.), an IA may be added in the initial 2 mos. of rx.	
	XDR-TB	Expert consultation strongly advised. See comments	18–24	Therapy requires administration of 4-6 drugs to which infecting organism is susceptible, including multiple second-line drugs (MMWR 56:250, 2007). Increased mortality seen primarily in HIV+ patients. Cure with outpatient therapy likely in non-HIV+ patients when regimens of 4 or 5 or more drugs to which organism is susceptible are employed (NEJM 359:563, 2008; CID 47:496, 2008). Successful sputum culture conversion correlates to initial susceptibility to FQs and kanamycin (CID 46:42, 2008). Bedaquiline (CID 60:188, 2015) and Linezolid are options.	

See page 2 for abbreviations   * Dosages are for adults (unless otherwise indicated) and assume normal renal function   † **DOT** = directly observed therapy

TABLE 12A (5)

CAUSATIVE AGENT/DISEASE; MODIFYING CIRCUMSTANCES	SUGGESTED REGIMENS		COMMENTS
	INITIAL THERAPY	CONTINUATION PHASE OF THERAPY (In vitro susceptibility known)	
III. Mycobacterium tuberculosis (continued)			
B. Extrapulmonary TB **Steroids:** see Comment	INH + RIF (or RFB) + PZA + EMB q24h times 2 mos Some add **pyridoxine** 25–50 mg po q24h	INH + RIF (or RFB)	IDSA recommends 6 mos for lymph node, pleural, pericardial, disseminated disease, genitourinary & peritoneal TB; 6–9 mos for bone & joint; 9-12 mos for CNS (including meningeal) TB; corticosteroids "strongly rec" only for meningeal TB; (MMWR 52(RR-11):1, 2003). Steroids not recommended for pericardial TB (NEJM 371:1121 & 1155, 2014).
C. Tuberculous meningitis Excellent summary of clinical aspects and therapy (including steroids): CMR 21:243, 2008. Also J Infect 59:167, 2009.	INH + RIF + EMB + PZA + prednisone 60 mg/day x 4 wks, then 30 mg/day x 4 wks, then 15 mg/day x 2 wks, then 5 mg/day x 1 wk	May omit EMB when susceptibility to INH and RIF established. Can D/C PZA after 2 months. Treat for total of 12 months. See Table 9, page 94. Initial reg of INH + RIF + SM + PZA also effective, even in patients with INH-resistant organisms.	3 drugs often rec for initial rx; we prefer 4 (J Infect 59:167, 2009) shown to ↓ complications & ↑ survival (for 1st mo). Infection with MDR-TB ↑ mortality & morbidity. **Dexamethasone** (for 1st mo) may be useful if started early (AAC 55:3244, 2011). FQs (Levo, Gati, CIP) may be useful if started early (AAC 55:3244, 2011).
D. Tuberculosis during pregnancy	INH + RIF + EMB for 9 mos		SM should not be substituted for EMB due to toxicity. AMK, capreomycin, kanamycin. FQs recommended for EMB for pregnant women in U.S. due to lack of safety data, although PZA has not been recommended for general use in U.S. due to lack of safety data, although PZA is not included in the WHO but has not been recommended for general use. Breast-feeding should not be discouraged if PZA is not included in the routine use in pregnant women by the WHO but has not reported adverse events. Breast-feeding should not be discouraged if been used in some US health jurisdictions without reported adverse events. Pyridoxine, 25 mg/day, should be administered.
E. Treatment failure or relapse. Usually due to poor compliance or resistant organisms, or suboptimal drug levels (CID 55:169, 2012).	Directly observed therapy (DOT). Check susceptibilities. (See section III. A, page 139.6 above)		= treatment failures. Failures may be due to non-compliance or resistant organisms. Confirm susceptibilities of original isolates and obtain susceptibility on current isolates. Non-compliance common, therefore institute DOT. If isolates show resistance, modify regimen to include at least 2 (preferably 3) new active agents, none that the patient has not previously received if at all possible. Patients with MDR-TB usually convert sputum within 12 weeks of successful therapy.
F. HIV infection or AIDS—pulmonary All HIV infected patients with TB should be treated with ARVs. If CD4 < 50, initiation of ARVs within 2 weeks of starting TB meds associated with improved survival (Ann Intern Med 163:32, 2015). If CD4 > 50 no proven survival benefit with early ARVs; initiate ARVs at 2-4 weeks. Immune reconstitution (IRIS) if trends to moderately severe or severe TB. 8-12 weeks for less severe TB.	INH + RIF (or RFB) + PZA q24h x 2 mos. Add **pyridoxine** 50 mg po q24h	INH + RIF (or RFB) q24h times 4 months (total 6 mos.) Treat up to 9 mos in pts with delayed response, cavitary disease. to regimens that include INH	1. Co-administration of RIF not recommended for these anti-retroviral drugs: nevirapine, etravirine, rilpivirine; maraviroc, elvitegravir (integrase inhibitor in the fixed combination Stribild®), all HIV protease inhibitors. Use RFB instead). 2. RIF may be coadministered with efavirenz; nucleoside reverse transcriptase inhibitors. Coadministration of RIF with raltegravir best avoided (use RFB instead) but if necessary increase raltegravir dose to 800 mg q12h; RIF + dolutegravir OK at 50 mg bid of latter. 3. Because of possibility of developing resistance to RIF or RFB in pts with low CD4 cell counts who receive weekly (2x/wk) therapy, daily dosing (preferred), or at a min 3x/wk dosing (failure likely higher) recommended for initial or continuation phase of rx. 4. Clinical & microbiologic response similar to that of HIV-neg patient 5. Post-treatment suppression not necessary for drug-susceptible strains. 6. Immune reconstitution inflammatory syndrome occurs in 10-20% of TB patients after initiation of ARVs.
Concomitant protease inhibitor (PI) therapy	INH 300 mg q24h + RFB (150 mcg q24h or 300 mg tiw) + EMB 15 mg/kg q24h + PZA 25 mg/kg q24h x 2 mos.; then INH + RFB times 4 mos. (up to 6 mos.)	INH + RFB x 4 mos. (7 mos in slow responders, cavitary disease)	Rifamycins induce cytochrome CYP450 enzymes (RIF > RFP > RFB) & reduce serum levels of PIs. Conversely, PIs inhibit CYP450 & cause toxicity ↑. RFB is the preferred rifamycin when concomitantly administered with PIs. If dose of RFB is not reduced, toxicity ↑.

* Dosages are for adults (unless otherwise indicated) and assume normal renal function   † **DOT** = directly observed therapy

See page 2 for abbreviations

TABLE 12A (6)

FIGURE 1 ALGORITHM FOR MANAGEMENT OF AT-RISK PATIENT WITH LOW OR HIGH SUSPICION OF ACTIVE TUBERCULOSIS WHILE CULTURES ARE PENDING *(modified from MMWR 52(RR-11):1, 2003).*

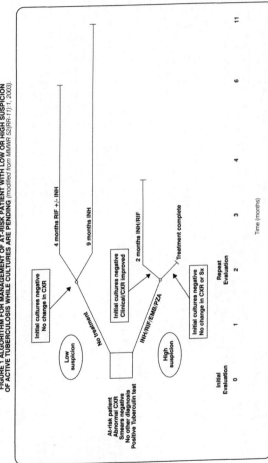

Patients at high clinical suspicion of active TB should be started on 4-drug therapy, pending results of cultures. If cultures are negative and there is no change in symptoms or CXR, the 4-drug regimen can be stopped and no further therapy is required. If cultures are negative and there is clinical or CXR improvement, continue INH/RIF for 2 additional months. For patients at low suspicion for active TB, treat for LTBI once cultures are negative.

* Dosages are for adults (unless otherwise indicated) and assume normal renal function   † **DOT** = directly observed therapy

See page 2 for abbreviations

TABLE 12A (7)
FIGURE 2 [Modified from MMWR 52(RR-11):1, 2003]

Treatment Algorithm for Tuberculosis

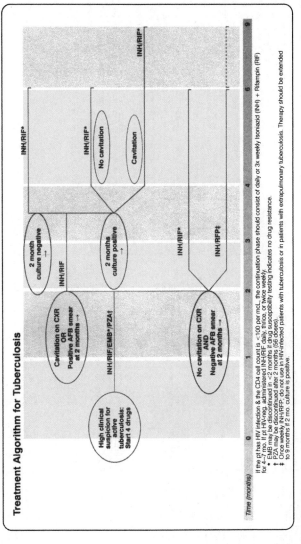

If the pt has HIV infection & the CD4 cell count is <100 per mcL, the continuation phase should consist of daily or 3x weekly Isoniazid (INH) + Rifampin (RIF) for 4–7 mo. If pt HIV-neg. administered INH/RIF daily, thrice, or twice weekly.

* EMB may be discontinued in <2 months if drug susceptibility testing indicates no drug resistance.
† PZA may be discontinued after 2 months (56 doses).
‡ Once weekly INH/RFP; do not use in HIV-infected patients with tuberculosis or in patients with extrapulmonary tuberculosis. Therapy should be extended to 9 months if 2 mo. culture is positive.

Time (months)

See page 2 for abbreviations.

TABLE 12A (8)

CAUSATIVE AGENT/DISEASE	MODIFYING CIRCUMSTANCES	SUGGESTED REGIMENS PRIMARY/ALTERNATIVE		COMMENTS
IV. Nontuberculous Mycobacteria (NTM) (See ATS Consensus: AJRCCM 175:367, 2007)				
A. M. bovis				The M. tuberculosis complex includes M. bovis and regimens effective for MTB (except PZA based) also likely to be effective for M. bovis. **All isolates resistant to PZA.** Isolation not required. Increased prevalence of extrapulmonary disease in U.S. born Hispanic populations and elsewhere (CID 47:168, 2008; EID 14:909, 2008; EID 17:457, 2011).
B. Bacillus Calmette-Guerin (BCG) (derived from M. bovis)	Only fever (>38.5°C) for 12–24 hrs.	INH 300 mg q24h times 3 months		Intravesical BCG effective in superficial bladder tumors and carcinoma in situ. With sepsis, persistent and adjective prednisolone. Also susceptible to RIFB, CIP, oflox, levo, moxi, strepto/m, amikacin (AAC 53:316, 2009). BCG may cause regional adenitis
	Systemic illness or sepsis	INH + RIF + EMB for 2 months then INH + RIF for 7 months		or pulmonary disease in HIV-infected children (CID 37:1226, 2003). **Resistant to PZA.**
		Same as for M. bovis.		
C. M. avium-intracellulare complex (MAC, MAI, or Battey bacillus) ATS/IDSA Consensus Statement: AJRCCM 175:367, 2007. See http://aidsinfo.nih.gov/guidelines/html/4/adult-and-adolescent-opportunistic-infection-prevention-and-treatment-guidelines/0 for updated CDC recommendations for AIDS patients.	**Immunocompetent patients**			See AJRCCM 175:367, 2007 for details of dosing and duration of therapy. Intermittent (tiw) therapy not recommended for patients with cavitary disease, patients who have been previously treated or patients with moderate of severe disease. Intermittent therapy may be an option in nodular bronchiectatic form of the disease (Am J Respir Crit Care Med 191:96, 2015). The primary microbiologic goal of therapy is 12 months of negative sputum cultures on therapy.
	Nodular/Bronchiectatic disease	[**Clarithro** 1000 mg or **azithro** 500 mg] tiw + **EMB** 25 mg/kg tiw + **RIF** 600 mg or **RFB** 300 mg] tiw		
	Cavitary or severe nodular/bronchiectatic disease	[dose for wt <50 kg] or **azithro** 250 mg] tiw + **EMB** 15 mg/kg/day + [**RIF** 600 mg/day or **RFB** 150–300 mg/day] ± **strep** or **AMK**]		**"Classic" pulmonary MAC:** Men 50–75, smokers, COPD. May be associated with hot tub use (Clin Chest Med 23:675, 2002).
		Clarithro 500–1000 mg/day (lower		**"New" pulmonary MAC:** Women 30–70, scoliosis, mitral valve prolapse, (bronchiectasis); pectus excavatum ("Lady Windermere syndrome") and fibronodular disease in elderly women (EID 16:1576, 2010). May also be associated with interferon gamma deficiency (AJM 113:756, 2002).
				For cervicofacial lymphadenitis (localized) in immunocompetent children, surgical excision is as effective as chemotherapy (CID 44:1057, 2007).
				Moxifloxacin and gatifloxacin, active in vitro & in vivo (AAC 51:4071, 2007).
	HIV infection: **Primary prophylaxis**—Pt's CD4 count <50–100 per mm³ Discontinue when CD4 count >100 per mm³ in response to ART	**Azithro** 1200 mg po weekly OR **Clarithro** 500 mg po bid	**RFB** 300 mg po q24h OR **Azithro** 1200 mg po weekly + **RIF** 300 mg po q24h	Many drug-drug interactions, see Table 22, page 237. Drug-resistant MAI disease seen in 29–58% of pts in whom disease develops while taking clarithro prophylaxis & in 11% of those on azithro but has not been observed with RFB prophylaxis. Clarithro resistance more likely in pts with extremely low CD4 counts at initiation Need to be sure no active MTB; RFB used for prophylaxis may promote selection of rifamycin-resistant MTB.
	Treatment: Either presumptive dx or after + culture of blood, bone marrow, or usually, sterile body fluids, eg liver	**Clarithro** 500 mg po bid + **EMB** 15 mg/kg/day ± **RFB** 300 mg po q24h * **Higher doses of clari (1000 mg bid) may be associated with ↑ mortality**	**Azithro** 500 mg po q24h + **EMB** 15 mg/kg/day +/- **RFB** 300–450 mg po/day	Adjust RFB dose as needed for drug interactions.

(continued on next page) |

See page 2 for abbreviations   * Dosages are for adults (unless otherwise indicated) and assume normal renal function   † **DOT** = directly observed therapy

TABLE 12A (9)

CAUSATIVE AGENT/DISEASE	MODIFYING CIRCUMSTANCES	SUGGESTED REGIMENS PRIMARY/ALTERNATIVE		COMMENTS

IV. Nontuberculous Mycobacteria (NTM) *(continued)*

C. M. avium-intracellulare complex *(continued)*				*(continued from previous page)*
				Addition of a third or fourth drug should be considered for patients with advanced immunosuppression (CD4+ count <50 cells/µL), high mycobacterial loads (>2 log CFU/mL of blood), or in the absence of effective ART: **AMK** 10-15 mg/kg IV daily, **Strep** 1 gm IV or IM daily, **Moxi** 400 mg PO daily. Testing of susceptibility to clarithromycin and azithromycin is recommended. Short term (4-8 weeks) of systemic corticosteroid (equivalent to 20-40 mg of prednisone) can be used for IRIS.
	Chronic post-treatment suppression—secondary prophylaxis	**Always necessary. Clarithro** (or azithro) + **EMB** 15 mg/kg/day *(dosage above)*	**Clarithro** or **azithro** or **RFB** *(dosage above)*	Recurrences almost universal without chronic suppression. Can discontinue if no signs and symptoms of MAC disease and sustained (>6 months) CD4 count >100 cells/µL in response to ART.
D. Mycobacterium celatum	Treatment; optimal regimen not defined	May be susceptible to **clarithro**. Treat as if MAC.		Isolated from pulmonary lesions and blood in AIDS patients. Easily confused with M. xenopi (and MAC).
E. Mycobacterium abscessus **Mycobacterium chelonae**	Treatment; Surgical excision may facilitate clarithro rx in subcutaneous abscess and is important adjunct to rx. For role of surgery in M. abscessus pulmonary disease, see *CID 52:565, 2011.*	Cutaneous: **Clarithro** 500 mg po bid x 6 months. Pulmonary/disseminated: 2 or 3 IV drugs (check susceptibility) (**Amikacin, IMP, Cefoxitin, Tigecycline**). Watch out for inducible resistance to Clarithro		M. abscessus susceptible in vitro to AMK (70%), clarithro (95%), cefoxitin (70%), CLO, cefmetazole, RFB, FQ, IMP: azithro, CIP, Doxy, Mino, tigecycline *(CID 42:1756, 2006; JIC 15:46, 2009)*. M. abscessus actually three species: M. abscessus, M. massiliense, M. bolletii. M. massiliense does not exhibit inducible resistance to macrolides and outcomes of medical therapy for infection with this organism may be better than with other species *(Int J Tuberc Lung Dis 18:1141, 2014).* Culture-conversion may not be achievable in M. abscessus pulmonary infection; suppressive therapy may be required to control disease progression. Tigecycline effective in combination with other drugs in salvage therapy *(J Antimicrob Chemother 69:1945, 2014).* Disseminated disease associated with auto-antibodies to interferon-γ *(Immunobiology 218: 762, 2013).* Tigecycline effective in combination with other drugs in salvage therapy *(J Antimicrob Chemother 69:1945, 2014).* In animal model, Cefoxitin & Tigecycline active *(JID 209:905, 2014).* M. chelonae susceptible to AMK (80%), clarithro, azithro, tobramycin (100%), IMP (60%), moxifloxacin, CIP, Mino, Doxy, linezolid (94%) *(CID 42:1756, 2006).* Resistant to cefoxitin, FQ. Tigecycline highly active in vitro and successfully used as salvage for M. chelonae infection in combination regimens *(J Antimicrob Chemother 69:1945, 2014).*
F. Mycobacterium fortuitum	Treatment; optimal regimen not defined. Surgical excision of infected areas.	**AMK + cefoxitin + probenecid** 2-6 wks, then po **TMP- SMX**, or **doxy** 2-6 mos. Usually responds to 6-12 mos of oral rx with 2 drugs to which it is susceptible.		**Resistant to all standard anti-TB: drugs.** Sensitive in vitro to doxycycline, minocycline, cefoxitin, IMP, AMK, TMP-SMX, ofloxa, azithro, clarithro, linezolid, tigecycline, but some strains resistant to azithromycin, rifabutin. For M. fortuitum pulmonary disease treat with at least 2 agents active in vitro until sputum cultures negative for 12 months *(AJRCCM 175:367, 2007).* Disseminated disease associated with auto-antibodies to interferon-γ *(Intern Med 53:1361, 2014).*
G. Mycobacterium haemophilum		Regimen(s) not defined in animal model. **clarithro + rifabutin** effective. Combination of **CIP + RFB + clarithro** reported effective but clinical experience limited *(CID 52:488, 2011).* Surgical debridement may be necessary.		Clinical: Ulcerating skin lesions, synovitis, osteomyelitis, cervicofacial lymphadenitis in children. Associated with permanent eyebrow makeup *(CID 52:488, 2011).* Lab: Requires supplemented media to isolate. Sensitive in vitro to: CIP, cycloserine, rifabutin, moxifloxacin. Over ½ resistant to: INH, RIF, EMB, PZA. For localized cervicofacial lymphadenitis in immunocompetent children, surgical excision as effective as chemotherapy *(CID 44:1057, 2007)* or watchful waiting *(CID 52:180, 2011).*

See page 2 for abbreviations   * Dosages are for adults (unless otherwise indicated) and assume normal renal function   † **DOT** = directly observed therapy

TABLE 12A (10)

CAUSATIVE AGENT/DISEASE	MODIFYING CIRCUMSTANCES	SUGGESTED REGIMENS PRIMARY/ALTERNATIVE		COMMENTS
IV. Nontuberculous Mycobacteria (NTM) *(continued)*				
H. Mycobacterium genavense	2 or more drugs: **Clarithro, EMB, RFB, CLO, Amikacin, Moxifloxacin** as alternatives.			Seen in AIDS patients with CD4 < 50 and in non-HIV severely immunocompromised hosts. *For review see Clin Microbiol Infect 19:432, 2013.*
I. Mycobacterium gordonae	Regimen(s) not defined, but consider **RIF + EMB + KM or CIP (or linezolid** *(AJRCCM 175:367, 2007)*			Frequent colonizer; not associated with disease. In vitro: sensitive to EMB, RIF, AMK, CIP, clarithro, linezolid. Surgical excision.
J. Mycobacterium kansasii	Q24h po: **INH** (300 mg) + **RIF** (600 mg) + **EMB** (25 mg per kg times 2 mos., then 15 mg per kg). Rx for 18 mos. (until culture-neg. sputum times 12 mos; 15 mos. if HIV+ pt.) *(See Comment)*	For **RIF** resistant organism: (**INH** 900 mg + **pyridoxine** 50 mg + **EMB** 25 mg/kg) po q24h + **Sulfamethoxazole** 1000 mg tid (if sulfamethoxazole is unavailable options include **TMP-SMX** two double strength tablets (320 mg **TMP** and 1600 mg **SMX**) bid OR **Clarithromycin** 500 mg po bid OR **Moxifloxacin** 400 mg once daily. Treat for 12-15 mos or until 12-15 mos of culture-negative sputum.		**All isolates are resistant to PZA.** Highly susceptible to linezolid in vitro (*AAC 47:1736, 2003*) and to clarithro and moxifloxacin (*AAC 55:950, 2005*). If HIV+ pt taking protease inhibitor, substitute either clarithro or RFB (150 mg per day) for RIF. Because of variable susceptibility to INH, some substitute clarithro for INH. Resistance to clarithro reported.
K. Mycobacterium marinum	Two active agents for 1-2 months after surgical incision. **Clarithro** 500 mg bid + **EMB** 25 mg/kg q24h or **RIF** 600 mg q24h + **EMB** 25 mg/kg q24h Surgical excision.			For deep tissue involvement a three drug combination therapy with Rifampin 600 mg q24h + Minocycline 100-200 mg q24h or Doxycycline 100-200 mg q24h) + Clarithromycin 500 mg bid. Monotherapy may be considered for minimal disease: Minocycline 100-200 mg q24h or Doxycycline 100-200 mg q24h or TMP-SMX 160/800 mg bid.
L. Mycobacterium scrofulaceum	Surgical excision. Chemotherapy seldom indicated. Although regimens not defined, **clarithro + CLO** with or **without EMB, INH, RIF, strep + cycloserine** have also been used.			
M.Mycobacterium simiae	Regimen(s) not defined. Start 4 drugs as for disseminated MAC			Most isolates resistant to all 1ˢᵗ line anti-Tbc drugs. Isolates often not clinically significant.
N. Mycobacterium ulcerans (Buruli ulcer)	WHO recommends **RIF + SM** for 8 weeks. **RIF + CIP** recommended as alternatives by WHO *(CMN 31:119, 2009).*			Susceptible in vitro to RIF, strep, CLO, clarithro, CIP, ofloxacin, amikacin, moxi, linezolid. Australian guidelines (*MJA 200:267, 2014*) recommend oral combination of RIF + Clarithro or RIF + a FQ (moxifloxacin or CIP). Surgery not required for cure and reserved for those declining or intolerant of antibiotic, debridement of necrotic tissue, large defects.
O. Mycobacterium xenopi	Regimen(s) not defined. **Clarithro** 500 mg bid + **RIF** 600 mg or **Rifabutin** 300 mg + **EMB** 15 mg/kg once daily + **INH** 300 mg once daily.			In vitro: sensitive to clarithro and many standard antimycobacterial drugs. MOXI active in vitro and may be an alternative.
V. Mycobacterium leprae (leprosy) Classification: *CID 44:1096, 2007; Overview: Lancet ID 11:464, 2011.*	There are 2 sets of therapeutic recommendations here: one from USA (National Hansen's Disease Programs [NHDP], Baton Rouge, LA) and one from WHO. Both are based on expert recommendations and neither has been subjected to controlled clinical trial.			

See page 2 for abbreviations   * Dosages are for adults (unless otherwise indicated) and assume normal renal function   † **DOT** = directly observed therapy

TABLE 12A (11)

Type of Disease	NHDP Regimen	WHO Regimen	COMMENTS
Paucibacillary Forms: (Intermediate, Tuberculoid, Borderline tuberculoid)	(**Dapsone** 100 mg/day + **RIF** 600 mg po/day) for 12 months	(**Dapsone** 100 mg/day (unsupervised) + **RIF** 600 mg 1x/mo (supervised)) for 6 mos	Side effects overall 0.4%
Single lesion paucibacillary	Treat as paucibacillary leprosy for 12 months.	Single dose ROM therapy: (RIF 600 mg + Oflox 400 mg + Mino 100 mg) (Ln 353:655, 1999).	
Multibacillary forms: Borderline Borderline-lepromatous Lepromatous *See Comment for erythema nodosum leprosum* Rev.: *Lancet* 363:1209, 2004	(**Dapsone** 100 mg/day + **CLO** 50 mg/day (both unsupervised)) + **RIF** 600 mg + **CLO** 300 mg once monthly (supervised)) Continue regimen for 12 months.	(**Dapsone** 100 mg/day + **CLO** 50 mg/day (both unsupervised)) + **RIF** 600 mg + **CLO** 300 mg once monthly (supervised)) Continue regimen for 12 months.	Side-effects overall 5.1%. For **erythema nodosum leprosum**: prednisone 60–80 mg/day or thalidomide 100–400 mg/day. Thalidomide available in US at 1-800-4-CELGENE. Altho thalidomide effective, WHO no longer rec because of potential toxicity however the majority of leprosy experts feel thalidomide remains drug of choice for ENL under strict supervision. **CLO (Clofazimine)** available from NHDP under IND protocol; contact at 1-800-642-2477. **Ethionamide** (250 mg q24h) or prothionamide (375 mg q24h) may be subbed for CLO. Etanercept effective in one case refractory to above standard therapy (CID 52:e133, 2011). Regimens incorporating clarithro, minocycline, dapsone monotherapy have been abandoned due to emergence of resistance (CID 52:e127, 2011), but older patients previously treated with dapsone monotherapy may remain on lifelong maintenance therapy. Moxi highly active in vitro and produces rapid clinical response (AAC 52:3113, 2008).

Alternative regimen: (**Dapsone** 100 mg/day + **RIF** 600 mg/day) for 24 mos of **CLO** is refused or unavailable.

* Dosages are for adults (unless otherwise indicated) and assume normal renal function   † **DOT** = directly observed therapy

See page 2 for abbreviations

TABLE 12B – DOSAGE AND ADVERSE EFFECTS OF ANTIMYCOBACTERIAL DRUGS

AGENT (TRADE NAME)[1]	USUAL DOSAGE*	ROUTE/[1]* DRUG RESISTANCE (RES) US*[1]	SIDE-EFFECTS, TOXICITY AND PRECAUTIONS	SURVEILLANCE
FIRST LINE DRUGS				
Ethambutol (Myambutol) (100, 400 mg tab)	25 mg/kg/day for 2 mos then 15 mg/kg/day q24h as 1 dose (<10% protein binding) [Bacteriostatic for both extracellular & intracellular organisms]	RES: 0.3% (0–0.7%) po 400 mg tab	**Optic neuritis** with decreased visual acuity, central scotomata, and loss of green and red perception; peripheral neuropathy and headache (~1%), rashes (rare), arthralgia (rare), hyperuricemia (rare). Anaphylactoid reaction (rare). *Comment:* Primarily used to inhibit resistance. Disrupts outer cell membrane in M. avium with ↑ activity to other drugs.	Monthly visual acuity & red/green with dose >15 mg/kg/day; ≥10% loss considered significant. Usually reversible if drug discontinued
Isoniazid (INH) (Nydrazid, Laniazid, Teebaconin) (50, 100, 300 mg tab)	Q24h dose: 5–10 mg/kg/day up to 300 mg/day as 1 dose or 2x/wk dose: 15 mg/kg (900 mg max dose) (<10% protein binding) [Bactericidal to both extracellular and intracellular organisms] Add pyridoxine in alcoholic, pregnant, or malnourished pts.	RES: 4.1% (2.6–8.5%) po 100 mg/mL in 10 mL (IV route not FDA-approved but has been used, esp. in AIDS)	Overall ~1%. Liver: **Hep** (children 10% mild) ↑ SGOT, normalizes with continued rx, age >20 yrs old, 20–34 yrs 1.2%, ≥50 yrs 2.3%) [also] ↑ with q24h alcohol & previous exposure to Hep. Usually asymptomatic (JID 126:799, 2003). May be fatal. With prodromal sx, stop, check urine ldo LFTs; discontinue if SGOT >3-5x normal. **Peripheral neuropathy** (17% on 6 mg/kg per day, less on 300 mg, incidence ↑ in slow acetylators); **pyridoxine** 10 mg q24h will **decrease incidence;** other neurologic sequelae, convulsions, optic neuritis, toxic encephalopathy, psychosis, muscle twitching, dizziness, coma (all rare); allergic skin rashes, fever, minor disulfiram-like reaction, flushing after Swiss cheese; blood dyscrasias (rare); + antinuclear (20%). **Drug-drug interactions** common, see Table 22.	Pre-rx liver functions. Repeat if symptoms (fatigue, weakness, malaise, anorexia, nausea or vomiting) >3 days (AJRCCM 152: 1705, 1995). Some recommend ↑ SGOT at 2, 4, 6 mos esp. if age >50 yrs. Clinical evaluation every mo.
Pyrazinamide (500 mg tab)	25 mg per kg per day (maximum 2.5 gm per day) q24h as 1 dose [Bactericidal for intracellular organisms]	po 500 mg tab	**Arthralgia; hyperuricemia** (with or without symptoms); hepatitis (not over 2% if recommended dose not exceeded); gastric irritation, photosensitivity (rare).	Pre-rx liver functions. Monthly SGOT, uric acid. Measure serum uric acid if symptomatic gouty attack occurs.
Rifamate* — combination tablet	2 tablets single dose q24h	po (1 hr before meal)	1 tablet contains 150 mg INH, 300 mg RIF	As with individual drugs
Rifampin (Rifadin, Rimactane, Rifocin) (150, 300, 450, 600 mg cap)	10.0 mg per kg per day up to 600 mg per day q24h 1 dose (60-90% protein binding) [Bactericidal to all populations of organisms]	RES: 0.2% (0–0.3%) po 600 mg cap (IV available, Merrell-Dow)	INH-RIF dc'd in ~3% for toxicity; gastrointestinal irritation, antibiotic-associated colitis, drug fever (1%), pruritus with or without rash (1%), anaphylactoid reactions in HIV+ pts, mental confusion, thrombocytopenia (1%), leukopenia, hemolytic anemia, transient **abnormalities in liver function. "Flu syndrome"** (fever, chills, headache, bone pain, shortness of breath) seen if RIF taken irregularly or if q24h dose restarted after an interval of no rx. **Discolors urine, tears, sweat, contact lens an orange-brownish color.** May cause drug-induced lupus erythematosus (Ln 349:1521, 1977).	Pre-rx liver function. Repeat if symptoms. **Multiple significant drug interactions,** see Table 22.
Rifater* — combination tablet (See Side-Effects)	Wt ≥55 kg, 6 tablets single dose q24h	po (1 hr before meal)	1 tablet contains 50 mg INH, 120 mg RIF, 300 mg PZA (25 mg per kg per day). Purpose is convenience in dosing, ↑ compliance (AnIM 122: 951, 1995) but cost 1.58 more. Side-effects = individual drugs.	As with individual drugs. PZA 25 mg per kg
Streptomycin (IV/IM sol'n)	15 mg per kg IM q24h, 0.75–1.0 gm per day initially for 60–90 days then (15 mg) 2–3 times per week (15 mg per kg per day) q24h as 1 dose	RES: 3.9% (2.7–7.6%) IM (or IV)	Overall 8%. **Ototoxicity:** vestibular dysfunction (vertigo); paresthesias; dizziness & nausea (all less in pts receiving 2–3 doses per week); tinnitus and high frequency loss (1%); nephrotoxicity; peripheral neuropathy; allergic skin rashes (4–5%); drug fever. Available from X-Gen Pharmaceuticals, 607-732-4411. Ref: IV—CID 9:1150, 1994. Toxicity similar with qd vs tid dosing (CID 38:1538, 2004).	Monthly audiogram. In older pts, serum creatinine or BUN at start of rx and weekly if pt stable

[1] Note: Malabsorption of antimycobacterial drugs may occur in patients with AIDS enteropathy. For review of adverse effects, see *AJRCCM 167:1472, 2003.*

[2] **RES** = % resistance of M. tuberculosis.

See page 2 for abbreviations.

* Dosages are for adults (unless otherwise indicated) and assume normal renal function   ' **DOT** = directly observed therapy

§ Mean (range) (higher in Hispanics, Asians, and patients <10 years old)

(TABLE 12B (2)

AGENT (TRADE NAME)[1]	USUAL DOSAGE*	ROUTE/[§] DRUG RESISTANCE (RES) US[‡,§]	SIDE-EFFECTS, TOXICITY AND PRECAUTIONS	SURVEILLANCE
SECOND LINE DRUGS (more difficult to use and/or less effective than first line drugs)				
Amikacin (Amikin (IV soln))	7.5–10.0 mg per kg q24h [Bacteriocidal for extracellular organisms]	RES: (est. 0.1%) IM/IV 500 mg vial	See Table 10B, pages 115 & 118	Monthly audiogram; Serum creatinine or BUN weekly if pt stable
Bedaquiline (Sirturo) (100 mg tab) Ref: JAC 69:2310, 2014; NEJM 371:723, 2014; CID 60:188, 2015.	Directly observed therapy (DOT): 400 mg once daily for 2 weeks, then 200 mg 3 times per week for 22 weeks, taken with food and always used in combination with other anti-TB medications.	Does not exhibit cross-resistance to other TB drugs; always use in combination with other TB drugs used in selection of resistant mutants	Most common: nausea, vomiting, arthralgia, headache, hyperuricemia. Elevated transaminases. Bedaquiline in clinical trials was administered as one component of a multiple drug regimen, so side-effects are common, yet difficult to assign to a particular drug.	Moderate QTc increases (average of 10-16 ms over the 24 weeks of therapy. Potential risks of pancreatitis, myopathy, myocardial injury, severe hepatotoxicity
Capreomycin sulfate (Capastat sulfate)	1 gm per day (15 mg per kg per day) q24h as 1 dose	RES: 0.1% (0–0.9%) IM/IV	Nephrotoxicity (36%), ototoxicity (auditory 11%), eosinophilia, skin rash, fever, hypokalemia, neuromuscular blockade.	Monthly audiogram, biweekly serum creatinine or BUN
Ciprofloxacin (Cipro) (250, 500, 750 mg tab)	750 mg bid	500 mg or 750 mg po IV 200-400 mg vial	TB not a FDA-approved indication for CIP. Desired CIP serum levels 4–6 mcg per mL. See Table 10A, page 110 & Table 10B, page 116 for adverse effects	None
Clofazimine (Lamprene) (50, 100 mg cap)	50 mg per day (unsupervised) + 300 mg 1 time per month supervised) 50-200 mg per day	50 mg (with meals)	Skin: **pigmentation (pink-brownish black)** 75–100%; dryness 20%, pruritus 5%. GI: abdominal pain 50% (rarely severe leading to exploratory laparoscopy), splenic infarction (VR), bowel obstruction (VR), GI bleeding (VR). Eye: conjunctival irritation, retinal crystal deposits.	None
Cycloserine (Seromycin) (250 mg tab)	750–1000 mg per day (15 mg per kg per day) 2-4 doses per day [Bacteriostatic for both extra-cellular & intracellular organisms]	RES: 0.1% (0–0.3%) 250 mg cap	Convulsions, **psychoses** (5–10% of those receiving 1.0 gm per day); headache; somnolence; hyperreflexia; increased CSF protein and pressure; **peripheral neuropathy**. 100 mg pyridoxine (or more) q24h should be given concomitantly. Contraindicated in epileptics.	None
Dapsone (25, 100 mg tab)	100 mg per day	100 mg tab	Blood: ↓ hemoglobin (1-2 gm), ↑ retics (2-12%), in most pts. Hemolysis in G6PD deficiency; ↑ hemolysis due to concomitant atazanavir (AAC 56:1081, 2012). Renal: albuminuria, nephrotic syndrome. Erythema nodosum leprosum in pts rx for leprosy (½ pts 1st year). Hypersensitivity syndrome in 0.5-3.6% (See Surveillance).	Hypersensitivity syndrome: fever, rash, eosinophilia, lymphadenopathy, hepatitis, pneumonitis. Genetic marker identified (NEJM 369:1620, 2013).
Ethionamide (Trecator-SC) (120, 250 mg tab)	500–1000 mg per day (15–20 mg per kg per day) divided 1-3 doses per day [Bacteriostatic for extracellular organisms only]	RES: 0.8% (0–1.5%) 250 mg tab	**Gastrointestinal irritation** (up to 50% on large dose); goiter; peripheral neuropathy (rare); convulsions (rare); changes in affect (rare); difficulty in diabetes control; rashes; hepatitis; purpura, stomatitis, gynecomastia, menstrual irregularly. Give drug with meals or antacids; 50–100 mg pyridoxine per day concomitantly; SGOT monthly. Possibly teratogenic.	Gastrointestinal irritation (up to 50% on large dose) and assume normal renal function

See page 2 for abbreviations.

* Dosages are for adults (unless otherwise indicated) and assume normal renal function
§ Mean (range) (higher in Hispanics, Asians, and patients <10 years old)

[1] **DOT** = directly observed therapy

TABLE 12B (3)

AGENT (TRADE NAME)[1]	USUAL DOSAGE*	ROUTE/1° DRUG RESISTANCE (RES) US[4,1]	SIDE-EFFECTS, TOXICITY AND PRECAUTIONS	SURVEILLANCE
SECOND LINE DRUGS (continued)				
Linezolid (Zyvox) (600 mg tab, oral suspension 100 mg/mL)	600 mg once daily	PO or IV	Not FDA-approved indication. High rate of adverse events (>80% with 4 months or longer of therapy: myelosuppression, peripheral neuropathy, optic neuropathy. Avoid tyramine-containing foods, soy products, adrenergic agents (e.g., pseudoephedrine, phenylpropanolamine) MAO inhibitors, SSRIs. 600 mg > 300 mg dose for toxicity; consider reducing dose to 300 mg for toxicity or after 4 mos of therapy or culture-conversion to reduce toxicity.	Baseline and monthly complete blood count, visual acuity checks, screen for symptoms of peripheral neuropathy, neurologic examination.
Moxifloxacin (Avelox) (400 mg tab)	400 mg qd	400 mg cap	Not FDA-approved indication. Concomitant administration of rifampin reduces serum levels of moxi (CID 45:1001, 2007).	None
Ofloxacin (Floxin) (200, 300, 400 mg tab)	400 mg bid	400 mg cap	Not FDA-approved indication. Overall adverse effects 11%, 4% discontinued due to side-effects. Gi: nausea 3%, diarrhea 1%. **CNS:** insomnia 3%, headache 1%, dizziness 1%.	None
Para-aminosalicylic acid (PAS, Paser) (Na⁺ or K⁺ salt) (4 gm cap)	4-6 gm bid (200 mg per kg per day) [Bacteriostatic for extracellular organisms only]	RES: 0.8% (0-1.5%) 450 mg tab (see Comment)	**Gastrointestinal irritation** (10-15%); goitrogenic action (rare); depressed prothrombin activity (rare); G6PD-mediated hemolytic anemia (rare); drug fever, rashes, hepatitis, myalgia, arthralgia. Retards hepatic enzyme induction, may ↓ INH hepatotoxicity. Available from CDC. (404) 639-3670, Jacobus Pharm. Co. (609) 921-7447.	None
Rifabutin (Mycobutin) (150 mg cap)	300 mg per day (prophylaxis or treatment)	150 mg tab	Polymyalgia, polyarthralgia, leukopenia, granulocytopenia. Anterior uveitis when given with concomitant clarithromycin; avoid 600 mg dose (NEJM 330:438, 1994). Uveitis reported with 300 mg per day (AnIM 12:510, 1994). Reddish urine, orange skin (pseudojaundice).	None
Rifapentine (Priftin) (150 mg tab)	600 mg twice weekly for 1ˢᵗ 2 mos., then 600 mg q week	150 mg tab	Similar to other rifabutins. (See RIF, RFB) Hyperuricemia seen in 21%. Causes red-orange discoloration of body fluids. Flu-like illness in pts given weekly Rifapentine + INH for latent MTB (CID 61:527, 2015).	None
Thalidomide (Thalomid) (50, 100, 200 mg cap)	100-300 mg po q24h (may use up to 400 mg po q24h for severe erythema nodosum leprosum)	50 mg tab	**Contraindicated in pregnancy. Causes severe life-threatening birth defects. Both male and female patients must use barrier contraceptive methods (Pregnancy Category X).** Frequently causes drowsiness or somnolence. May cause peripheral neuropathy (AJM 108:487, 2000) For review, see Ln 363:1803, 2004.	In US: contact Celgene (800-4-CELGENE)

See page 2 for abbreviations.

* Dosages are for adults (unless otherwise indicated) and assume normal renal function   † **DOT** = directly observed therapy
§ Mean (range) (higher in Hispanics, Asians, and patients <10 years old)

TABLE 13A– TREATMENT OF PARASITIC INFECTIONS

- **See Table 13D for sources for antiparasitic drugs not otherwise commercially available.**
- The following resources are available through the Centers for Disease Control and Prevention (CDC) in Atlanta. Website is www.cdc.gov. General advice for parasitic diseases other than malaria:
  (+1) (404) 718-4745 (day), (+1) (770) 488-7100 (after hours). For CDC Drug Service 8:00 a.m. – 4:30 p.m. EST: (+1) (404) 639-3670; fax: (+1) (404) 639-3717. See www.cdc.gov/laboratory/drugservice/index.html
  For malaria: Prophylaxis advice (+1) (770) 488-7788; or after hours (+1) (770) 488-7100; toll-free (US) 1-(855)-856-4713; www.cdc.gov/malaria
- **NOTE: All dosage regimens are for adults with normal renal function unless otherwise stated.** Many of the suggested regimens are not FDA approved.
- For licensed drugs, suggest checking package inserts to verify dosage and side-effects. Occasionally, post-licensure data may alter dosage as compared to package inserts.

INFECTING ORGANISM	SUGGESTED REGIMENS		COMMENTS
	PRIMARY	ALTERNATIVE	
PROTOZOA—INTESTINAL (non-pathogenic: E. hartmanni, E. dispar, E. coli, Iodamoeba butschlii, E. moshkovskii, Endolimax nana, Chilomastix mesnili)			
Balantidium coli	Tetracycline 500 mg qid x 10 days	**Alternatives: Iodoquinol** 650 mg po tid x 20 days or **Metronidazole** 750 mg po tid times 5 days	Another alternative: Iodoquinol 650 mg po tid x 20 days.
Blastocystis hominis Ref.: *Trends Parasitol 28:305, 2012*	Metronidazole 1.5 gm 1x/day x 10 days or 750 mg po bid x 10 days (need to treat is dubious)	**TMP-SMX-DS**, one bid x 7 days or **Nitazoxanide** 500 mg po x 3 days	Role as pathogen unclear; may serve as marker of exposure to contaminated food/water. Some genotypes may be more virulent.
Cryptosporidium parvum & hominis Treatment is unsatisfactory Ref.: *Curr Opin Infect Dis 23:494, 2010*	**Immunocompetent—No HIV: Nitazoxanide** 500 mg po bid x 3 days (expensive)	**HIV with immunodeficiency:** Effective antiretroviral therapy best therapy. **Nitazoxanide** no clinical or parasite response compared to placebo.	**Nitazoxanide:** Approved in liquid formulation for rx of children & 500 mg tabs for adults who are immunocompetent. Ref.: *CID 40:1173, 2005.* *C. hominis* assoc. with 1 in post-infection eye & joint pain, recurrent headache, & dizzy spells (*CID 39:504, 2004*)
Cyclospora cayetanensis; cyclosporiasis *Clin Micro Rev 23:218, 2010)*	**Immunocompetent pts: TMP-SMX-DS** tab 1 po bid x 7–10 days. Other options: see Comments.	**AIDS pts: TMP-SMX-DS** tab 1 po qid for up to 3–4 wks. Immunocompromised pts: may require suppressive rx with **TMP-SMX-DS** 1 tab 3x/wk.	If sulfa-allergic: **CIP** 500 mg po bid x 7 days but results inconsistent. Anecdotal success with nitazoxanide. Biliary disease described in HIV pts.
Dientamoeba fragilis See *AAC 58:651, 2010;* *Clin Micro Int 14:601, 2008.*	**Iodoquinol** 650 mg po tid x 20 days or **Paromomycin** 25–35 mg/kg/day po in 3 div doses x 7 days or **Metronidazole** 750 mg tid x 10 days.	For treatment failures: **Tetracycline** 500 mg po qid x 10 days + **Iodoquinol** 650 mg po tid x 10 days OR (**Iodoquinol** + **Paromomycin***) May try second course of Iodoquinol	**Metronidazole** failed in prospective random placebo-control DB study (*CID 58:1692, 2014*). In vitro tinidazole, metronidazole most active. *AAC 56:487, 2012*
Entamoeba histolytica; amebiasis. If available, use stool PCR for diagnosis.			Note: E. hartmanni and E. dispar are non-pathogenic.
Asymptomatic cyst passer	**Paromomycin*** 25–35 mg/kg/day po in 3 divided doses x 7 days **OR Iodoquinol*** 650 mg po tid x 20 days	**Diloxanide furoate*** (Furamide) 500 mg po x 10 days.	Colitis can mimic ulcerative colitis; ameboma can mimic adenocarcinoma of colon.
Patient with diarrhea/dysentery; mild/moderate disease. Oral therapy possible	**Metronidazole** 500–750 mg po bid x 7–10 days or **tinidazole** 2 gm po daily x 3 days, followed by: Either [**paromomycin*** 25–35 mg/kg/day po divided in 3 doses x 7 days] or [**Iodoquinol*** 650 mg po tid x 20 days] to clear intestinal cysts. *See comment.*		**Nitazoxanide** 500 mg po bid x 3 days may be effective (*JID 184:381, 2001 & Tran R Soc Trop Med & Hyg 101:1025, 2007*).
Severe or extraintestinal infection, e.g. hepatic abscess	**Metronidazole** 750 mg **iv to po** tid x 10 days or **tinidazole** 2 gm 1x/day x 5 days or **Iodoquinol*** 650 mg po tid x 20 days + (**metronidazole** or tinidazole 25–35 mg/kg/day po divided in 3 doses x 7 days)		**Serology positive (antibody present) with extraintestinal disease.**
Giardia intestinalis also known as **Giardia lamblia, Giardia duodenalis.**	(**Tinidazole** 2 gm po x 1) OR (**nitazoxanide** 500 mg po bid x 3 days). **Metro & Paromomycin** are alternatives	**Metronidazole** 250 mg po tid x 5 days; Albendazole 400 mg po once daily with food x 5 days, Cochrane Database Syst Rev 2012 Dec 12; 12:CD007789. **Pregnancy: Paromomycin*** 25–35 mg/kg/day po in 3 divided doses x 5–10 days.	**Refractory pts:** (metro 750 mg po + quinacrine 100 mg po) or (Paromomycin 10 mg/kg po 3x/day x 3 wks (*CID 33:22, 2001*) giardia genetically heterogeneous (*J Clin Invest 123:2346, 2013*)

* For source of drug, see *Table 13D, page 165.*

TABLE 13A (2)

INFECTING ORGANISM	SUGGESTED REGIMENS		COMMENTS
	PRIMARY	ALTERNATIVE	
PROTOZOA—INTESTINAL (continued)			
Cystoisospora belli (formerly Isospora belli) (AIDS ref: MMWR 58 (RR-4):1, 2009)	**Immunocompetent: TMP-SMX-DS tab 1 po bid x 10 days; Immunocompromised: TMP-SMX-DS qid for up to 3-4 wks (see Comment);** need ART.	**CIP** 500 mg po bid x 7 days is second-line alternative (AnIM 132:885, 2000) OR **Pyrimethamine** 50-75 mg/day + **Folinic acid** 10-25 mg/day (po).	**Chronic suppression in AIDS pts:** either **TMP-SMX-DS** 1 tab 3x/wk OR **TMP-SMX-DS** tab 1 po daily OR **(pyrimethamine 25 mg/day po + folinic acid** 10 mg/day po) OR as 2nd-line alternative: **CIP** 500 mg po 3x/wk.
Microsporidiosis			
Ocular: Encephalitozoon hellum or cuniculi, Vittaforma (Nosema) corneae, Nosema ocularum	For HIV pts: antiretroviral therapy key **Albendazole** 400 mg po bid x 3 wks plus fumagillin eye drops (see Comment).	For HIV - pts reports of response of E. hellum to **fumagillin** (NEJM 351:42, 2004). For V. corneae, may need keratoplasty.	To obtain fumagillin: 800-292-6773 or www.leiterx.com. Neutropenia & thrombo-cytopenia serious adverse events. Dx: Most labs use modified trichrome stain. Need electron micrographs for species identification. FA and PCR methods in development. Peds dose ref: PIDJ 23:915, 2004.
Intestinal (diarrhea): Enterocytozoon bieneusi, Encephalitozoon (Septata) intestinalis	**Albendazole** 400 mg po bid x 3 wks; peds dose: 15 mg/kg per day div. into 2 daily doses x 7 days for E. intestinalis. Fumagillin equally effective.	Oral **fumagillin 20 mg po tid** reported effective for E. bieneusi (NEJM 346:1963, 2002).	For Trachipleistophora sp., try itraconazole + albendazole (NEJM 351:42, 2004). Other pathogens: Brachiola vesiculatum & algerae (NEJM 351:42, 2004).
Disseminated: E. hellum, cuniculi or intestinalis; Pleistophora sp., others in 20 mg po tid (not available in US) Comment. Ref: JCM 52:3839, 2014.	**Albendazole** 400 mg po bid x 3 wks. Fumagillin 20 mg po tid (not available in US)	No established rx for Pleistophora sp.	
PROTOZOA—EXTRAINTESTINAL			
Amebic meningoencephalitis (Clin Infect Dis 51:e7, 2010 (Balamuthia)) Milfefosine available from CDC for all species of free-living ameba. contact CDC Emergency Operations Center at 770-488-7100			
Acanthamoeba sp.— no proven rx Rev: FEMS Immunol Med Micro 50:1, 2007.	Iv therapy. (Pentamidine + Fluconazole or itraconazole) + Milfefosine + Fluconazole. Metronidazole, and a Macrolide	May add TMP-SMX, Metronidazole, and Fluconazole	For Acanthamoeba keratitis: milfefosine or voriconazole.
Balamuthia mandrillaris	**Pentamidine + Albendazole + (Fluconazole or itraconazole) + Milfefosine + Fluconazole**		
Naegleria fowleri >95% mortality. Ref: MMWR 57:573, 2008.	**Amphotericin B** 1.5 mg/kg/day ÷ 2 IV/po intrathecal + Rifampin 10 mg/kg/day + Fluconazole 10 mg/kg/day IV/po + Milfefosine 50 mg po tid		
Babesia microti (US) and **Babesia divergens** (EU) (NEJM 366:2397, 2012)	For **mild/moderate disease: Atovaquone** 750 mg po bid + **Azithro** 500 mg po on day 1, then 250-1000 mg po/day for total of 7-10 days. If relapse, treat x 6 wks & until blood smear neg x 2. wks.	For **severe babesiosis: (Clindamycin** 600 mg tid) + **(quinine** 650 mg po tid) x 7-10 days For adults, can give **clinda** IV as 1.2 gm bid.	Overwhelming infection in asplenic patients. In immunocompromised patients, treat for 6 or more weeks (CID 46:370, 2008). Transfusion related cases occur.
Leishmaniasis (Suggest consultation—CDC (+1) 404-718-4745) Note: Milfefosine available directly from Profounda, Inc. (+1 407-270-7790), www.Impavido.com. CDC IND does not cover			
leishmaniasis Ref: Med Lett 56:89, 2014.	**Mild Disease:** Paromomycin* ointment bid x 20 days (investigational) cryotherapy (freeze up to 3x with liquid nitrogen), intralesional Antimony 20 mg/kg into lesions weekly x 8-10. wks. CDC antimony IND does not cover intralesional use. Leave outside US. **Milfefosine** (w/food) 50 mg (wt 30-44 kg): 50 mg tid (wt ≥ 45 kg). Treat for 28 days. Response in	**Moderate Disease: Sodium stibogluconate*** (Pentostam) or **Meglumine antimoniate** (Glucantime) 20 mg/kg/day IV/IM x 20 days. Dilute in 120 mL of D5W and infuse over 2 hrs. **Alternatives: Fluconazole** 200 mg po daily x 6 weeks (for L. mexicana, L. panamensis, L. major) or **Ketoconazole** 600 mg po daily x 30 days (for L. mexicana) or **Milfefosine** (dose as for mild disease) Some experts use **liposomal amphotericin B** (regimens vary) with total cumulative dose of 20-60 mg/kg.	Oral therapy. Topical paromomycin* & other topical treatment only when low potential for mucosal spread. Active for L. braziliensis or L. guyanensis cutaneous lesions. Generic pentavalent antimony varies in quality and safety. Leishmania in travelers frequently responds to observation and local therapy (CID 57:370, 2013). Milfefosine is preg cat D (do not use in pregnancy).
Cutaneous: Mild Disease (< 4 lesions, none > 5 cm diameter, no lesions in cosmetically sensitive area, no lesions over joints) Otherwise, consider Moderate Disease			

* For source of drug, see Table 13D, page 165.

TABLE 13A (3)

INFECTING ORGANISM	SUGGESTED REGIMENS		COMMENTS
	PRIMARY	ALTERNATIVE	
PROTOZOA—EXTRAINTESTINAL (continued)			
Leishmaniasis, Mucosal (Espundia). All cutaneous lesions due to L. braziliensis. High cure rate with Lipo Ampho B (Trans R Soc Trop Med Hyg 108:176, 2014).	**Pentavalent antimony (Sb)*** 20 mg/kg/day IV or IM x 28 days or use of **liposomal amphotericin B** (regimens vary) or **amphotericin B** 0.5-1 mg/kg IV daily or qod to total dose of 20-40 mg/kg. See J Am Acad Dermatol 68:284, 2013.	**Miltefosine*** (w/food) 50 mg po bid (wt 30-44 kg); 50 mg po tid (wt ≥ 45 kg). Treat for 28 days. Complete resolution in 62% of pts.	Antimony available from CDC drug service; miltefosine FDA approved for leishmania in 2014 but not marketed in US at present. See Table 13D for contact information.
Visceral leishmaniasis – Kala-Azar – New World & Old World. L. donovani: India, Africa. L. infantum: Mediterranean. L. chagasi: New World	Immunocompetent: **Liposomal ampho B** 3 mg/kg once daily days 1-5 & days 14, 21 or **Miltefosine** (w/food) 50 mg po bid (wt 30-44 kg); 50 mg po tid (wt ≥ 45 kg). Treat for 28 days. HIV/AIDS: **Liposomal Ampho B** 4 mg/kg qd on days 1-5, 10, 17, 24, 31, 38 (Curr Opin Infect Dis 26:1, 2013).	**Standard Ampho B** 1 mg/kg IV daily x 15-20 days or qod x 8 wks (to total of 15-20 mg/kg) or **Miltefosine** (w/food) 50 mg po bid (wt 30-44 kg); 50 mg po tid (wt ≥ 45 kg). Treat for 28 days. HIV/AIDS: **Liposomal Ampho B** 4 mg/kg qd on days 1-5, 10, 17, 24, 31, 38 (Curr Opin Infect Dis 26:1, 2013), OR **pentavalent antimony** 20 mg/kg/day IV/IM x 28 days.	In HIV patients, may need lifelong suppression with Amphotericin B q 2-4 wks
Malaria (Plasmodia species) —NOTE: CDC Malaria info— prophylaxis/treatment (770) 488-7788. After hours: 770-488-7100. US toll-free 1-855-856-4713. CDC offers species confirmation and drug resistance testing. Refs: JAMA 297:2251, 2264 & 2285, 2007. Websites: www.cdc.gov/malaria; http://www.who.int/ith/ITH_chapter_/_pdf/ua—1 Review of rapid diagnostic tests: CID 54:1637, 2012. Prophylaxis—Drugs plus personal protection: screens, nets, 30-35% DEET skin repellent (avoid > 50% DEET) (Med Lett 54:75, 2012), permethrin spray on clothing and mosquito nets. Country risk in CDC Yellow Book.			
For areas free of chloroquine (CQ-resistant) P. falciparum. Central America (west of Panama Canal), Caribbean, Korea, Middle East (most)	**CQ** phosphate 500 mg (300 mg base) po per wk 1x/wk up to 300 mg (5 mg/kg of base) po 1x/wk up to 300 mg (5 mg/kg of base) po starting 1-2 wks before travel, during travel, & 4 wks post-travel or **atovaquone-proguanil (AP)** 1 adult tab po q day (1 day prior to, during, & 7 days post-travel). Another option for P. vivax only countries: **primaquine (PQ)** 30 mg base po daily in non-pregnant, G6PD-normal travelers'; >92% effective vs P. vivax (CID 33:1990, 2001). Note: **CQ** may exacerbate psoriasis.	**CQ Peds dose:** 8.3 mg/kg (5 mg/kg of base) po 1x/wk up to 300 mg. Adult dose of AP (peds tabs): 11-20 kg, 1 tab; 21-30 kg, 2 tabs; 31-40 kg, 3 tabs; >40 kg, 1 adult tab per day. **Adults:** Doxy or MQ as below.	CQ safe during pregnancy. **The areas free of CQ-resistant falciparum malaria continue to shrink.** See CDC or WHO maps for most current information on CQ resistance. **Doxy AEs:** photosensitivity, candida vaginitis, gastritis.
For areas with CQ-resistant P. falciparum	**Atovaquone 250 mg—proguanil 100 mg (Malarone)** comb. tablet, 1 per day with food 1-2 days prior to, during, & 7 days post-travel. Malarone preferred for trips of a week or less; expense may preclude use for longer trips. Native population: intermittent pregnancy prophylaxis/treatment programs in a few countries. Fansidar 1 tab po 3 times during pregnancy (Expert Rev Anti Infect Ther 8:569, 2010).	**Doxycycline** 100 mg po daily for adults & children > 8 yrs of age.' Take 1-2 days before, during, & for 4 wks after travel. **OR Mefloquine (MQ)** 250 mg (228 mg base) po once per wk, 1-2 wks before, during, & 4 wks after travel. Peds dose in footnote' **Doxy AEs:** photosensitivity, candida vaginitis, gastritis.	**Pregnancy: MQ** current best option. Insufficient data with **Malarone.** Avoid **Doxycycline** and primaquine. **Primaquine: Can cause hemolytic anemia if G6PD deficiency present. MQ not recommended** if cardiac conduction abnormalities, seizures, or psychiatric disorders, e.g., depression, psychosis. MQ outside U.S. 275 mg tab, contains 250 mg of base. If used, can start 3 wks before travel to assure tolerability.

¹ **Peds prophylaxis dosages:** Mefloquine weekly dose by **weight** in kg: <9 kg = 5 mg/kg weekly dose by weight; 10-19 kg = ¼ adult tab weekly; 20-30 kg = ½ adult tab weekly; 31-45 kg = ¾ adult tab weekly; >45 kg = 1 tab weekly. **Atovaquone/proguanil** by **weight** in kg, single daily dose using peds tabs (62.5 mg atovaquone & 25 mg proguanil): 5-8 kg, 1/2 tab; 8-10 kg, 3/4 tab; 11-20 kg, 1 tab; 21-30 kg, 2 tabs; 31-40 kg, 3 tabs; ≥41 kg, one adult tab. **Doxycycline,** ages >8-12 yrs: 2 mg per kg per day up to 100 mg/day. Continue daily x 4 wks after leaving risk area.

* For source of drug, see Table 13D, page 165.

TABLE 13A (4)

INFECTING ORGANISM		SUGGESTED REGIMENS		COMMENTS
	PRIMARY		ALTERNATIVE	

PROTOZOA—EXTRAINTESTINAL/Malaria (Plasmodia species) *(continued)*

Treatment of Malaria. Diagnosis is by microscopy. Alternative: rapid antigen detection test (Binax NOW); detects 96-100% of P. falciparum and 50% of other plasmodia *(CID 49:908, 2009; CID 54:1637, 2012).* Need microscopy to speciate. Can stay positive for over a month after successful treatment.

Clinical Severity/ Plasmodia sp.		Suggested Treatment Regimens (Drug)		
	Region Acquired	Adults	Peds	Comments
Uncomplicated/ P. falciparum (or species not identified) 2015 WHO Guidelines suggest artemisinin combination therapy for adults (except in pregnancy) for all malaria species. E.g. Artemether- lumefantrine.	Cen. Amer., west of Panama Canal; Haiti, Dom. Repub., & most of Mid-East **CQ-sensitive**	**CQ phosphate** 1 gm salt (600 mg base) po, then 0.5 gm in 6 hrs, then 0.5 gm daily x 2 days. Total: 2500 mg salt	**Peds: CQ** 10 mg/kg of base po; then 5 mg/kg of base at 6, 24, & 48 hrs. Total: 25 mg/kg base	Other chloroquine salts available in some countries, total dose may differ. **Peds dose should never exceed adult dose. CQ + MQ prolong QTc. Doses > 2x recommended may be fatal.**
	CQ-resistant or unknown resistance. Note: If >5% parasitemia or Hb <7, treat as severe malaria regardless of clinical findings or lack thereof.	**Adults: Atovaquone-proguanil** 1 gm—400 mg (4 adult tabs) po 1x/day x 3 days w/food **OR [QS** 650 mg po tid x 3 days (7 days if SE Asia)] + **[Doxy** 100 mg po bid) or (**tetra** 250 mg po qid)] x 7 days] **OR Artemether-lumefantrine** tabs 20/120 mg. 4 tabs po (at 0, 8 hrs) then bid x 2 days (total 6 doses); take with food **OR** a less desirable adult alternative, **mefloquine** 750 mg po x 1 dose, then 500 mg po x 1 dose 6-12 hr later. **MQ** is 2nd line alternative due to neuropsychiatric reaction and cannot use in SE Asia due to resistance. Clinda or tetracycline only if doxy not available.	**Peds: (QS** 10 mg/kg po tid x 3 days) —both x7 days. Use doxy >8 yrs of age 2.2 mg/kg/ bid up to 100 mg per dose OR **Atovaquone-proguanil** (all once daily x 3 d) by weight: 5-8 kg; 2 peds tabs; 9-10 kg; 3 peds tabs, 11-20 kg; 1 adult tab; 21-30 kg; 2 adult tabs; 31-40 kg; 3 adult tabs; >40 kg 4 adult tabs OR **MQ Salt:** 15 mg/kg x 1, then 6-12 hrs later, 10 mg/kg ALL po. OR **Artemether-lumefantrine** • 5 kg to < 15 kg: 1 tablet (20 mg/ 120 mg) as a single dose, then 1 tablet again after 8 hours, then 1 tablet every 12 hours for 2 days • 15 kg to < 25 kg: 2 tablets (40 mg/ 240 mg) as a single dose, then 2 tablets again after 8 hours, then 2 tablets every 12 hours for 2 days • 25 kg to < 35 kg: 3 tablets (60 mg/ 360 mg) as a single dose, then 3 tablets again after 8 hours, then 3 tablets every 12 hours for 2 days • ≥35 kg: as per adult dose	**Pregnancy:** • Artemether-lumefantrine 4 tablets (80 mg/480 mg) as a single dose, then 4 tablets again after 8 hours, then 4 tablets every 12 hours for 2 days (take with food). Drug of choice in 2nd/3rd trimester. Artemether-lumefantrine is safer than quinine in the first trimester of pregnancy. *Malar J. 13:197, 2014* OR • Quinine sulfate 10 mg/kg po tid x 3 days (7 days if SE Asia)) + Clindamycin 20 mg/kg/day divided tid x 7 days • Do not delay therapy if quinine available and artemether-lumefantrine is not in U.S. QS is only available as quinine 324 mg capsule, thus hard to use to treat children. **Note: Oral Artemether-lumefantrine tabs FDA-approved but not widely stocked. Call 1-800-COARTEM to obtain.** Wt-based dose of Artesunate IV in children: Wt < 20 kg: 3 mg/kg; Wt > 20 kg: 2.4 mg/kg.
Uncomplicated / P. malariae or P. knowlesi *(JID 199: 1107 & 1143, 2009).*	All regions – **CQ-sensitive**	**CQ** as above. Adults & peds. In South Pacific, beware of P. knowlesi: looks like P. malariae, but behaves like P. falciparum *(CID 46:165, 2007).*	**Artemether-lumefantrine** (20/120 mg tab) 4 tabs po x 1 dose, repeat in 8 hrs, then repeat q12h x 2 days (take with food) OR **Atovaquone-proguanil** (1000/400 mg) 4 adult tabs po daily x 3 days	

* For source of drug, see *Table 13D, page 165.*

TABLE 13A (5)

PROTOZOA—EXTRAINTESTINAL/Malaria (Plasmodia species)/Treatment of Malaria (continued)

INFECTING ORGANISM		SUGGESTED REGIMENS		COMMENTS
		PRIMARY	ALTERNATIVE	
Clinical Severity/ Plasmodia sp.	Region Acquired	Suggested Treatment Regimens (Drug)		Comments
		Adults	Peds	
Uncomplicated/ P. vivax or P. ovale	CQ-sensitive (except Papua New Guinea, Indonesia which are CQ-resistant-see below)	CQ as above + PQ base: 30 mg po once daily x 14 days. Each primaquine phosphate tab is 26.3 mg of salt and 15 mg of base. 30 mg of base = 2 26.3 mg tabs prim. phos.	CQ as above + PQ base 0.5 mg po once daily x 14 days	PQ added to eradicate latent parasites in liver. **Screen for G6PD def. before starting PQ;** if G6PD deficient dose PQ as 45 mg once weekly x 8 wks. **Note: rare severe reactions.** Avoid PQ in pregnancy. If P. vivax or P. ovale, after pregnancy check for G6PD deficiency & give PQ 30 mg po daily times14 days.
Uncomplicated/ P. vivax	**CQ-resistant:** Papua, New Guinea & Indonesia	**[QS + (doxy or tetra) + PQ]** as above or **Artemether-Lumefantrine** (same dose as for P. falciparum)	**MQ + PQ** as above **Peds** (<8 yrs old) **QS** alone x 7 days or **MQ** alone. If latter fail, add **doxy** or **tetra**	Rarely acute. Lung injury and other serious complications: LnID 8:449, 2008.

Clinical Severity/ Plasmodia sp.	Region Acquired	Suggested Treatment Regimens (Drug)		Comments
		Primary—Adults	Alternative & Peds	
Uncomplicated Malaria/Alternatives for Pregnancy Ref: LnID 7:118 & 136, 2007	CQ-sensitive areas ----- CQ-resistant P. falciparum ----- CQ-resistant P. vivax intermittent pregnancy treatment (empiric)	**CQ** as above ----- **QS + clinda** ----- **QS** 650 mg po tid x 7 days ----- Give treatment dose of [Sulfadoxine 500 mg + Pyrimethamine 25 mg (Fansidar) po] at 3 times during pregnancy to decrease material & fetal morbidity & mortality	If failing or intolerant: **QS + doxy**	Doxy or tetra used if benefits outweigh risks. No controlled studies of AP in pregnancy. If P. vivax or P. ovale, after pregnancy check for G6PD deficiency & give PQ 30 mg po daily times 14 days.
Severe malaria, i.e., impaired consciousness, severe anemia, renal failure, pulmonary edema, ARDS, DIC, jaundice, acidosis, seizures, parasitemia >5%. One or more of latter **Almost always P. falciparum.** Ref: NEJM 358:1829, 2008; Science 320:30, 2008.	All regions Note: •IV Artesunate is drug of choice but not FDA-approved. Available from CDC Drug Service under specific conditions, need to state quinidine not available or not tolerated. •IV quinidine uncommonly available. Possible emergency availability from Eli Lilly.	**Quinidine gluconate** in normal saline 10 mg/kg (salt) IV over 1 hr then 0.02 mg/kg/min by constant infusion OR 24 mg/kg IV over 4 hrs & then 12 mg/kg over 4 hrs q8h. Continue until parasite density <1% & can take po. **QS** 650 mg po tid x 3 days (7 days if SE Asia) + (**Doxy** 100 mg IV q12h x 7 days) OR (**Doxy** 100 mg IV q12h) **Artesunate** "2.4 mg/kg IV at 0, 12, 24, 48 hrs, and Doxy 100 mg IV q12h x 7 days")	**Peds: Quinidine gluconate IV**—same mg/kg dose as for adults **PLUS** (**Doxy:** if <45 kg, 4 mg per kg IV q12h; ≥45 kg, dose as for adults) OR **Clinda, Clindamycin** 10 mg/kg IV loading dose, then 5 mg/kg IV q8h (as tolerated) q8h x 7 days. **Follow IV artesunate with a complete oral course of one of:** **Doxycycline, Atovaquone/proguanil, Artemether/lumefantrine,** or **Dihydroartemisinin/piperaquine (not available in US)**	During quinidine IV, monitor BP, EKG (prolongation of QTc), & blood glucose (hypoglycemia). Exchange transfusion no longer recommended. Switch to QS po + (Doxy or Clinda) when patient able to take oral meds. **Steroids not recommended for cerebral malaria.** IV artesunate from CDC (8 hr transport time post-approval), see Table 13D (Ref: CID 44:1067 & 1075, 2007). Can cause motile threatening, but transfusion requiring, hemolytic anemia up to 15 days post-therapy (AnIM 163:498, 2015).

* For source of drug, see Table 13D, page 165

TABLE 13A (6)

INFECTING ORGANISM	SUGGESTED REGIMENS		COMMENTS
	PRIMARY	ALTERNATIVE	
PROTOZOA—EXTRAINTESTINAL/Malaria (Plasmodia species) Treatment of Malaria (continued)			
Malaria—self-initiated treatment: Only for people at risk who do not have ready access to medical care and when professional medical care is not available within 24 hrs. Give a reliable supply of Coartem for self-administered treatment (to avoid counterfeit meds). Use only if travel is lab-diagnosed and no available reliable meds	**Artemether-lumefantrine** (20/120 mg tab) 4 tabs po (take with food). OR **Atovaquone-proguanil (AP)**	**Peds:** Using adult AP tabs for 3 consecutive days: Peds tabs 62.5 mg/25 mg, 5-8 kg: 2 tabs, 9-10 kg: 3 tabs, 11-20 kg: 1 adult tab, 21-30 kg: 2 adult tabs, 31-40 kg: 3 adult tabs, >40 kg: 4 adult tabs. For Peds dosing of Artemether-lumefantrine, see *Uncomplicated* P. falciparum, page 154.	Do not use for renal insufficiency pts. Do not use if weight <11 kg, pregnant, or breast-feeding. **Artemether** same caution as Malarone (EU) and Coartem (US & elsewhere).
Toxoplasma gondii (Reference: Ln 363:1965, 2004)			
Immunologically normal patients (For pediatric doses, see reference)			
Acute illness w/ lymphadenopathy. Acq via transfusion or lab accident	No specific rx unless severe/persistent symptoms or evidence of vital organ damage		
Active chorioretinitis: meningitis; lowered resistance due to steroids or cytotoxic drugs	Treat as for active chorioretinitis		For congenital Toxo, Toxo meningitis in adults, & chorioretinitis, **add prednisone 1 mg/kg/day in 2 div. doses** until CSF protein conc. falls or vision-threatening inflammation subsides.
Acute in pregnant women. Ref: CID 47:554, 2008	**Pyrimethamine** (pyri) 200 mg po once on 1st day, then 50-75 mg/day 1-1.5 gm po qid) + **leucovorin (folinic acid)** 5-20 mg 3x/wk) + **sulfadiazine** (see footnote[2]) 5-20 mg 3x/wk)—see Comment. Treat 1-2 wks beyond resolution of signs/symptoms; continue leucovorin 1 wk after stopping pyri.		Adjust folinic acid dose by following CBC results. Screen patients with IgG/IgM serology at commercial lab. IgG+/IgM neg = remote past infection; IgG+/IgM+ = serology positive. For Spiramycin, consult with Palo Alto Medical Foundation Toxoplasma Serology Lab: 650-853-4828 or toxlab@pamf.org. Details in Ln 363:1965, 2004. **Consultation advisable.**
Fetal/congenital	**if <18 wks gestation at diagnosis:** Spiramycin 1 gm po q8h until amniotic fluid PCR is negative. Positive PCR treat as below. **if >18 wks gestation & documented fetal infection (positive amniotic fluid PCR): Pyrimethamine** 75 mg/kg po x 1 dose, then 50 mg/kg q12h (max 50 mg po q12h x 2 days, then 50 mg/day + **sulfadiazine** 4 gm/day) + **folinic acid** 10-20 mg po daily for minimum of 4 wks or for duration of pregnancy		
	Mgmt complex. Combo rx with pyrimethamine + sulfadiazine + leucovorin—see Comment		
AIDS			
Cerebral toxoplasmosis Ref: MMWR 58/RR-4:1, 2009	[**Pyrimethamine** (pyri) 200 mg x 1 po, then 75 mg/day po] + **sulfadiazine** (Wt based dose: 1 gm if <60 kg, 1.5 gm if ≥60 kg) po q6h) + **(folinic acid** 10-25 mg/day po) for minimum of 6 wks after resolution of signs/ symptoms, and then suppression rx (see below) OR **TMP-SMX** (TMP-SMX-DS 1 tab po q24h or 3x/wk) OR (**TMP-SMX-SS** 1 tab po q24h)	[**Pyri + folinic acid** (as in primary regimen)] + the following alternatives: **Clinda** 600 mg po/IV q6h or (2) **TMP-SMX** 5/25 mg/kg/day po or IV q12h or (3) **atovaquone** 750 mg po q6h. Treat 4-6 wks after resolution of signs/symptoms, then suppression.	Use alternative regimen for pts with severe sulfa allergy. If multiple ring-enhancing lesions (CT or MRI), >85% of pts respond to 7-10 days of empiric rx. Pyri penetrates brain even if no inflammation; folinic acid prevents pyri-related hematologic toxicity. Consult MMWR 58/RR-4:1, 2009. **Another alternative:** (Dapsone 200 mg/day + pyri 75 mg po q24h + folinic acid 25 mg po q24h) once weekly.
Primary prophylaxis AIDS pts—IgG Toxo antibody + CD4 count <100 per mcL	**TMP-SMX-DS**, 1 tab po q24h. OR **(folinic acid** 25 mg po q24h or 3x/wk) OR **atovaquone** 1500 mg	**(Dapsone** 50 mg po q24h) + [**pyri** 50 mg q wk) + (**folinic acid** 25 mg po q wk.)] OR **atovaquone** 1500 mg	(Pyri + sulfa) prevents PCP and Toxo. (Pyri + dapsone) also effective vs Toxo. Ref: MMWR 58/RR-4:1, 2009. Atovaquone active vs Toxo and PCP.
Suppression after rx of cerebral Toxo	[**Sulfadiazine** 2-4 gm po divided in 2-4 doses/day) + **pyri** 25-50 mg po q24h) + **folinic acid** 10-25 mg po q24h]. DC if CD4 count >200 x 3 mos	[**Clinda** 600 mg po q8h) + (**pyri** 25-50 mg po q24h) + (**folinic acid** 10-25 mg po q24h)] OR **atovaquone** 750 mg po q6-12h po	Alternative to Toxo only. Additional drug needed to prevent PCP.
Trichomonas vaginalis	See Vaginitis, Table 1, page 26		

---

[2] Sulfonamides for Toxo. Sulfadiazine now commercially available. Sulfisoxazole much less effective.

* For source of drug, see *Table 13D, page 165.*

TABLE 13A (7)

INFECTING ORGANISM	SUGGESTED REGIMENS		COMMENTS
	PRIMARY	ALTERNATIVE	
PROTOZOA—EXTRAINTESTINAL/Toxoplasma gondii/AIDS (continued)			
Trypanosomiasis. Ref.: Ln 362:1469, 2003. **Note: Drugs for African trypanosomiasis may be obtained free from WHO or CDC. See Table 13D, page 165, for source information.**			
West African sleeping sickness (T. brucei gambiense)			
Early: Blood/lymphatic—CNS OK	Pentamidine 4 mg/kg IV/IM daily x 7-10 days	In US, free from CDC drug service **Suramin** * 100 mg IV (test dose); then 1 gm IV on days 1, 3, 7, 14, & 21. Peds dose is 20 mg/kg.	Suramin effective but avoid if possible due to possible co-infection with O. volvulus in W. Africa. See Table 13D, page 165, for source information.
Late: Encephalitis	**Combination of IV eflornithine** 400 mg/kg/day IV divided q12h x 7 days, plus **nifurtimox** 15 mg/kg/day po, divided q6h x 10 days (abbreviated NECT) now WHO standard of care (Lancet 374:56, 2009, CID 56:195 2013)	Melarsoprol 2.2 mg/kg/day IV x 10 days; toxic arsenical now superseded by NECT	
East African sleeping sickness (T. brucei rhodesiense)			
Early: Blood/lymphatic	**Suramin** * 100 mg IV (test dose), then 1 gm IV on days 1, 3, 7, 14, & 21	Peds: Suramin * 2 mg/kg test dose, then 20 mg/kg IV on days 1, 3, 7, 14 & 21.	Suramin & Melarsoprol: CDC Drug Service or WHO (at no charge) (see Table 13D).
Late: Encephalitis (prednisolone may prevent encephalitis) Pre-treatment with Suramin advised by some.	**Melarsoprol** 2.2 mg/kg/day IV x 10 days (PLoS NTD 6:e1695, 2012)	**Melarsoprol** (from 2-3 schedules) per day IV over 3 days; repeat 3.6 mg/kg after 7 days & for 3rd time at 3.6 mg/kg 7 days after 2nd course	If Suramin resistant or toxic, use pentamidine 4 mg/kg/day IV/IM x 1-2 doses. Does not enter CSF.
T. cruzi—**Chagas disease** or acute American trypanosomiasis Ref: NEJM 373:456, 2015. For chronic disease: no benefit in established cardiopathy (NEJM 373:1295, 2015)	Adult (Age ≥12 years): **Benznidazole** 5-7 mg/kg/day in 2 doses (q12h) x 60 days Pediatric (Age <12 years): **Benznidazole** 7.5 mg/kg/day in 2 doses (q12h) x 60 days	**Nifurtimox** 8-10 mg/kg po per day div 4x/day after meals x 120 days Ages 11-16 yrs: 12.5-15 mg/kg per day div. qid po x 90 days Children <11yrs: 15-20 mg/kg/day qid po x 90 days	Due to adverse effects may give Benznidazole 300 mg per day for 60 days, regardless of body weight OR give 300 mg per day but prolong treatment to complete the total dose corresponding to 5 mg/kg per day for 60 days. N Engl J Med 373:456, 2015. Immunosuppression of heart transplant can reactivate chronic Chagas disease. Can transmit by organ/transfusions. Do not use benznidazole in pregnancy.
NEMATODES—INTESTINAL (Roundworms) Ascaris simplex (**anisakiasis**) Anisakiasis differentiated from Anisakidosis (CID 51:806, 2010). Other A. physalary Pseudoterranova decipiens	Physical removal by endoscope or surgery Anecdotal report of apparent benefit from Albendazole 400 mg po bid x 21 days No antimicrobial therapy.	Think Strongyloides, toxocaria and filariasis: CID 34:407, 2006; 42:1781 & 1655, 2006— See Table 13C. Anecdotal report of possible benefit from Albendazole (Ln 360:54, 2002; CID 41:1825, 2005)	
Ascaris lumbricoides (**ascariasis**) Ln 367:1521, 2006	**Albendazole** 400 mg po daily x 3 days or **mebendazole** 100 mg po bid x 3 days	**Ivermectin** 150-200 mcg/kg po x 1 dose	Review of efficacy of single dose: JAMA 299:1937, 2008
Capillaria philippinensis (**capillariasis**)	**Albendazole** 400 mg po bid x 10 days	**Mebendazole** 200 mg po bid x 20 days	Albendazole preferred
Enterobius vermicularis (**pinworm**)	**Mebendazole** 100 mg po x 1, repeat in 2 wks OR **Pyrantel pamoate** 11 mg/kg base (to max. dose of 1 gm) po x 1 dose, repeat in 2 wks	**Albendazole** 400 mg po x 1 dose, repeat in 2 wks.	Side-effects in Table 13B, page 164. Treat whole household
Gongylonemiasis (adult worms in oral mucosa)	Surgical removal		
Hookworm (Necator americanus and Ancylostoma duodenale)	**Albendazole** 400 mg po daily x 3 days	**Mebendazole** 100 mg po bid x 3 days OR **Pyrantel pamoate** 11 mg/kg po daily x 3 days	NOTE: Ivermectin not effective. Single dose therapy as used in public health programs has lower cure rates and 3-day regimen superior to 3-day Mebendazole. PLoS One 6:e25003, 2011
Strongyloides stercoralis (**strongyloidiasis**) (Hyperinfection, See Comment)	**Ivermectin** 200 mcg/kg po per day x 2 days	**Albendazole** 400 mg po bid x 7 days - less effective	**For hyperinfections,** repeat in 15 days. For hyperinfection, veterinary ivermectin given subcutaneously or rectally (CID 49:1411, 2009).

* For source of drug, see Table 13D, page 165.

TABLE 13A (8)

INFECTING ORGANISM	SUGGESTED REGIMENS		COMMENTS
	PRIMARY	ALTERNATIVE	
NEMATODES—INTESTINAL (Roundworms) _(continued)_			
Trichostrongylus orientalis, T. colubriformis	**Pyrantel pamoate** 11 mg/kg (max. 1 gm) po x 1	**Albendazole** 400 mg po x 1 dose	**Mebendazole** 100 mg bid x 3 days
Trichuris trichiura (whipworm) _NEJM 376:610, 2014; PLoS One 6:e25003 2011_	**Mebendazole** 100 mg po bid x 3 days	**Albendazole** 400 mg po qd x 3 days or **ivermectin** 200 mcg/kg po qd x 3 days	**Mebendazole** clearly superior for trichuris _(PLoS One 6:e25003, 2011; N Engl J Med 370:610, 2014)_
NEMATODES—EXTRAINTESTINAL (Roundworms)			
Ancylostoma braziliense & caninum: causes **cutaneous larva migrans**	**Albendazole** 400 mg po bid x 3-7 days _(Ln ID 8:302, 2008)._	**Ivermectin** 200 mcg/kg po x 1 dose/day x 1-2 days (not in children wt < 15 kg)	Also called "creeping eruption"; dog and cat hookworm. Ivermectin cure rate 81-100% (1 dose) to 97% (2-3 doses) _(CID 31:493, 2000)._
Angiostrongylus cantonensis (**Angiostrongyliasis**); causes eosinophilic meningitis	Mild/moderate disease: Analgesics, serial LPs (if necessary). Prednisone 60 mg/day x 14 days reduces headache & need for LPs.	Adding **Albendazole** 15 mg/kg/day po to prednisone 60 mg/day both for 14 days may reduce duration of headaches and need for repeat LPs.	**Do not use Albendazole without prednisone,** see _TRSMH 102:990, 2008._ Gnathostoma and Baylisascaris also cause eosinophilic meningitis.
Baylisascariasis (Raccoon roundworm); eosinophilic meningitis	No drug proven efficacious. Try **albendazole**, Peds: 25-50 mg/kg po, Adults: 400 mg po with corticosteroids. Treat for one month.		_Clin Microbiol Rev 18:703, 2005._ Other causes of eosinophilic meningitis: Gnathostoma & Angiostrongylus
Dracunculus medinensis: **Guinea worm** _[trans R Soc Trop Med Hyg 108:249, 2014]_	Slow extraction of pre-emergent worm over several days	No drug effective. Oral analgesics, anti-inflammatory drugs, topical antiseptics/antibiotic ointments to alleviate symptoms and facilitate worm removal by gentle manual traction over several days.	
Filariasis: Determine if co-infection with either Loa loa or Onchocerca			
Lymphatic filariasis (Elephantiasis) Etiologies: Wuchereria bancrofti, Brugia malayi, Brugia timori	_Mono-infection:_ **Diethylcarbamazine**"(**DEC**)* 6 mg/kg/day po in 3 divided doses x 12 days + **Doxy** 200 mg/day po x 6 wks	_Dual infection with Onchocerca:_ Treat Onchocerciasis first, then **DEC** as for mono-infection. _Dual infection with Loa Loa:_ DEC drug of choice for both but can cause severe encephalopathy if >5000 Loa microfilaria/mL in blood. Refer to expert center for apheresis pre-DEC or prednisone + small doses of DEC. If <5000 microfilaria/mL, start regular dose of **DEC.**	Doxy x 6 wks may improve mild/moderate lymphedema & kill adult worm (macrofilaricidal) independent of parasite infection _(CID 55:621, 2012)._ **Note: DEC can cause irreversible eye damage if concomitant Onchocerciasis.**
Loiasis Loa loa, eye worm disease. **Look for dual infection with either Onchocerciasis or Lymphatic filariasis**	_Mono-infection with <5000 L. loa microfilaria/mL:_ **DEC** 8-10 mg/kg/day po x 21 days _Mono-infection with >5000 L. loa microfilaria/mL:_ Refer to expert center for apheresis prior to DEC therapy; alternatively, **Albendazole** 200 mg bid x 21 days	_Dual infection with Lymphatic filariasis:_ See Lymphatic filariasis, above _Dual infection with Onchocerciasis:_ Treat Onchocerciasis first with **ivermectin**, then treat L. loa with **DEC**	If >5000 L. loa microfilaria/mL in blood & given ivermectin for Onchocerciasis, can facilitate entry of L. loa into CNS with severe encephalopathy.
Onchocerca volvulus (Onchocerciasis), river blindness. **Look for dual infection with either Loa loa or Lymphatic filariasis**	_Mono-infection:_ **Ivermectin** 150 mcg/kg x 1 dose, then repeat every 3-6 months until asymptomatic + **Doxy** 200 mg/day x 6 wks. No accepted alternative therapy.	_Dual infection with Lymphatic filariasis:_ See Lymphatic filariasis, above _Dual infection with L. loa:_ Treat Onchocerciasis first with **ivermectin**, then treat L. loa with **DEC.** If >5000 L. loa microfilaria/mL in blood. Refer to expert center for apheresis before starting DEC	Onchocerciasis and Loa loa are mildly co-endemic in West and Central Africa.

ª May need antihistamine or corticosteroid for allergic reaction from disintegrating organisms
* For source of drug, see Table 13D, page 165.

TABLE 13A (9)

INFECTING ORGANISM	SUGGESTED REGIMENS		COMMENTS
	PRIMARY	ALTERNATIVE	
NEMATODES—EXTRAINTESTINAL (Roundworms)/Filariasis *(continued)*			
Mansonella perstans	In randomized trial, doxy 200 mg po once daily x 6 weeks cleared microfilaria from blood in 67 of 69 patients *(NEJM 361:1448, 2009).*	**Albendazole** in high dose x 3 weeks.	Efficacy of doxy believed to be due to inhibition of endosymbiont *wolbachia*. Ivermectin has no activity. Ref: *Trans R Soc Trop Med Hyg 100:458, 2006.*
Mansonella streptocerca	**Ivermectin** 150 μg/kg x 1 dose.		May need antihistamine or corticosteroid for allergic reaction from disintegrating organisms. Chronic pruritic hypopigmented lesions that may be confused with leprosy. Can be asymptomatic.
Mansonella ozzardi	**Ivermectin** 200 μg/kg x 1 dose may be effective. Limited data but no other option. *Am J Trop Med Hyg 90:1170, 2014*		Usually asymptomatic. Articular pain, pruritus, lymphadenopathy reported. May have allergic reaction from dying organisms.
Dirofilariasis: Heartworm			
D. immitis, dog heartworm	No effective drugs; surgical removal only option		Can lodge in pulmonary artery → coin lesion. *Eosinophilia rare.*
D. tenuis (raccoon), D. ursi (bear), D. repens (dogs, cats)	No effective drugs		Worms migrate to conjunctivae, subcutaneous tissue, scrotum, breasts, extremities. D. repens emerging throughout Europe *Clin Microbiol Rev 25:507, 2012*
Gnathostoma spinigerum			
Cutaneous larva migrans	**Albendazole** 400 mg po q24h or bid times 21 days	**Ivermectin** 200 μg/kg/day po x 2 days.	Other etiology of larva migrans: *Ancylostoma sp, see page 158*
Eosinophilic meningitis	Supportive care: monitor for cerebral hemorrhage	Case reports of steroid use: both benefit and harm from Albendazole or ivermectin *(EIN 17:1174, 2011).*	Other causes of eosinophilic meningitis: *Angiostrongylus (see page 158)* & *Baylisascaris (see page 158)*
Toxocariasis *(Ann Trop Med Parasit 103:3, 2010)*	**Rx directed at relief of symptoms as infection self-limited, e.g., steroids & antihistamines; use of anthelmintics controversial.**		
Visceral larval migrans	**Albendazole** 400 mg po bid x 5 days ± **Prednisone** 60 mg/day	**Mebendazole** 100–200 mg po bid times 5 days	Severe lung, heart or CNS disease may warrant steroids *(Clin Micro Rev 16:265, 2003).* Differential dx of larval migrans syndromes: *Toxocara canis & catis, Ancylostoma spp, Gnathostoma spp., Spirometra spp.* No added benefit of anthelmintic drugs. Rx of little effect after 4 wks. Some use steroids *Clin Microbiol Rev 16:265, 2003).*
Ocular larval migrans	First 4 wks of illness: (Oral **prednisone** 30–60 mg po q24h + subtenon **triamcinolone** 40 mg/wk) x 2 wks (Surgery is sometimes necessary) Concomitant **prednisone** 40–60 mg po q24h		
Trichinella spiralis (**Trichinellosis**) — muscle infection *(Review: Clin Micro Rev 22:127, 2009).*	**Albendazole** 400 mg po bid x 8–14 days	**Mebendazole** 200–400 mg po tid x 3 days, then 400–500 mg po tid x 10 days	Use albendazole/mebendazole with caution during pregnancy (1 IgG, 1 CPK, ESR 0, massive eosinophilia: >5000/μL.
TREMATODES (Flukes) – Liver, Lung, Intestinal. All flukes have snail intermediate hosts; transmitted by ingestion of metacercariae on plants, fish or crustaceans.			
Liver flukes: Clonorchis sinensis, Metorchis conjunctus, Colsthorchis viverrini	**Praziquantel** 25 mg/kg po tid x 2 days	**Albendazole** 10 mg/kg per day po x 7 days	Same dose in children
Fasciola hepatica (sheep liver fluke), Fasciola gigantica	**Triclabendazole** once, may repeat after 12-24 hrs. 10 mg/kg x 1 dose. Single 20 mg/kg po dose effective in treatment failures.		
Intestinal flukes: Fasciola buski, Heterophyes heterophyes, Metagonimus yokogawai, Nanophyetus salmincola	**Praziquantel** 25 mg/kg po tid x 1 days		Same dose in children

* For source of drug, see Table 13D, page 165.

TABLE 13A (10)

INFECTING ORGANISM	SUGGESTED REGIMENS		COMMENTS
	PRIMARY	ALTERNATIVE	
TREMATODES (Flukes) – Liver, Lung, Intestinal *(continued)*			
Lung fluke: Paragonimus sp.	**Praziquantel** 25 mg/kg po tid x 2 days	**Triclabendazole*** 10 mg/kg po x 2 doses over 12-24 hrs.	Same dose in children
Schistosoma haematobium, GU bilharziasis,	**Praziquantel** 40 mg/kg po on the same day (one dose of 40 mg/kg or two doses of 20 mg/kg).		Same dose in children
Schistosoma mansoni	**Praziquantel** 20 mg/kg po on the same day in 1 or 2 doses		Same dose in children
Schistosoma japonicum, Oriental schisto	**Praziquantel** 60 mg/kg po on the same day (3 doses of 20 mg/kg)		Same dose in children. Cures 60-90% pts
Schistosoma mansoni (intestinal bilharziasis)	**Praziquantel** 40 mg/kg po on the same day (one dose of 40 mg/kg or two doses of 20 mg/kg)		Praziquantel: Same dose for children and adults. Cures 60-90% pts. No advantage to splitting dose in 2 Cochrane Database Syst Rev, 8:CD000053, 2014
Schistosoma mekong	**Praziquantel** 60 mg/kg po on the same day (3 doses of 20 mg/kg)		Same dose for children
Toxemic schisto; Katayama fever	**Praziquantel** 20 mg/kg po bid with short course of high dose prednisone. Repeat Praziquantel in 4-6 wks after *(Clin Micro Rev 16:223, 2010).*		Reaction to onset of egg laying 4-6 wks after infection exposure in fresh water.
CESTODES (Tapeworms)			
Echinococcus granulosus (hydatid disease) *(LnID 12:871, 2012; Int Dis Clin No Amer 26:421, 2012)*	**Liver cysts:** Meta-analysis supports percutaneous aspiration-injection-reaspiration **(PAIR)** + albendazole for uncomplicated single liver cysts. Before & after drainage **albendazole** 260 mg, 400 mg bid or < 60 kg, 15 mg/kg per day div. bid. with meals. After 1-2 days puncture (P) & needle aspirate (A) cyst content. Instill 20% hypertonic saline (15-30%) or absolute alcohol. Wait 20-30 min, then re-aspirate (R) with final irrigation. **Continue albendazole for at least 30 days.** Cure in 96% as comp to 90% pts with surgical resection. Albendazole ref: *Acta Tropica 114:1, 2010.*		
Echinococcus multilocularis (alveolar cyst disease) *(COID 16:437, 2003)*	**Albendazole** efficacy not clearly demonstrated; can try in dosages noted above for hydatid disease. Wide surgical resection only reliable rx; technique evolving. Post-surgical resection or if inoperable Albendazole for several years *(Acta Tropic 114:1, 2010).*		
Intestinal tapeworms			
Diphyllobothrium latum (fish), Dipylidium caninum (dog), Taenia saginata (beef), & Taenia solium (pork)	**Praziquantel** 5-10 mg/kg po x 1 dose for children and adults.	**Niclosamide*** 2 gm po x 1 dose	Niclosamide from: Expert Compounding Pharm, see Table 13D.
Hymenolepis diminuta (rats) and H. nana (humans)	**Praziquantel** 25 mg/kg po x 1 dose for children and adults.	**Niclosamide*** 2 gm po daily x 7 days	
	NOTE: Treat concomitant T. solium intestinal tapeworms, if present, with **praziquantel** 5-10 mg/kg po x 1 dose after starting steroid.		
Neurocysticercosis (NCC): Larval form of T. solium Ref.: *AJTMH 72:3, 2005*			
Parenchymal NCC			
1-20 "viable" or degenerating cysts by CT/MRI.	**Albendazole** 15 mg/kg/d po + **Praziquantel** 50 mg/kg/d po + **dexamethasone** 0.1 mg/kg/d po. Start steroid 1 day before antiparasitics. Treat for 10 days. May need seizure meds for 1 yr.	**Albendazole** alone 800 mg per day plus **Dexamethasone** 0.1 mg/kg per day ± Anti-seizure medication). See *Comment*	Ref: *LnID 14:687, 2014.* Steroids decrease serum levels of praziquantel so shouldn't use alone without albendazole. NIH reports methotrexate at < 30 mg/wk allows a reduction in steroid use *(CID 44:449, 2007).*
Meta-analysis (treatment assoc with cyst resolution, ↓ seizures and ↓ seizure recurrence. Ref.: *Neurology 80:1424, 2013.*			
Dead calcified cysts	**No treatment indicated**		
Subarachnoid NCC	(Albendazole + **steroids** as above) + shunting for hydrocephalus prior to drug therapy. Ref: *Expert Rev Anti Infect Ther 9:123, 2011*		
Intraventricular NCC	Neuroendoscopic removal is treatment of choice with or without albendazole. If surgery not possible, **albendazole** + **dexamethasone; observe closely for evidence of obstruction of flow of CSF.**		

* For source of drug, see Table 13D, page 165

TABLE 13D (1)

INFECTING ORGANISM		SUGGESTED REGIMENS		COMMENTS
DISEASE	INFECTING ORGANISM	PRIMARY	ALTERNATIVE	

CESTODES (Tapeworms)/Neurocysticercosis (NCC) (continued)

Sparganosis (Spirometra mansonoides) — Surgical resection. No antiparasitic therapy. Can inject alcohol into subcutaneous masses.
Larval cysts, source—frogs/snakes.

ECTOPARASITES. Ref.: CID 36:1355, 2003; Ln 363:889, 2004. **NOTE: Due to potential neurotoxicity and risk of aplastic anemia, lindane not recommended.**

Head lice	Pediculus humanus, var. capitis	**Permethrin** 1% lotion: Apply to shampooed dried hair for 10 min.; repeat in 9–10 days. **OR Malathion** 0.5% lotion: Apply to dry hair for 8–12 hrs, then shampoo. 2 doses 7–9 days apart. **OR Spinosad** 0.9% suspension, wash off after 10 min (86% effective). Repeat in 7 days, if needed. Use nit comb initially & repeat in 7–10 days.	**Ivermectin** 200–400 µg/kg po once; 3 doses at 7 day intervals effective in 95% (JID 193:474, 2006). Topical ivermectin 0.5% lotion, 75% effective. **Malathion:** Report that 1–2 20-min. applications 98% effective (Ped Derm 21:670, 2004). In alcohol—potentially flammable. **Benzyl alcohol:** 76% effective	**Permethrin:** success in 78%. Resistance increasing. No advantage to 5% permethrin. **Spinosad** is effective, but expensive. Wash hats, scarves, coats & bedding in hot water, then dry in hot dryer for 20+ minutes.
Pubic lice (crabs)	Phthirus pubis	**Pubic hair: Permethrin OR malathion** as for head lice. Shave pubic hair.	**Eyelids: Petroleum jelly** applied qid x 10 days **OR yellow oide of mercury** 1% qid x 14 days	**Do not use lindane.** Treat sex partners of the last 30 days.
Body lice	Pediculus humanus, var. corporis	No drugs for the patient. Organism lives in & deposits eggs in seams of clothing. Discard clothing; if not possible, treat clothing with 1% malathion powder or 0.5% permethrin powder. Success with ivermectin in homeless shelter. 12 mg po on days 0, 7, & 14 (JID 193:474, 2006)		
Myiasis Due to larvae of flies		Usually cutaneous/subcutaneous nodule with central punctum. Treatment: Occlude punctum to prevent gas exchange with petrolatum, fingernail polish, makeup cream or bacon. When larva migrates, manually remove. Ref. Clin Microbiol Rev 25:79, 2012.		
Scabies Immunocompetent patients Refs: MMWR 59(RR-12):89, 2010; NEJM 362:717, 2010.	Sarcoptes scabiei	**Permethrin** 5% cream (ELIMITE) under nails (finger and toe). Apply entire skin from chin down to and including under fingernails and toenails. Leave on 8–14 hrs. Repeat in 1–2 wks. Safe for children age >2 mos.	**Ivermectin** 200 µg/kg po with food x 1, then second dose in 2 wks. **Less effective: Crotamiton** 10% cream, apply x 24 hr, rinse off, then reapply x 24 hr	Trim fingernails. Reapply cream to hands after handwashing. Treat close contacts; wash and heat dry linens. Pruritus may persist times 2 wks after mites gone.
AIDS and HIV-infected patients (CD4 <150 per mm³), debilitated or developmentally disabled patients (**Norwegian scabies**—see Comments)		For Norwegian crusted scabies: **Permethrin** 5% cream daily x 7 days, then twice weekly until cured. Add **ivermectin** po (dose in Alternative)	**Ivermectin** 200 mcg/kg po on days 1, 2, 8, 9 & 15+ **Permethrin** cream. May need addt'l doses of ivermectin on days 22 & 29.	Norwegian scabies in AIDS pts. Extensive, crusted. Can mimic psoriasis. Not pruritic. Highly contagious—isolate!

* For source of drug, see Table 13D, page 165.

TABLE 13B – DOSAGE AND SELECTED ADVERSE EFFECTS OF ANTIPARASITIC DRUGS

Doses vary with indication. For convenience, drugs divided by type of parasite; some drugs used for multiple types of parasites, e.g., albendazole.

CLASS, AGENT, GENERIC NAME (TRADE NAME)	USUAL ADULT DOSAGE	ADVERSE REACTIONS/COMMENTS
Antiprotozoan Drugs		
Intestinal Parasites		
Diloxanide furoate[NUS] (Furamide) Iodoquinol (Yodoxin)	500 mg po tid x 10 days Adults: 650 mg po tid (or 30-40 mg/kg/day div. tid); children: 40 mg/kg per day div. tid.	*Source: See Table 13D, page 165.* Flatulence, N/V, diarrhea. Rarely causes nausea, abdominal cramps, rash, acne. **Contraindicated if iodine intolerance** (contains 64% bound iodine). Can cause iododerma (papular or pustular rash) and/or thyroid enlargement.
Metronidazole **Nitazoxanide** (Alinia)	Side-effects similar for all. See metronidazole in Table 10B, page 116, & Table 10A, page 112. Adults: 500 mg po q12h. Children 4-11: 200 mg susp. po q12h. Take with food. Expensive.	*CID 40:1173, 2005; Expert Opin Pharmacother 7:953, 2006.* Abdominal pain 7.8%, diarrhea 2.1%. Rev: *CID 40:1173, 2005; Expert Opin Pharmacother 7:953, 2006.*
Paromomycin (Humatin) Aminosidine IV in U.K.	Up to 750 mg po qid (250 mg tabs). Source: See Table 13D	Headaches, rarely yellow sclera (resolves after treatment). **Aminoglycoside similar to neomycin;** if absorbed due to concomitant inflammatory bowel disease can result in oto/nephrotoxicity. Doses >3 gm daily are associated with nausea, abdominal cramps, diarrhea.
Quinacrine[NUS] (Atabrine, Mepacrine)	100 mg po tid x 5 days. No longer available in U.S.; www.expertpharmacy.com; www.fagron.com	**Contraindicated for pts with history of psychosis or psoriasis. Yellow staining of skin.** Dizziness, headache, vomiting, toxic psychosis (1.5%), hemolytic anemia, leukopenia, thrombocytopenia, urticaria, rash, fever, minor disulfiram-like reactions.
Tinidazole (Tindamax)	250-500 mg tabs, with food. Regimen varies with indication.	**Chemical structure similar to metronidazole but better tolerated.** Seizures/peripheral neuropathy reported. **Adverse effects:** Metallic taste 4-6%, nausea 3-5%, anorexia 2-3%.
Antiprotozoan Drugs: Non-Intestinal Protozoa		
Extraintestinal Parasites		
Antimony compounds[NUS] Stibogluconate sodium (Pentostam) from CDC or Meglumine antimoniate (Glucantime) —French trade name	For IV use: vials with 100 mg antimony/mL. Dilute selected dose in 50 mL of D5W shortly before use. Infuse over at least 10 minutes.	**AEs in 1st 10 days:** headache, fatigue, elevated lipase/amylase, clinical pancreatitis. After 10 days: elevated AST/ALT/ALK/PHOS. **NOTE: Reversible T wave changes in 30-60%. Risk of QTc prolongation.** **Renal excretion; modify dose if renal insufficiency.** Metabolized in liver; lower dose if hepatic insufficiency. Generic drug may have increased toxicity due to antimony complex formation.
Artemether-Lumefantrine, po (Coartem, FDA-approved)	Tablets contain 20 mg Artemether and 120 mg Lumefantrine. Take with food. Can be crushed and mixed with a few teaspoons of water	**Can prolong QTc:** avoid in patients with congenital long QTc, family history of sudden death or long QTc, or need for drugs known to prolong QTc *(see list under fluoroquinolones, Table 10A, page 111).* Artemether induces CYP3A4 and both Artemether & Lumefantrine are metabolized >30% of adults: headache, anorexia, dizziness, arthralgia and myalgia. Non-life threatening, but translation requiring, hemolytic anemia can occur up to 15 days post-therapy *(AnIM 163:498, 2015).*
Artesunate, IV Ref: *NEJM 358:1829, 2008*	Available from CDC Malaria Branch. 2.4 mg/kg IV at 0, 12, 24, 48 hrs.	**More effective than quinine & safer than quinidine.** Contact CDC at 770-488-7758 or 770-488-7100 after hours. No dosage adjustment for hepatic or renal insufficiency. No known drug interactions.
Atovaquone (Mepron) Ref: *AAC 46:1163, 2002*	Suspension: 1 tsp (750 mg) po bid 750 mg/5 mL.	No. pts stopping rx due to side-effects was 9%; rash 22%, GI 20%, insomnia 10%, fever 14%
Atovaquone and proguanil (Malarone) For prophylaxis of P. falciparum; little data on P. vivax. Generic available in US.	**Prophylaxis:** 1 tab po (250 mg + 100 mg) q24h with food **Treatment:** 4 tabs po (1000 mg + 400 mg) once daily with food x 3 days Adult tab: 250/100 mg, Peds tab 62.5/25 mg. Peds dosage: *prophylaxis footnote 1 page 153*; *treatment see comment, page 154*	N/V 12%, N/V 12%, headache 10%, dizziness 5%. Rx stopped in 1%. Asymptomatic mild 1 in ALT/AST. Children—cough, headache, anorexia, vomiting, abd. pain. See *drug interactions, Table 22.* Safe in G6PD-deficient pts. Can crush tabs for children and give with milk or other liquid nutrients. Renal insufficiency: contraindicated if CrCl <30 mL per min.

NOTE: Drugs available from CDC Drug Service indicated by "CDC". Call (+1) (404) 639-3670 (or 2888 [Fax]). **See Table 13D, page 165 for sources and contact information for hard-to-find antiparasitic drugs.**

TABLE 13B (2)

CLASS, AGENT, GENERIC NAME (TRADE NAME)	USUAL ADULT DOSAGE	ADVERSE REACTIONS/COMMENTS
Antiprotozoan Drugs: Non-Intestinal Protozoa/Extraintestinal Parasites *(continued)*		
Benznidazole (CDC Drug Service)	7.5 mg/kg per day po, 100 mg tabs. May use 100 mg per day for 60 days, regardless of body weight. Give 300 mg per day but prolong treatment to complete the total dose corresponding to 5 mg/kg per day for 60 days.	Photosensitivity in 50% of pts. GI: abdominal pain, nausea/vomiting/anorexia. CNS: disorientation, insomnia, twitching/seizures, paresthesias, polyneuritis. **Contraindicated in pregnancy**
Chloroquine phosphate (Aralen)	Dose varies—see *Malaria Prophylaxis and rx, pages 153-154.*	Minor - anorexia/nausea/vomiting, headache, dizziness, blurred vision, pruritus in dark-skinned pts. Major: protracted rx in rheumatoid arthritis can lead to retinopathy. Can exacerbate psoriasis. Can block response to rabies vaccine. **Contraindicated in pts with epilepsy.**
Dapsone *See Comment re methemoglobinemia*	100 mg po q24h	Usually tolerated by pts with rash after TMP-SMX. **Dapsone is common etiology of acquired methemoglobinemia** (*NEJM 364:957, 2011*). Metabolite of dapsone converts heme iron to +3 charge (no O2 transport) Normal blood level 1%, cyanosis at 10%, headache, fatigue, tachycardia, dizziness at 30-40%, acidosis & coma at 60%, death at 70-80%. Low G6PD is a risk factor. Treatment: methylene blue 1-2 mg/kg IV over 5 min x 1 dose.
Eflornithine (Ornidyl) (WHO or CDC drug service)	200 mg/kg IV (slowly) q12h x 7 days for African trypanosomiasis	Diarrhea in ½ pts, vomiting, abdominal pain, anemia/leukopenia in ½ pts, seizures, alopecia, jaundice, ↓ hearing. Contraindicated in pregnancy
Fumagillin	Eyedrops + po. 20 mg po tid. Leiter's: 800-292-6772.	Adverse events. Neutropenia & thrombocytopenia
Mefloquine	One 250 mg tab/wk for **malaria prophylaxis**; for rx, 1250 mg x 1 or 750 mg x 1 & then 500 mg in 6-8 hrs. In U.S. 250 mg tab = 228 mg base; outside U.S. 275 mg tab = 250 mg base.	Side-effects in roughly 3%. Minor: headache, irritability, insomnia, weakness, diarrhea. **Toxic psychosis, seizures can occur.** Do not use with quinine, quinidine, or halofantrine. Rare: Prolonged QT interval and toxic epidermal necrolysis (*Ln 349:101, 1997*). **Not used for self-rx due to neuropsychiatric side-effects.**
Melarsoprol (Mel B, Arsobal) (CDC)	See Trypanosomiasis for adult dose. Peds dose: 0.36 mg/kg IV, then gradual ↑ to 3.6 mg/kg q1-5 days for up to 9-10 doses.	Post-rx encephalopathy (2-10%) with 50% mortality overall, risk of death is 8-14%. Prednisolone 1 mg per kg per day po may ↓ encephalopathy. Other: Heart damage, albuminuria, abdominal pain, vomiting, peripheral neuropathy. Herxheimer-like reaction, pruritus
Miltefosine (Impavido) *Med J 56:69, 2014, but no commercialization in US at present*	50 mg po bid (wt 33-44 kg); 50 mg po tid (wt ≥45 kg). Treat for 28 days	Pregnancy—No: teratogenic. Side-effects vary. Kala-azar pts, vomiting in up to 40%, diarrhea in 17% "motion sickness", headache & increased creatinine. Metabolized by excretion, virtually no urinary excretion.
Nifurtimox (Lampit) (CDC) (Manufactured in Germany by Bayer)	8-10 mg/kg per day po div. 4 x per day for 90-120 days	Side-effects in 40-70% of pts. GI: abdominal pain, nausea/vomiting. CNS: polyneuritis (1/3), disorientation, insomnia, twitching, seizures. Skin rash. Hemolysis with G6PD deficiency.
Pentamidine (NebuPent)	300 mg via aerosol q month. Also used IM.	Hypotension, hypoglycemia, hypocalcemia, pancreatitis. Neutropenia (15%), thrombocytopenia. Nephrotoxicity. Others: nausea/vomiting, ↑ liver tests, rash.
Primaquine phosphate	26.3 mg (= 15 mg base) of base po daily.	In G6PD def, pts, can cause hemolytic anemia with hemoglobinuria, esp. African, Asian peoples. Methemoglobinemia. Nausea/abdominal pain if pt. fasting. Pregnancy: No.
Pyrimethamine (Daraprim, Malocide) Also combined with sulfadoxine as **Fansidar** (25-500 mg)	100 mg, then 25 mg/day. Very expensive: $79,000 for 100 tabs (25 mg) (Sep 2015, US price)	Major problem is hematologic: megaloblastic anemia, ↓ WBC, ↓ platelets, ↓ bone marrow depression and not interfere with antitoxoplasmosis effect. If high-dose pyrimethamine, ↑ folinic acid to 10-50 mg/day. Pyrimethamine + sulfadiazine can cause mental changes due to carnitine deficiency (AJM 95:112, 1993). Other: Rash, vomiting, diarrhea, xerostomia.
Quinidine gluconate Cardiotoxicity ref: *LnID 7:549, 2007*	Loading dose of 10 mg (equiv to 6.2 mg of quinidine base) / kg IV over 1-2 hr, then constant infusion of 0.02 mg/kg quinidine gluconate / kg per minute. May be available for compassionate use from Lilly.	Adverse reactions of quinidine/quinine similar: (1) IV bolus injection can cause fatal hypotension, (2) hypoglycemia, esp. in pregnancy, (3) ↓ rate of infusion if IV quinidine gluconate if QTc interval ↑ 25% of baseline, (4) reduce dose 30-50% after day 3 due to ↓ renal clearance and ↓ vol. of distribution.

NOTE: Drugs available from CDC Drug Service indicated by "CDC". Call (+1) (404) 639-3670 (or -2888 (Fax)). **See Table 13D, page 165 for sources and contact information for hard-to-find antiparasitic drugs.**

TABLE 13B (3)

CLASS, AGENT, GENERIC NAME (TRADE NAME)	USUAL ADULT DOSAGE	ADVERSE REACTIONS/COMMENTS
Antiprotozoan Drugs: Non-Intestinal Protozoa/Extraintestinal Parasites *(continued)*		
Quinine sulfate (Qualaquin)	324 mg tabs. No IV prep. in US. Oral rx of chloroquine-resistant falciparum malaria: 624 mg po bid x 3 days, then (tetracycline 250 mg po qid or doxy 100 mg bid) x 7 days	Cinchonism; tinnitus, headache, nausea, abdominal pain, blurred vision. Rarely: blood dyscrasias, drug fever, asthma, hypoglycemia. Transient blindness in < 1% of 500 pts (*AnIM* 136:339, 2002). **Contraindicated if prolonged QTc, myasthenia gravis, optic neuritis or G6PD deficiency.**
Spiramycin (Rovamycin)	1 gm po q8h *(see Comment)*.	GI and allergic reactions have occurred. Available at no cost after consultation with Palo Alto Medical Foundation Toxoplasma Serology Lab 650-853-4828 or from U.S. FDA 301-796-1600.
Sulfadiazine	1–1.5 gm po q6h.	See *Table 10A*, page 113, for *sulfonamide side-effects*.
Sulfadoxine & pyrimethamine combination (Fansidar)	Contains 500 mg sulfadoxine & 25 mg pyrimethamine	Long half-life of both drugs: Sulfadoxine 169 hrs, pyrimethamine 111 hrs allows weekly dosage. In African, used empirically in pregnancy for intermittent preventative treatment (ITPp) against malaria: dosing at 3 set times during pregnancy. Reduces material and fetal mortality if HIV+. See *Expert Rev Anti Infect Ther* 8:589, 2010. **Fatalities reported due to Stevens-Johnson syndrome and toxic epidermal necrolysis.** Renal excretion—caution if renal impairment.
DRUGS USED TO TREAT NEMATODES, TREMATODES, AND CESTODES		
Albendazole (Albenza)	Doses vary with indication. Take with food; fatty meal increases absorption.	**Pregnancy Cat. C;** give after negative pregnancy test. Abdominal pain, nausea/vomiting, alopecia, ↑ serum transaminase. Rare leukopenia.
Diethylcarbamazine (CDC)	Used to treat filariasis.	Headache, dizziness, nausea, fever. Host may experience inflammatory reaction to death of adult worms: fever, urticaria, asthma, GI upset (**Mazzotti reaction**). **Pregnancy—No.**
Ivermectin (Stromectol, Mectizan) (3 mg tab & topical 0.5% lotion for head lice). Take on empty stomach.	Strongyloidiasis dose: 200 μg/kg/day po x 2 days Onchocerciasis: 150 μg/kg x 1 dose Scabies: 200 μg/kg po x 1; if AIDS, wait 14 days & repeat	Mild side-effects: fever, pruritus, rash. In rx of onchocerciasis, can see tender lymphadenopathy, headache, bone/joint pain. Host may experience inflammatory reaction to death of adult worms: fever, urticaria, asthma, GI upset (**Mazzotti reaction**).
Mebendazole (Vermox) Not available in US, but widely available elsewhere.	Doses vary with indication.	Rarely causes abdominal pain, nausea, diarrhea. Contraindicated in pregnancy & children < 2 yrs old.
Praziquantel (Biltricide)	Doses vary with parasite; see *Table 13A*	Mild dizziness/drowsiness; N/V, rash, fever. **Only contraindication is ocular cysticercosis.** Potential exacerbation of neurocysticercosis. Metab.-induced by anticonvulsants and steroids; can negate effect with cimetidine 400 mg po x 1 dose. Reduce dose if advanced liver disease.
Pyrantel pamoate (over-the-counter)	Oral suspension. Dose for all ages: 11 mg/kg to max. of 1 gm) x 1 dose	Rare GI upset, headache, dizziness, rash
Suramin (Germanin) (CDC)	Drug powder mixed to 10% solution with 5 mL water and used within 30 min. First give test dose of 0.1 gm IV. Try to avoid pregnancy.	Does not cross blood-brain barrier; no effect on CNS infection. Side-effects: vomiting, pruritus, urticaria, fever, paresthesias; albuminuria (discontinue drug if casts appear). Do not use if renal/liver disease present. Deaths from vascular collapse reported.
Triclabendazole (Egaten) (CDC)	Used for fasciola hepatica liver infection. 10 mg/kg po x 1 dose. May repeat in 12-24 hrs. 250 mg tabs	AEs ≥ 10%: sweating and abdominal pain. AEs 1-10%: weakness, chest pain, fever, anorexia, nausea, vomiting. **Note: use with caution if G6PD def. or impaired liver function.**

NOTE: Drugs available from CDC Drug Service indicated by "CDC." Call (+1) (404) 639-3670 (or -2888 (Fax)). **See *Table 13D*, page 165 for sources and contact information for hard-to-find antiparasitic drugs.**

TABLE 13C – PARASITES THAT CAUSE EOSINOPHILIA (EOSINOPHILIA IN TRAVELERS)

Frequent and Intense (>5000 eos/mcL)	Moderate to Marked During Early Infections	During Larval Migration; Absent or Mild During Chronic Infections	Other
Strongyloides (absent in compromised hosts); Lymphatic Filariasis; Toxocaria (cutaneous larva migrans)	Ascaris; Hookworm; Clonorchis; Paragonimis	Opisthorchis	Schistosomiasis; Cysticercosis; Trichuris; Angiostrongylus; Non-lymphatic filariasis; Gnathostoma; Capillaria Trichostrongylus

TABLE 13D – SOURCES FOR HARD-TO-FIND ANTIPARASITIC DRUGS

Source	Drugs Available	Contact Information
CDC Drug Service	Artesunate, Benznidazole, Diethylcarbamazine (DEC), Eflornithine, Melarsoprol, Nifurtimox, Sodium stibogluconate, Suramin, Triclabendazole	www.cdc.gov/laboratory/drugservice/index.html (+1) 404-639-3670
WHO	Drugs for treatment of African trypanosomiasis	simarrop@who.int; (+41) 794-682-726, (+41) 227-911-345 franco@who.int; (+41) 796-198-535, (+41) 227-913-313
Compounding Pharmacies, Specialty Distributors, Others		
Expert Compounding Pharmacy	Quinacrine, Iodoquinol, niclosamide	www.expertpharmacy.org 1-800-247-9767, (+1) 818-988-7979
Fagron Compounding Pharmacy (formerly Gallipot)	Quinacrine, Iodoquinol, Paromomycin, Diloxanide	www.fagron.com 1-800-423-6967, (+1) 651-681-9517
Leiter's Pharmacy	Fumagillin	www.leiterrx.com 1-800-292-6772, +1-408-292-6772
Profounda, Inc.	Miltefosine	www.impavido.com; +1 407-270-7790
Victoria Apotheke Zurich will ship worldwide if sent physicians prescription.	Paromomycin (oral and topical). Triclabendazole. Other hard to find anti-parasitic drugs	www.pharmaworld.com (+41) 43-344-6060
Palo Alto Medical Foundation, Toxoplasma Serology Lab	Spiramycin (consultation required for release)	(+1) 650-853-4828; toxlab@pamf.org

TABLE 14A - ANTIVIRAL THERAPY*

For HIV, see *Table 14C*; for Hepatitis, see *Table 14E. For Antiviral Activity Spectra, see Table 4C, page 79*

VIRUS/DISEASE	DRUG/DOSAGE	SIDE EFFECTS/COMMENTS
Adenovirus: Cause of RTIs including fatal pneumonia in children & young adults and 60% mortality in transplant pts *(CID 43.331, 2006)*. Frequent cause of cystitis in transplant patients. Adenovirus 14 associated with severe pneumonia in otherwise healthy young adults *(MMWR 56(45):1181, 2007)*. **Findings include:** fever, ↑ liver enzymes, leukopenia, thrombocytopenia, diarrhea, or hemorrhagic cystitis.	In severe cases of pneumonia or post HSCT¹: **Cidofovir** • 5 mg/kg/wk x 2 wks, then q 2 wks + **probenecid** • 1.25 gm/M² given 3 hrs before cidofovir and 3 & 9 hrs after each infusion • Or 1 mg/kg IV 3x/wk. For adenovirus hemorrhagic cystitis *(CID 40:199, 2005; Transplantation 2006; 81:1398)*. Intravesical **cidofovir** (5 mg/kg in 100 mL saline instilled into bladder).	Cidofovir successful in 3/8 immunosuppressed *children with HSCT (CID 41: 1812, 2005)*. ↓ in virus load predicted response to cidofovir. Ribavirin has mixed activity, appears restricted to group C serotypes. Vidarabine and Ganciclovir with in vitro activity against adenovirus, little to no clinical data. **Brincidofovir** (CMX001-Chimerix) oral cidofovir prodrug in Phase III. Adenovirus specific T-cell (Cytovir) infusions under development.*(Cytotherapy 16.4: S22, 2014)*
Bunyaviridae. Severe fever with thrombocytopenia virus (SFTSV) Possibly transmitted by *Haemaphysalis longicornis* tick	No therapy recommended. Ribavirin ineffective. Clinical symptoms: Fever, weakness, myalgias, GI symptoms	Lab: Elevated LDH (> 1200) and CPK (> 800) associated with higher mortality rates. Initially thought to be an anaplasma infection, but serology showed a new virus.
Coronavirus—SARS-CoV Severe acute respiratory syndrome *(NEJM 348:1953, 1967, 2003)* **MERS-CoV:** Middle East respiratory syndrome *(LnID 14:1090, 2014)*	**SARS:** • Ribavirin—ineffective. • Interferon ± steroids—small case series. • Pegylated IFN-α effective in monkeys. • Low dose steroids alone successful in one Beijing hospital. High dose steroids ↑ serious fungal infections. • inhaled nitric oxide improved oxygenation & improved chest x-ray *(CID 39:1531, 2004)*. **MERS:** increased 14 day survival with **Ribavirin** po + **PEG-IFN** 180 mcg/kg sc x 2 wks *(LnID 14:1090, 2014)*. Other therapies: *LnID 14:1136, 2014*.	**SARS: Transmission by close contact: (mask [changed frequently],** eye protection, gown, gloves) key to stopping transmission. **MERS:** Suspected reservoirs are camels and perhaps other animals. *Review: Clin Micro Rev. 28:465, 2015.*
Enterovirus—Meningitis: most common cause of aseptic meningitis. Rapid CSF PCR test is accurate, reduces costs and hospital stay for infants *(Peds 120:489, 2007)*	**No rx currently recommended;** however, **pleconaril** (VP 63843) still under investigation.	No clinical benefit from Pleconaril in double-blind placebo-controlled study in 21 infants with enteroviral aseptic meningitis *(PIDJ 22:335, 2003)*. Some improvement among those with severe headache *(AAC 2006 50:2409-14)*. Severe respiratory illness with enterovirus D68 *(MMWR 63:798 & 901, 2014)*
Hemorrhagic Fever Virus Infections: Review: *LnID 6.203, 2006*. **Congo-Crimean Hemorrhagic Fever** (HF) Tick-borne, symptoms include IV.V. fever, headache, myalgias, stupor. (3). Signs: conjunctival injection, hepatomegaly, petechiae. ↓ WBC, ↓ platelets, ↓ WBC, ↑ ALT, AST, LDH & CPK (100%).	Oral **ribavirin, 30 mg/kg** as initial loading dose & 15 mg/kg q6h x 4 days then 7.5 mg/kg q8h x 6 days (WHO recommendation) *(see Comment)*. Reviewed *Antiviral Res 78:125, 2008*.	3/3 healthcare workers in Pakistan had complete recovery *(Ln 346:472, 1995)*. & 61/69 (89%) with confirmed CCHF rx with ribavirin in Iran *(CID 36:1613, 2003)*. Shorter time of hospitalization among ribavirin treated pts (7.7 vs. 10.3 days), but no difference in mortality or transfusion needs in study in Turkey *(J Infection 52: 207-215, 2006)*. Suggested benefit from ribavirin & dexamethasone (281 pts) *(CID 57:1270, 2013)*.

¹ HSCT = Hematopoietic stem cell transplant
* See page 2 for abbreviations. NOTE: All dosage recommendations are for adults (unless otherwise indicated) and assume normal renal function.

TABLE 14A (2)

VIRUS/DISEASE	DRUG/DOSAGE	SIDE EFFECTS/COMMENTS
Hemorrhagic Fever Virus Infections (continued)		
Ebola/Marburg HF (Central Africa) Largest ever documented outbreak of Ebola virus (EVD), West Africa, 2014. Diagnostic testing at U.S. CDC. Within a few days of symptom onset, diagnosis is most commonly made by antigen-capture enzyme linked immunosorbent assay (ELISA), IgM antibody ELISA, NAAT or viral culture. (Update). See http://emergency.cdc.gov/han/han00365.asp http://www.bt.cdc.gov/han/han00364.asp	**No effective antiviral rx** (J Virol 77: 9733, 2003). Investigational antibody treatment "ZMapp" used as compassionate use in a few selected patients (Mapp Biopharmaceutical; http://mappbio.com/). ZMapp is a 3 in one monoclonal antibody preparation, derived from convalescent serum from pts who have recovered is approved by the WHO (BMJ 349:g5539, 2014). GS-5734 (Gilead) active in animal models.	**Abrupt onset of symptoms typically 8-10 days after exposure (range 2-21 days).** Fever may be an early symptom, which may include fever, chills, myalgias, and malaise. Fever, anorexia, asthenia/weakness are the most common signs and symptoms. Patients may develop a diffuse erythematous maculopapular rash (days 5-7) (usually involving the face, neck, trunk, and arms) that can desquamate. EVD can **often be confused with** other common infectious diseases such as malaria, typhoid fever, and other bacterial infections (e.g., pneumonia). **Gastrointestinal symptoms:** severe watery diarrhea, nausea, vomiting and abdominal pain. **Other:** chest pain, shortness of breath, headache or confusion, may also develop. Patients often have conjunctival injection. Hiccups reported. Seizures may occur, and cerebral edema reported. Bleeding is not universally present but can manifest later in the course as petechiae, ecchymoses/bruising, or oozing from venipuncture sites and mucosal hemorrhage. Frank hemorrhage is less common. Pregnant women may experience spontaneous miscarriages.
With pulmonary syndrome: Hantavirus pulmonary syndrome, "sin nombre virus"	**No benefit from ribavirin demonstrated** (CID 39:1307, 2004). Early recognition of disease and supportive (usually ICU) care is key to successful outcome.	Acute onset of fever, headache, myalgias, non-productive cough, thrombocytopenia, increased PT and non-cardiogenic pulmonary edema with respiratory insufficiency following exposure to droppings of infected rodents.
With renal syndrome: Lassa, Venezuelan, Korean, HF, Sabia, Argentinian HF, Bolivian HF, Junin, Machupo. (> 90% occur in China 59:1040, 2014)	**Oral ribavirin, 30 mg/kg** as initial loading dose & 15 mg/kg q6h x 4 days then 7.5 mg/kg x 6 days (WHO recommendation) (see Comment).	Toxicity low, hemolysis reported but recovery when treatment stopped. No significant changes in WBC, platelets, hepatic or renal function. See CID 36:1254, 2003.
Dengue and dengue hemorrhagic fever (DHF) http://www.cdc.gov/ncidod/dvbid/dengue/dengue-hcp.htm Think dengue in travels to tropics or subtropics (incubation period usually 4-7 days) with fever, bleeding, thrombocytopenia, or hemoconcentration with shock. Dx by viral isolation or serology: serum to CDC (telephone 787-706-2399).	**No data on antiviral rx.** Fluid replacement with careful hemodynamic monitoring critical. Rx of **DHF** with colloids effective: 6% hydroxyethyl starch preferred in 1 study (NEJM 353:9, 2005). Review in Semin Ped Infect Dis 16: 60-65, 2005.	Of 77 cases dx at CDC (2001-2004), recent (2-wks) travel to Caribbean island 30%, Asia 17%, Central America 15%, S. America 15%, 5 pts with severe DHF rx with dengue antibody-neg. gamma globulin 500 mg/kg q24H IV for 3-5 days; rapid ↑ in platelet counts (CID 36:1623, 2003). Diagnosis: ELISA detects IgM antibody. Has some cross-reactivity with West Nile Fever. Should only be used in pts with symptoms c/w Dengue Fever.
West Nile virus (JAMA 310:308, 2013) A flavivirus transmitted by mosquitoes, blood transfusions, transplanted organs & breast-feeding. Birds (>200 species) are main host with humans & horses incidental hosts. The US epidemic continues.	**No proven rx to date.** Reviewed in Lancet Neurology 6: 171-181, 2007.	Usually nonspecific febrile illness develops but 1/150 cases develops meningo-encephalitis, aseptic meningitis or polio-like paralysis (AnIM 104:545, 2004; JCI 113: 1102, 2004). Long-term sequelae (neuromuscular weakness & psychiatric) (NEJM 43:723, 2006). Diagnosis: Increased IgM antibody in serum & CSF or CSF PCR (contact State Health Dept./CDC). Blood supply now tested in U.S. Increased serum tulare in 11/17 cases (NEJM 352:420, 2005).
Yellow fever	**No data on antiviral rx** **Guidelines for use of preventative vaccine:** (http://www.cdc.gov/mmwr/preview/mmwrhtml/mm6423a5.htm) (http://www.cdc.gov/mmwr/preview/mmwrhtml/rr5701a_w)	Reemergence in Africa & S. Amer. due to urbanization of susceptible population (Lancet Inf I:5604, 2005). Vaccination Diagnosis: increased IgM antibody in serum and effective in HIV patients, especially in those with suppressed VL and higher CD4 counts (CID 48:659, 2009). Purified whole-virus, inactivated, alum-adjuvanted cell-culture–derived vaccine (XRX-001) using the 17D strain proven safe and resulted in neutralizing antibodies after 2 doses in a de-escalation, phase I study. (N Engl J Med 2011 Apr 7; 364:1326)
Chikungunya fever: brake bone fever. A self-limited arbovirus illness spread by Aedes mosquito. High epidemic potential (Caribbean).	**No antiviral therapy.** Fluids, analgesics, anti-pyretics	Clinical presentation: high fever, severe myalgias & headache, macular papular rash with occ. thrombocytopenia. Rarely hemorrhagic complications. Dx mostly clinical: definitive diagnosis by PCR (NEJM 372:1231, 2015).
SFTSV (Severe fever with thrombocytopenia syndrome virus)	**See** Bunyaviridae, page 166	
Hepatitis Viral Infections	See Table 14E (Hepatitis A & B), Table 14F (Hepatitis C)	

* See page 2 for abbreviations. NOTE: All dosage recommendations are for adults (unless otherwise indicated) and assume normal renal function.

TABLE 14A (3)

VIRUS/DISEASE	DRUG/DOSAGE	SIDE EFFECTS/COMMENTS
Herpesvirus Infections **Cytomegalovirus (CMV)** At risk pts: HIV/AIDS, cancer chemotherapy, post-transplant Ref: *Transplantation* 96:333, 2013; *Am J Transplant* 13(Suppl 4):93, 2013	**Primary prophylaxis** not generally recommended except in certain transplant populations (see *TABLE 15E*). **Preemptive therapy** in pts with ↑ CMV DNA (see *TABLE 15E*). **Mild:** If used: **valganciclovir** 900 mg po q12h (*CID 32: 783, 2001*). Authors rec: primary prophylaxis be dc if response to ART with ↑ CD4 >100 for 6 mos (*MMWR 53:98, 2004*).	Risk for developing CMV disease correlates with quantity of CMV DNA in plasma; each log$_{10}$ ↑ associated with 3.1-fold ↑ in disease (*CID 28:758, 1999*). Resistance demonstrated in 5% CMV transplant recipients receiving primary prophylaxis (*J Antimicrob Chemother 65:2628 2010*). Consensus guidelines: *Transplantation 96:333, 2013*.
CMV: Colitis, Esophagitis, Gastritis Symptoms relate to site of disease	**Mild: Valganciclovir** 900 mg po bid with food x 14-21 days **Severe: Ganciclovir** 5 mg/kg IV q12h x 14-21 days OR **Foscarnet** (60 mg/kg IV q8h or 90 mg/kg q12h) x 14-21 days **Post-treatment suppression: Valganciclovir** 900 mg po once daily until CD4 > 100 x 6 mos. Treat as for colitis, esophagitis, gastritis above	Diagnosis: Elevated whole blood quantitative PCR & histopathology. Severe bouts of Inflammatory Bowel Disease (IBD) colitis may be complicated by CMV. Rx of CMV in this setting is recommended (*European J Clin Micro & Inf Dis 34:13, 2015*). Rx of CMV in less severe bouts of IBD unclear.
CMV: Neurologic disease, Encephalitis Myelitis, polyradiculopathy, peripheral neuropathy Symptoms relate to site of disease	Treat as for colitis, esophagitis, gastritis above	Diagnosis: Elevated whole blood and/or CSF quantitative PCR Note: **Severe or fatal IRIS** has occurred in CMV pts, suggest delay starting ART for 2 wks after initiation of CMV therapy.
CMV: Pneumonia At risk: 1st 6 months post-transplant & 3 months post-stopping prophylaxis Diagnosis: CMV in whole blood quantitative PCR and/or positive lung biopsy histopathology Ref: *Transplantation 96:333, 2013*; *Am J Transplant 13(Suppl 4):93, 2013*	**Viremic but no/mild symptoms: Valganciclovir** 900 mg po bid (*Am J Transplant 7:2106, 2007*) **Severe in lung transplant or AIDS pts: Ganciclovir** 5 mg/kg IV q12h (adjust for renal insufficiency). Treat until clinical resolution & neg blood PCR; min duration: 2 wks If Ganciclovir-resistant: **Foscarnet** (60 mg/kg q8h or 90 mg/kg q12h) IV (adjust for renal insufficiency). Try to reduce immunosuppression	Post-treatment suppression: Valganciclovir 900 mg po once daily x 1-3 months if high risk of relapse. Suspect resistant CMV if treatment failure or relapse (*CID 16:1018, 2013*). Note: IVIG or CMV specific immunoglobulin did not improve overall or attributable mortality in retrospective study of 421 bone marrow transplant pts (*CID 61:31, 2015*).
CMV: Retinitis Most common ocular complication of HIV/AIDS. Rare in pts on ART with CD4 >200. If not on ART, wait to start until after 2 wks of CMV therapy. Ref: aidsinfo.nih.gov/guidelines **CMV immune recovery retinitis:** new retinitis after starting ART. Do not stop ART or Valganciclovir. No steroids	**Not sight-threatening: Valganciclovir** 900 mg po bid with food x 14-21 days, then 900 mg po q12h (CD4 >100 x 6 months **Sight-threatening** (see Comment): **Valganciclovir** + intravitreal **Ganciclovir** 2 mg (1-4 doses over 7-10 days).	Sight-threatening: <1500 microns from fovea or next to head of optic nerve. It can I use Valganciclovir, Ganciclovir 5 mg/kg IV q12h x 14-21 days, then 5 mg/kg IV once daily If suspect Ganciclovir resistance: Foscarnet (60 gm/kg q8h or 90 mg/kg q12h) x 14-21 days. Ganciclovir ocular implants no longer available.
CMV in Transplant patients: See Table 15E for discussion of prophylaxis. CMV disease can manifest as CMV syndrome with or without end-organ disease. **Guidelines for CMV therapy** (*Transplantation 2013: 96(4):333*) and *Am J Transplant 2013: 13 Suppl 4:93*. Treatment options. (1) Oral Valganciclovir 900 mg po q12h and IV Ganciclovir 900 mg po q12h (Am J Transplant 7:2106, 2007) are effective treatment options. Treatment duration should be individualized. Continue treatment until (1) CMV PCR is negative or undetectable, (2) clinical evidence of disease has resolved, and (3) at least 2-3 weeks of treatment (Am J Transplant 13(Suppl 4):93, 2013; Blood 113:5711, 2009). Secondary prophylaxis (Valganciclovir 900 mg po once daily) should be considered for 1-3 month course in patients recently treated with high-dose immunosuppression such as lymphocyte depleting antibodies, those with severe CMV disease, or those with >1 episode of CMV disease. In HSCT recipients, secondary prophylaxis should be considered in similar cases balancing the risk of recurrent infection and drug toxicity		
CMV in pregnancy: Hyperimmune globulin 200 IU/kg maternal weight as single dose during pregnancy (early), administered IV reduced complications of CMV in infant at one year of life. (*CID 55: 497, 2012*).		
CMV: Congenital/Neonatal Symptomatic	Valganciclovir 16 mg/kg po bid x 6 mos	Better outcome after 6 mos compared to 6 wks with no difference in AEs (*NEJM 372:933, 2015*).

* See page 2 for abbreviations. NOTE: *All dosage recommendations are for adults (unless otherwise indicated) and assume normal renal function.*

TABLE 14A (4)

VIRUS/DISEASE	DRUG/DOSAGE	SIDE EFFECTS/COMMENTS
Herpesvirus Infections (continued)		
Epstein Barr Virus (EBV) — Mononucleosis (Ln D 3:131, 2003)	**No treatment.** Corticosteroids for tonsillar obstruction, CNS complications, or threat of splenic rupture.	**Etiology of atypical lymphocytes: EBV, CMV, Hep A, Hep B, Toxo, measles, mumps, drugs** (Int Pediat 18:20, 2003).
HHV-6—implicated as cause of roseola (exanthem subitum) & other febrile diseases of childhood (NEJM 352:768, 2005). Fever & rash documented in transplant pts (JID 179:311, 1999). Reactivation in 47% of 110 U.S. hematopoietic stem cell transplant pts assoc. with delayed monocytes & platelet engraftment (CID 40:932, 2005). Recognized in assoc. with meningoencephalitis in immunocompetent adults. Diagnosis made by pos. PCR in CSF; ↑ viral copies in CSF is second line therapy (Bone Marrow Transplantation (2008) 42, 227–240).		Reactivation in assoc. with thrombotic microangiopathy (Am J Hemato 76:156, 2004). Cidofovir & valganciclovir responded to ganciclovir (Blood 103/1632, 2004) & valganciclovir (JID 2006).
HHV-7—ubiquitous virus (>90% of the population is infected by age 3 yrs). No relationship to human disease. Infects CD4 lymphocytes via CD4 receptor; transmitted via saliva.		
HHV-8—The agent of Kaposi's sarcoma, Castleman's disease, & body cavity lymphoma. Associated with diabetes in sub-Saharan Africa (JAMA 299:2770, 2008).	**No antiviral treatment.** Effective anti-HIV therapy may help.	Localized lesions: radiotherapy, laser surgery or intralesional chemotherapy. Systemic: chemotherapy. Castleman's disease responded to ganciclovir (Blood 103/1632, 2004) & valganciclovir (JID 2006).
Herpes simplex virus (HSV Types 1 & 2) **Bell's palsy** H. simplex, most implicated etiology. Other etiologic considerations: VZV, HHV-6, Lyme disease.	As soon as possible after onset of palsy: **Prednisone** 1 mg/kg po divided bid x 5 days then taper to 5 mg tid over the next 5 days (total of 10 days prednisone). Alternate: **Prednisone** (dose as above) + **Valacyclovir** 500 mg bid x 5 days	Prospective randomized double blind placebo controlled trial compared prednisolone vs acyclovir vs. (prednisolone + acyclovir) vs placebo. Best result with prednisolone 85% recovery with placebo, 96% recovery with prednisolone. 93% with combination of acyclovir & prednisolone (NEJM 357:1598 & 1653, 2007). **Large meta-analysis confirms: Steroids alone, effective; antiviral drugs alone, not effective: steroids + antiviral drugs, no more effective than steroids alone** (JAMA 302: 985, 2009).
Encephalitis (Excellent reviews: CID 35: 254, 2002; UK experience (EID 9:234, 2003; Eur J Neurol 12:331, 2005; Antiviral Res: 71:141-148, 2006). HSV-1 is most common cause of sporadic encephalitis. 63% survival & recovery normal neurological sequelae dependent on mental status at time of initiation of rx. **Early dx and rx imperative.** NEJM 371:68, 2014.	**Acyclovir** 10 mg/kg IV infuse over 1 hr) q8h x 14-21 days 20 mg/kg q8h in children <12 yrs. Dose calculation in obese patients uncertain. To lessen risk of nephrotoxicity with larger doses seems reasonable to infuse each dose over more than 1 hour. In morbid obesity, use actual body weight.	Mortality rate reduced from >70% to 19% with acyclovir rx. PCR analysis of CSF for HSV-1 DNA is 100% specific & 75–98% sensitive. 8/33 (25%) CSF samples drawn before day 3 were neg. by PCR; neg. PCR assoc. with ↓ protein & < 10 WBC per mm³ in CSF (CID 36:335, 2003). All were + after 3 days. Relapse after successful rx reported in 7/27 (27%) children. Relapse was associated with a lower total dose of initial acyclovir rx (285 ± 82 mg per kg vs 462 ± 149 mg per kg, p <0.03) (CID 30:185, 2000; Neuropediatrics 35:37, 2004). Series in 106 adults J Clin Virol 60:112, 2014.
Genital Herpes: Sexually Transmitted Treatment Guidelines 2010: MMWR 59 (RR-12), 2010. **Primary (initial episode)**	**Acyclovir** (Zovirax or generic) 400 mg po tid x 7–10 days OR **Valacyclovir** (Valtrex) 1000 mg po bid x 7-10 days. OR **Famciclovir** (Famvir) 250 mg po tid x 7-10 days	↓ by 2 days time to resolution of signs & symptoms, ↓ by 4 days time to healing of lesions, ↓ by 7 days duration of viral shedding. Does not prevent recurrences. For severe cases only: 5 mg per kg IV q8h times 5–7 days. An ester of acyclovir, which is well absorbed, bioavailability 3–5 times greater than acyclovir. Metabolized to penciclovir, which is active component. Side effects and activity similar to acyclovir. **Famciclovir 250 mg po bid equal to acyclovir 200 mg 5 times per day.**
Episodic recurrences	**Acyclovir** 800 mg po tid **x 2 days** or 400 mg po tid po bid **x 5 days**, or 800 mg po **bid x 5 days** or **Valacyclovir** 500 mg po bid **x 3 days** or 1 gm po daily **x 5 days** For HIV patients, see Comment	For episodic recurrences in HIV patients: **Acyclovir** 400 mg po tid x 5–10 days or **Famciclovir** 500 mg po bid x 5–10 days or **Valacyclovir** 1 gm po bid x 5–10 days

* See page 2 for abbreviations. NOTE: All dosage recommendations are for adults (unless otherwise indicated) and assume normal renal function.

TABLE 14A (5)

VIRUS/DISEASE	DRUG/DOSAGE	SIDE EFFECTS/COMMENTS
Herpesvirus Infections/Herpes simplex virus (HSV) Types 1 & 2) (continued)		
Chronic daily suppression	Suppressive therapy reduces the frequency of genital herpes recurrences by 70–80% among pts who have frequent recurrences (i.e. >6 recurrences per yr) & many report no symptomatic outbreaks. **acyclovir** 400 mg po bid or tid or **famciclovir** 250 mg po bid or **valacyclovir** 1 gm po q24h and then use per yr or could use 500 mg po q24h if breakthrough at 500 mg. For HIV patients, See Comment	For chronic suppression in HIV patients: (all regimens equally efficacious: Cochrane Database System Rev 8:CD009036, 2014). Suppressive rx with acyclovir (400 mg bid) reduced recurrences of ocular HSV from 32% to 19% (NEJM 339:300, 1998). **acyclovir** 400–800 mg po bid or **famciclovir** 500 mg po bid or **valacyclovir** 500 mg po bid
Genital, immunocompetent		
Gingivostomatitis, primary (children)	**Acyclovir** 15 mg/kg po 5x/day x 7 days	Efficacy in randomized double-blind placebo-controlled trial (BMJ 314:1800, 1997).
Keratoconjunctivitis and recurrent epithelial keratitis	**Trifluridine** (Viroptic), 1 drop 1% solution q2h (max. 9 drops per day) for max. of 21 days (see Table 1, page 13)	
Mollaret's recurrent "aseptic" meningitis (usually HSV-2) (Ln 363:1772, 2004)	No controlled trials of antiviral rx & resolves spontaneously. If therapy is to be given, **acyclovir** (15–30 mg/kg/day IV) or **valacyclovir** 1-2 gm po qid should be used	Pos. PCR for HSV in CSF confirms dx (EJCMID 23:560, 2004). Daily suppression rx might ↓ frequency of recurrence but no clinical trials. Oral Valacyclovir ref: JAC 47:855, 2001.
Mucocutaneous (for genital see previous page) **Normal host**	Start rx with prodrome symptoms (tingling/burning) before lesions appear	Penciclovir (AAC 46: 2848, 2002). Oral acyclovir 5% cream (AAC 46:2238, 2002). Oral fam-ciclovir 5% cream (0.05% Lidex gel) q8h times 5 days in combination with famciclovir (JID 181:1906, 2000). Acyclovir 5% cream + 1% hydrocortisone (Xerese) superior to acyclovir alone (AAC 58:1273, 2014).
Oral labial, "fever blisters": See Ann Pharmacotherapy 38:705, 2004; JAC 53:703, 2004	**Drug** / **Dose** / **Sx Decrease** Oral: **Valacyclovir** 2 gm po q12h x 1 day ↓ 1 day **Famciclovir** 500 mg po bid x 7 days ↓ 2 days **Acyclovir** 400 mg po 5 x per day ↓ ½ day (q4h while awake) x 5 days) Topical: **Penciclovir** 1% cream q2h during day x 4 days ↓ 1 day **Acyclovir** 5% cream 6x/day (q3h) x 7 days ↓ ½ day See Table 1, page 27	
Herpes Whitlow		
Oral labial or genital: Immunocompromised (includes pts with AIDS) and critically ill pts in ICU setting/large necrotic ulcers in perineum or face (See Comment) Primary HSV in pregnancy: increased risk of dissemination, including severe hepatitis. Risk greatest in 3rd trimester (NEJM 370:2211, 2014).	**Acyclovir** 5 mg per kg IV (infused over 1 hr) q8h times 14–21 days. In HIV setting 400 mg po 5 times per day times 14–21 days (see Comment if suspect Acyclovir-resistant) OR **Famciclovir** In HIV infected, 500 mg po bid for 7 days for recurrent episodes of genital herpes **Valacyclovir****: In HIV-infected, 500 mg po bid for 5–10 days for recurrent episodes of genital herpes or 500 mg po bid for chronic suppressive rx.	**Acyclovir-resistant HSV: IV foscarnet** 90 mg/kg IV q12h x 7 days. Suppressive therapy with famciclovir (500 mg po bid), valacyclovir (500 mg po bid) or acyclovir (400–800 mg po bid) reduces viral shedding and clinical recurrences.

² FDA approved only for HIV pts
³ Approved for immunocompromised pts
* See page 2 for abbreviations. NOTE: All dosage recommendations are for adults (unless otherwise indicated) and assume normal renal function.

TABLE 14A (6)

VIRUS/DISEASE	DRUG/DOSAGE	SIDE EFFECTS/COMMENTS
Herpesvirus Infections/ Herpes simplex virus (HSV Types 1 & 2): Mucocutaneous *(continued)*		
Pregnancy and genital H. simplex	Acyclovir safe even in first trimester. No proof that acyclovir at delivery reduces risk/severity of neonatal Herpes. In contrast, C-section in women with active lesions reduces risk of transmission. Ref. *Obstet Gyn 106:845, 2006*	
Herpes simiae (Herpes B virus): **Monkey bite** *CID 35:1191, 2002*	**Postexposure prophylaxis: Valacyclovir** 1 gm po q8h times 14 days or acyclovir 800 mg po 5 times per day times 14 days. **Treatment of disease:** (1) CNS symptoms absent: **Acyclovir** 12.5–15 mg per kg IV q8h or ganciclovir 5 mg per kg IV q12h. (2) CNS symptoms present: **Ganciclovir** 5 mg per kg IV q12h.	Fatal human cases of myelitis and hemorrhagic encephalitis have been reported following bites, scratches, or eye inoculation of saliva from monkeys. Initial sx include fever, headache, myalgias and diffuse adenopathy; incubation period of 2–14 days (*EID 9:246, 2003*). In vitro ACV and Valacyclovir less active than other nucleosides (ganciclovir or 5-ethyldeoxyuridine may be more active; clinical data needed) (*AAC 51:2028, 2007*).
Varicella-Zoster Virus (VZV)		
Varicella: Vaccination has markedly ↓ incidence of varicella & morbidity (*MMWR 61:609, 2012*). Guidelines for VZV vaccine (*MMWR 56(RR-4) 2007*).		
Normal host (chickenpox)		
Child (2–12 years)	**In general, treatment not recommended.** Might use oral **acyclovir** for healthy persons at ↑ risk for moderate to severe varicella, i.e., > 12 yrs of age, chronic cutaneous or pulmonary diseases; chronic salicylate rx (↑ risk of Reye syndrome), **acyclovir** dose: 20 mg/kg po qid x 5 days (start within 24 hrs of rash) or **valacyclovir** 20 mg/kg tid x 5 days.	Acyclovir slowed development and ↓ duration of disease in children; 9 to 7.6 days (*PIDJ 21:739, 2002*). Oral dose of acyclovir in children should not exceed 80 mg per kg per day or 3200 mg per day.
Adolescents, young adults	Start within 24 hrs of rash: **Valacyclovir** 1000 mg po tid x 5–7 days or **Famciclovir** 500 mg po tid (probably effective, but data lacking)	↓ duration of fever, time to healing, and symptoms.
Pneumonia or chickenpox in 3rd trimester of pregnancy	**Acyclovir** 800 mg po 5 times per day or 10 mg per kg IV q8h times 5 days. Risks and benefits to fetus and mother still unknown. Many experts recommend rx, especially in 3rd trimester. Some would add VZIG (varicella-zoster immune globulin).	Varicella pneumonia associated with 41% mortality in pregnancy. Acyclovir ↓ incidence and severity (*JID 185:422, 2002*). If varicella-susceptible mother exposed and respiratory symptoms develop within 10 days after exposure, start acyclovir
Immunocompromised host	**Acyclovir** 10–12 mg per kg (500 mg per M²) IV (infused over 1 hr) q8h times 7 days	Disseminated 1° varicella infection reported during treatment with infliximab rx of rheumatoid arthritis (*J Rheum 31:2517, 2004*). Continuous infusion of high-dose acyclovir (2 mg per kg per hr) successful in 1 pt with severe hemorrhagic varicella (*NEJM 336:732, 1997*).
Prevention—Postexposure prophylaxis Varicella deaths still occur in unvaccinated persons (*MMWR 56 (RR-4) 1-40, 2007*)	**CDC Recommendations for Prevention:** Since <5% of cases of varicella (but >50% of varicella-related deaths occur in adults >20 yrs of age, the CDC recommends a more aggressive approach in this age group: **1st, varicella-zoster immune globulin** (VZIG) (125 units/10 kg (22 lbs) body weight IM up to a max. of 625 units; minimum dose is 125 units) is recommended for postexposure prophylaxis in susceptible persons at greater risk for complications (immunocompromised such as HIV, malignancies, pregnancy, and steroid therapy) as soon as possible after exposure (<96 hrs). If varicella develops, initiate treatment quickly (<24 hrs of rash) with **acyclovir** as below. Many would rx presumptively with acyclovir in high-risk pts. **2nd,** susceptible adults should be vaccinated. Check antibody in adults with negative or uncertain history of varicella (10–30% will be AB-neg), and vaccinate those who are Ab-neg. **3rd,** susceptible children should receive vaccination. Recommended routinely before age 12–18 mos. but OK at any age.	

* See page 2 for abbreviations. NOTE: All dosage recommendations are for adults (unless otherwise indicated) and assume normal renal function.

TABLE 14A (7)

VIRUS/DISEASE	DRUG/DOSAGE	SIDE EFFECTS/COMMENTS
Herpes zoster (shingles) (See NEJM 369:255, 2013) **Normal host** • Effective therapy most evident in pts >50 yrs *(For treatment of post-herpetic neuralgia, see CID 36: 877, 2003; Ln 374:1252, 2009)* • Vaccination; herpes zoster & post-herpetic neuralgia (NEJM 352: 2271, 2005; JAMA 292:157, 2006). Reviewed in J Am Acad Derm 58:361, 2008 • Analgesics for acute pain associated with Herpes zoster (NEJM 369:255, 2013)	**[NOTE: Trials showing benefit of therapy: only in pts treated within 3 days of onset of rash]** **Valacyclovir** 1000 mg po tid times 7 days (adjust dose for renal failure) (See Table 17A) **OR** **Famciclovir** 500 mg po tid x 7 days. Adjust for renal failure (see Table 17A) **OR** **Acyclovir** 800 mg po 5 times per day times 7-10 days Add **Prednisone** in pts over 50 yrs old to decrease discomfort during acute phase of zoster. Does not decrease incidence of post-herpetic neuralgia. Dose: 30 mg po bid days 1-7, 15 mg bid days 8-14 and 7.5 mg bid days 15-21.	Increasing recognition of risk of stroke during 6 mos after episode of Shingles. Oral antivirals during clinical H. zoster infection may have protective effect (CID 58: 1497, 1504, 2014). VZV found in wall of cerebral and temporal arteries of pts with giant cell arteritis (Neurology 84:1948, 2015; JID 51:537, 2015). Time to healing more rapid. Reduced incidence of post-herpetic neuralgia (PHN) vs placebo in pts >50 yrs of age. Famciclovir similar to acyclovir in reduction of acute pain and incidence of PHN (J Micro Immunol Inf 37:75, 2004). A meta-analysis of 4 placebo-controlled trials (691 ptts): acyclovir accelerated by approx. 2-fold pain resolution and reduced incidence of post-herpetic neuralgia at 3 & 6 mos (CID 22:341, 1996); med. time to resolution of pain 41 days vs 101 days in those > 50 yrs. In post-herpetic neuralgia, controlled trials demonstrated effectiveness of **gabapentin**, the **lidocaine patch** (5%) & **opioid analgesic** in controlling pain (Drugs 64:937, 2004; J Clin Virol 29:248, 2004). **Nortriptyline & amitriptyline** are equally effective but nortriptyline is better tolerated (CID 36:877, 2003). Role of antiviral drugs in rx of PHN unproven (Neurol 64:21, 2005) but 8 of 15 pt improved with IV acyclovir 10 mg/kg q 8 hrs x 14 days followed by oral valacyclovir 1 gm 3x a day for 1 month (Arch Neur 63:940, 2006). Review: NEJM 371:1526, 2014; Expert Opin Pharmacotherapy 15:61, 2014
Immunocompromised host Not severe	**Acyclovir** 800 mg po 5 times per day times 7 days. **(Options: Famciclovir** 750 mg po q24h or 500 mg bid or 250 mg 3 times per day times 7 days **OR valacyclovir** 1000 mg po tid times 7 days, though both are not FDA-approved for this indication)	If progression, switch to IV. RA pts on TNF-alpha inhibitors at high risk for VZV. Zoster more severe, but less post-herpetic neuralgia (JAMA 301:737, 2009).
Severe: >1 dermatome, trigeminal nerve or disseminated	**Acyclovir** 10-12 mg po/kg IV (infusion over 1 hr) q8h times 7-10 days. In older pts, ↓ to 7.5 mg per kg q8h. If nephrotoxicity and pt improving, ↓ to 5 mg per kg q8h.	A common manifestation of immune reconstitution following HAART in HIV-infected children (J All Clin Immun 113:742, 2004). Rx must be begun within 72 hrs. For Acyclovir-resistant VZV in HIV+ pts previously treated with acyclovir: **Foscarnet** (40 mg per kg IV q8h for 14-26 days).
Human T-cell Leukotrophic Virus-1 (HTLV-1) Causes illness in only 5% of infected persons. Two are associated with HTLV-1: Adult T-cell leukemia/lymphoma (NEJM 367:552, 2012) and HTLV-1-associated myelopathy (HAM), also known as tropical spastic paraparesis (TSP).	No proven therapy. Some nucleoside antiretroviral therapies used with limited success	Laboratory diagnosis is by blood and CSF. Anti-HTLV-1 antibodies are detected by ELISA antibody testing. Western Blot is used for confirmation (Focus Diagnostics or Quest Diagnostics). HTLV DNA can be detected by PCR in circulating CD4 cells. One tube multiplex qPCR highly specific / sensitive (Retrovirology 11(Suppl): P105, 2014).

TABLE 14A (8)

Influenza A & B and novel influenza viruses Refs: *http://www.cdc.gov/flu/professionals/antivirals/index.htm http://www.cdc.gov/flu/weekly/; NEJM 370:789, 2014. Vaccine Info (http://www.cdc.gov/flu/professionals/acip/index.htm); Med Lett 56:97, 2014; MMWR 63:691, 2014.*

- **Oseltamivir and zanamivir are recommended drugs.** Amantadine and rimantadine should not be used because of widespread resistance.
  - Novel H1N1 (referred to as pandemic H1N1, pH1N1, H1N1pdm and formerly swine flu) emerged in 2009 and now is the dominant H1N1 strain worldwide. Old distinction from seasonal H1N1 is still sometimes used but not relevant
- Rapid influenza tests are can be falsely negative in 20-50%. PCR is gold standard test.
- Initiate therapy as close to the onset of symptoms as possible, and certainly within 48 hrs of onset of symptoms. Starting therapy after 48 hours of onset of symptoms is associated with reduced therapeutic benefit. However, starting therapy up to 5 days after onset in patients who are hospitalized is associated with improved survival (*Clin Infect Dis 55:1198, 2012*).
- Empiric therapy should be started for all patients who are hospitalized, have severe or progressive influenza or are at higher risk of complications due to age or underlying medical conditions.
- Look for concomitant bacterial pneumonia.
- Other important influenza viruses causing human disease
  - **H3N2v influenza:** 159 cases of influenza A/H3N2v reported over the summer of 2012. Most of the cases of influenza A/H3N2v occurred in children under the age of 10 with direct contact with pigs. This variant is susceptible to the neuraminidase inhibitors, oseltamivir and zanamivir. See MMWR 61:619, 2012.
  - **Avian influenza H5N1:** Re-emerged in Asia in 2003 and human cases detected in 15 countries mostly in Asia as well as Egypt, Nigeria and Djibouti. Circulation associated with massive poultry die off. Imported cases rare – one in Canada. As of January 2014, 648 confirmed cases and 384 deaths (59%). Human infection associated with close contact with poultry; very limited human to human transmission. Mortality associated with high viral load, disseminated virus and high cytokine activity (*Nature Medicine 12:1203-1207 2006*). Sensitive to oseltamivir but oseltamivir resistance has emerged on therapy (*NEJM 353:267-272 2005*). Use oseltamivir and consider IV zanamivir
  - **Avian influenza H7N9:** Emerged in Eastern China in March 2013 and 132 cases documented during Spring 2013 with 44 deaths (33%). Cases appeared again in early winter 2013-2014 and continue to increase. Infection associated with close contact with live bird markets, extremely limited human to human transmission to date. Mortality highest among older persons and those with medical conditions. Oseltamivir active against most but not all strains. No zanamivir resistance documented to date.

Virus/Disease	Susceptible to: (Recommended Drug/Dosage):	Resistant to:	Alternatives/Side Effects/Comments
A/H1N1 (current seasonal resembles pandemic H1N1) Influenza B Influenza A (A/H3N2, A/H3N2v*, A/H5N1, A/H7N9**)	**Oseltamivir** Adult: Oseltamivir 75 mg po bid x 5 days Pediatric (child age 1-12 years): Infant 2 wks–11 months: 3 mg/kg bid x 5 days ≤15 kg: 30 mg bid x 5 days >15 kg to 23 kg: 45 mg bid x 5 days >23 kg to 40 kg: 60 mg bid x 5 days >40 kg: 75 mg bid x 5 days **or** **Zanamivir** 2 inhalations (5 mg each) bid x 5 days or Peramivir 600 mg IV once daily x 5–10 days For IV Zanamivir, see Comment	Amantadine and rimantadine (100%) * A/H3N2v strain are susceptible ** A/H7N9 resistant to oseltamivir (rarely)	- **A/H1N1:** Higher dose (150 mg bid) **not** more effective for H1N1 - **Zanamivir** not recommended for children < 7 years or those with reactive airway disease - **IV zanamivir** is available under compassionate use IND and clinical trials for hospitalized influenza patients with suspected or known gastric stasis, gastric malabsorption, gastrointestinal bleeding, or for patients suspected or confirmed with oseltamivir-resistant influenza virus infection. For compassionate use, contact GlaxoSmithKline at (+1) 919-315-5215 or email: gskclinicalsupportHD@GSK.com. - **Influenza B:** One study suggested virologic benefit to higher dose oseltamivir for critically ill patients with influenza B. - **A/H5N1:** Given high mortality, consider obtaining investigational drug. Zanamivir retains activity against most oseltamivir resistant H5N1 - Association between corticosteroid rx & increased mortality (*JID 212:183, 2015*). For now, avoid steroids unless indicated for another reason.

* See page 2 for abbreviations. NOTE: All dosage recommendations are for adults (unless otherwise indicated) and assume normal renal function.

TABLE 14A (9)

VIRUS/DISEASE	DRUG/DOSAGE	SIDE EFFECTS/COMMENTS
Measles Increasing reports of measles in unvaccinated children and adults (MMWR 63:781, 2014; NEJM 371:358, 2014).		
Children	No therapy or **vitamin A** 200,000 units po daily times 2 days	Vitamin A may ↓ severity of measles.
Adults	No rx or **ribavirin** IV: 20–35 mg per kg per day times 7 days	↓ severity of illness in adults (CID 20:454, 1994).
Metapneumovirus (HMPV) A paramyxovirus isolated from pts of all ages, with mild bronchiolitis/bronchospasm to pneumonia. Review: Sem Resp Crit Care Med 32:447, 2011.	**No proven antiviral therapy** (intravenous ribavirin used anecdotally with variable results) Investigational Agents Reviewed (Clin Vaccine Immunol 22:8 & 858, 2015)	Human metapneumovirus isolated from 6–21% of children with RTIs (NEJM 350:443, 2004). Dual infection with RSV assoc. with severe bronchiolitis (JID 191:382, 2005).
Monkey pox (orthopox virus) (see LnID 4:17, 2004) Outbreak from contact with ill prairie dogs. Source likely imported Gambian giant rats (CID 58:260, 2014)	**No proven antiviral therapy.** Cidofovir is active in vitro & in mouse model	Incubation period of 12 days, then fever, headache, cough, adenopathy, & a vesicular papular rash that pustulates, umbilicates, & crusts on the head, trunk, & extremities. Transmission in healthcare setting rare.
Norovirus (Norwalk-like virus, or NLV) Vast majority of outbreaks of non-bacterial gastroenteritis (NEJM 368:1121, 2013).	**No antiviral therapy.** Replete volume. Transmission by contaminated food, fecal-oral contact with contaminated surfaces, or fomites.	Sudden onset of nausea, vomiting, and/or watery diarrhea lasting 12–60 hours. Ethanol-based hand rubs effective (J Hosp Inf 60:144, 2005).
Papillomaviruses: Warts **External Genital Warts** Also look for warts in anal canal (MMWR 64(3):1, 2015)	**Patient applied:** **Podofilox** (0.5% solution or gel): apply 2x/day x 3 days, 4th day no therapy, repeat cycle 4x; OR **Imiquimod** 5% cream: apply once daily 3x/wk for up to 16 wks. **Sinecatechins** Apply to external genital warts only 3x/day until effect or adverse effect **Provider administered:** Cryotherapy with liquid nitrogen: repeat q1-2 wks; OR **Trichloroacetic acid** (TCA): repeat weekly as needed; OR surgical removal.	**Podofilox:** Inexpensive and safe (pregnancy safety not established). Mild irritation after treatment. **Imiquimod:** Mild to moderate redness & irritation. Topical imiquimod effective for treatment of vulvar intraepithelial neoplasms (NEJM 358:1465, 2008). Safety in pregnancy not established. **Sinecatechins:** Local irritation, redness, pain, and itching **Cryotherapy:** Blistering and skin necrosis common. **Podophyllin resin:** No longer recommended as other less toxic regimens available. **TCA:** Caustic. Can cause severe pain on adjacent normal skin. Neutralize with soap or sodium bicarbonate.
Warts on cervix	Need evaluation for evolving neoplasia	Gynecological consult advised
Vaginal warts	Cryotherapy with liquid nitrogen or **TCA**	
Urethral warts	Cryotherapy with liquid nitrogen	
Anal warts	Cryotherapy with liquid nitrogen or **TCA** or surgical removal	Advise anoscopy to look for rectal warts.
Skin papillomas	**Topical α-lactalbumin**. **Oleic acid** (from human milk) applied 1x/day for 3 wks	↓ lesion size & recurrence vs placebo (p <0.001) (NEJM 350:2663, 2004). Further studies warranted.

*See page 2 for abbreviations. NOTE: All dosage recommendations are for adults (unless otherwise indicated) and assume normal renal function.

TABLE 14A (10)

VIRUS/DISEASE	DRUG/DOSAGE	SIDE EFFECTS/COMMENTS
Parvo B19 Virus (Erythrovirus B19). *Review: NEJM 350:586, 2004. Wide range of manifestation.* **Treatment options for common symptomatic infections:**		
Erythema infectiosum	Symptomatic treatment only	Diagnostic tools: IgM and Igb antibody titers. Perhaps better: blood parvovirus PCR.
Arthritis/arthralgia	Nonsteroidal anti-inflammatory drugs (NSAID)	Dose of IVIG not standardized; suggest 400 mg/kg IV of commercial IVIG daily x 5 days, or 1 gm/kg IV x 3 days.
Transient aplastic crisis	Transfusions and oxygen	Most dramatic anemias in pts with pre-existing hemolytic anemia.
Fetal hydrops	Intrauterine blood transfusion	Bone marrow shows erythrocyte maturation arrest with giant pronormoblasts. *(Rev Med Virol 25:224, 2015)*
Chronic infection with anemia	**IVIG** and transfusion *(CID 56:968, 2013)* For dose, see Comment	
Chronic infection without anemia	Perhaps **IVIG**	
Papovavirus/Polyomavirus		
Progressive multifocal leukoencephalopathy (PML)	No specific therapy for JC virus. Two general approaches:	Failure of treatment with interferon alfa-2b, cytarabine and topotecan. Immunosuppressive **natalizumab** temporarily removed from market due to reported associations with PML. Most likely
Serious demyelinating disease due to JC virus in immunocompromised pts.	1. In HIV pts: HAART. Cidofovir may be effective. 2. Stop or decrease immunosuppressive therapy.	effective on **cidofovir**. Mixed reports on **cidofovir**.
BK virus induced nephropathy in immunocompromised pts and hemorrhagic cystitis	Decrease immunosuppression if possible. Suggested antiviral therapy based on anecdotal data. If progressive renal dysfunction: 1. **Fluoroquinolone** first; 2. **IVIG** 500 mg/kg IV; 3. **Leflunomide** 100 mg po daily x 3 days, then 10-20 mg po daily; 4. **Cidofovir** only if refractory to all of the above *(see Table 14B for dose)*.	Use PCR to monitor viral "load" in urine and/or plasma. Report of cidofovir as potentially effective for BK hemorrhagic cystitis *(CID 49:233, 2009).*
Rabies *(see Table 20B, page 233; diagnosis and management)*		
Rabid dogs account for 50,000 cases per yr worldwide. Most cases in the U.S. are cryptic; 70% assoc. with 2 rare bat species *(EID 9:151, 2003).* An organ donor with early rabies infected 4 recipients (2 kidneys, liver & artery) all died avg. 13 days after transplant *(NEJM 352:1103, 2005)*	No specific therapy for JC virus. Two general approaches: **Mortality 100% with only survivors those who receive rabies vaccine before the onset of illness/symptoms** *(CID 36:61, 2003).* A 15-year-old female who developed rabies 1 month post-bat bite survived after drug induction of coma (+ other rx) for 7 days; did not receive immunoprophylaxis *(NEJM 352:2508, 2005).* For post-exposure prophylaxis: www.cdc.gov/rabies	Corticosteroids ↑ mortality rate and ↓ incubation time in mice. Therapies that have failed after symptoms develop include rabies vaccine, rabies immunoglobulin, rabies virus neutralizing antibody, ribavirin, alfa interferon, & ketamine. For post-exposure prophylaxis, see Table 20B, page 233.
Respiratory Syncytial Virus (RSV)	All ages: Hydration, O₂ as needed. If wheezing, trial of beta-agonist.	In adults, RSV accounted for 10.6% of hospitalizations for pneumonia, 11.4%
Major cause of morbidity in neonates/infants.	Corticosteroids: children-no; adults-maybe	of AECB, 7.2% for asthma & 5.4% for CHF in pts >65 yrs of age *(NEJM
Treatment of RSV	**Nebulized Ribavirin**: no benefit in children, adults *(CID 57:1731, 2013).*	352:1749, 2005).* RSV caused 11% of clinically important respiratory illnesses
Prevention of RSV *(1)*	**Nebulized Ribavirin + RSV immune globulin:** immunocompromised adults *(HSCT) (CID 56:258, 2013).*	in military recruits *(CID 41:311, 2005)*
(1) Children <24 mos. old with chronic lung disease of prematurity (formerly bronchopulmonary dysplasia) requiring supplemental O₂,or	**Palivizumab** (Synagis) 15 mg per kg IM q month Nov-Apr. *See Pediatrics 126:e16, 2010.*	Expense argues against its use. Guidance from the Academy of Pediatrics recommends use of Palivizumab only in newborn infants born at 29 weeks gestation (or earlier) and in special populations (e.g., those infants with
(2) Premature infants (<32 wks gestation) and <6 mos. old at start of RSV season or		significant heart disease) *(Pediatrics 2014;134:415-420)*
(3) Children with selected congenital heart diseases		

* See page 2 for abbreviations. NOTE: All dosage recommendations are for adults (unless otherwise indicated) and assume normal renal function.

TABLE 14A (11)

VIRUS/DISEASE	DRUG/DOSAGE	SIDE EFFECTS/COMMENTS
Respiratory Syncytial Virus (RSV) *(continued)*		
Rhinovirus (Colds) See *Ln 361:51, 2003* Found in 1/2 of children with community-acquired pneumonia, role in pathogenesis unclear *(CID 39:681, 2004).* High rate of rhinovirus identified in children with significant lower resp tract infections *(Ped Int Dis 28:337, 2009)*	No antiviral rx indicated *(Ped Ann 34:53, 2005).* Symptomatic rx: • **Ipratropium bromide** nasal (2 sprays per nostril tid) • **Clemastine** 1.34 mg 1–2 tab po bid–tid (OTC). • Oral zinc preparations reduce duration of symptoms by ~ 1 day; does not reduce severity of symptoms *(JAMA 311:1440, 2014).* Avoid intranasal zinc products *(see Comment).*	Sx relief: ipratropum nasal spray ↓ rhinorrhea and sneezing vs placebo *(AviM 125:89, 1996).* Clemastine (an antihistamine) ↓ sneezing, rhinorrhea but associated with dry nose, mouth & throat in 6–19% *(CID 22:656, 1996).* **Echinacea** didn't work *(CID 38:1367, 2004 & 40:807, 2005)*—put to rest! Public health advisory advising that three over-the-counter cold remedy products containing **zinc** (e.g., Zicam) should not be used because of multiple reports of permanent anosmia *(www.fda.gov/Safety/MedWatch/Safety/Information/ SafetyAlertsforHumanMedicalProducts/ucm166996.htm).*
Rotavirus: Leading recognized cause of diarrhea-related illness among infants and children worldwide and kills ½ million children annually.	**No antiviral rx available;** oral hydration life-saving.	**Two live-attenuated vaccines highly effective (85 and 98%)** and safe in preventing rotavirus diarrhea and hospitalization *(NEJM 354: 1 & 23, 2006).* ACIP recommends either of the two vaccines, RV1 or RV5, for infants *(MMWR 58(RR02): 1, 2009).*
Smallpox *(NEJM 346:1300, 2002).*	Smallpox vaccine (if within 4 days of exposure) + cidofovir (dosage uncertain but likely similar to CMV (5 mg/kg IV once weekly for 2 weeks followed by once weekly dosing. Must be used with hydration and Probenecid. *contact CDC: 770-488-7100.*	
Contact vaccinia: See page 167	From vaccination. Progressive vaccinia—vaccinia immune globulin may be of benefit. To obtain immune globulin, contact CDC: 770-488-7100. *(CID 39:759, 776 & 819, 2004)*	
West Nile virus: See page 167		
Zika Virus: Mosquito (Aedes sp.) transmitted flavivirus CDC Interim Guidance: *MMWR 65:30, January 22, 2016.* Travel advisory for pregnant women.	No treatment available. Symptomatic support (avoid aspirin, NSAIDs until Dengue ruled out Most serious manifestation of infection is **congenital birth defect(s)**: microcephaly and fetal demise	3–7 day incubation. Asymptomatic infection most often; when symptoms occur, usually consists of low grade fever, arthralgias, morbilliform rash, and / or conjunctival redness (non-purulent conjunctivitis). Duration of symptoms ranges from a few days to one week. Rare Guillain-Barré syndrome. Hospitalization very infrequent, fatalities are very rare.

TABLE 14B – ANTIVIRAL DRUGS (NON-HIV)

DRUG NAME(S) GENERIC (TRADE)	DOSAGE/ROUTE IN ADULTS*	COMMENTS/ADVERSE EFFECTS
CMV (See SANFORD GUIDE TO HIV/AIDS THERAPY)		
Cidofovir (Vistide)	5 mg per kg IV, once weekly for 2 weeks, then once every other week. **Properly timed IV prehydration with normal saline & Probenecid must be used with each cidofovir infusion:** 2 gm po 3 hrs before each dose and further 1 gm given 2 & 8 hrs after completion of the cidofovir infusion. Renal function (serum creatinine and urine protein) must be monitored prior to each dose (see *pkg insert for details*). Contraindicated if creatinine >1.5 mg/dL, CrCl ≤55 mL/min or urine protein ≥ 100 mg/dL.	**Adverse effects: Nephrotoxicity:** dose-dependent proximal tubular injury (Fanconi-like syndrome): proteinuria, glycosuria, bicarbonaturia, phosphaturia, polyuria, nephrogenic diabetic insipidus; ↑ creatinine. Concomitant saline prehydration, probenecid, extended dosing intervals allow use but still highly nephrotoxic. Other major toxicities: neutropenia (give G-CSF as needed); even monthly intra-ocular pressure. Dc cidofovir if pressure decreases 50% or uveitis occurs. **Black Box warning.** Renal impairment can occur after ≤2 doses. Contraindicated in pts receiving concomitant nephrotoxic agents. Monitor for ↓ WBC. In animals, carcinogenic, teratogenic (causes ↓ sperm and ↓ fertility). FDA indication only CMV retinitis in HIV pts. **Comment:** Dose must be reduced or discontinued if changes in renal function occur during rx. For ↑ of 0.3-0.4 mg per dL in serum creatinine, cidofovir dose must be ↓ from 5 to 3 mg per kg; discontinue cidofovir if ↑ of 0.5 mg per dL above baseline or 3+ proteinuria develops (for 2+ proteinuria, observe pts carefully and consider discontinuation).
Foscarnet (Foscavir)	Induction: 90 mg per kg IV, over 1.5-2 hours, q12h **OR** 60 mg per kg IV, over 1 hour, q8h Maintenance: 90 –120 mg per kg IV, over 2 hours, q24h Dosage adjustment with renal dysfunction.	Use infusion pump to control rate of administration. **Adverse effects: Major toxicity is renal impairment (1/3 of patients).** Can cause infusion-related ionized hypocalcemia: manifests as arrhythmia, tetany, paresthesia, changes in mental status. Slow infusion rate and avoid drugs that lower Ca++, e.g., pentamidine. --↑ creatinine, proteinuria, nephrogenic diabetes insipidus, ↓K+, ↓Ca++, ↓Mg++. Adequate hydration may ↓ toxicity. Other: headache, mild (100%), fatigue (100%), fever (25%), nausea (80%). Hemato↓ WBC, ↓ Hgb. Hepatic: liver function tests ↑. Neuropathy. Penile and oral ulcers.
Ganciclovir (Cytovene)	IV: 5 mg per kg q12h times 14 days (induction) 5 mg per kg IV q24h or 6 mg per kg 5 times per wk (maintenance) Dosage adjust. with renal dysfunction (see *Table 17A*)	**Adverse effects: Black Box warnings:** mutagenic, carcinogenic/teratogenic & aspermia in animals. Absolute neutrophil count dropped below 500 per mm³ in 15%, thrombocytopenia 21%, anemia 6%. Fever 48%. GI 50%: nausea, vomiting, diarrhea, abdominal pain 19%, rash 10%. Confusion, headache, psychiatric disturbances and seizures. Neutropenia may respond to granulocyte colony stimulating factor (G-CSF) or GM-CSF). Severe myelosuppression may be ↑ with coadministration of zidovudine or azathioprine 32% dc/interrupted rx, principally for neutropenia. Avoid extravasation.
Valganciclovir (Valcyte)	450 mg tablets; take with food. Oral solution: 50 mg/mL. Adult dose 900 mg. Treatment (induction): 900 mg po q12h with food. Prophylaxis (maintenance): 900 mg po q24h. Dosage adjustment for renal dysfunction (See *Table 17A*).	A prodrug of ganciclovir with better bioavailability than oral ganciclovir. 60% with food. Preg cat: C (may be teratogenic, contraceptive precaution for females). **Adverse effects:** Similar to ganciclovir. May cause dose limiting neutropenia, anemia, thrombocytopenia. Diarrhea (16-41%), nausea (8-30%), vomiting (3-21%). **CMV retinitis** (sight-threatening lesions): 900 mg po q12h + intravitreal Ganciclovir: 900 mg q12h x 14-21 days, then 900 mg po q24h for maintenance
Herpesvirus Acyclovir (Zovirax) or generic	Doses: see *Table 14A* for various indications 400 mg or 800 mg tab 200 mg cap Suspension 200 mg per 5 mL Ointment or cream 5% IV injection Dosage adjustment for renal dysfunction (See *Table 17A*).	**po:** Generally well-tolerated with occ. diarrhea, vertigo, arthralgia. Less frequent rash, fatigue, insomnia, fever, menstrual abnormalities, acne, sore throat, muscle cramps, lymphadenopathy. **IV:** Phlebitis, caustic with vesicular lesions → obstructive uropathy (rapid infusion, dehydration, renal insufficiency and ↑ dose ↑ risk). Adequate pre-hydration may prevent such nephrotoxicity. Hepatic: ↑ ALT, AST. Uncommon: neutropenia, rash, diaphoresis, hypotension, headache, nausea. **Neurotoxicity:** hallucination, death delusions, involuntary movements. To avoid, lower dose if renal impairment (AJM 128, 692, 2015).

See page 2 for abbreviations. NOTE: All dosage recommendations are for adults (unless otherwise indicated) and assume normal renal/renal function.

TABLE 14B (2)

DRUG NAME(S) GENERIC (TRADE)	DOSAGE/ROUTE IN ADULTS*	COMMENTS/ADVERSE EFFECTS
Herpesvirus *(continued)*		
Famciclovir (Famvir)	125 mg, 250 mg, 500 mg tabs Dosage depends on indication *(see label and Table 14A).*	Metabolized to penciclovir. **Adverse effects:** similar to acyclovir, included headache, nausea, diarrhea, and dizziness, but incidence does not differ from placebo. May be taken without regard to meals. Dose should be reduced if CrCl <60 mL per min *(see package insert & Table 17A, page 169 & Table 17A, page 225).*
Penciclovir (Denavir) Trifluridine (Viroptic)	Topical 1% cream. Topical 1% solution: 1 drop q2h (max. 9 drops/day) until corneal re-epithelialization, then dose is ↓ for 7 more days (one drop q4h for at least 5 drops/day), not to exceed 21 days total rx.	May be taken with or without food. Apply to area of recurrence of herpes labialis with start of sx, then q2h while awake times 4 days. Well tolerated. Mild burning (5%), palpebral edema (3%), punctate keratopathy, stromal edema. For HSV keratoconjunctivitis or recurrent epithelial keratitis.
Valacyclovir (Valtrex)	500 mg, 1 gm tabs Dosage depends on indication and renal function *(see label, Table 14A & Table 17A).*	An ester pro-drug of acyclovir that is well-absorbed, bioavailability 3–5 times greater than acyclovir. **Adverse effects** similar to acyclovir. Thrombotic thrombocytopenic purpura/hemolytic uremic syndrome reported in pts with advanced HIV disease and transplant recipients participating in clinical trials at doses of 8 gm per day. Death delusion with high serum levels.
Valganciclovir (Valcyte)	450 mg tablets; take with food. Oral solution: 50 mg/mL. Adult dose 900 mg (Treatment induction): 900 mg po q12h with food: 900 mg (maintenance): 900 mg po q24h Dosage adjustment for renal dysfunction *(See Table 17A).*	A prodrug of ganciclovir. May cause dose limiting neutropenia, anemia, thrombocytopenia. Ganciclovir with better bioavailability than oral ganciclovir. 60% with food. Preg Cat: C (may be teratogenic, contraceptive precaution for females). **Adverse effects:** Similar to ganciclovir. Diarrhea (16–41%), nausea (8–30%), vomiting (3–21%). Acute renal failure may occur. **CMV retinitis** (sight-threatening lesions): 900 mg po q12h ÷ intravitreal Ganciclovir: 900 mg po q12h x 14–21 days, then 900 mg po q24h for maintenance
Hepatitis B Adefovir dipivoxil (Hepsera)	10 mg po q24h (with normal CrCl) 10 mg tab	It is an acyclic nucleotide analog with activity against hepatitis B (HBV) at 0.2–2.5 mM (IC₅₀). *See Table 5 for Cmax, &* IC_{50}. Active against lamivudine-resistant HBV strains and in vitro vs. entecavir- resistant strains. To minimize resistance: use in combination with treatment. For lamivudine-resistant lamivudine/adefovir therapy if viral load remains >1000 copies/mL when starting treatment. Primarily renal excretion—adjust dose. No food interactions. Generally few side effects, but **Black Box warning** regarding lactic acidosis/hepatic steatosis with nucleoside analogs. At risks for renal impairment, esp. in pts with pre-existing renal dysfunction. Monitor renal function, and other risks for renal impairment *(see Table 17A, page 224)*. **Hepatitis may exacerbate when treatment discontinued:** Up to 25% of pts developed ALT ↑ times normal within 12 wks; usually responds to re-treatment or self-limited, but hepatic decompensation has occurred. **Do not use adefovir in HIV infected patients**
Entecavir (Baraclude)	0.5 mg q24h, if refractory or resistant to lamivudine or telbivudine. 1 mg per day. Tabs: 0.5 mg & 1 mg. Oral solution: 0.05 mg/mL. Administer on an empty stomach.	A nucleoside analog active against HBV including lamivudine-resistant mutants. Minimal adverse effects reported: headache, fatigue, dizziness, & nausea reported in 22% of pts. Alopecia, anaphylactoid reactions reported. **Black Box warning** regarding lactic acidosis and exacerbation of HepB at discontinuation **(Black Box warning).** Do not use as single anti-retroviral agent in HIV/HBV co-infected pts, M184 mutation can emerge *(NEJM 356:2614, 2007)*. Adjust dose in renal impairment *(see Table 17A, page 224).*
Lamivudine (3TC) (Epivir-HBV)	HBV dose: 100 mg po q24h Dosage adjustment with renal dysfunction *(see label).* Tabs 100 mg and oral solution 5 mg/mL.	**Black Box warnings:** caution, dose is lower than HIV dose. So must include co-infection with HIV before using this formulation; lactic acidosis/hepatic steatosis; severe exacerbation of liver disease can occur on d/c. YMDD-mutants resistant to lamivudine may emerge on treatment. **Adverse effects:** See Table 14C.
Telbivudine (Tyzeka)	HBV: 600 mg orally q24h, without regard to food Dosage adjustment with renal dysfunction. Ccr < 50 mL/min *(see label).* 600 mg tabs; 100 mg per 5 mL solution.	Oral nucleoside analog approved for Rx of Hep B. It has ↑ rates of response and superior viral suppression than lamivudine *(NEJM 357:2576, 2007)*. **Black Box warnings** regarding lactic acidosis/hepatic steatosis with nucleosides and potential for severe exacerbation of HepB on d/c. Generally well-tolerated but ↑ mitochondrial toxicity vs other nucleosides. Dose limiting toxicity observed *(Medical Letter 49:11, 2007)*. Myalgias, myopathy and rhabdomyolysis reported. Peripheral neuropathy. Genotypic resistance rate was 4.4% by one yr, 21.6% by 2 yrs of rx at eKg+ pts. Selects for YMDD mutation like lamivudine. Combination with lamivudine was inferior to monotherapy *(Hepatology 45:507, 2007).*
Tenofovir (TDF/TAF)	See page 193	

*See page 2 for abbreviations. NOTE: All dosage recommendations are for adults (unless otherwise indicated) and assume normal renal function.

DRUG NAME(S) GENERIC (TRADE)	DOSAGE/ROUTE IN ADULTS*	COMMENTS/ADVERSE EFFECTS
Hepatitis C		
Daclatasvir (Daklinza)	60 mg 1 tab po once daily (dose adjustment when used with CYP 3A4 inhibitors / inducers)	Contraindicated with strong CYP3A inducers, e.g., phenytoin, carbamazepine, Rifampin, St. John's wort. Most common AE: headache and fatigue. Bradycardia when administered in combination with Sofosbuvir and Amiodarone **Co-administration with Amiodarone not recommended.** If used, cardiac monitoring advised.
Interferon alfa is available as alfa-2a (Roferon-A), alfa-2b (Intron-A)	For HCV combination therapy, usual Roferon-A and Intron-A doses are 3 million international units 3x weekly subQ.	Depending on agent, available in pre-filled syringes, vials of solution, or powder. **Black Box warnings:** (can cause/aggravate psychiatric illness; autoimmune disorders, ischemic events, infection. Withdraw therapy if any of these sustained.) A **flu-like syndrome** is common, esp. during 1st wk of rx: fever 98%, fatigue 89%, myalgia 73%, headache 71%. **Adverse effects: Git:** anorexia 46%, diarrhea 29%. **CNS:** dizziness 21%. Hemorrhagic or ischemic stroke. Rash 18%, may progress to Stevens-Johnson or exfoliative dermatitis. Alopecia. ↑ TSH, autoimmune thyroid disorders with ↓- or ↑- thyroidism. **Hemat:** ↓ WBC 49%, ↓ Hgb 27%, ↓ platelets 35%. Post-marketing reports of antibody-mediated pure red cell aplasia in patients receiving interferon/ribavirin with erythropoiesis-stimulating agents.
PEG interferon alfa-2b (PEG-Intron)	0.5-1.5 mcg/kg subQ q wk	
Pegylated-40k interferon alfa-2a (Pegasys)	180 mcg subQ q wk	Acute reversible hearing loss &/or tinnitus in up to 1/3 (*Ln 343:1134, 1994*). Optic neuropathy (retinal hemorrhage, cotton wool spots, ↓ in color vision) reported (*AIDS 18:1805, 2004*). Doses may require adjustment (or dc) based on individual response or adverse events, and can vary by product, indication (eg, HCV or HBV) and mode of use (mono- or combination-rx). (Refer to labels of individual products and to ribavirin if used in combination for details of use.)
Ledipasvir + Sofosbuvir (Harvoni)	Combination formulation (Ledipasvir 90 mg + Sofosbuvir 400 mg) 1 tab po once daily	NS5A/NS5B inhibitor combination for Genotype 1 HCV. First agent for HCV treatment without Ribavirin or Interferon. No adjustment for mild/moderate renal or hepatic impairment. Most common AEs: fatigue (16%), headache (14%), nausea (7%), diarrhea (7%), insomnia (5%). Antacids and H2 blockers interfere with absorption of ledipasvir. The drug solubility decreases as pH increases. Recommended to separate administration of ledipasvir and antacid Rx by at least 4 hours.
Ribavirin (Rebetol, Copegus)	For use with an interferon for hepatitis C. Available as 200 mg caps and 40 mg/mL oral solution (Rebetol) or 200 mg and 400 mg tabs (Copegus) (See Comments regarding dosage).	**Black Box warnings:** ribavirin monotherapy of HCV is ineffective; hemolytic anemia may precipitate cardiac events; teratogenic/embryocidal (**Preg Category X**). Drug may persist for 6 mos. avoid pregnancy for 6 mos after end of use in women or their partners. Only approved Rx for pts with severe heart disease or hemoglobinopathies. ARDS reported (*Chest 124:406, 2003*). **Adverse effects:** hemolytic anemia (may require dose reduction or dc), dental/periodontal disorders, and all adverse effects of concomitant interferon used (see above). Postmarketing: retinal detachment, ↓ hearing, hypersensitivity reactions. See **Table 14A** for specific regimens, but dosing depends on: interferon used, weight, HCV genotype, and is modified based on side effects (especially degree of hemolysis, with different criteria in those with/without cardiac disease). **Rebetol dose with Intron A (interferon alfa-2b) is wt-based:** 400 mg po am & 600 mg po pm for wt < 75 kg, and 600 mg po am & 600 mg pm for wt > 75 kg with meals. Doses and duration of **Copegus with peg-interferon alfa-2a** are less in pts with genotype 2 or 3 (800 mg/day divided into 2 doses for 24 wks) than with genotypes 1 or 4 (1000 mg for wt < 75 kg, and 1200 mg for wt > 75 kg, divided into 2 doses for 48 wks). In HIV/HCV co-infected pts, dose is 800 mg per day regardless of genotype (See individual labels for details, including initial dosing and criteria for dose modification in those with/without cardiac disease.)
Partaprevir/ritonavir + Ombitasvir + Dasabuvir (P+O/D)(Viekira Pak); Partaprevir/ritonavir + Ombitasvir (Technivie)	Ombitasvir 12.5 mg, Partaprevir 75 mg, and Ritonavir 50 mg co-packaged with tablets of Dasabuvir 250 mg (Viekira Pak); or without Dasabuvir (Technivie)	Do not co-administer with drugs that are highly dependent on CYP3A for clearance, strong inducers of CYP3A and CYP2C8, and strong inhibitors of CYP2C8. Do not use if known hypersensitivity to Ritonavir (e.g., toxic epidermal necrolysis, Stevens-Johnson syndrome). If used with Ribavirin: fatigue, nausea, pruritus, other skin reactions, insomnia and asthenia. When used without Ribavirin: nausea, pruritus and insomnia. **Warning: Hepatic decompensation and hepatic failure, including liver transplantation or fatal outcomes, have been reported** mostly in patients with advanced cirrhosis.
Simeprevir (Olysio)	150 mg 1 cap po once daily with food + both Ribavirin and Interferon	NS3/4A inhibitor. Need to screen patients with HCV genotype 1a for the Q80K polymorphism; if present consider alternative therapy. Contraindicated in pregnancy and in men whose female partners are pregnant (risk category X). No dose adjustment required in patients with mild, moderate or severe renal impairment. Most common AE: rash, pruritus, nausea. CYP3A inhibitors affect plasma concentration of Simeprevir.

TABLE 14B (4)

DRUG NAME(S) GENERIC (TRADE)	DOSAGE/ROUTE IN ADULTS*	COMMENTS/ADVERSE EFFECTS
Hepatitis C *(Continued)*		
Sofosbuvir (Solvadi)	400 mg 1 tab po once daily with food + both PegIntron Interferon and Ribavirin. For combination formulation, see Ledipasvir.	NS5B inhibitor for Genotypes 1, 2, 3, 4 HCV. Efficacy established in patients awaiting liver transplant and in patients with HIV-1/HCV co-infection. Most common AEs (in combination with interferon and ribavirin): fatigue, headache, nausea, insomnia, anemia. Rifampin and St. John's wort may alter plasma concentrations of Sofosbuvir.
Influenza A		
Amantadine (Symmetrel) or Rimantadine (Flumadine) Influenza B intrinsically resistant.	**Amantadine** 100 mg caps, tabs: 50 mg/mL oral solution & syrup. Treatment or prophylaxis: 100 mg po bid (or q12h) for adults; for age ≥65, 100 mg po once daily. **Rimantadine** 100 mg tabs, 50 mg/5 mL syrup. Treatment or prophylaxis: 100 mg bid, or 100 mg daily in elderly nursing home pts, or severe hepatic disease, or CrCl ≤ 10 mL/min. For children, amantadine only approved for prophylaxis.	**Side-effects/toxicity: CNS** (can be mild: nervousness, anxiety, difficulty concentrating, and lightheadedness). Serious: delirium, hallucinations, and seizures—are associated with high plasma drug levels resulting from renal insufficiency, esp. in older pts, those with prior seizure disorders, or psychiatric disorders.
Influenza A and B—For both drugs, initiate within 48 hrs of symptom onset		
Zanamivir (Relenza) For pts ≥ 7 yrs of age (treatment) or ≥ 5 yrs (prophylaxis)	Powder is inhaled by specially designed inhalation device. Each blister contains 5 mg zanamivir. **Treatment:** two inhalations (10 mg) bid for 5 days. **Prophylaxis:** 2 blisters (10 mg) once daily for 10 days (household outbreak) or for 28 days (community outbreak).	Active by inhalation against neuraminidase of both influenza A and B and inhibits release of virus from epithelial cells of respiratory tract. Approx. 4–17% of inhaled dose reaches lower respiratory tract. Excreted by kidney but with low absorption, dose reduction not necessary in renal impairment. AEs: <3% cough, sinusitis, diarrhea, nausea and vomiting. **Reports of respiratory adverse events in pts with or without h/o airways disease, should be avoided in pts with underlying respiratory disease.** Allergic reactions and neuropsychiatric events have been reported. **Caution: do not reconstitute zanamivir powder for use in nebulizers or mechanical ventilators** (MedWatch report of death). **Zanamivir for IV** administration is available for compassionate use through an emergency IND application. Contact GSK (301-796-5215) for forms, then contact FDA (301-796-1500 or 301-796-9900).
Oseltamivir (Tamiflu) For pts ≥ 1 yr (treatment or prophylaxis)	75 mg caps, powder for oral suspension. For adults: **Treatment,** 75 mg po bid for 5 days; 150 mg bid for severe infection. In morbidly obese patients but this dose is not FDA-approved. **Prophylaxis,** 75 mg po once daily for 10 days to 6 wks. (See label for pediatric weight-based dosing.) Adjust doses for CrCl ≤30 mL/min. 30 mg, 45 mg, 75 mg caps, powder for oral suspension	Well absorbed (80% bioavailable) from GI tract and metabolized to active compound GS 4071. T½ 6–10 hrs; excreted unchanged by kidney. Adverse effects include diarrhea, nausea, vomiting, headache. Nausea and vomiting can be reduced by taking oral dose with food. Rarely, severe skin reactions (toxic epidermal necrolysis, Stevens-Johnson syndrome, erythema multiforme). **Delirium** & abnormal behavior reported (CID 48:1003, 2009). No benefit from higher dose in non- critically ill; not recommended (CID 57:1511, 2013).
Peramivir (Rapivab)	600 mg IV single dose	FDA indication is for single dose use in acute uncomplicated influenza. No approved dose for hospitalized patients but 200–400 mg IV daily for 5 days used in trial. Flu with H275Y oseltamivir resistance has moderate resistance to peramivir
Respiratory Syncytial Virus (RSV) monoclonal antibody		
Palivizumab (Synagis) Used for prophylaxis of RSV infection in high-risk children	15 mg per kg IM q month throughout RSV season Single dose 100 mg vial	A monoclonal antibody directed against the surface F glycoprotein. **AEs:** uncommon, occ. ↑ ALT. Anaphylaxis <1/10⁵ pts; acute hypersensitivity reaction <1/1000; otitis media, fever, URI pts, injection site reactions. Postmarketing reports: URI, otitis media, fever. Preferred over polyclonal immune globulin in high risk infants & children.
Warts Regimens are from drug labels specific for external genital and/or perianal condylomata acuminata only. (See specific labels for indications, regimens, age limits)		
Interferon alfa-2b (IntronA)	Injection of 0.05 mL into base of lesion, up to 0.5 mL total per session, twice weekly for up to 8 weeks.	**Black box warning:** Flu-like illness and other systemic effects. 88% had at least one adverse effect. Alpha interferons may cause or aggravate neuropsychiatric, autoimmune, ischemic or infectious disorders.
Interferon alfa-N3 (Alferon N)	Injection of 0.05 mL into base of each wart, up to 0.5 mL total per session, twice weekly for up to 8 weeks.	Flu-like syndrome and hypersensitivity reactions. Contraindicated with allergy to mouse IgG, egg proteins, or neomycin.
Imiquimod (Aldara) (Zyclara)	5% cream. Thin layer applied at bedtime, washing off after 6–10 hr 3 x/wk for up to 16 wks. 3.75% cream: apply q day.	Erythema, itching & burning, erosions. Flu-like syndrome, increased susceptibility to sunburn (avoid UV).
Podophyllotoxin (Condylox)	0.5% solution or gel. Apply to warts twice daily for 3 days, no therapy for 4 days; can repeat up to 4 cycles.	Local reactions—pain, burning, inflammation in 50%. Can ulcerate. Limit surface area treated as per label.
Sinecatechins (Veregen)	15% ointment. Apply 0.5 cm strand to each wart three times per day until healing but not more than 16 weeks.	Application site reactions, which may result in ulcerations, phimosis, meatal stenosis, superinfection.

See page 2 for abbreviations. NOTE: All dosage recommendations are for adults (unless otherwise indicated) and assume normal renal function.

TABLE 14C – ANTIRETROVIRAL THERAPY (ART) IN TREATMENT-NAIVE ADULTS *(continued)*

A. Overview

- Antiretroviral therapy (ART) in treatment-naive adult patients.
- Guidelines: www.aidsinfo.nih.gov and IAS-USA in *JAMA* 312:410, 2014.
- Design a regimen consisting of:
  - **Dual-nucleoside/-nucleotide reverse transcriptase inhibitor (NRTI component) PLUS either a:**
    - **Non-nucleoside reverse transcriptase inhibitor (NNRTI) OR**
    - **Protease inhibitor (PI) OR**
    - **Strand-Transfer Integrase inhibitor (STII)**
- Selection of components is influenced by many factors, including:
  - Results of viral resistance testing
  - Pregnancy (e.g., avoid Efavirenz—pregnancy risk category D)
  - HIV status (e.g., Nevirapine CONTRAINDICATED in women with CD4 >250 cells/µL and men with CD4 >400 cells/µL)
  - Potential drug interactions or adverse drug effects; special focus on tolerability (even low grade side effects can profoundly affect adherence)
  - Co-morbidities (e.g., lipid effects of PIs, liver or renal disease, cardiovascular disease risk, chemical dependency, psychiatric disease)
  - Convenience of dosing. Co-formulations increase convenience, but sometimes prescribing the two constituents individually is preferred, as when dose-adjustments are needed for renal disease.
  - HLA-B5701 testing required prior to using Abacavir (ABC)
  - Co-receptor tropism assay if considering Maraviroc (MVC)

B. Preferred Regimens (Non-pregnancy)

Single tablet Combinations	**Atripla** (Tenofovir/Emtricitabine/Efavirenz) 1 tablet once daily qhs OR **Genvoya** (Elvitegravir/Cobicistat/Emtricitabine/Tenofovir alafenamide (TAF)) 1 tablet once daily with food OR **Stribild** (use only if **Genvoya** not available): (Elvitegravir/Cobicistat/Emtricitabine/Tenofovir) 1 tablet once daily OR **Complera/Eviplera** (Emtricitabine/Tenofovir/Rilpivirine) 1 tablet once daily with food(avoid when VL > 100,000 cells/mL) OR **Triumeq** (Abacavir/3TC/Dolutegravir) 1 tablet each once daily (see Warnings below)
NNRTI Multi-tablet regimens (Select one)	**Truvada** (Tenofovir/Emtricitabine) + **Efavirenz** 1 tablet each once daily qhs OR **Epzicom/Kivexa** (Abacavir/3TC) + **Efavirenz** 1 tablet each once daily qhs (see Warnings below)
Ritonavir-boosted PI Multi-tablet regimens (Select one)	**Truvada** (Tenofovir/Emtricitabine) + **Atazanavir/r** 1 tablet each once daily OR **Epzicom/Kivexa** (Abacavir/3TC) + **Atazanavir/r** 1 tablet each once daily (see Warnings below) OR **Truvada** (Tenofovir/Emtricitabine) + **Darunavir/r** 1 tablet each once daily OR
INSTI Multi-tablet regimens	**Truvada** (Tenofovir/Emtricitabine) + **Raltegravir** 1 tablet each once daily OR **Truvada** (Tenofovir/Emtricitabine) + **Dolutegravir** 1 tablet each once daily OR **Epzicom/Kivexa** (Abacavir/3TC) + **Dolutegravir** 1 tablet each once daily (see Warnings below) OR

NNRTI = non-nucleoside reverse transcriptase inhibitor, PI = protease inhibitor, INSTI = Strand transfer integrase inhibitor, /r = ritonavir boosted

- **Warnings:**
  - **Epzicom/Kivexa** (Abacavir/3TC) containing regimens: Use only in patients who are HLA-B5701 negative. Use Abacavir with caution in those with HIV RNA < 100,000 c/mL at baseline (this does not apply when Dolutegravir is the anchor drug of the regimen)
  - **DO NOT** use Efavirenz when Ct count > 250 cells/µL for women, > 400 cells/µL for men. Can result in life-threatening hypersensitivity reaction
  - Co-formulations increase convenience, but sometimes prescribing the two components individually is preferred, as when dose adjustments are needed for renal disease.
  - Rilpivirine is best used for patients with viral load < 100,000.
  - Raltegravir 800 mg once daily is not quite as effective as 400 mg bid.

TABLE 14C (2)

C. Alternative Regimens (Non-pregnancy)

NNRTI Multi-tablet regimens (Select one)	• **Epzicom/Kivexa** (Abacavir/3TC) + **Rilpivirine** 1 tablet each once daily (see Warnings) OR • **Epzicom/Kivexa** (Abacavir/3TC) + **Nevirapine** 1 tablet each once daily (see Warnings) OR • **Truvada** (Tenofovir/Emtricitabine) + **Nevirapine** 1 tablet each once daily (see Warnings) OR
Boosted PI Multi-tablet regimens (Select one) */c = cobicistat* */r = ritonavir*	• **Epzicom/Kivexa** (Abacavir/3TC) + **Atazanavir/c** 1 tablet each once daily OR • **Truvada** (Tenofovir/Emtricitabine) + **Atazanavir/c** 1 tablet each once daily OR • **Truvada** (Tenofovir/Emtricitabine) + **Darunavir/c** 1 tablet each once daily OR • **Epzicom/Kivexa** (Abacavir/3TC) + **Darunavir/c** 1 tablet each once daily (see Warnings) OR • **Epzicom/Kivexa** (Abacavir/3TC) + **Darunavir/r** 1 tablet each once daily (see Warnings) OR • **Epzicom/Kivexa** (Abacavir/3TC) one tablet daily + **Kaletra** (Lopinavir/r) 4 tablets once daily (see Warnings) OR • **Truvada** (Tenofovir/Emtricitabine) 1 tablet once daily + **Kaletra** (Lopinavir/r) 4 tablets once daily
Nucleoside sparing (or limited) regimens	• **Darunavir/r** 1 tablet once daily with food + Raltegravir 400 mg bid OR • **Kaletra** (Lopinavir/r) 4 tablets once daily + Raltegravir 400 mg bid OR • **Kaletra** (Lopinavir/r) 4 tablets once daily + Lamivudine 1 tablet each once daily

• Nevirapine 400 mg (Viramune XR) is the preferred formulation.
• Nevirapine should be used with caution with Abacavir owing to possible overlap of idiosyncratic hypersensitivity.
• Etravirine and Rilpivirine are options for some patients who have NNRTI resistance mutations, e.g., K103N, at baseline. Expert consultation is recommended.
• Boosted PIs can be administered once or twice daily.
• Cobicistat is now available as a PI-boosting agent
• Non-boosted PIs are no longer recommended
• Maraviroc is no longer recommended for initial treatment but may be used in cases of resistant viruses and as second line therapy (or beyond)
• Kaletra can be given as 2 tablets twice daily (must be given twice daily if multiple PI mutations present)

D. Pregnancy Regimens

| • Timing of initiation of therapy and drug choice must be individualized
• Viral resistance testing should be performed
• Long-term effects of agents is unknown
• Certain drugs are hazardous or contraindicated (Didanosine, Stavudine, Efavirenz) | • **Combivir** (Zidovudine/Lamivudine) 1 tablet bid + **Nevirapine** 1 tablet bid (fed or fasting)] after 14-day lead-in period or 1 tablet each once daily OR
• **Combivir** (Zidovudine/Lamivudine) 1 tablet bid + **Kaletra** 2 tablets bid (without regard to food) |

E.

Selected Characteristics of Antiretroviral Drugs (*CPE = CSF penetration effectiveness)

TABLE 14C (3)

1. **Selected Characteristics of Nucleoside or Nucleotide Reverse Transcriptase Inhibitors (NRTIs)**
All agents have Black Box warning: Risk of lactic acidosis/hepatic steatosis. Also, risk of fat redistribution/accumulation. For combinations, see warnings for component agents.

* CPE (CNS Penetration Effectiveness) value: 1 = Low Penetration; 2 - 3 = Intermediate Penetration; 4 = Highest Penetration into CNS (AIDS 25;357, 2011)

Generic/ Trade Name	Pharmaceutical Prep.	Usual Adult Dosage & Food Effect	% Absorbed, po	Serum T½, hrs	Intracellular T½, hrs	CPE*	Elimination	Major Adverse Events/Comments (See Table 14D)
Abacavir (ABC, Ziagen)	300 mg tabs or 20 mg/mL oral solution	300 mg po bid or 600 mg po q24h. Food OK	83	1.5	20	1	Liver metab., renal excretion of metabolites, 82%	**Hypersensitivity reaction:** fever, rash, N/V, malaise, diarrhea, abdominal pain, respiratory symptoms. (Severe reactions may be ↑ with subsequent doses.) **Do not rechallenge!** Report to 800-270-0425. **Test HLA-B*5701 before use.** **See Comment Table 14D.** Studies raise concerns re ABC/3TC regimens in pts with VL ≥ 100,000 (www.niaid.nih.gov/news/newsreleases/2008/actg52 02bulletin.htm). Controversy re increased CV events with use of ABC. Large meta-analysis shows no increased risk (JAIDS 61, 441, 2012)
Abacavir/lamivudine (Epzicom or Kivexa)	Film coated tabs: ABC 600 mg + 3TC 300 mg	1 tab once daily (not recommended)					(See for individual components)	(See for individual components) **Black Box warning**— limited data for VL > 100,000 copies/mL. Not recommended as initial therapy because of inferior virologic efficacy.
Abacavir/lamivudine (3TC)/dolutegravir (DTV)(Triumeq)	Film coated tabs: ABC 600 mg + 3TC 300 mg + DTV 50 mg	1 tab po once daily						
Abacavir (ABC)/ lamivudine (3TC)/ zidovudine (AZT) (Trizivir)	Film-coated tabs: ABC 300 mg + 3TC 150 mg + ZDV 300 mg	1 tab po bid (not recommended for wt < 40 kg or CrCl < 50 mL/min or impaired hepatic function)						
Didanosine (ddI; Videx or Videx EC)	125, 200, 250, 400 mg enteric-coated caps; 100, 167, 250 mg powder for oral solution.	≥60 kg: Usually 400 mg enteric-coated po q24h 0.5 hr before or 2 hrs after meal. Do not crush. <60 kg: 250 mg EC po q24h.* Food ↓ ddI levels. See Comment	30-40	1.6	25-40	2	Renal excretion, 50%	**Pancreatitis**, peripheral neuropathy, lactic acidosis & hepatic steatosis (rare but life-threatening, esp. combined with stavudine in pregnancy). Retinal optic nerve changes. **The combination ddI + TDF is generally avoided, but if used,** reduce dose of ddI-EC from 400 mg to 250 mg EC q24h (or from 250 mg EC to 200 mg EC for adults <60 kg). **Monitor for ↑ toxicity & possible ↓ in efficacy of this combination; may result in ↓ CD4.**

TABLE 14C (4)

E. Selected Characteristics of Antiretroviral Drugs (*CPE = CSF penetration effectiveness; 1-4)

1. Selected Characteristics of Nucleoside or Nucleotide **Reverse Transcriptase Inhibitors (NRTIs)** *(continued)*

Generic/ Trade Name	Pharmaceutical Prep.	Usual Adult Dosage & Food Effect	% Absorbed, po	Serum T½, hrs	Intracellular T½, hrs	CPE*	Elimination	Major Adverse Events/Comments (See Table 14D)
Emtricitabine (FTC, Emtriva)	200 mg caps, 10 mg per mL oral solution.	200 mg po q24h. Food OK.	93 (caps), 75 (oral sol'n)	Approx. 10	39	3	Renal excretion 86%	Well tolerated; headache, nausea, vomiting & diarrhea occasionally, skin rash rarely. Skin hyperpigmentation. Differs only slightly in structure from lamivudine (5-fluoro substitution). **Exacerbation of Hep B reported in pts after stopping FTC.** Monitor at least several months after stopping FTC in Hep B pts; some may need anti-HBV therapy.
Emtricitabine/ tenofovir disoproxil fumarate (Truvada)	Film-coated tabs: FTC 200 mg + TDF 300 mg	1 tab po q24h for CrCl ≥50 mL/min Food OK	92/25	10/17	—	(See individual components)	Primarily renal/renal	See Comments for individual agents **Black Box warning—Exacerbation of HepB after stopping FTC;** but preferred therapy for those with Hep B/HIV co-infection.
Emtricitabine/ tenofovir/efavirenz (Atripla)	Film-coated tabs: FTC 200 mg + TDF 300 mg + efavirenz 600 mg	1 tab po q24h on an empty stomach, preferably at bedtime. Do not use if CrCl <50 mL/min			(See individual components)			Not recommended for pts <18 yrs. See warnings for individual components. **Exacerbation of Hep B** reported in pts discontinuing component drugs; some need anti-HBV therapy (tenofovir preferred). **Pregnancy category D.** Efavirenz may cause fetal harm. Avoid in pregnancy or in women who may become pregnant.
Emtricitabine/ tenofovir/rilpivirine (Complera/ Eviplera)	Film-coated tabs: FTC 200 mg + TDF 300 mg + RPL 25 mg	1 tab po q24h with food			(See individual components)	(See individual components)	Primarily renal/renal	Preferred use in pts with HIV RNA level < 100,000 c/mL. Should not be used with PPI agents.
Lamivudine (3TC, Epivir)	150, 300 mg tabs; 10 mg/mL oral solution	150 mg po bid or 300 mg po q24h. Food OK	86	5-7	18	2	Renal excretion, minimal metabolism	Use HIV dose, not Hep B dose. Usually well tolerated. **Risk of exacerbation of Hep B after stopping 3TC.** Monitor at least several months after stopping 3TC in Hep B pts; some may need anti-HBV therapy.
Lamivudine/ abacavir (Epzicom)	Film-coated tabs 3TC 300 mg + abacavir 600 mg	1 tab po q24h. Food OK Not recommended for CrCl <50 mL/min or impaired hepatic function	86/86	5-7/1.5	16/20	(See individual components)	Primarily renal/ metabolism	See Comments for individual agents. Note **abacavir hypersensitivity Black Box warnings** (severe reactions more frequent with 600 mg dose) and 3TC Hep B warnings. Test HLA-B*5701 before use.
Lamivudine/ zidovudine (Combivir)	Film-coated tabs 3TC 150 mg + ZDV 300 mg	1 tab po bid. Not recommended for CrCl <50 mL/min or impaired hepatic function Food OK	86/64	5-7/ 0.5-3	—	(See individual components)	Primarily renal/ metabolism with renal excretion of glucuronide	See Comments for individual agents **Black Box warning**—exacerbation of Hep B in pts stopping 3TC

TABLE 14C (b)

Generic/Trade Name	Pharmaceutical Prep.	Usual Adult Dosage & Food Effect	% Absorbed po	Serum T½, hrs	Intracellular T½, hrs	CPE*	Elimination	Major Adverse Events/Comments (See Table 14D)
E. Selected Characteristics of Antiretroviral Drugs (*CPE = CSF penetration effectiveness: 1-4)								
1. Selected Characteristics of Nucleoside or Nucleotide Reverse Transcriptase Inhibitors (NRTIs) (continued)								
Stavudine (d4T, Zerit)	15, 20, 30, 40 mg capsules; 1 mg per mL oral solution	≥60 kg: 40 mg po bid <60 kg: 30 mg po bid Food OK	86	1.2-1.6	3.5	2	Renal excretion, 40%	Not recommended by DHHS as initial therapy because of adverse reactions. **Highest incidence of lipoatrophy, hyperlipidemia, & lactic acidosis of all NRTIs.** Pancreatitis. Peripheral neuropathy. (See didanosine comments.)
Tenofovir disoproxil fumarate (TDF; Viread)—a nucleotide	300 mg tabs	CrCl ≥50 mL/min: 300 mg po q24h. Food OK; high-fat meal ↑ absorption	39 (with food) 25 (fasted)	17	>60	1	Renal excretion	Headache, N/V. **Cases of renal dysfunction reported:** check renal function before using (dose reductions necessary if CrCl <50 cc/min); avoid concomitant nephrotoxic agents. One study found ↑ renal function at 48-wk in pts receiving TDF with a PI (mostly lopinavir/ritonavir) than with a NNRTI (JID 197:102, 2008). Avoid concomitant ddI. Atazanavir & lopinavir/ritonavir ↑ tenofovir concentrations: monitor for adverse effects. **Black Box warning—exacerbations of Hep B reported after stopping tenofovir.** Monitor liver enzymes if TDF stopped on HBV pts.
Tenofovir alafenamide (TAF)	25 mg (10 mg when used with Cobi or RTV)	CrCl >30 ml/min Food OK; high-fat meal ↑ absorption						
Zidovudine (ZDV, AZT, Retrovir)	100 mg caps, 300 mg tabs; 10 mg per mL IV solution; 10 mg/mL oral syrup	300 mg po q12h. Food OK	64	1.1	11	4	Metabolized to glucuronide & excreted in urine	Bone marrow suppression, GI intolerance, headache, insomnia, malaise, myopathy.
2. Selected Characteristics of Non-Nucleoside Reverse Transcriptase Inhibitors (NNRTIs)								
Delavirdine (Rescriptor)	100, 200 mg tabs	400 mg po three times daily. Food OK	85	5.8	3		Cytochrome P450 (3A inhibitor). 51% excreted in urine (<5% unchanged)	Rash severe enough to stop drug in 4.3%. ↑ AST/ALT, headaches. **Use of this agent is not recommended.**

TABLE 14C (6)

E. **Selected Characteristics of Antiretroviral Drugs** (*CPE = CSF penetration effectiveness: 1-4*)

2. **Selected Characteristics of Non-Nucleoside Reverse Transcriptase Inhibitors (NNRTIs)** *(continued)*

Generic/ Trade Name	Pharmaceutical Prep.	Usual Adult Dosage & Food Effect	% Absorbed, po	Serum T½, hrs	Intracellular T½, hrs	CPE	Elimination	Major Adverse Events/Comments (See Table 14D)
Efavirenz (Sustiva) New Guidelines indicate is OK to use in pregnant women (WHO Guidelines) or continue EFV in pregnant as pregnant (HHS Guidelines).	50, 100, 200 mg capsules; 600 mg tablet	600 mg po q24h at bedtime, without food. Food may ↑ serum conc. which can lead to ↑ in risk of adverse events.	42	40-55 See Comment	3		Cytochrome P450 2B6 (3A mixed inducer/ inhibitor); 14-34% excreted in urine as glucuroni-dated metabolites, 16-61% in feces	Severe rash in 1.7%. High frequency of CNS AEs: somnolence, dreams, confusion, agitation. Serious psychiatric symptoms. Certain CYP2B6 polymorphisms may predict exceptionally high plasma levels with standard doses (*CID 45:1230, 2007*). False-pos. cannabinoid screen. Very long tissue T½. **If rx to be discontinued, stop efavirenz 1-2 wks before stopping companion drugs.** Otherwise, risk of developing efavirenz resistance, as after 1-2 days only efavirenz may be present. Some bridge this gap by adding a PI to the NRTI backbone after efavirenz is discontinued (*CID 42:401, 2006*)
Etravirine (Intelence)	100 mg tabs 200 mg tabs	200 mg twice daily after a meal. May also be given as 400 mg once daily.	Unknown (↓ systemic exposure if taken fasting)	41	2		Metabolized by CYP 3A4 (inducer) & 2C9, 2C19 (inhibitor). Fecal extraction.	For pts with HIV-1 resistant to NNRTIs & others. Active in vitro against most such isolates. Rash common, but rarely can be severe. Potential for multiple drug interactions. Generally, multiple mutations are required for high-level resistance. *See Table 14D, page 193 for specific mutations and effects.* Because of interactions, do not use with boosted atazanavir, boosted tipranavir; unboosted PIs, or other NNRTIs.
Nevirapine (Viramune) Viramune XR	200 mg tabs; 50 mg per 5 mL oral suspension; XR 400 mg tabs	200 mg po q24h x 14 days & then 200 mg po bid (see comments & **Black Box warning**) Food OK. **If using Viramune XR, Still need the lead in dosing of 200 mg q24h prior to using 400 mg/d**	>90	25-30	4		Cytochrome P450 (3A, 2B6) inducer; 80% excreted in urine as glucuronidat-ed metabolites, 10% in feces	**Black Box warning—fatal hepatotoxicity.** Women with CD4 >250 esp. vulnerable, inc. pregnant women. Avoid in this group unless benefits clearly > risks (*www.fda.gov/cderdrug/advisory/nevirapine.htm*) Intensive monitoring for liver toxicity required. Men with CD4 >400 also at ↑ risk. Severe rash in 7%, **severe or life-threatening skin reactions** in 2%. Do not restart if any suspicion of such reactions. Because of long T½, consider continuing companion agents for several days if nevirapine is discontinued

TABLE 14C (7)

Generic/ Trade Name	Pharmaceutical Prep.	Usual Adult Dosage & Food Effect	% Absorbed, po	Serum T½, hrs	Intracellular T½, hrs	Elimination	Major Adverse Events/Comments (See Table 14D)

E. **Selected Characteristics of Antiretroviral Drugs** (*CPE = CSF penetration effectiveness: 1-4)

2. **Selected Characteristics of Non-Nucleoside Reverse Transcriptase Inhibitors (NNRTIs)** *(continued)*

Generic/ Trade Name	Pharmaceutical Prep.	Usual Adult Dosage & Food Effect	% Absorbed po	Serum T½, hrs	Intracellular T½, hrs	Elimination	Major Adverse Events/Comments (See Table 14D)
Rilpivirine (Edurant)	25 mg tabs	25 mg daily with food	absolute bio-availability unknown; 40% lower Cmax in fasted state	50	unknown	Metabolized by Cyp3A4 in liver; 25% excreted unchanged in feces.	QTc prolongation with doses higher than 50 mg per day. Common AEs: depression, insomnia, headache, and rash. Do not co-administer with carbamazepine, phenobarbitol, phenytoin, rifabutin, rifampin, rifapentine, proton pump inhibitors, or multiple doses of dexamethasone. A fixed dose combination of rilpivirine + TDF/FTC (Complera/Eviplera) is approved. **Needs stomach acid for absorption. Do not administer with PPI.**

3. **Selected Characteristics of Protease Inhibitors (PIs)**

All PIs: Glucose metabolism: new diabetes mellitus or deterioration of glucose control; fat redistribution; possible hemophilia bleeding; hypertriglyceridemia or hypercholesterolemia. Exercise caution re: potential drug interactions & contraindications. QTc prolongation has been reported in a few pts taking PIs, some PIs can block HERG channels in vitro (Lancet 365:682, 2005).

Generic/ Trade Name	Pharmaceutical Prep.	Usual Adult Dosage & Food Effect	% Absorbed, po	Serum T½, hrs	CPE*	Elimination	Major Adverse Events/Comments (See Table 14D)
Atazanavir (Reyataz)	100, 150, 200, 300 mg capsules	400 mg q24h with food. Ritonavir-boosted dose (atazanavir 300 mg po q24h + ritonavir 100 mg po q24h), with food, is recommended for ART-experienced pts. Use boosted dose when combined with either efavirenz 600 mg po q24h or TDF 300 mg po q24h. If used with buffered ddI, take with food 2 hrs po or 1 hr post ddI.	Good oral bioavailability, food enhances bioavailability & ↓ pharmacokinetic variability. Absorption ↓ by antacids, H₂-blockers, proton pump inhibitors. Avoid unboosted drug with PPIs/H2-blockers. Boosted drug can be used with or >10 hr after H2-blockers or >12 hr after a PPI, if limited doses of the acid agents are used.	Approx. 7	2	Cytochrome P450 (3A4, 1A2 & 2C9 inhibitor) & UGT1A1 inhibitor; 13% excreted in urine (7% unchanged), 79% excreted in feces (20% unchanged)	Lower potential for ↑ lipids. Asymptomatic unconjugated hyperbilirubinemia common; jaundice especially likely in Gilbert's syndrome (JID 192:1381, 2005). Headache, rash, GI symptoms. Prolongation of PR interval (1st degree AV block) reported. Caution in pre-existing conduction system disease. Efavirenz & tenofovir ↓ atazanavir exposure: use atazanavir/ritonavir regimen; also, atazanavir ↑ tenofovir concentrations—watch for adverse events. In rx-experienced pts taking TDF and needing H2 blockers, atazanavir 400 mg with ritonavir 100 mg can be given; do not use PPIs. Rare reports of renal stones.
Darunavir (Prezista)	400 mg, 600 mg, 800 mg tablets	[600 mg darunavir + 100 mg ritonavir] po bid, with food or [800 mg darunavir (two 400 mg tabs or one 800 mg tab) + 100 mg ritonavir] po once daily with food (Preferred regimen in ART naïve pts)	82% absorbed (taken with ritonavir). Food ↑ absorption.	Approx 15 hr (with ritonavir)	3	Metabolized by CYP3A and is a CYP3A inhibitor	Contains sulfa moiety. Rash, nausea, headaches seen. Coadmin of certain drugs cleared by CYP3A is contraindicated (see label). Use with caution in pts with hepatic dysfunction. (FDA warning about occasional hepatic dysfunction early in the course of treatment). Monitor carefully, esp. first several months of therapy in pts with pre-existing liver disease. May cause hormonal contraception failure.

TABLE 14C (8)

E. Selected Characteristics of Antiretroviral Drugs (*CPE = CSF penetration effectiveness): 1-4)
3. Selected Characteristics of Protease Inhibitors (PIs) *(continued)*

Generic/ Trade Name	Pharmaceutical Prep.	Usual Adult Dosage & Food Effect	% Absorbed, po	Serum T½, hrs	CPE*	Elimination	Major Adverse Events/Comments (See Table 14D)
Fosamprenavir (Lexiva)	700 mg tablet, 50 mg/mL oral suspension	1400 mg fosamprenavir po bid **OR** with ritonavir: [1400 mg fosamprenavir (2 tabs) + ritonavir 100 mg or 200 mg] po q24h **OR** [700 mg fosamprenavir (1 tab) + ritonavir 100 mg] po bid	Bioavailability not established. Food OK	7.7 Amprenavir	3	Hydrolyzed to amprenavir, then acts as cytochrome P450 (3A4 substrate, inhibitor, inducer)	Amprenavir prodrug. Contains sulfa moiety. Potential for serious drug interactions (see label). Rash, including Stevens-Johnson syndrome. Once daily regimens: (1) not recommended for PI-experienced pts; (2) additional ritonavir needed if given with efavirenz (see label). Boosted twice daily regimen is recommended for PI-experienced pts. Potential for PI cross-resistance with darunavir.
Indinavir (Crixivan)	100, 200, 400 mg capsules. Store in original container with desiccant	Two 400 mg caps (800 mg) po q8h, without food or with light meal. Can take with enteric-coated Videx. [If taken with ritonavir (e.g., 800 mg indinavir + 100 mg ritonavir po q12h), no food restrictions]	65	1.2–2	4	Cytochrome P450 (3A4 inhibitor)	Maintain hydration. Nephrolithiasis, nausea, inconsequential ↑ of indirect bilirubin (jaundice in Gilbert syndrome). ↑ AST/ALT, headache, asthenia, blurred vision, metallic taste, hemolysis. ↑ urine WBC (>100/hpf) has been assoc. with nephritis/ medullary calcification, cortical atrophy.
Lopinavir + ritonavir (Kaletra)	(200 mg lopinavir + 50 mg ritonavir), and (100 mg lopinavir + 25 mg ritonavir) tablets. Tabs do not need refrigeration. Oral solution: (80 mg lopinavir + 20 mg ritonavir) per mL. Refrigerate, but can be kept at room temp. (≤77°F) x 2 mos.	(400 mg lopinavir + 100 mg ritonavir)—2 tabs po bid. Higher dose may be needed in non-rx-naive pts when used with efavirenz, nevirapine, or unboosted fosamprenavir. [Dose adjustment in concomitant drugs may be necessary: see Table 22B.]	No food effect with tablets.	5–6	3	Cytochrome P450 (3A4 inhibitor)	Nausea/vomiting/diarrhea (worse when administered with zidovudine). ↑ AST/ALT, pancreatitis. Oral solution 42% alcohol. Lopinavir + ritonavir can be taken as a single daily dose of 4 tabs (total 800 mg lopinavir + 200 mg ritonavir), except in treatment-experienced pts or those taking concomitant efavirenz, nevirapine, amprenavir, or nelfinavir. Possible PR and QT prolongation. Use with caution in those with cardiac conduction abnormalities or when used with drugs with similar effects.
Nelfinavir (Viracept)	625, 250 mg tabs; 50 mg/gm oral powder	Two 625 mg tabs (1250 mg) po bid, with food	20–80 Food ↑ exposure & ↓ variability	3.5–5	1	Cytochrome P450 (3A4 inhibitor)	Diarrhea. Coadministration of drugs with life-threatening toxicities & which are cleared by CYP34A is contraindicated. Not recommended in initial regimens because of inferior virologic efficacy; **prior concerns about EMS now resolved. Acceptable choice in pregnant women although it has inferior virologic efficacy than most other ARV anchor drugs.**

TABLE 14C (9)

E. Selected Characteristics of Antiretroviral Drugs

3. Selected Characteristics of Protease Inhibitors (PIs), (continued)

Generic/ Trade Name	Pharmaceutical Prep.	Usual Adult Dosage & Food Effect	% Absorbed, po	CPE	Serum T½, hrs	Elimination	Major Adverse Events/Comments (See Table 14D)
Ritonavir (Norvir)	100 mg capsules; 600 mg per 7.5 mL oral solution. Refrigerate caps but not solution. Room temperature for 1 mo. is OK.	Full dose not recommended (see comments). **With rare exceptions, used exclusively to enhance pharmacokinetics of other PIs, using lower ritonavir doses.**	Food ↑ absorption	1	3–5	Cytochrome P450. Potent 3A4 & 2 d6 inhibitor	Nausea/vomiting/diarrhea, extremity & circumoral paresthesias, hepatitis, pancreatitis, taste perversion, ↑ CPK & uric acid. **Black Box warning**—potentially fatal drug interactions. Many drug interactions— see Table 22A–Table 22B.
Saquinavir (Invirase—hard gel caps or tabs) + **ritonavir**	Saquinavir 200 mg caps, 500 mg film-coated tabs; ritonavir 100 mg caps	[2 tabs saquinavir (1000 mg) + 1 cap ritonavir (100 mg)] po bid with food	Erratic, 4 (saquinavir alone). Much more reliably absorbed when boosted with ritonavir.	1	1–2	Cytochrome P450 (3A4 inhibitor)	Nausea, diarrhea, headache, ↑ AST/ALT. Avoid rifampin with saquinavir + ritonavir; hepatitis risk. **Black Box warning**—Invirase to be used only with ritonavir. Possible QT prolongation. Use with caution in those with cardiac conduction abnormalities or when used with drugs with similar effects.
Tipranavir (Aptivus)	250 mg caps. Refrigerate unopened bottles. Use opened bottles within 2 mo. 100 mg/mL solution	[500 (two 250 mg caps) + ritonavir 200 mg] po bid with food	Absorption low, ↑ with high fat meal, ↓ with Al⁺⁺⁺ & Mg⁺⁺ antacids.	1	5.5–6	Cytochrome 3A4 but ritonavir, most of drug is eliminated in feces.	Contains sulfa moiety. **Black Box warning—reports of fatal/nonfatal intracranial hemorrhage, hepatitis, fatal hepatic failure.** Use cautiously in liver disease, esp. hepB, hepC; contraindicated in Child-Pugh class B-C. Monitor LFTs. Coadministration of certain drugs contraindicated (see label). **For highly ART-experienced pts or for multiple-PI resistant virus.** Do not use tipranavir and etravirine together owing to 76% reduction in etravirine levels.

4. Selected Characteristics of Fusion Inhibitors

Generic/ Trade Name	Pharmaceutical Prep.	Usual Adult Dosage	% Absorbed	CPE*	Serum T½, hrs	Elimination	Major Adverse Events/Comments (See Table 14D)
Enfuvirtide (T20, Fuzeon)	Single-use vials of 90 mg/mL when reconstituted. Vials should be stored at room temperature. Reconstituted vials can be refrigerated for 24 hrs only.	90 mg (1 mL) subcut. bid. Rotate injection sites, avoiding those currently inflamed.	84	1	3.8	Catabolism to its constituent amino acids with subsequent recycling of the amino acids in the body pool. Elimination pathway(s) have not been performed in humans. Does not alter the metabolism of CYP3A4, CYP 2 d6, CYP1A2, CYP2C19 or CYP2E1 substrates.	Local reaction site reactions 98%, 4% discontinue; erythema/induration—80–90%, nodules/cysts ~80%. **Hypersensitivity reactions reported** (fever, rash, chills, N/V, ↓ BP, & or ↑ AST/ALT)—do not restart if occur. Including background regimens, peripheral neuropathy 8.9%, insomnia 11.3%, ↓ appetite 6.3%, myalgia 5%, lymphadenopathy 2.3%, eosinophilia ~10%. ↑ incidence of bacterial pneumonias.

TABLE 14C (10)

Selected Characteristics of Antiretroviral Drugs (*CPE = CSF penetration effectiveness: 1-4) (continued)

Generic/ Trade Name	Pharmaceutical Prep.	Usual Adult Dosage & Food Effect	% Absorbed	Serum $T_{1/2}$, hrs	CPE	Elimination	Major Adverse Events/Comments (See Table 14D)
5. Selected Characteristics of CCR-5 Co-receptor Antagonists							
Maraviroc (Selzentry)	150 mg, 300 mg film-coated tabs	Without regard to food. –150 mg bid if concomitant meds include CYP3A inhibitors including PIs (except tipranavir/ritonavir) and delavirdine (with/without CYP3A inducers) –300 mg bid without significantly interacting meds including NRTIs, tipranavir/ritonavir, nevirapine –600 mg bid if concomitant meds include CYP3A inducers, including efavirenz (without strong CYP3A inhibitors)	Est. 33% with 300 mg dosage	14-18	3	CYP3A and P-glycoprotein substrate. Metabolites (via CYP3A) excreted feces > urine	**Black Box Warning-Hepatotoxicity;** may be preceded by rash, ↑ eos or IgE. NB: no hepatotoxicity was noted in MVC trials. Black box inserted owing to concern about potential CCR5 class effect. Data lacking in hepatic/renal insufficiency; ↑ concern with either could ↑ risk of IBP. Currently for treatment-experienced patients with multi-resistant strains. **Document CCR-5-tropic virus before use, as treatment failures assoc. with appearance of CXCR-4 or mixed-tropic virus.**
6. Selected Characteristics of Strand Transfer Integrase Inhibitors							
Raltegravir (Isentress)	400 mg film-coated tabs	400 mg po bid, without regard to food	Unknown	~ 9	3	Glucuronidation via UGT1A1, with excretion into feces and urine. (Therefore does NOT require ritonavir boosting)	For naive patients and treatment experienced pts with multiply-resistant virus. Well-tolerated. Nausea, diarrhea, headache, fever similar to placebo. CK↑ & rhabdomyolysis reported: unclear relationship. Increased depression in those with a history of depression. Low genetic barrier to resistance. Increase in CPK, myositis, rhabdomyolysis have been reported. Rare Stevens Johnson Syndrome. Better oral absorption if chewed (CID 57:480, 2013).
Elvitegravir/ cobicistat (Stribild)	150 mg - 150 mg	150 mg -150 mg once daily with or without food	<10%	12.9 (Cobi), 3.5 (ELV)	Un-known	The majority of **elvitegravir** metabolism is mediated by CYP3A enzymes. Elvitegravir also undergoes glucuronidation via UGT1A1/3 enzymes. **Cobicistat** is metabolized by CYP3A and to a minor extent by CYP2D6	For both treatment naive patients and treatment experienced pts with multiply-resistant viruses. Generally well-tolerated. Use by-products inhibit proximal tubular enzyme; this does not result in reduction in true GFR but will result in apparent reduction in eGFR by MDRD or Cockcroft Gault calculations. Usual AEs are similar to those observed with ritonavir (cobi) and tenofovir/FTC.

TABLE 14C (11)

Generic/ Trade Name	Pharmaceutical Prep.	Usual Adult Dosage & Food Effect	% Absorbed	CPE	Serum T½, hrs	Elimination	Major Adverse Events/Comments (See Table 14D)
6. Selected Characteristics of Strand Transfer Integrase Inhibitors (continued)							
Elvitegravir (Vitekta)(EVG)	85 mg, 150 mg tabs	• EVG85 mg once daily + ATV/r 300/100 mg po once daily • EVG85 mg once daily + LPV/r 400/100 mg po bid • EVG150 mg once daily + DRV/r 600/100 mg po bid • EVG150 mg once daily + FOS/r 700/100 mg po bid • EVG150 mg once daily + TPV/r 500/200 mg bid	ND	No	8.7	Hepatobiliary, metabolized by CYP3A	Well tolerated, mild diarrhea
Dolutegravir (Tivicay)	50 mg	50 mg po once daily 50 mg po BID (if STFI resistance present or if co-admin with EFV, FOS. TIP or Rif)	Unknown	4	14	Glucuronidation via UGT1A1 (therefore does not require ritonavir or cobicistat boosting)	Hypersensitivity (rare). Most common: insomnia (3%) headache (2%), N/V (1%), rash (<1%). Watch for IRIS; Watch for elevated LFTs in those with HCV

F. Other Considerations in Selection of Therapy

Caution: Initiation of ART may result in immune reconstitution syndrome with significant clinical consequences. See Table 11B of Sanford Guide to HIV/AIDS Therapy (AIDS Reader 16:199, 2006).

1. **Resistance testing:** Given current rates of resistance, resistance testing is recommended in all patients prior to initiation of therapy, including those with acute infection syndrome (may initiate therapy while waiting for test results and adjusting Rx once results return). at time of change of therapy owing to antiretroviral failure, when suboptimal virologic response is observed, and in pregnant women. **Resistance testing NOT recommended if pt is off ART for > 4 weeks or if HIV RNA is < 1000 c/mL.** See Table 6F of SANFORD GUIDE TO HIV/AIDS THERAPY.

2. Drug-induced disturbances of glucose & lipid metabolism (see Table 14D).
3. Drug-induced lactic acidosis & other FDA "box warnings" (see Table 14D).
4. Drug-drug interactions (see Table 22B).
5. Risk in pregnancy (see Table 8).
6. Use in women & children (see Table 14C).
7. Dosing in patients with renal or hepatic dysfunction (see Table 17A & Table 17B).

* CPE (CNS Penetration Effectiveness) value: 1 = Low Penetration; 2 - 3 = Intermediate Penetration; 4 = Highest Penetration into CNS (AIDS 25:357, 2011).

192

TABLE 14D – ANTIRETROVIRAL DRUGS & ADVERSE EFFECTS
(www.aidsinfo.nih.gov)

DRUG NAME(S): GENERIC (TRADE)	MOST COMMON ADVERSE EFFECTS	MOST SIGNIFICANT ADVERSE EFFECTS
Nucleoside Reverse Transcriptase Inhibitors (NRTI) Black Box warning for all nucleoside/nucleotide RTIs: **lactic acidosis/hepatic steatosis, potentially fatal.** Also carry Warnings that fat redistribution and immune reconstitution syndromes (including autoimmune syndromes) with delayed onset) have been observed		
Abacavir (Ziagen)	Headache 7–13%, nausea 7–19%, diarrhea 7%, malaise 7–12%	**Black Box warning–Hypersensitivity reaction (HR)** in 8% with malaise, fever, GI upset, rash, lethargy & respiratory symptoms most commonly reported; myalgia, arthralgia, edema, paresthesia less common. **Discontinue immediately if HR suspected. Rechallenge contraindicated; may be life-threatening.** Severe HR may be more common with once-daily dosing. **HLA-B*5701 allele** predicts ↑ risk of HR in Caucasian pop., excluding pts w/ B*5701 ↓ HR incidence (*NEJM 358:568, 2008; CID 46:1111-1118, 2008*). DHHS guidelines recommend testing for B*5701 and use of abacavir-containing regimens only if HLA-B*5701 negative. Vigorous essential in all groups. Possible ↑ increased risk of MI with use of abacavir had been suggested (*JID 201:318, 2010*). Other studies found no increased risk of MI (*CID 52: 929, 2011*). A meta-analysis of randomized trials by FDA also did not show increased risk of MI (www.fda.gov/drugs/drugsafety/ucm245164.htm). Nevertheless, care is advised to optimize potentially modifiable risk factors when abacavir is used.
Didanosine (ddl) (Videx)	Diarrhea 28%, nausea 6%, rash 9%, headache 7%, fever 12%, hyperuricemia 2%	**Pancreatitis 1–9%. Black Box warning—Cases of fatal & nonfatal pancreatitis** have occurred in pts receiving ddl, especially when in combination with d4T or d4T + hydroxyurea. Fatal lactic acidosis in pregnancy with ddl + d4T. Peripheral neuropathy in 20%, 12% required dose reduction. ↑ toxicity if used with ribavirin. Use with TDF generally avoided (but would require dose reduction of ddl) because of ↑ toxicity and possible ↓ efficacy; may result in ↓ CD4. Rarely, retinal changes or optic neuropathy. Diabetes mellitus and rhabdomyolysis reported in post-marketing surveillance. Possible increased risk of MI under study (www.fda.gov/CDER, JID 201:318, 2010). Non-cirrhotic portal hypertension with ascites, varices, splenomegaly reported in post-marketing surveillance. See also Clin Infect Dis 49:626, 2009; Amer J Gastrointestinal 104:1707, 2009.
Emtricitabine (FTC) (Emtriva)	Well tolerated. Headache, diarrhea, nausea, rash, skin hyperpigmentation	Potential for lactic acidosis (as with other NRTIs). Also in Black Box—**severe exacerbation of hepatitis B on stopping drug component—monitor clinical/labs for several months after stopping in pts with hepB.** Anti-HBV rx may be warranted if FTC stopped.
Lamivudine (3TC) (Epivir)	Well tolerated. Headache 35%, nausea 33%, diarrhea 18%, abdominal pain 9%, insomnia 11% (all in combination with ZDV). Pancreatitis more common in pediatrics.	**Black Box warning.** Make sure to use HIV dosage, not Hep B dosage. **Exacerbation of hepatitis B on stopping drug. Patients with hepB who stop lamivudine require close clinical/lab monitoring for several months.** Anti-HBV rx may be warranted if 3TC stopped.
Stavudine (d4T) (Zerit)	Diarrhea, nausea, vomiting, headache	**Peripheral neuropathy** 15–20%. Pancreatitis 1%. Appears to produce lactic acidosis, hepatic steatosis and lipoatrophy/lipodystrophy more commonly than other NRTIs. **Black Box warning—Fatal & nonfatal pancreatitis with d4T + ddl.** Use with TDF generally avoided (but would require dose reduction of ddl) because of ↑ toxicity and possible ↓ efficacy; may result in ↓ CD4. Rarely, retinal changes or optic neuropathy. Diabetes mellitus and rhabdomyolysis reported in post-marketing surveillance. **Fatal lactic acidosis/steatosis in pregnant women receiving d4T + ddl.** Fatal and non-fatal lactic acidosis and severe hepatic steatosis can occur in pts receiving d4T. Use with particular caution in patients with risk factors for liver disease, but lactic acidosis can occur even in those without known risk factors. Possible ↑ toxicity if used with ribavirin. Motor weakness in the setting of lactic acidosis mimicking the clinical presentation of Guillain-Barré syndrome (including respiratory failure) (rare).
Zidovudine (ZDV, AZT) (Retrovir)	Nausea 50%, anorexia 20%, vomiting 17%, **headache 62%**. Also reported: asthenia, insomnia, myalgias, nail pigmentation. Macrocytosis expected with all dosage regimens.	**Black Box warning—hematologic toxicity, myopathy. Anemia** (<8 gm, 1%), granulocytopenia (<750, 1.8%) toxicity ↑ with ribavirin. Co-administration with Ribavirin and epoetin alfa erythropoietin levels are ≤500 mlllU/mL. Possible ↑ toxicity if used with ribavirin. Hepatic decompensation may occur in HIV/HCV co-infected patients receiving zidovudine with interferon alfa ± ribavirin.

DRUG NAME(S): GENERIC (TRADE)	MOST COMMON ADVERSE EFFECTS	MOST SIGNIFICANT ADVERSE EFFECTS

Nucleoside Reverse Transcriptase Inhibitor (NRRT) Black Box warning for all nucleoside/nucleotide RTIs: lactic acidosis/hepatic steatosis, potentially fatal. Also carry Warnings that fat redistribution and immune reconstitution syndromes (including autoimmune syndromes with delayed onset) have been observed *(continued)*

| Tenofovir disoproxil fumarate (TDF) (Viread); Tenofovir alafenamide (TAF) | Diarrhea 11%, nausea 8%, vomiting 5%, flatulence 4% (generally well tolerated) | Black Box Warning—Severe exacerbations of hepatitis B reported in pts who stop tenofovir. Monitor carefully if drug is stopped; anti-HBV rx may be warranted if TDF stopped. Reports of renal injury from TDF, including Fanconi syndrome and diabetes insipidus reported with TDF → ddI *(AIDS Reader 19:114, 2009)*. Modest decline in renal function appears greater with TDF than with NRTIs *(CID 51:296, 2010)* or TAF and may be greater in those receiving TDF with a PI instead of an NNRTI *(JID 197:102, 2008; AIDS 26:567, 2012)*. In a VA study that followed >10,000 HIV-infected individuals, TDF exposure was significantly associated with increased risk of proteinuria, a more rapid decline in renal function and chronic kidney disease *(AIDS 26:867, 2012)*. Monitor Ccr, serum phosphate and urinalysis, especially carefully in those with pre-existing renal dysfunction or nephrotoxic medications. TDF, but not TAF, also appears to be associated with increased risk of bone loss. In a substudy of an ACTG comparative treatment trial, those randomized to TDF-FTC experienced greater decreases in spine and hip bone mineral density (BMD) at 96 weeks compared with those treated with ABC-3TC *(JID 203:1791, 2011)*. Consider monitoring BMD in those with history of pathologic fractures, or who have risks for osteoporosis or bone loss. |

Non-Nucleoside Reverse Transcriptase Inhibitors (NNRTI). Labels caution that fat redistribution and immune reconstitution can occur with ART.

Delavirdine (Rescriptor)	Nausea, diarrhea, headache	Skin rash has occurred in 18%, can continue or restart drug in most cases. Stevens-Johnson syndrome & erythema multiforme have been reported rarely. ↑ in liver enzymes in <5% of patients.
Efavirenz (Sustiva)	CNS side effects 52%, symptoms include dizziness, insomnia, somnolence, impaired concentration, psychiatric sx, & abnormal dreams; symptoms are worse after 1st or 2nd dose & improve over 2–4 weeks; discontinuation rate 2.6%. Rash 26% (vs. 17% in comparators); often improves with oral antihistamines; discontinuation rate 1.7%. Can cause false-positive urine test results for cannabinoid with CEDIA DAU multi-level THC assay. Metabolite can cause false-positive urine screening test for benzodiazepines *(CID 48:1787, 2009)*.	Caution: CNS effects may impair driving and other hazardous activities. Serious neuropsychiatric symptoms reported, including severe depression (2.4%) & suicidal ideation (0.7%). Elevation in liver enzymes. Fulminant hepatic failure reported *(see FDA label)*. Teratogenicity reported in primates; pregnancy category D—may cause fetal harm, avoid in pregnant women or those who might become pregnant. NOTE: No single method of contraception is 100% reliable Barrier + 2nd method of contraception advised, continued 12 weeks after stopping efavirenz. Contraindicated with certain drugs metabolized by CYP3A4. Slow metabolism in those homozygous for the CYP-2B6 G516T allele can result in exaggerated toxicity and intolerance. This allele much more common in blacks and women *(CID 42:408, 2006)*. Stevens-Johnson syndrome and erythema multiforme reported in post-marketing surveillance.
Etravirine (Intelence)	Rash 9%, generally mild to moderate and spontaneously resolving; 2% dc clinical trials for rash. Nausea 5%.	Severe rash (erythema multiforme, toxic epidermal necrolysis, Stevens-Johnson syndrome) has been reported. Hypersensitivity reactions can occur with rash, constitutional symptoms and organ dysfunction, including hepatic failure *(see FDA label)*. Potential for CYP450-mediated drug interactions. Rhabdomyolysis has been reported in post-marketing surveillance.
Nevirapine (Viramune)	Rash 37%, usually occurs during 1st 6 wks of therapy. Follow recommendations for 14-day lead-in period to ↓ risk of rash *(see Table 14C)*. Women experience 7-fold ↑ in risk of severe rash *(CID 32:124, 2001)*. 50% resolve with 2 wks of dc of drug & 80% by 1 month. 6.7% discontinuation rate.	Black Box warning—Severe life-threatening skin reactions reported: Stevens-Johnson syndrome, toxic epidermal necrolysis, & hypersensitivity reaction or drug rash with eosinophilia & systemic symptoms (DRESS) *(ArIM 161:2501, 2001)*. For severe rashes, dc drug immediately & do not restart. In a clinical trial, the use of prednisone ↑ the risk of rash. Overall 1% develops hepatitis. Pts with pre-existing ↑ in ALT or AST &/or history of chronic Hep B or C ↑ susceptible *(Hepatol 35:182, 2002)*. Black Box warning—Life-threatening hepatotoxicity reported, 2/3 during the first 12 wks of rx. Women with CD4 >250, including pregnant women, at ↑ risk. Avoid in this group unless no other option. Men with CD4 >400 also at ↑ risk. Monitor pts intensively (clinical & LFTs), esp. during the first 12 wks of rx. If clinical hepatotoxicity, severe skin or hypersensitivity reactions occur, dc drug & never rechallenge.

TABLE 14D (3)

DRUG NAME(S): GENERIC (TRADE)	MOST COMMON ADVERSE EFFECTS	MOST SIGNIFICANT ADVERSE EFFECTS
Non-Nucleoside Reverse Transcriptase Inhibitors (NNRTI) *(continued)*		
Rilpivirine (Edurant)	Headache (3%), rash (3%, led to discontinuation in 0.1%) insomnia (3%), depressive disorders (4%). Psychiatric disorders led to discontinuation in 1%. Increased liver enzymes observed.	Drugs that induce CYP3A or increase gastric pH may decrease plasma concentration of rilpivirine and co-administration with rilpivirine should be avoided. Among these are certain anticonvulsants, rifamycins, PPIs, dexamethasone and St. John's wort. At supra-therapeutic doses, rilpivirine can increase QTc interval; use with caution with other drugs known to increase QTc. May cause depressive disorder, including suicide attempts or suicidal ideation. Overall, appears to cause fewer neuropsychiatric side effects than efavirenz (*AIDS* 60:33, 2012).
Protease inhibitors (PI)		
	Diarrhea is common AE (**crofelemer** 125 mg bid may help, but expensive). Abnormalities in glucose metabolism, dyslipidemias, fat redistribution syndromes are potential problems. Pts taking PI may be at increased risk for developing osteopenia/osteoporosis. Spontaneous bleeding episodes have been reported in HIV+ pts with hemophilia being treated with PI. Rheumatoid complications have been reported (*An Rheum Dis* 61:82, 2002). Potential for QTc prolongation (*Lancet* 365:682, 2005). **Caution for all PIs**—Coadministration with drugs dependent on CYP3A or other enzymes for elimination & for which ↑ levels can cause serious toxicity may be contraindicated. ART may result in immune reconstitution syndromes, which may include early or late presentations of autoimmune syndromes. Increased premature births among women receiving ritonavir-boosted PIs as compared with those receiving other antiretroviral therapy, even after accounting for other potential risk factors (*CID* 54: 1348, 2012).	
Atazanavir (Reyataz)	Asymptomatic unconjugated hyperbilirubinemia in up to 60% of pts, jaundice in 7-9% [especially with Gilbert syndrome (*JID* 192: 1381, 2005)]. Moderate to severe events: Diarrhea 1-3%, nausea 6-14%, abdominal pain 4%, headache 6%, rash 20%.	Prolongation of PR interval (1st degree AV block; rarely 2° AV block. QTc increase and torsades reported (*CID* 44:e67, 2007). Acute interstitial nephritis (*Am J Kid Dis* 44:E81, 2004) and urolithiasis (atazanavir stones) reported (*AIDS* 20:2131, 2006; *NEJM* 355:2158, 2006). Potential ↑ transaminases in pts co-infected with HBV or HCV. Severe skin eruptions (Stevens-Johnson syndrome, erythema multiforme, and toxic eruptions, or DRESS syndrome) have been reported.
Darunavir (Prezista)	With background regimens, headache 15%, nausea 18%, diarrhea 20%, ↑ amylase 17%. Rash in 10% of treated; 0.5% discontinuation.	Hepatitis in 0.5%, some with fatal outcome. Use caution in pts with HBV or HCV co-infections or other hepatic dysfunction. Monitor for clinical symptoms and LFTs. Stevens-Johnson syndrome, toxic epidermal necrolysis, erythema multiforme. Contains sulfa moiety. Potential for major drug interactions. May cause failure of hormonal contraceptives.
Fosamprenavir (Lexiva)	Skin rash — 20% (moderate or worse in 3-8%), nausea, headache, diarrhea.	Rarely Stevens-Johnson syndrome, hemolytic anemia. Pro-drug of amprenavir. Contains sulfa moiety. Angioedema and nephrolithiasis reported in post-marketing experience. Potential increased risk of MI (*see FDA label*). Angioedema, oral paresthesias, myocardial infarction and nephrolithiasis reported in post-marketing experience. Elevated LFTs seen with higher than recommended doses; increased risk in those with pre-existing liver abnormalities. Acute hemolytic anemia reported with amprenavir.
Indinavir (Crixivan)	↑ indirect bilirubin 10-15% (≥2.5 mg/dL with overt jaundice especially likely in those with Gilbert syndrome (*JID* 192: 1381, 2005). Nausea 12%, vomiting 4%, diarrhea 5%. Metallic taste. Paronychia and ingrown toenails reported (*CID* 32:140, 2001).	**Kidney stones.** Due to indinavir crystals in collecting system. Nephrolithiasis in 12% of adults, higher in pediatrics. Minimize risk with good hydration (at least 48 oz. water/day) (*AAC* 42:332, 1998). Tubulointerstitial nephritis/renal cortical atrophy reported in association with asymptomatic ↑ urine WBC. Severe hepatitis reported in 3 cases (*Ln* 349:924, 1997). Hemolytic anemia reported.
Lopinavir/Ritonavir (Kaletra)	GI: **diarrhea** 14-24%, nausea 2-16%. More diarrhea with q24h dosing.	Lipid abnormalities in up to 20-40%. Possible increased risk of MI with cumulative exposure (*JID* 201:318, 2010). ↑ PR interval, 2° or 3° heart block described. Post-marketing reports of ↑ QTc and torsades. Avoid use in congenital QTc prolongation or in other circumstances that prolong QTc or increase susceptibility to torsades. Hepatitis, with hepatic decompensation; caution especially in those with pre-existing liver disease. Pancreatitis. Inflammatory edema of legs (*AIDS* 16:673, 2002). Stevens-Johnson syndrome & erythema multiforme reported. Note high drug concentration in oral solution. Toxic potential of oral solution (contains ethanol and propylene glycol) in neonates.
Nelfinavir (Viracept)	Mild to moderate **diarrhea** 20%. Oat bran tabs, calcium, or oral anti-diarrheal agents (e.g., loperamide, diphenoxylate/atropine sulfate) can be used to manage diarrhea.	Potential for drug interactions. Powder contains phenylalanine.

DRUG NAME(S): GENERIC (TRADE)	MOST COMMON ADVERSE EFFECTS	MOST SIGNIFICANT ADVERSE EFFECTS
Protease Inhibitors (PI) *(continued)*		
Ritonavir (Norvir) (Currently, primary use is to enhance levels of other anti-retrovirals, because of ↑ toxicity/interactions with full-dose ritonavir)	GI: bitter aftertaste ↓ by taking with chocolate milk, Ensure, or Advera. nausea 23%, ↓ by initial dose esc (titration) regimen; vomiting 13%, diarrhea 15%. Circumoral paresthesias 5–6%. Dose >100 mg bid assoc. with ↑ GI side effects & ↑ in lipid abnormalities.	**Black Box** warning relates to many important drug-drug interactions—inhibits P450 CYP3A & CYP2D6 system—may be life-threatening (see *Table 32b, p. 198*). Several cases of iatrogenic Cushing's syndrome reported with concomitant use of ritonavir and corticosteroids, including dosing of the latter by inhalation, epidural injection or a single IM injection. Rarely Stevens-Johnson syndrome, toxic epidermal necrolysis and anaphylaxis. Primary A-V block (and higher) and pancreatitis have been reported. Hepatic reactions, including fatalities. Monitor LFTs carefully during therapy, especially in those with pre-existing liver disease, including HBV and HCV.
Saquinavir (Invirase hard cap, tablet)	**Diarrhea,** abdominal discomfort, nausea, headache	**Warning—Use Invirase only with ritonavir.** Avoid garlic capsules (may reduce SQV levels) and use cautiously with proton-pump inhibitors (increased SQV levels possible). Use of saquinavir/ritonavir can prolong QTc interval or may rarely cause 2° or 3° heart block; torsades reported. Contraindicated in patients with prolonged QTc or those taking drugs of who have other conditions (e.g., low K+ or Mg++) that pose a risk with prolonged QTc interval. Contraindicated in patients with complete AV block, or those at risk, who do not have a pacemaker. Hepatic toxicity encountered in patients with pre-existing liver disease or in individuals receiving concomitant rifampin. Rarely, Stevens Johnson syndrome *(http://www.fda.gov/drugs/DrugSafety/ucm230096.htm, accessed May 25, 2011)*.
Tipranavir (Aptivus)	Nausea & vomiting, diarrhea, abdominal pain. Rash in 8–14%, more common in women, & 33% in women taking ethinyl estradiol. Major lipid effects.	**Black Box Warning—associated with hepatitis & fatal hepatic failure.** Risk of hepatotoxicity increased in hepB or hepC co-infection. Possible photosensitivity & ↑ serum transaminases). Contraindicated in Child-Pugh Class B or C hepatic impairment. **Associated with fatal/nonfatal intracranial hemorrhage (can inhibit platelet aggregation).** Caution in those with bleeding risks. Potential for major drug interactions. Contains sulfa moiety and vitamin E.
Fusion Inhibitor		
Enfuvirtide (T20, Fuzeon)	Local injection site reactions (98%, at least ↑ local ISR, 4% dc because of ISR (pain & discomfort, induration, erythema, nodules & cysts, pruritus, & ecchymosis). Diarrhea 32%, nausea 23%, fatigue 20%.	↑ Rate of bacterial pneumonia (3.2 pneumonia events/100 yrs). hypersensitivity reactions <1% (rash, fever, nausea & vomiting, chills, rigors, hypotension, & ↑ serum liver transaminases), can occur with reexposure. Cutaneous amyloid deposits containing enfuvirtide peptide reported in skin plaques persisting after discontinuation of drug *(J Cutan Pathol 39:220, 2012)*.
CCR5 Co-receptor Antagonists		
Maraviroc (Selzentry)	With ARV background: Cough 13%, fever 12%, rash 10%, abdominal pain 8%. Also, dizziness, myalgia, arthralgias. ↑ Risk of URI, HSV infection.	**Black box warning–Hepatotoxicity.** May be preceded by allergic features (rash, ↑eosinophils or IgE levels). Use with caution in pt with HepB or C. Cardiac ischemia/infarction 1.3%. May cause ↓BP, orthostatic syncope, especially in patients with renal dysfunction. Significant interactions with CYP3A inducers/inhibitors. Long-term risk of malignancy unknown. Stevens-Johnson syndrome reported post-marketing. Generally favorable safety profile during trial of ART-naive individuals *(JID 201: 803, 2010)*.
Integrase Inhibitors		
Raltegravir (Isentress)	Diarrhea, headache, insomnia, nausea. LFT ↑ may be more common in pts co-infected with HBV or HCV.	Hypersensitivity reactions can occur. Rash, Stevens-Johnson syndrome. toxic epidermal necrolysis reported. Hepatic failure reported. ↑CK, myopathy and rhabdomyolysis reported *(AIDS 22:1382, 2008)*. ↑ of preexisting depression reported in 4 pts; all could continue raltegravir after adjustment of psych. meds *(AIDS 22:1890, 2008)*. Chewable tablets contain phenylalanine.
Elvitegravir + Cobicistat (Stribild), Elvitegravir (Vitekta)	Nausea and diarrhea are the two most common AEs. ↑ serum creatinine 0.1–0.15 mg/dL due to inhibition of prox. tubular enzymes by cobicistat with no decrease in GFR	Same **Black Box warnings as ritonavir and tenofovir** (TDF and TAF). Rare lactic acidosis syndrome. Owing to renal toxicity, should not initiate Rx when pre-Rx eGFR is < 70 cc/min. Monitor serum creatinine and urinary protein and glucose. Discontinue drug if serum Cr rises > 0.4 mg/dl above baseline value.
Dolutegravir (Tivicay)	Insomnia and headache (2–4%)	Rash, liver injury reported. Increased ALT/AST in 20%. Competition with creatinine for tubular secretion increased serum creatinine by a mean of 0.1 mg/dL with no change in GFR.

TABLE 14E – HEPATITIS A & HBV TREATMENT

For HBV Activity Spectra, see *Table 4C, page 79*

Hepatitis A Virus (HAV)

1. **Drug/Dosage:** No therapy recommended. If within 2 wks of exposure, prophylactic IVIG 0.02 mL per kg IM times 1 protective. Hep A vaccine equally effective as IVIG in randomized trial and is emerging as preferred Rx *(NEJM 357:1685, 2007).*

2. **HAV Superinfection:** 40% of pts with chronic Hepatitis C virus (HCV) infection who developed superinfection with HAV developed fulminant hepatic failure *(NEJM 338:286, 1998)*. Similar data in pts with chronic Hepatitis B virus (HBV) infection that suffer acute HAV *(Ann Trop Med Parasitol 93:745, 1999)*. **Hence, need to vaccinate all HBV and HCV pts with HAV vaccine.**

HBV Treatment

	ALT	HBV DNA	HBe Ag	Recommendation
Immune-Tolerant Phase	Normal	> 1x106 IU/ml	Positive	**Monitor:** ALT levels be tested at least every 6 months for adults with immunetolerant CHB to monitor for potential transition to immune-active or -inactive CHB. **NB: For those over 40 years of age + liver fibrosis, TREAT as Immune Active (below)**
HBeAg+ Immune Active Phase	Elevated	> 20,000 IU/ml	Positive	**TREAT (Duration of therapy+):** Tenofovir (indefinitely; esp. if fibrosis) OR Entecavir (indefinitely; esp. if fibrosis) OR Peg-IFN++ (48 weeks of Rx)
Inactive CHB Phase	Normal	< 2,000 IU/ml	Negative	**Monitor:** ALT levels at least once / year
HBeAg-neg Immune Reactivation Phase	Elevated	> 2,000 IU/ml	Negative	**TREAT (Duration of therapy+):** Tenofovir (indefinitely); esp. if fibrosis) OR Entecavir (indefinitely; esp. if fibrosis) OR Peg-IFN++ (48 weeks of Rx)

+ Duration of therapy largely unknown; most experts favor indefinite Rx, esp. among those with moderate to advanced fibrosis or inflammation (liver biopsy)

++ Peg-INF contraindicated in patients with decompensated cirrhosis, autoimmune disease, uncontrolled psychiatric disease, cytopenias, severe cardiac disease, and uncontrolled seizures

For details of therapy, especially in special populations (e.g., pregnant women, children) see updated AASLD Guidelines *(Hepatology, 2015 Nov 13. doi: 10.1002/hep.2)*

HBV Treatment Regimens. Single drug therapy is usually sufficient; combination therapy for HIV co-infection.

	Drug/Dose	Comments
Preferred Regimens	**Pegylated-Interferon-alpha 2a** 180 µg sc once weekly OR **Entecavir** 0.5 mg po once daily OR **Tenofovir** 300 mg po once daily OR **Tenofovir alfenamide** 25 mg po once daily	PEG-IFN: Treat for 48 weeks Entecavir: Do not use Entecavir if Lamivudine resistance present. Entecavir/Tenofovir: Treat for at least 24-48 weeks after seroconversion from HBeAg to anti-HBe (if no mod-adv fibrosis present). Indefinite chronic therapy for HBeAg negative patients. Renal impairment dose adjustments necessary.
Alternative Regimens	**Lamivudine** 100 mg po once daily OR **Telbivudine** 600 mg po once daily OR **Emtricitabine** 200 mg po once daily (investigational) OR **Adefovir** 10 mg po once daily	These alternative agents are rarely used except in combination. When used, restrict to short term therapy owing to high rates of development of resistance. Not recommended as first-line therapy. Use of Adefovir has mostly been replaced by Tenofovir.
Preferred Regimen for HIV-HBV Co-Infected Patient	**Truvada** (Tenofovir 300 mg + Emtricitabine 200 mg) po once daily + another anti-HIV drug	ALL patients if possible as part of a fully suppressive anti-HIV/anti-HBV regimen. Continue therapy indefinitely.

TABLE 14F – HCV TREATMENT REGIMENS AND RESPONSE

For HCV Activity Spectra, see Table 4C, page 79

- **Indications for Treatment.** Treatment is indicated for all patients with chronic HCV. Rx should be initiated urgently for those with more advanced fibrosis (F3 / F4) and those with underlying co-morbid conditions due to HCV. Type and duration of Rx is based on genotype. Pegylated interferon (Peg-IFN) is no longer a recommended regimen; all DAA regimens with or without ribavirin are the preferred choice.

- **Definitions of Response to Therapy.**

End of Treatment Response (ETR)	Undetectable at end of treatment.
Relapse	Undetectable at end of therapy (ETR) but rebound (detectable) virus within 12 weeks after therapy stopped.
Sustained Virologic Response (SVR)	CURE! Still undetectable at end of therapy and beyond 12 weeks after therapy is stopped.

- **HCV Treatment Regimens**

  - Biopsy is a 'gold standard' for staging HCV infection and is helpful in some settings to determine the ideal timing of HCV treatment. When bx not obtained, 'non-invasive' tests are often employed to assess the relative probability of advanced fibrosis or cirrhosis. Fibroscan (elastography) is now approved in the US and most of the world as a means of assessing liver fibrosis. Elastography values of > 10 kPa (Kilopascals) correlates with significant fibrosis (F3 or F4 disease).

  - Resistance tests: Genotypic resistance assays are available that can determine polymorphisms associated with reduction in susceptibility to some DAAs (Direct Acting Agents, e.g., protease inhibitors). **However, resistance tests are recommended only for those who have failed treatment with a prior NS5A or protease inhibitor regimen.**

  - **Patients with decompensated cirrhosis should only be treated by hepatologists owing to the risk of rapid clinical deterioration while receiving treatment for HCV.**

  - **IMPORTANT NOTE REGARDING TREATMENT DECISION-MAKING:** Newer drugs are in development and options for Rx are changing rapidly (i.e., several times per year). Monitor updates at *webedition.sanfordguide.com* or *hcvguidelines.org*.

INITIAL TREATMENT FOR PATIENTS WITH CHRONIC HCV

For retreatment and special populations (e.g., decompensated cirrhotics) see www.hcvguidelines.org.

Drug	Abbreviation	Formulation/Dose
Daclatasvir	DCL	60 mg tablet once daily (dose adjustment needed for CYP3A4 inhibitors or inducers)
Dasabuvir	DBV	250 mg tablet po twice daily
Paritaprevir + Ritonavir + Ombitasvir	PTV/r/OBV	Fixed dose combination tablet (Paritaprevir 150 mg + Ritonavir 100 mg + Ombitasvir 25 mg) po once daily
Pegylated Interferon (alfa 2a)	PEG-IFN	180 mcg sc per week
Ribavirin	RBV	Weight based dosing: 1000 mg (< 75 kg) or 1200 mg (> 75 kg)) po twice daily
Simeprevir	SMV	150 mg tablet po once daily
Sofosbuvir	SOF	400 mg tablet po once daily
Sofosbuvir + Ledipasvir	SOF/LDV	Fixed dose combination tablet (Sofosbuvir 400 mg + Ledipasvir 90 mg) po once daily

TABLE 14F (2)

Genotype	Recommended	Alternative	Not Recommended
1a	• **(Harvoni)** SOF/LDV x 12 weeks OR • DCL / **SOF** x 12 weeks (24 wks +/- RBV if cirrhosis) OR • **(Viekira Pak)** PTV/r/OBV + DBV + **RBV X** 12 weeks OR • **SOF/SMV** ± RBV x 12 weeks	None	• SOF + RBV x 24 weeks • SOF + PEG-IFN/RBV x 12 weeks • SMV + PEG-IFN/RBV X 24 or 48 weeks (RGT) TVR + PEG-IFN/RBV x 24 or 48 weeks (RGT) • BOC + PEG-IFN/RBV x 28 or 48 weeks (RGT) • PEG-IFN/RBV x 48 weeks • Monotherapy with PEG-IFN, RBV, a DAA Do not treat with PEG-IFN or combination DAA regimens. See www.hcvguidelines.org
1b	• **(Harvoni)** SOF/LDV x 12 weeks * OR • DCL / **SOF** x 12 weeks (24 wks +/- RBV if cirrhosis) OR • **(Viekira Pak)** PTV/r/OBV + DBV ± **RBV** (cirrhosis) X 12 weeks OR • SOF + SMV x 12 weeks	None	
2	• **SOF** + RBV x 12-16 weeks (if cirrhosis: extend course) OR • DCL / **SOF** x 12 weeks	None	• PEG-IFN/RBV x 24 weeks • Monotherapy with PEG-IFN, RBV or a DAA • Any regimen with TVR, BOC or SMV
3	• DCL / **SOF** x 12 weeks (24 wks +/- RBV if cirrhosis) OR • SOF + RBV x 24 weeks	SOF + PEG-IFN/RBV x 12 weeks	• PEG-IFN/RBV x 24-48 weeks • Monotherapy with PEG-IFN, RBV or a DAA • Any regimen with TVR, BOC or SMV
4	• **(Technivie)** PTV/r/OBV + RBV x 12 weeks OR • **SOF** + RBV x 24 weeks OR • **(Harvoni)** SOF/LDV x 12 weeks	• **SOF +** PEG-**IFN/RBV** x 12 weeks • **SOF/SMV** +/- RBV x 12 weeks	• SMV x 12 weeks + PEG-IFN/RBV x 24-48 weeks • SMV x 12 weeks + PEG-IFN/RBV x 24-48 weeks • Monotherapy with PEG-IFN, RBV, or a DAA • Any regimen with TVR or BOC
5	SOF + PEG-IFN + RBV x 12 weeks	PEG-IFN + RBV x 48 weeks	• Monotherapy with PEG-IFN, RBV, or a DAA • Any regimen with TVR or BOC
6	**(Harvoni)** SOF/LDV x 12 weeks	SOF + PEG-IFN + RBV x 12 weeks	

* 8 weeks of therapy can be used in selected patients (see www.hcvguidelines.org); not applicable to those with HIV-HCV coinfection

The regimens will change. For updates go to: webedition.sanfordguide.com and www.hcvguidelines.org

TABLE 15A – ANTIMICROBIAL PROPHYLAXIS FOR SELECTED BACTERIAL INFECTIONS

CLASS OF ETIOLOGIC AGENT/DISEASE/CONDITION	PROPHYLAXIS AGENT/DOSE/ROUTE/DURATION	COMMENTS
Group B streptococcal disease (GBS), neonatal: Approaches to management [CDC Guidelines, *MMWR 59 (RR-10):1, 2010*]:		
Pregnant women—Intrapartum antimicrobial prophylaxis procedures:		**Regimens for prophylaxis against early-onset group B streptococcal disease in**
1. Screen all pregnant women with vaginal & rectal swab for GBS at 35–37 wks gestation (unless other indications for prophylaxis exist: GBS bacteriuria during this pregnancy or previously delivered infant with invasive GBS disease; even then cultures may be useful for susceptibility testing). Use transport medium; GBS survive at room temp. up to 96 hrs. **Rx during labor if swab culture positive.**		**neonate used during labor:** **Penicillin** G 5 million Units IV (initial dose) then 2.5 to 3 million Units IV q4h until delivery Alternative: **Ampicillin** 2 gm IV (initial dose) then 1 gm IV q4h until delivery Penicillin-allergic patients: • Patient not at high risk for anaphylaxis: **Cefazolin** 2 gm IV (initial dose) then 1 gm IV q8h until delivery • Patient at high risk for anaphylaxis from β-lactams:
2. Rx during labor if previously delivered infant with invasive GBS infection, or if any GBS bacteriuria during this pregnancy.		□ If organism is both clindamycin- and erythromycin-susceptible, **or** is erythromycin-resistant, but clindamycin-susceptible confirmed by D-zone test
3. Rx if GBS status unknown but if any of the following are present: (a) delivery at <37 wks gestation [see *MMWR 59 (RR-10): 1, 2010* algorithms for preterm premature rupture of membranes]; or (b) duration of ruptured membranes ≥18 hrs; or (c) intrapartum temp. ≥100.4ºF (≥38.0ºC). If amnionitis suspected, broad-spectrum antibiotic coverage should include an agent active vs. group B streptococcus.		(or equivalent) showing lack of inducible resistance: **Clindamycin** 900 mg IV q8h until delivery □ If susceptibility of organism unknown, lack of inducible resistance to clindamycin has not been excluded, or patient is allergic to clindamycin: **Vancomycin** 1 gm IV q12h until delivery
4. Rx if positive intra-partum NAAT for GBS.		
5. Rx not indicated if: negative vaginal/rectal cultures at 35–37 wks gestation or C-section performed before onset of labor with intact amniotic membranes (use standard surgical prophylaxis).		
Neonate of mother given prophylaxis	See detailed algorithm in MMWR 59 (RR-10):1, 2010	
Pre-term, premature rupture of the membranes: Grp B strep-negative women Cochrane Database Rev 12:CD00:1058, 2013; *Obstet Gyn* 124:515;2014; *Am J Ob-Gyn* 207:475, 2012.	(**AMP** 2 gm IV q6h + **Erythro** 250 mg IV q6h) x 48 hrs, then (**Amox** 250 mg po q8h + **Erythro base** 333 mg po q8h) x 5 days	
Post-splenectomy bacteremia. Usually encapsulated bacteria: pneumococci, H. flu type B, bacteremia: meningococci, Enterobacter, S. aureus, Capnocytophaga, P. aeruginosa. Also at risk for fatal malaria, severe babesiosis	Protein conjugate pneumococcal (followed by polysaccharide vaccine at least 8 wks later in those age 2 yrs or older); H. influenza type B and meningococcal vaccine (CID 58:309, 2014); persons age 10 yrs or older should also receive meningococcal B vaccine (MMWR 64:608, 2015). Daily Prophylaxis in asplenic child (daily until age 5 yrs or minimum of 1 yr): **Amox** 125 mg po bid (age 2mo-3yr); **Amox** 250 mg po bid (age >3yr-5 yr). If allergic, e.g rash only: **Cephalexin** 250 mg po bid. If IgE-mediated reaction, i.e. CID 52:e18; 2011. In Children & Adults: **AM-CL** 875/125 po bid (adult), 90 mg/kg po div bid (child); Alternative: (**Levo** 750 mg po or **Moxi** 400 mg po) once daily. Some recommend **Amox** 2 gm po before sinus or airway procedures.

TABLE 15A (2)

CLASS OF ETIOLOGIC AGENT/DISEASE/CONDITION	PROPHYLAXIS AGENT/DOSE/ROUTE/DURATION	COMMENTS
Sexual Exposure		
Sexual assault survivor [likely agents and risks; see CDC Guidelines at *MMWR* 64(RR-3):1, 2015]. For review of overall care: *NEJM* 365:834, 2011.	[**Ceftriaxone** 250 mg IM + **Azithro** 1 gm po once + **Metro** 2 gm po once or **Tinidazole** 2 gm po once)]. Can delay Metro/Tinidazole if alcohol was recently ingested.	• Obtain expert individualized advice re: forensic exam and specimens; pregnancy (incl. emergency contraception); physical trauma, psychological support • Test for chlamydia and gonorrhea at sites of penetration or attempted penetration by NAATs. Obtain molecular tests for Trichomonas and check vaginal secretions for BV and candidiasis. • Serological evaluation for syphilis, HIV, HBV, HCV • Initiate post-exposure protocols for HBV vaccine, HIV post-exposure prophylaxis as appropriate • HPV vaccine recommended for females 9-26 or males 9-21, if not already immunized • Follow-up in 1-2 weeks to review results; repeat negative tests in 1-2 weeks to detect infections not detected previously; repeat syphilis testing 4-6 weeks and 3 months, repeat HIV testing 6 weeks and 3-6 months. • Check for anogenital warts at 1-2 months. Notes: If ceftriaxone not available, can use cefixime 400 mg po once in its place for prevention of gonorrhea, but the latter is less effective for pharyngeal infection and against strains with reduced susceptibility to cephalosporins. For non-pregnant individuals who cannot receive cephalosporins, treatment with (Gemi 320 mg po once + azithro 2 gm po once) or (gent 240 mg IM once + azithro 2 gm po once) can be substituted for ceftriaxone/ azithro.
Contact with specific sexually transmitted diseases	See comprehensive guidelines for specific pathogens in *MMWR* 59 (RR-10):1, 2010.	
Syphilis exposure		Presumptive Rx for exposure within 3 mos., as tests may be negative. *See Table 1, page 24.* If exposure occurred > 90 days prior, establish dx or treat empirically (*MMWR* 59 (RR-12): 1, 2010).
Sickle-cell disease. Likely agent: S. pneumoniae (see post-splenectomy, above) Ref. 2009 Red Book Online, Amer Acad Pediatrics	Children <5 yrs: **Penicillin V** 125 mg po bid ≥5 yrs: **Penicillin V** 250 mg po bid. (Alternative in children: Amoxicillin 20 mg per kg per day)	Start prophylaxis by 2 mos. Prophylaxis in infants age < 3 mos. must be individualized. Age-appropriate vaccines, including pneumococcal, Hib, influenza, meningococcal. Treating infections, consider possibility of penicillin non-susceptible pneumococci.

TABLE 15B – ANTIBIOTIC PROPHYLAXIS TO PREVENT SURGICAL INFECTIONS IN ADULTS*

2013 Guidelines; Am J Health Syst Pharm 70:195, 2013

General Comments:
• To be optimally effective, antibiotics must be started within 60 minutes of the surgical incision. Vancomycin and FQs may require 1-2 hr infusion time, so start dose 2 hrs before the surgical incision.
• Most applications employ a single preoperative dose or continuation for less than 24 hrs.
• For procedures lasting > 2 half-lives of prophylactic agent, intraoperative supplementary dose(s) may be required.
• Dose adjustments may be desirable in pts with BMI > 30.
• Prophylaxis does carry risk, e.g., difficile colitis, allergic reactions
• Active S. aureus screening, decolonization & customized antimicrobial prophylaxis demonstrated efficacious in decreasing infections after hip, knee & cardiac surgery (*JAMA* 313:2131 & 2162, 2015).
• In general, recommendations are consistent with those of the Surgical Care Improvement Project (SCIP)

Use of Vancomycin:
• For many common prophylaxis indications, vancomycin is considered an alternative to β-lactams in pts allergic to or intolerant of the latter.
• Vancomycin use may be justifiable in centers where rates of post-operative infection with methicillin-resistant staphylococci are high or in pts at high risk for these.
• Unlike β-lactams in common use, vancomycin has no activity against gram-negative organisms. **When gram-negative bacteria are a concern following specific procedures, it may be necessary or desirable to add a second agent with appropriate in vitro activity.** This can be done using cefazolin with vancomycin in the non-allergic pt, or in pts intolerant of β-lactams using vancomycin with another gram-negative agent (e.g., aminoglycoside, fluoroquinolone, possibly aztreonam, if pt not allergic; local resistance patterns & pt factors would influence choice).
• Infusion of vancomycin, especially too rapidly, may result in hypotension or other manifestations of histamine release (red person syndrome). Does not indicate an allergy to vancomycin.

TYPE OF SURGERY	PROPHYLAXIS	COMMENTS
Cardiovascular Surgery Antibiotic prophylaxis in cardiovascular surgery has been proven beneficial in the following procedures: • Procedures that involve a groin incision • Any vascular procedure that inserts prosthesis/foreign body • Lower extremity amputation for ischemia • Cardiac surgery • Permanent Pacemakers (*Circulation 121:458, 2010*) • Heart transplant • Implanted cardiac defibrillators	**Cefazolin** 1–2 gm IV as a single dose or 3 gm (Wt >120 kg) IV as a single dose or q8h for 1–2 days or **cefuroxime** 1.5 gm IV as a single dose or q12h for total of 6 gm or **vancomycin** 1 gm IV as single dose or q12h for pts weighing ≥90 kg, use vanco 1.5 gm IV as a single dose or q12h for 1–2 days. Re-dose cefazolin q4h if CrCl >30 mL/min or q8h if CrCl ≤30 mL/min Consider **intranasal mupirocin** evening before, day of surgery & bid for 5 days post-op in pts with pos. nasal culture for S. aureus. Mupirocin resistance has been encountered.	**Timing & duration:** Single infusion just before surgery as effective as multiple doses. No prophylaxis needed for cardiac catheterization. For prosthetic heart valves, customary to stop prophylaxis either after removal of retrosternal drainage catheters or just a single dose after stop prophylaxis either after removal of retrosternal drainage catheters. For MRSA in high-risk pts, those colonized with MRSA or for Pen-allergic pts. **Vancomycin** 1 gm IV as single dose is another alternative for Pen-allergic or Vanco-allergic pt. Clindamycin 900 mg IV is another alternative for Pen-allergic or Vanco-allergic pt. Clindamycin 900 mg IV is another alternative for Pen-allergic or Vanco-allergic pt. Clindamycin 900 mg IV is another alternative for Pen-allergic or Vanco-allergic pt. See *JAC 70:325, 2015.*
Gastric, Biliary and Colonic Surgery **Gastroduodenal/Biliary** Gastroduodenal, includes percutaneous endoscopic gastrostomy (high risk only), pancreaticoduodenectomy (Whipple procedure).	**Cefazolin** (1–2 gm IV) or **cefoxitin** (1–2 gm IV) or **cefotetan** (1–2 gm IV) or **ceftriaxone** (2 gm IV) as a single dose (some give additional doses q12h for 2–3 days). See *Comment*	Gastroduodenal (PEG placement): High-risk: marked obesity, obstruction, ↓ gastric acid or ↓ motility. Re-dose cefazolin q4h and cefoxitin q2h if CrCl >30 mL/min; q8h and q4h, respectively, if CrCl ≤30 ml/min
Biliary, includes laparoscopic cholecystectomy.	Low risk, laparoscopic: No prophylaxis Open cholecystectomy: **cefazolin, cefoxitin, cefotetan, ampicillin-sulbactam**	Biliary high-risk or open procedure: age >70, acute cholecystitis, non-functioning gallbladder, obstructive jaundice or common duct stones. With cholangitis, treat as infection, not prophylaxis.
Endoscopic retrograde cholangiopancreatography	No rx without obstruction. If obstruction: **Ciprofloxacin** 500–750 mg po or 400 mg IV 2 hrs prior to procedure or **PIP-TZ** 4.5 gm IV 1 hr prior to procedure	Most studies show that achieving adequate drainage will prevent post-procedural cholangitis or sepsis and no further benefit from prophylactic antibiotics; greatest benefit likely when complete drainage cannot be achieved. See *Gastroint Endosc 67:791, 2008; Gut 58:868, 2009.*
Colorectal Recommend combination of: • Mechanical bowel prep • PO antibiotic (See Comment) • IV antibiotic	**Parenteral regimens** (emergency or elective): [**Cefazolin** 1–2 gm IV + **metronidazole** 0.5 gm IV (see *Comment*)] or **cefoxitin** or **cefotetan** 1–2 gm IV (if available) or **Ceftriaxone** 2 gm IV + Metro 0.5 gm IV or **ERTA** 1 gm IV Beta-lactam allergy, see *Comment*	**Oral regimens: Neomycin + erythromycin.** Pre-op day: (1) 10 am 4L polyethylene glycol electrolyte solution (Colyte, GoLYTELY) po over 2 hr. (2) Clear liquid diet only. (3) 1 pm, 2 pm & 11 pm, neomycin 1 gm + erythro base 1 gm po. (4) NPO after midnight. GoLYTELY 1–6 pm; then neomycin 2 gm po + metronidazole 2 gm po at 7 pm & 11 pm. Alternative regimens have been less well studied. Oral regimen as effective as parenteral; parenteral in addition to oral not required but often used (*Am J Surg 189:395, 2005*). Study found **Ertapenem** more effective than cefotetan, but associated with non-significant ↑ risk of C. difficile (*NEJM 355:2640, 2006*). **Beta lactam allergy: Clindamycin** 900 mg IV + (**Gentamicin** 5 mg/kg or **Aztreonam** 2 gm IV or **Ciprofloxacin** 400 mg IV)

Ruptured viscus: See *Peritoneum/Peritonitis, Secondary, Table 1, page 47.*

TABLE 15B (3)

TYPE OF SURGERY	PROPHYLAXIS	COMMENTS
Head and Neck Surgery		
	Cefazolin 2 gm IV (Single dose) (some add **metronidazole** 500 mg IV) **OR Clindamycin** 600–900 mg IV (single dose) ± **gentamicin** 5 mg/kg IV (single dose) (See Table 10D for weight-based dose calculation).	Antimicrobial prophylaxis in head & neck surg appears efficacious only for procedures involving oral/pharyngeal mucosa (e.g., laryngeal or pharyngeal tumor) but even with prophylaxis, wound infection rate can be high. **Clean, uncontaminated head & neck surg does not require prophylaxis.** Re-dose cefazolin q4h if CrCl >30 mL/min or q8h if CrCl ≤50 mL/min
Neurosurgical Procedures		
Clean, non-implant; e.g. elective craniotomy	**Cefazolin** 1–2 gm IV once. Alternative: **vanco** 1 gm IV once; for pts weighing > 90 kg, use vanco 1.5 gm IV as single dose.	**Clindamycin** 900 mg IV is alternative for vanco-allergic or beta-lactam allergic pt. Re-dose cefazolin q4h if CrCl >30 mL/min or q8h if CrCl ≤50 mL/min
Clean, contaminated (cross sinuses, or naso/oropharynx)	**Clindamycin** 900 mg IV (single dose)	British recommend amoxicillin-clavulanate 1.2 gm IV^a,d or (cefuroxime 1.5 gm IV + metronidazole 0.5 gm IV)
CSF shunt surgery, intrathecal pumps:	**Cefazolin** 1–2 gm (Wt < 120 kg) or 3 gm (Wt > 120 kg) IV once. Alternative: **vanco** 1 gm IV once; for pts weighing > 90 kg, use vanco 1.5 gm IV as single dose OR **Clindamycin** 900 mg IV	Randomized study in a hospital with high prevalence of infection due to methicillin-resistant staphylococci showed vancomycin was more effective than cefazolin in preventing CSF shunt infections (J Hosp Infect 69:337, 2008). Re-dose cefazolin q4h if CrCl >30 mL/min or q8h if CrCl ≤50 mL/min
Obstetric/Gynecologic Surgery		
Vaginal or abdominal hysterectomy	**Cefazolin** 1–2 gm or **cefoxitin** 1–2 gm or **cefotetan** 1–2 gm or **ampicillin-sulbactam** 3 gm IV 30 min. before surgery.	Alternative: (**Clindamycin** 900 mg IV or **Vancomycin** 1 gm IV) + (**Gentamicin** 5 mg/kg x 1 dose or **Aztreonam** 2 gm IV or **Ciprofloxacin** 400 mg IV) OR (**Metronidazole** 500 mg IV + **Ciprofloxacin** 400 mg IV)
Cesarean section for premature rupture of membranes or active labor	**Cefazolin** 1–2 gm IV (See Comments). Alternative: **Clindamycin** 900 mg IV + (**Gentamicin** 5 mg/kg IV or **Tobramycin** 5 mg/kg IV) x 1 dose	Prophylaxis decreases risk of endometritis and wound infection. Traditional approach had been to administer antibiotics after cord is clamped to avoid exposing infant to antibiotic. However, studies suggest that administering prophylaxis before the skin incision results in fewer surgical site infections (Obstet Gynecol 115:187, 2010; Amer J Obstet Gynecol 199:301.e1 and 310.e1, 2008) and endometritis (Amer J Obstet Gynecol 196:455.e1, 2007). Meta-analysis showed benefit of antibiotic prophylaxis in all risk groups.
Surgical Abortion (1st trimester)	1st trimester: **Doxycycline** 300 mg po: 100 mg 1 hr before procedure + 200 mg post-procedure.	
Orthopedic Surgery		
Hip arthroplasty, spinal fusion	Same as cardiac surgery	Customarily stopped after "Hemovac" removed. 2013 Guidelines recommend stopping prophylaxis within 24 hrs of surgery (Am J Health Syst Pharm 70:195, 2013).
Total joint replacement (other than hip)	**Cefazolin** 1–2 gm IV pre-op (± 2nd dose) or **vancomycin** 1 gm IV. For pts weighing > 90 kg, use vanco 1.5 gm IV as single dose or **Clindamycin** 900 mg IV	2013 Guidelines recommend stopping prophylaxis within 24 hrs of surgery (Am J Health Syst Pharm 70:195, 2013). Usual to administer before tourniquet inflation. Intranasal mupirocin if colonized with S. aureus.
Open reduction of closed fracture with internal fixation	**Ceftriaxone** 2 gm IV once	3.6% (ceftriaxone) vs 8.3% (for placebo) infection found in Dutch trauma trial (Ln 347:1133, 1996). Several alternative antimicrobials can ↓ risk of infection (Cochrane Database Syst Rev 2010: CD 000244).

TABLE 15B (4)

TYPE OF SURGERY	PROPHYLAXIS	COMMENTS
Orthop. Surgery, (contd) Prophylaxis to protect prosthetic joints from hematogenous infection related to distant procedures (patients with plates, pins and screws only are not considered to be at risk)		• A prospective, case-control study concluded that antibiotic prophylaxis for dental procedures did not decrease the risk of hip or knee prosthesis infection (*Clin Infect Dis 50:8, 2010*). • An expert panel of the American Dental Association concluded that, in general, prophylactic antibiotics are not recommended prior to dental procedures to prevent prosthetic joint infection (*J Amer Dental Assoc. 146: 11, 2015*). • Individual circumstances should be considered, when there is planned manipulation of tissues thought to be actively infected, antimicrobial therapy for the infection is likely to be appropriate.
Peritoneal Dialysis Catheter Placement	**Vancomycin** single 1 gm IV dose 12 hrs prior to procedure	Effectively reduced peritonitis during 14 days post-placement in 221 pts: vanco 1%, cefazolin 7%, placebo 12% (p=0.02) (*Am J Kidney Dis 36:1014, 2000*).
Urologic Surgery/Procedures • See **Best Practice Policy Statement** of Amer. Urological Assoc. (AUA) (*J Urol 179: 1379, 2008*) and 2013 Guidelines (*Am J Health Syst Pharm. 70:195, 2013*). • Selection of agents targeting urinary pathogens may require modification based on local resistance patterns; † TMP-SMX and/or fluoroquinolone (FQ) resistance among enteric gram-negative bacteria is a concern.		
Cystoscopy	• Prophylaxis generally not necessary if urine is sterile (however, AUA recommends FQ or TMP-SMX for those with several potentially adverse host factors (e.g. advanced age, immunocompromised state, anatomic abnormalities, etc.) • Treat patients with UTI prior to procedure using an antimicrobial active against pathogen isolated	
Cystoscopy with manipulation	**Ciprofloxacin** 500 mg po or **TMP-SMX** 1 DS tablet po may be an alternative in populations with low rates of resistance	Procedures mentioned include ureteroscopy, biopsy, fulguration, TURP, etc. Treat UTI with targeted therapy before procedure if possible
Transrectal prostate biopsy	**Ciprofloxacin** 500 mg po 12 hrs prior to biopsy and repeated 12 hrs after 1st dose. See *Comment*.	Bacteremia 7% with **CIP** & 37% with **gentamicin** (*JAC 39:115, 1997*). **Levofloxacin** 500 mg 30-60 min before procedure was effective in low risk pts; additional doses were given for † risk (*J Urol 168:1021, 2002*). Serious bacteremias due to FQ-resistant organisms have been encountered in patients receiving FQ prophylaxis. Screening stool cultures pre-procedure for colonization with FQ-resistant organisms is increasingly utilized to inform choice of infection with culture-directed antimicrobial prophylaxis (*Clin Infect Dis 60: 979, 2015*). One study showed non-significant decrease in risk of infection with culture-directed antimicrobial prophylaxis (*Urology 146: 11, 2015*). Pre-operative prophylaxis should be determined on an institutional basis based on susceptibility profiles of prevailing organisms. Although 2nd or 3rd generation Cephalosporins or addition of single-dose gentamicin has been suggested, infections due to ESBL-producing and multi-resistant organisms have been encountered (*Urol 74:332, 2009*).
Other Breast surgery, herniorrhaphy	**Cefazolin** 1-2 gm IV x 1 dose or **Ampicillin-sulbactam** 3 gm IV x 1 dose or **Clindamycin** 900 mg IV x 1 dose or **Vancomycin** 1 gm IV x 1 dose (1.5 gm if wt > 90 kg)	*Am J Health Syst Pharm 70:195, 2013.*

TABLE 15C – ANTIMICROBIAL PROPHYLAXIS FOR THE PREVENTION OF BACTERIAL ENDOCARDITIS IN PATIENTS WITH UNDERLYING CARDIAC CONDITIONS*

In 2007, the American Heart Association guidelines for the prevention of bacterial endocarditis were updated. The resulting document (*Circulation 2007; 116:1736-1754* and *http://circ.ahajournals.org/cgi/reprint/116/15/1736*), which was also endorsed by the Infectious Diseases Society of America, represents a significant departure from earlier recommendations.

- Antibiotic prophylaxis for dental procedures is now directed at individuals who are likely to suffer the most devastating consequences should they develop endocarditis.
- Prophylaxis to prevent endocarditis is no longer specified for gastrointestinal or genitourinary procedures. The following is adapted from and reflects the new AHA recommendations.

See original publication for explanation and precise details.

SELECTION OF PATIENTS FOR ENDOCARDITIS PROPHYLAXIS

FOR PATIENTS WITH ANY OF THESE HIGH-RISK CARDIAC CONDITIONS ASSOCIATED WITH ENDOCARDITIS:	WHO UNDERGO DENTAL PROCEDURES INVOLVING:	WHO UNDERGO INVASIVE RESPIRATORY PROCEDURES INVOLVING:	WHO UNDERGO INVASIVE PROCEDURES OF THE GI OR GU TRACTS:	WHO UNDERGO PROCEDURES INVOLVING INFECTED SKIN AND SOFT TISSUES:
Prosthetic heart valves Previous infective endocarditis Congenital heart disease with any of the following: • Completely repaired cardiac defect using prosthetic material (Only for 1st 6 months) • Partially corrected but with residual defect near prosthetic material • Uncorrected cyanotic congenital heart disease • Surgically constructed shunts and conduits Valvulopathy following heart transplant	Any manipulation of gingival tissue, dental periapical regions, or perforating the oral mucosa. **PROPHYLAXIS RECOMMENDED‡** *(See Dental Procedures Regimens table below)* (Prophylaxis is not recommended for routine anesthetic injections (unless through infected area), dental x-rays, shedding of primary teeth, adjustment of orthodontic appliances or placement of orthodontic brackets or removable appliances.)	Incision of respiratory tract mucosa **CONSIDER PROPHYLAXIS** *(see Dental Procedures Regimens table)* Or For treatment of established infection: **PROPHYLAXIS RECOMMENDED** *(See Dental Procedures Regimens table but include anti-staphylococcal coverage when S. aureus is of concern).*	PROPHYLAXIS is no longer recommended solely to prevent endocarditis, **but the following approach is reasonable:** For patients with enterococcal UTIs • treat before elective GU procedures • include enterococcal coverage in perioperative regimen for non-elective procedures† For patients with existing GU or GI infections or those who receive perioperative antibiotics to prevent surgical site infections or sepsis • it is reasonable to include agents with anti-enterococcal activity in perioperative coverage†	Include coverage against staphylococci and β-hemolytic streptococci in treatment regimens

† Agents with anti-enterococcal activity include penicillin, ampicillin, amoxicillin, vancomycin and others. Check susceptibility if available. *(See Table 5 for highly resistant organisms).*
‡ 2008 AHA/ACC focused update of guidelines on valvular heart disease use term "is reasonable to reflect level of evidence *(Circulation 118:887, 2008).*

PROPHYLACTIC REGIMENS FOR DENTAL PROCEDURES

SITUATION	AGENT	REGIMEN†
Usual oral prophylaxis	Amoxicillin	Adults 2 gm, children 50 mg per kg, orally, 1 hour before procedure.
Unable to take oral medications	Ampicillin²	Adults 2 gm, children 50 mg per kg, IV or IM, within 30 min before procedure.
Allergic to penicillins	Cephalexin³ OR	Adults 2 gm, children 50 mg per kg, orally, 1 hour before procedure.
	Clindamycin OR	Adults 600 mg, children 20 mg per kg, orally, 1 hour before procedure
	Azithromycin or clarithromycin	Adults 500 mg, children 15 mg per kg, orally, 1 hour before procedure.
Allergic to penicillins and unable to take oral medications	Cefazolin³ OR	Adults 1 gm, children 50 mg per kg, IV or IM, within 30 min before procedure
	Clindamycin	Adults 600 mg, children 20 mg per kg, IV or IM, within 30 min before procedure

¹ Children's dose should not exceed adult dose. AHA document lists all doses as 30-60 min before procedure.
² AHA lists cefazolin or ceftriaxone IM or IV as alternatives here.
³ Cephalosporins should not be used in individuals with immediate-type hypersensitivity reaction (urticaria, angioedema, or anaphylaxis) to penicillins or other β-lactams. AHA proposes ceftriaxone as potential alternative to cefazolin, and other 1st or 2nd generation cephalosporin in equivalent doses as potential alternatives to cephalexin.

TABLE 15D – MANAGEMENT OF EXPOSURE TO HIV-1 AND HEPATITIS B AND C*

OCCUPATIONAL EXPOSURE TO BLOOD, PENILE/VAGINAL SECRETIONS OR OTHER POTENTIALLY INFECTIOUS BODY FLUIDS OR TISSUES WITH RISK OF TRANSMISSION OF HEPATITIS B/C AND/OR HIV-1 (E.G., NEEDLESTICK INJURY)

Free consultation for occupational exposures, call (PEPline) 1-888-448-4911. *[Information also available at www.adsinfo.nih.gov]*

General steps in management:

1. Wash clean wounds/flush mucous membranes immediately (use of caustic agents or squeezing the wound is discouraged; data lacking regarding antiseptics).
2. Assess risk by doing the following: (a) Characterize exposure; (b) Determine/evaluate source of exposure by medical history, risk behavior, & testing for hepatitis B/C, HIV; (c) Evaluate and test exposed individual for hepatitis B/C & HIV.

Hepatitis B Occupational Exposure Prophylaxis *(MMWR 62(RR-10):1-19, 2013)*

Exposed Person Vaccine Status	Exposure Source		
	HBs Ag+	HBs Ag–	Status Unknown or Unavailable for Testing[†]
Unvaccinated	Give HBIG 0.06 mL per kg IM & initiate HB vaccine	Initiate HB vaccine	Initiate HB vaccine
Vaccinated (antibody status unknown)	Do anti-HBs on exposed person: If titer ≥10 milli-international units per mL, no rx If titer <10 milli-international units per mL, give HBIG + 1 dose HB vaccine**	No rx necessary	Do anti-HBs on exposed person: If titer ≥10 milli-international units per mL, no rx § If titer <10 milli-international units per mL, give 1 dose of HB vaccine**

[†] Persons previously infected with HBV are immune to reinfection and do not require postexposure prophylaxis.

For known vaccine series responder (titer ≥10 milli-international units per mL), monitoring of levels or booster doses not currently recommended. Known non-responder (<10 milli-international units per mL) to 1° series HB vaccine & exposed to either HBsAg+ source or suspected high-risk source—rx with HBIG & re-initiate vaccine series **or** give 2 doses HBIG 1 month apart. For non-responders after a 2nd vaccine series, 2 doses HBIG 1 month apart is preferred approach to new exposure.

§ If known high risk source, treat as if source were HBsAG positive
** Follow-up to assess vaccine response or address completion of vaccine series.

Hepatitis B Non-Occupational Exposure & Reactivation of Latent Hepatitis B
Non-Occupational Exposure *(MMWR 59(RR-10):1, 2010)*

- Exposure to blood or sexual secretion of HBsAg-positive person
  - Percutaneous (bile, needlestick)
  - Sexual assault
- Initiate immunoprophylaxis within 24 hrs or sexual exposure & no more than 7 days after parenteral exposure
- Use Guidelines for occupational exposure for use of HBIG and HBV vaccine

TABLE 15D (2)

Hepatitis B Non-Occupational Exposure & Reactivation of Latent Hepatitis B (continued)

Reactivation of Latent HBV (Eur J Cancer 49:3486, 2013; Seminar of Liver Dis 33:167, 2013; Crit Rev Oncol-Hematol 87:12, 2013)

- Patients requiring administration of anti-CD 20 monoclonal antibodies as part of treatment selected malignancies, rheumatoid arthritis and vasculitis are at risk for reactivation of latent HBV
- Two FDA-approved anti-CD 20 drugs: ofatumumab (Arzerra) & rituximab (Rituxan)
- Prior to starting anti-CD 20 drug, test for latent HBV with test for HBsAg and Anti IgG HB core antibody
- If pt has latent HBV & anti-CD 20 treatment is necessary, treatment should include an effective anti-HBV drug

Hepatitis C Exposure

Determine antibody to hepatitis C for both exposed person &, if possible, exposure source. If source + or unknown and exposed person test negative, follow-up HCV testing for HCV RNA (detectable in blood in 1-3 weeks) and HCV antibody (90% who seroconvert will do so by 3 months) is advised. **No recommended prophylaxis;** immune serum globulin not effective. Monitor for early infection, as therapy may ↓ risk of progression to chronic hepatitis. Persons who remain viremic 8-12 weeks after exposure should be treated with a course of pegylated interferon (*Gastro 130:632, 2006 and Hot 43:923, 2006*). See *Table 14F*. Case-control study suggested risk factors for occupational HCV transmission include percutaneous exposure to needle that had been in artery or vein, deep injury, male sex of HCW, & was more likely when source VL >6 log10 copies/mL.

HIV: Occupational exposure management [Adapted from CDC recommendations, Infect Control Hosp Epi 34: 875, 2014]

- The decision to initiate postexposure prophylaxis (PEP) for HIV is a clinical judgment that should be made in concert with the exposed healthcare worker (HCW). It is based on:
  1. Likelihood of the source patient having HIV infection: ↑ with history of high-risk activity—injection drug use, sexual activity with multiple partners (either hetero- or homosexual), receipt of blood products 1978–1985, ↑ with clinical signs suggestive of advanced HIV (unexplained wasting, night sweats, thrush, seborrheic dermatitis, etc.).
  2. Type of exposure (approx. 1 in 300–400 needlesticks from infected source will transmit HIV).
  3. Limited data regarding efficacy of PEP (*Cochrane Database Syst Rev. Jan 24; (1):CD002835, 2007*).
  4. Significant adverse effects of PEP drugs & potential for drug interactions.

     Substances considered potentially infectious include: blood, tissues, semen, vaginal secretions, CSF, synovial, pleural, pericardial and amniotic fluids; and other visibly bloody fluids. Fluids normally considered low risk for transmission, unless visibly bloody, include: urine, vomitus, stool, sweat, saliva, nasal secretions, tears and sputum.

- If source person is **known positive for HIV** or **likely to be infected** and **status of exposure warrants PEP,** antiretroviral drugs should be started **immediately.** If source person is HIV antibody negative, drugs can be stopped **unless source is suspected of having acute HIV infection.** The HCW should be re-tested at **3–4 weeks, 3 & 6 months whether PEP is used or not** (the vast majority of seroconversions will occur by 3 months, delayed conversions after 6 months are considered exceedingly rare). Tests for HIV RNA should not be used for dx of HIV infection in HCW because of false-positives (esp. at low titers) & these tests are only approved for dx of established HIV infection (a possible exception is if pt develops signs of acute HIV (mononucleosis-like) syndrome within the 1st 4–6 wks of exposure when antibody tests might still be negative.]
- PEP for HIV is usually given for **4 wks** and monitoring of adverse effects include: baseline **complete blood count, renal and hepatic panel** is repeated at 2 weeks. 50–75% of HCW on PEP demonstrates mild side-effects (nausea, diarrhea, myalgias, headache, etc.) but in up to ½ severe enough to discontinue PEP. Consultation with infectious diseases/ HIV specialist valuable when questions regarding PEP arise. **Seek expert help in special situations, such as pregnancy, renal impairment, treatment-experienced source.**

TABLE 100 (5)

3 Steps to HIV Postexposure Prophylaxis (PEP) After Occupational Exposure: *[Latest CDC recommendations available at www.aidsinfo.nih.gov]*

Step 1: Determine the exposure code (EC)

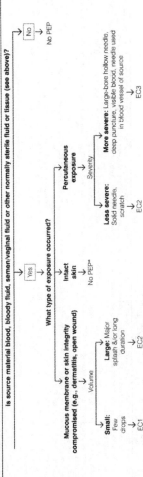

Is source material blood, bloody fluid, semen/vaginal fluid or other normally sterile fluid or tissue (see above)?

→ **Yes**

What type of exposure occurred?

Mucous membrane or skin integrity compromised (e.g., dermatitis, open wound)

Volume

Small: Few drops
→ EC1

Large: Major splash &/or long duration
→ EC2

Intact skin
→ No PEP*

Percutaneous exposure

Severity

Less severe: Solid needle, scratch
→ EC2

More severe: Large-bore hollow needle, deep puncture, visible blood, needle used in blood vessel of source
→ EC3

→ **No** → No PEP

* Exceptions can be considered when there has been prolonged, high-volume contact.

Step 2: Determine the HIV Status Code (HIV SC)

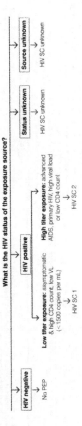

What is the HIV status of the exposure source?

HIV negative
→ No PEP

HIV positive

Low titer exposure: asymptomatic & high CD4 count, low VL (<1500 copies per mL)
→ HIV SC 1

High titer exposure: advanced AIDS, primary HIV, high viral load or low CD4 count
→ HIV SC 2

Status unknown
→ HIV SC unknown

Source unknown
→ HIV SC unknown

TABLE 15D (4)

3 Steps to HIV Postexposure Prophylaxis (PEP) After Occupational Exposure *(continued)*

Step 3: Determine Postexposure Prophylaxis (PEP) Recommendation

EC	HIV SC	PEP
1	1	Consider basic regimen[a]
1	2	Recommend basic regimen[a,b]
2	1	Recommend basic regimen[b]
2	2	Recommend expanded regimen[b]
3	1 or 2	Recommend expanded regimen[b]
1, 2, 3	Unknown	If exposure setting suggests risks of HIV exposure, consider basic regimen[c]

[a] Based on estimates of ↓ risk of infection after mucous membrane exposure in occupational setting compared with needlestick.

[b] Or, consider expanded regimen[a].

[c] In high risk circumstances, consider expanded regimen on case-by-case basis.

**Around the clock, urgent expert consultation available from: National Clinicians'
Postexposure Prophylaxis Hotline (PEPline) at 1-888-HIV-4911 (1-888-448-4911) and on-line
at http://www.ucsf.edu/hivcntr**

Regimens: (Treat for 4 weeks; monitor for drug side-effects every 2 weeks)

Basic regimen: ZDV + 3TC or FTC + TDF, or as an alternative d4T + 3TC.

Expanded regimen: Basic regimen + one of the following: lopinavir/ritonavir *(preferred)*,
or *(as alternatives)* atazanavir/ritonavir or fosamprenavir/ritonavir. Efavirenz can be considered
(except in pregnancy or potential for pregnancy—**Pregnancy Category D**), but CNS
symptoms might be problematic. [**Do not use nevirapine**; serious adverse reactions
including hepatic necrosis reported in healthcare workers.]

Other regimens can be designed. If possible, use antiretroviral drugs for which resistance is
unlikely based on susceptibility data of source pt (if known). Seek expert
consultation if ART-experienced source or potential for pregnancy.

NOTE: Some authorities feel that an expanded regimen should be employed whenever PEP
is indicated. Expanded regimens are likely to be advantageous with ↑ numbers of ART-
experienced source pts or when there is doubt about exact extent of exposures in decision
algorithm. Mathematical model suggests that under some conditions, completion of full course
basic regimen is better than prematurely discontinued expanded regimen. However, while
expanded PEP regimens have ↑ adverse effects, there is not necessarily ↑ discontinuation.

[down arrow]

POSTEXPOSURE PROPHYLAXIS FOR NON-OCCUPATIONAL EXPOSURES TO HIV-1
[Adapted from CDC recommendations, MMWR 54 (RR2), 2005, available at www.cdc.gov/mmwr/indrr_2005.html]

Because the risk of transmission of HIV via sexual contact or sharing needles may reach or exceed that of occupational needlestick exposure, it is reasonable to consider PEP in
persons who have had a non-occupational exposure to blood or other potentially infected fluids (e.g., genital/rectal secretions, breast milk) from an HIV+ source. Risk of HIV acquisition per exposure
varies with the act (for needle sharing and receptive anal intercourse, ≥0.5%; approximately 10-fold lower with insertive vaginal or anal intercourse, 0.05–0.07%). Overt or occult traumatic lesions
may ↑ risk in survivors of sexual assault.

For pts at risk of HIV acquisition through non-occupational exposure to HIV+ source material having occured ≤72 hours before evaluation, DHHS recommendation is to treat for 28 days with an antiretroviral **expanded regimen**, using preferred regimens [efavirenz *(not in pregnancy or pregnancy risk—Pregnancy Category D)* + (3TC or FTC) + (ZDV or TDF)] **or** lopinavir/ritonavir + (3TC or FTC) +
ZDV] or one of several alternative regimens *(see Table 14C & MMWR 54(RR-2):1, 2005].* Failures of prophylaxis have been reported, and may be associated with longer interval from exposure to start
of PEP; this supports prompt initiation of PEP if it is to be used.

Areas of uncertainty: (1) expanded regimens are not proven to be superior to 2-drug regimens, (2) while PEP not recommended for exposures >72 hours before evaluation, it may possibly be effective
in some cases, (3) when HIV status of source patient is unknown, decision to treat and treatment selection must be individualized based on assessment of specific circumstances.

Evaluate for exposures to Hep B, Hep C *(see Occupational PEP above)*, and bacterial sexually-transmitted diseases *(see Table 15A)* and treat as indicated. DHHS recommendations for sexual exposures
to HepB and bacterial pathogens are available in MMWR 55(RR-11), 2006. Persons who are unvaccinated or who have not responded to full HepB vaccine series should receive hepB immune globulin
preferably within 24-hours of percutaneous or mucosal exposure to blood or body fluids of an HBsAg-positive person, along with hepB vaccine, with follow-up to complete vaccine series. Unvaccinated
or not-fully-vaccinated persons exposed to a source with unknown HepBsAg-status should receive vaccine and complete vaccine series. See MMWR 55(RR-11), 2006 for details and recommendations
in other circumstances.

TABLE 15E – PREVENTION OF SELECTED OPPORTUNISTIC INFECTIONS IN HUMAN HEMATOPOIETIC CELL TRANSPLANTATION (HCT) OR SOLID ORGAN TRANSPLANTATION (SOT) IN ADULTS WITH NORMAL RENAL FUNCTION.

General comments: Medical centers performing transplants will have detailed protocols for the prevention of opportunistic infections which are appropriate to the infections encountered, patients represented and resources available at those sites. Regimens continue to evolve and protocols adopted by an institution may differ from those at other centers. Care of transplant patients should be guided by physicians with expertise in this area.

References:

For HCT: Expert guidelines endorsed by the IDSA, updating earlier guidelines (*MMWR 49 (RR-10):1, 2000*) in: *Biol Blood Marrow Transpl 15:1143, 2009*. These guidelines provide recommendations for prevention of additional infections not discussed in this table and provide more detailed information on the infections included here.

For SOT: Recommendations of an expert panel of The Transplantation Society for management of CMV in solid organ transplant recipients in: *Transplantation 89:779, 2010*. Timeline of infections following SOT in: *Amer J Transpl 9 (Suppl 4):S3, 2009*.

OPPORTUNISTIC INFECTION	TYPE OF TRANSPLANT	PROPHYLACTIC REGIMENS
CMV (Recipient + **or** Donor +/Recipient –) Ganciclovir resistance: risk, detection, management (*CID 56:1018, 2013*)	SOT	**Prophylaxis: Valganciclovir** 900 mg po q24h Alternatives include **Ganciclovir** 1000 mg po 3 x/day, **Valacyclovir** 2 gm po 4 x/day *(kidney only, see comment)*; CMV IVIG or IVIG. **Also consider preemptive therapy** (monitor weekly for CMV viremia by PCR (or antigenemia) for 3-6 months post-transplant. If viremia detected, start Valganciclovir 900 mg po bid or Ganciclovir 5 mg/kg IV q12h until clearance of viremia, but for not less than 2 weeks followed by secondary prophylaxis or preemptive approach. Prophylaxis vs pre-emptive rx compared: *CID 58:785, 2014.* CMV hyper IVIG is as adjunct to prophylaxis in high-risk lung, heart/lung, heart, or pancreas organ transplant recipients. Dosing: 150 mg/kg within 72 hrs of transplant and at 2, 4, 6 and 8 weeks; then 100 mg/kg at weeks 12 and 16.
	HCT	Preemptive Strategy: Monitor weekly for CMV viremia by PCR (or antigenemia) for 3-6 months post-transplant with consideration for more prolonged monitoring in patients at risk for late-onset CMV disease (chronic GVHD), requiring systemic treatment, patients receiving high-dose steroids, T-cell depleted or cord blood transplant recipients, and CD4 < 100 cells/mL). Start treatment with identification of CMV viremia or antigenemia as above. Consider prophylaxis (beginning post-engraftment) with **Valganciclovir** 900 mg po q24h or **Ganciclovir** 900 mg po q24h. *National Comprehensive Cancer Network Guidelines on Prevention and Treatment of Cancer-Related Infections, Version 1 2013, Blood 113:5711, 2009, and Biol Blood Marrow Transpl 15:1143, 2009.*
Hepatitis B	SOT	For anti-viral agents with activity against HBV, see Table 14B, page 178. For discussion of prevention of HBV re-infection after transplantation and prevention of donor-derived infection see *Am J Transplant 9: S116, 2013*
	HCT	Patients who are anti-HBC positive, and anti-HBs positive, but without evidence of active viral replication, can be monitored for ↑LFTs and presence of ++HBV-DNA, and given pre-emptive therapy at that time. Alternatively, prophylactic anti-viral therapy can be given, commencing before transplant. (*See guidelines for other specific situations: Biol Blood Marrow Transpl 15:1143, 2009.*) These guidelines recommend Lamivudine 100 mg po q24h as an anti-viral.
Herpes simplex	SOT	**Acyclovir** 400 mg po bid, starting early post-transplant (*Clin Microbiol Rev 10:86, 1997*)
	HCT	**Acyclovir** 250 mg per meter-squared iv q12h **or Acyclovir** 400 mg po to 800 mg po bid, from conditioning to engraftment or resolution or mucositis. For those requiring prolonged suppression of HSV, the higher dose (Acyclovir 800 mg po bid) is recommended to minimize the risk of emerging resistance.

* See page 2 for abbreviations

TABLE 15E (2)

OPPORTUNISTIC INFECTION	TYPE OF TRANSPLANT	PROPHYLACTIC REGIMENS
		PROPHYLACTIC REGIMENS
Aspergillus spp.	SOT	Lung and heart/lung transplant: Inhaled **Amphotericin B** and/or a mold active oral azole are commonly used, but optimal regimen not defined. Aerosolized **Amphotericin B** 6 mg q8h (or 25 mg/day) OR aerosolized **LAB** 25 mg/day q24h OR **Voriconazole** 200 mg po bid OR **Itraconazole** 200 mg po bid. 59% centers employ universal prophylaxis for 6 months in lung transplant recipients with 97% targeting Aspergillus. Most use Voriconazole alone or in combination with inhaled Amphotericin B (Am J Transplant 11:361, 2011). Consider restarting prophylaxis during periods of intensified immune suppression. Liver transplant: Consider only in high-risk, re-transplant and/or those requiring renal-replacement therapy. Recommendations on aspergillus prophylaxis in SOT can be found at (Am J Transplant 13:228, 2013).
	HCT/Heme malignancy	Indications for prophylaxis against aspergillus include AML and MDS with neutropenia and HCT with GVHD. Posaconazole 200 mg po tid approved for this indication (NEJM 356:335, 2007 and NEJM 356:348,2007). Posaconazole ER tablets, also approved for prophylaxis (300 mg po BID x 1 day, then 300 daily). **Fluconazole** 400 mg daily for 4 weeks post-transplant. Retrospective analysis suggests that Voriconazole would have efficacy in steroid-treated patients with GVHD (Bone Marrow Transpl 45:662, 2010), but is not approved for this indication. Amphotericin B and echinocandins are alternatives as well.
Candida spp.	SOT	Consider in select, high risk patients (liver, small bowel, pancreas): Consider in select, high-risk patients (re-transplants, dialysis). **Fluconazole** 400 mg daily for 4 weeks post-transplant. (Amer J Transpl 13:200, 2013).
	HCT	**Fluconazole** 400 mg po or iv once daily from day 0 to engraftment or when ANC consistently >1000, or **Posaconazole** solution 200 mg po tid or Posa ER tablets (300 mg po BID x 1 day, then 300 daily). Approved for high-risk patients (e.g., with GVHD or prolonged neutropenia), or Micafungin 50 mg iv once daily.
Coccidioides immitis	Any	**Fluconazole** 200-400 mg po q24h (Transpl Inf Dis 5:3, 2003; Am J Transpl 6:340, 2006). See CID 21-45, 2008 for approach at one center in endemic area; e.g., for positive serology without evidence of active infection, Fluconazole 400 mg q24h for first year post-transplant, then 200 mg q24h thereafter.
Pneumocystis jiroveci	SOT	**TMP-SMX**: 1 single-strength tab po q24h or 1 double-strength tab po once daily for 3 to 7 days per week. Duration: kidney: 6 mos to 1 year (Amer J Transpl 9 (Suppl 3): S59, 2009); heart, lung, liver: ≥ 1 year to life-long (Amer J Transpl 4 (Suppl 10): 135, 2004).
	HCT	**TMP-SMX**: 1 single-strength tab po q24h or 1 double-strength tab po once daily or once a day for 3 days per week, from engraftment to ≥ 6 mos post transplant.
Toxoplasma gondii	SOT	**TMP-SMX** (1 SS tab po q24h or 1 DS tab po once daily) x 3-7 days/wk for 6 mos post-transplant. (See Clin Micro Infect 14:1089, 2008).
	HCT	**TMP-SMX**: 1 single-strength tab po q24h or 1 double-strength tab po once daily or once a day for 3 days per week. from engraftment to ≥ 6 mos post transplant for seropositive allogeneic transplant recipients.
Trypanosoma cruzi	Heart	May be transmitted from organs or transfusions (CID 48:1534, 2009). Inspect peripheral blood of suspected cases for parasites (MMWR 55:798, 2006). Risk of reactivation during immunosuppression is variable (JAMA 298:2171, 2007; JAMA 299:1134, 2008; J Cardiac Fail 15:249, 2009). If known Chagas disease in donor or recipient, contact CDC for treatment options (phone 770-488-7775 or in emergency 770-488-7100). Am J Transplant 11:672, 2011

TABLE 16 – PEDIATRIC DOSING (AGE > 28 DAYS)

Editorial Note
There are limited data on when to switch adolescents to adult dosing. In general, pediatric weight based dosing is appropriate through mid puberty (Tanner 3) if no maximum dose is specified. Some change to adult dosing at 40 kg. If in doubt, when treating serious infections in peri-pubertal adolescents with drugs that have large margins of safety (e.g. Beta lactams and carbapenems) it may be safer to err on the side of higher doses.

DRUG	DOSE (AGE >28 DAYS) (Daily maximum dose shown, when applicable)
ANTIBACTERIALS	
Aminoglycosides	
Amikacin	15-20 mg/kg/day (once daily); 15-22.5 mg/kg/day (divided q8h)
Gentamicin	5-7 mg/kg/day once daily 2.5 mg/kg q8h
Tobramycin	5-7 mg/kg/day once daily 2.5 mg/kg q8h. Max per day: 8 gm
Beta-Lactams	
Carbapenems	
Ertapenem	30 mg/kg/day (divided q12h). Max per day: 1 gm
Imipenem	60-100 mg/kg/day (divided q6-8h). Max per day: 2-4 gm
Meropenem	60 mg/kg/day (divided q8h); Meningitis: 120 mg/kg/day (divided q8h). Max per day: 2-4 gm
Cephalosporins (po)	
Cefaclor	20-40 mg/kg/day (divided q8-12h). Max per day: 1 gm
Cefadroxil	30 mg/kg/day (divided q12h). Max per day: 2 gm
Cefdinir	14 mg/kg/day (divided q12-24h)
Cefixime	8 mg/kg/day (divided q12-24h)
Cefpodoxime	10 mg/kg/day (divided q12h). Max per day: 400 mg
Cefprozil	15-30 mg/kg/day (divided q12h) -- use 30 for AOM
Ceftibuten	9 mg/kg/day (divided q12-24h). Max per day: 1 gm
Cefuroxime axetil	20-30 mg/kg/day (divided q12h) -- use 30 for AOM. Max per day: 1 gm
Cephalexin	25-100 mg/kg/day (divided q6h). Max per day: 4 gm
Loracarbef	15-30 mg/kg/day (divided q12h). Max per day: 800 mg
Cephalosporins (IV)	
Cefazolin	50-150 mg/kg/day (divided q6-8h). Max per day: 6 gm
Cefepime (non-Pseudomonal)	100 mg/kg/day (divided q8h)
Cefepime (Pseudomonal)	150 mg/kg/day (divided q8h)
Cefotaxime	150-200 mg/kg/day (divided q6-8h); Meningitis: 300 mg/kg/day (divided q6h)
Cefotetan	60-100 mg/kg/day (divided q12h). Max per day: 6 gm
Cefoxitin	80-160 mg/kg/day (divided q6-8h)
Ceftazidime	150-200 mg/kg/day (divided q8h); CF: 300 mg/kg/day (divided q8h). Max per day: 6 gm
Ceftizoxime	150-200 mg/kg/day (divided q6-8h)
Ceftriaxone	50-100 mg/kg/day q24h; Meningitis: 50 mg/kg q12h
Cefuroxime	150 mg/kg/day (divided q8h); Meningitis: 80 mg/kg q8h
Penicillins	
Amoxicillin	25-50 mg/kg/day (divided q8h)
Amoxicillin (AOM, pneumonia)	80-100 mg/kg/day (divided q8-12h; q12h for AOM)
Amoxicillin-clavulanate 7:1 formulation	45 mg/kg/day (divided q12h)
Amoxicillin-clavulanate 14:1 (AOM)	90 mg/kg/day (divided q12h) for wt <40 kg
Ampicillin (IV)	200 mg/kg/day (divided q6h); Meningitis: 300-400 mg/kg/day (divided q6h)
Ampicillin-sulbactam	100-300 mg/kg/day (divided q6h)
Cloxacillin (PO)	If <20 kg: 25-50 mg/kg/day (divided q6h); Otherwise dose as adult
Dicloxacillin (mild - moderate)	12.5-25 mg/kg/day (divided q6h)
Dicloxacillin (osteo articular infection)	100 mg/kg/day (divided q 6h)
Flucloxacillin	Age 2-10: 50% of adult dose; Age<2: 25% of adult dose
Nafcillin	150-200 mg/kg/day (divided q6h)
Oxacillin	150-200 mg/kg/day (divided q6h)
Penicillin G	150,000-300,000 units/kg/day (divided q4-6h). Max per day: 12-20 million units
Penicillin VK	25-75 mg/kg/day (divided q6-8h)
Piperacillin-tazobactam	300 mg/kg/day (divided q6h)
Temocillin	25 mg/kg q12h
Fluoroquinolones * Approved only for CF, anthrax, and complicated UTI	
Ciprofloxacin (PO)	20-40 mg/kg/day (divided q12h) *. Max per day: 1.5 gm
Ciprofloxacin (IV)	20-30 mg/kg/day (divided q12h) *. Max per day: 1.2 gm
Levofloxacin (IV/PO)	16-20 mg/kg/day (divided q12h) *. Max per day: 750 mg

TABLE 16 (2)

DRUG	DOSE (AGE >28 DAYS) (Daily maximum dose shown, when applicable)
Lincosamides	
Clindamycin (PO)	30-40 mg/kg/day (divided q6-8h)
Clindamycin (IV)	20-40 mg/kg/day (divided q6-8h)
Lincomycin	10-20 mg/kg/day (divided q8-12h)
Lipopeptides	
Daptomycin	6-10 mg/kg/day (once daily)
Macrolides	
Azithromycin (po)	5-12 mg/kg/day (once daily)
Azithromycin (IV)	10 mg/kg/day (once daily)
Clarithromycin	15 mg/kg/day (divided q12h). Max per day: 1 gm
Erythromycin (po, IV)	40-50 mg/kg/day (divided q6h)
Monobactams	
Aztreonam	90-120 mg/kg/day (divided q8h). Max per day: 8 gm
Tetracyclines	
Doxycycline (po/IV, age >8 yrs)	2-4 mg/kg/day (divided q12h). Max per day: 200 mg
Fosfomycin (PO)	2 gm once
Fusidic acid (PO)	Age 1-5: 250 mg q8h Age 6-12: 250-500 mg q8h
Minocycline (PO, age >8)	4 mg/kg/day (divided q12h)
Tetracycline	Age >8: 25-50 mg/kg/day (divided q6h). Max per day: 2 gm
Other	
Chloramphenicol (IV)	50-100 mg/kg/day (divided q6h). Max per day: 2-4 gm
Colistin	2.5-5 mg/kg/day (divided q6-12h) CF: 3-8 mg/kg/day (divided q8h)
Linezolid (up to age 12 yrs)	30 mg/kg/day IV/po (divided q8h)
Methenamine hippurate (age 6-12)	500-1000 mg q12h
Methenamine mandelate	Age >2 to 6: 50-75 mg/kg/day (divided q6-8h) Age 6-12: 500 mg q6h
Metronidazole (PO)	30-40 mg/kg/day (divided q6h)
Metronidazole (IV)	22.5-40 mg/kg/day (divided q6h)
Nitrofurantoin (PO Cystitis)	5-7 mg/kg/day (divided q 6h)
Nitrofurantoin (PO UTI prophylaxis)	1-2 mg/kg/day (once daily)
Polymyxin B (age 2 and older)	2.5 mg/kg (load), then 1.5 mg/kg q12h
Rifampin (meningococcal prophylaxis)	10 mg/kg q12h x2 days
Tinidazole (age >3 for Giardia, amebiasis)	50 mg/kg q24h x1-5 days. Max per day: 2 gm
Sulfadiazine	120-150 mg/kg/day (divided q4-6h). Max per day: 6 gm
TMP-SMX (UTI and other)	8-12 mg TMP/kg/day (divided q12h)
TMP-SMX (PCP)	15-20 mg TMP/kg/day (divided q12h)
Trimethoprim	4 mg/kg/day (divided q12h)
Vancomycin (IV)	40-60 mg/kg/day (divided q6-8h)*
Vancomycin (PO for C. difficile)	40 mg/kg/day (divided q6h)
ANTIMYCOBACTERIALS	
Capreomycin	15-30 mg/kg/day (divided q12-24h). Max per day: 1 gm
Cycloserine	10-15 mg/kg/day (divided q12h). Max per day: 1 gm
Ethambutol	15-25 mg/kg/day (once daily). Max per day: 2.5 gm
Ethionamide	15-20 mg/kg/day (divided q12h). Max per day: 1 gm
Isoniazid (daily dosing)	10-15 mg/kg/day (once daily). Max per day: 300 mg
Isoniazid (2 x/week)	20-30 mg/kg twice weekly. Max per day: 900 mg
Kanamycin	15 -30 mg/kg/day (divided q12-24h). Max per day: 1 gm
Para-aminosalicylic acid	200-300 mg/kg/day (divided q6-12h)
Pyrazinamide (daily)	15-30 mg/kg/day (once daily). Max per day: 2 gm
Pyrazinamide (2 x/week)	50 mg/kg/day (2 days/week). Max per day: 2 gm
Rifabutin (MAC prophylaxis)	5 mg/kg/day (once daily). Max per day: 300 mg
Rifabutin (active TB)	10-20 mg/kg/day (once daily). Max per day: 300 mg
Rifampin	10-20 mg/kg/day (divided q12-24h). Max per day: 600 mg
Streptomycin (age 2 and older)	20-40 mg/kg/day (once daily). Max per day: 1 gm
ANTIFUNGALS	
Amphotericin B deoxycholate	0.5-1 mg/kg/day (once daily)
Amphotericin B lipid complex	5 mg/kg/day (once daily)
Anidulafungin	1.5-3 mg/kg loading dose then .75-1.5 mg/kg/day (once daily)
Caspofungin	70 mg/m2 loading dose then 50 mg/m2 (once daily)

TABLE 16 (3)   213

DRUG	DOSE (AGE >28 DAYS) (Daily maximum dose shown, when applicable)
ANTIFUNGALS (continued)	
Fluconazole	6 mg/kg/day for oral/esophageal Candida; 12 mg/kg/day for invasive disease
Isavuconazole	Not known; adult dose 372 mg q8h x 3 doses loading dose then 744 mg/day (divided q12h)
Itraconazole	5-10 mg/kg/day (divided q12h)
Ketoconazole	3.3-6.6 mg/kg/day (once daily)
Micafungin	Age >4 mon: 2 mg/kg q24h (max 100 mg) for candidiasis; for EC use 3 mg/kg q24h if <30 kg, 2.5 mg/kg q24h (max 150 mg) if >30 kg
Posaconazole	Not known; adult dose 300 mg bid loading dose then 300 mg/day (extended release)
Terbinafine	< 20 kg 67.5 mg/day; 20-40 kg 125 mg/day; >40 kg 250 mg/day (adult dose)
Voriconazole	12-20 mg/kg/day (divided q12h) *
ANTIVIRALS	
Acyclovir (IV) neonatal herpes simplex	60 mg/kg/day (divided q8h)
Acyclovir (IV) HSV encephalitis >3 months	30-45 mg/kg/day (divided q8h)
Acyclovir (IV) varicella immunocompromised	<1 year 30 mg/kg/day (divided q8h); > 1 year 30 mg/kg/day or 1500 mg/M2/day (divided q8h)
Acyclovir (IV) HSV immunocompromised	30 mg/kg/day (divided q8h)
Cidofovir	Induction 5 mg/kg once weekly; suppressive therapy 3 mg/kg once weekly (all with hydration and probenecid)
Foscarnet	120-180 mg/kg/day (divided q8-12h)
Ganciclovir	Symptomatic congenital CMV 12 mg/kg/day (divided q12h) CMV treatment or first 2 weeks after SOT 10 mg/kg/day (divided q12h) suppressive therapy or prophylaxis 5 mg/kg/day (divided q24h)
Oseltamivir <1 year old	6 mg/kg/day (divided q12h)
Oseltamivir ≥ 1 year old	< 15 kg 30 mg bid; > 15 to 23 kg 45 mg bid; >23 - 40 kg 60 mg bid; > 40 kg 75 mg bid (adult dose)
Peramivir	Not studied
Valacyclovir (Varicella or Herpes Zoster)	20 mg/kg/day (divided q8h). Max per day: 3 gm
Valganciclovir	Symptomatic congenital CMV 32 mg/kg/day (divided q12h); Prevention of CMV after SOT: 7 mg x BSA x CrCl (once daily; use Schwartz formula for CrCl)
Zanamivir (age >7 years)	10 mg (two 5-mg inhalations) twice daily

TABLE 17A – DOSAGE OF ANTIMICROBIAL DRUGS IN ADULT PATIENTS WITH RENAL IMPAIRMENT

- For listing of drugs with NO need for adjustment for renal failure, see *Table 17B*.
- Adjustments for renal failure are based on an estimate of creatinine clearance (CrCl) which reflects the glomerular filtration rate.
- **Different methods for calculating estimated CrCl are suggested for non-obese and obese patients.**
  - Calculations for ideal body weight (IBW) in kg
    - Men: 50 kg plus 2.3 kg/inch over 60 inches height.
    - Women: 45 kg plus 2.3 kg/inch over 60 inches height.
  - Obese is defined as 20% over ideal body weight or body mass index (BMI) >30

- Calculations of estimated CrCl *(References, see (NEJM 354:2473, 2006 (non-obese), AJM 84:1053, 1988 (obese))*
  - **Non-obese patient—**
    - Calculate ideal body weight (IBW) in kg (as above)
    - Use the following formula to determine estimated CrCl

$$\frac{(140 \text{ minus age}) \times (\text{IBW in kg})}{72 \times \text{serum creatinine}} = \begin{array}{l} \text{CrCl in mL/min for men.} \\ \textbf{Multiply answer by 0.85} \\ \textbf{for women (estimated)} \end{array}$$

  - **Obese patient—**
    - Weight ≥20% over IBW or BMI >30
    - Use the following formulas to determine estimated CrCl

$$\frac{(137 \text{ minus age}) \times [(0.285 \times \text{wt in kg}) + (12.1 \times \text{ht in meters}^2)]}{51 \times \text{serum creatinine}} = \text{CrCl (obese male)}$$

$$\frac{(146 \text{ minus age}) \times [(0.287 \times \text{wt in kg}) + (9.74 \times \text{ht in meters}^2)]}{60 \times \text{serum creatinine}} = \text{CrCl (obese female)}$$

- If estimated CrCl ≥90 mL/min, *see Tables 10A and 10D for dosing.*
- What weight should be used to calculate dosage on a mg/kg basis?
  - If less than 20% over IBW, use the patient's actual weight for all drugs.
  - **For obese patients** (≥20% over IBW or BMI >30):
    - **Aminoglycosides:** IBW plus 0.4(actual weight minus IBW) = adjusted weight.
    - **Vancomycin:** actual body weight whether non-obese or obese.
    - **All other drugs:** insufficient data *(Pharmacotherapy 27:1081, 2007).*

- For slow or sustained extended daily dialysis **(SLEDD)**, over 6-12 hours, adjust does as for CRRT. For details, see *CiD 49:433, 2009; CCM 39:560, 2011.*
- General reference: Drug Prescribing in Renal Failure, 5th ed. Aronoff, et al (eds) *(Amer College Physicians, 2007 and drug package inserts).*

TABLE 17A (2)

ANTIMICROBIAL	Half-life, hrs (renal function normal)	Half-life, hrs (ESRD)	Dose (renal function normal)	CrCl >50-90	CrCl 10-50	CrCl <10	Hemodialysis	CAPD	CRRT
ANTIBACTERIAL ANTIBIOTICS **AMINOGLYCOSIDES , MDD**									
Amikacin[1,2]	2-3	30-70	7.5 mg/kg IM/IV q12h (once-daily dosing below)	7.5 mg/kg q12h	7.5 mg/kg q24h	7.5 mg/kg q48h	7.5 mg/kg q48h (+ extra 3.25 mg/kg AD)	15-20 mg lost per L of dialysate/day	7.5 mg/kg q24h
Gentamicin, Netilmicin NUS, Tobramycin[1,2,3]	2-3	30-70	1.7-2.0 mg/kg IM/IV q8h	1.7-2.0 mg/kg q8h	1.7-2.0 mg/kg q12-24h	1.7-2.0 mg/kg q48h	1.7-2.0 mg/kg q48h (+ extra 0.85-1.0 mg/kg AD)	3-4 mg lost per L of dialysate/day	1.7-2.0 mg/kg q24h
AMINOGLYCOSIDES, ODD (see Table 10D)									
			Dose for CrCl >80 (mg/kg q24h)	CrCl 60-80 (mg/kg q24h)	CrCl 40-60 (mg/kg q24h)	CrCl 30-40 (mg/kg q24h)	CrCl 20-30 (mg/kg q48h)	CrCl 10-20 (mg/kg q48h)	CrCl 0-10 (mg/kg q72h and AD)
Gentamicin, Tobramycin	2-3	30-70	5.1	4	3.5	2.5	4	3	2
Amikacin, Kanamycin, Streptomycin	2-3	30-70	15	12	7.5	4	7.5	4	3
Isepamicin NUS	2-3	30-70	8	8	8	8 mg/kg q48h	8	8 mg/kg q72h	8 mg/kg q96h
Netilmicin NUS	2-3	30-70	6.5	5	4	2	3	2.5	2
BETA-LACTAMS **Carbapenems**									
Doripenem	1	18	500 mg IV q8h	500 mg q8h	CrCl 30-50: 250 mg q8h; CrCl 10-30: 250 mg q12h	No data	No data	No data	500 mg q8h (JAC 69:2508, 2014)
Ertapenem	4	>4	1 gm IV q24h	1 gm q24h	CrCl <30: 0.5 gm q24h	0.5 gm q24h	0.5 gm q24h (+ 150 mg AD if given within 6 hr prior to HD)	0.5 gm q24h	0.5-1 gm q24h
Imipenem	1	4	500 mg IV q6h	250-500 mg q6-8h	250 mg q8-12h	125-250 mg q12h	125-250 mg q12h (give one of the dialysis day doses AD)	125-250 mg q12h	0.5-1 gm q12h (AAC 49:2421, 2005)
Meropenem	1	10	1 gm IV q8h	1 gm q8h	CrCl 25-50: 1 gm q12h; CrCl 10-25: 0.5 gm q12h	0.5 gm q24h	0.5 gm q24h (give dialysis day dose AD)	0.5 gm q24h	1 gm q12h

TABLE 17A (3)

ANTIMICROBIAL	Half-life, hrs (renal function normal)	Half-life, hrs (ESRD)	Dose (renal function normal)	CrCl >50-90	CrCl 10-50	CrCl <10	Hemodialysis	CAPD	CRRT
Cephalosporins, IV, 1st gen									
Cefazolin	1.9	40-70	1-2 gm IV q8h	1-2 gm q8h	1-2 g q12h	1-2 gm q24-48h	1-2 gm q24-48h (+ extra 0.5-1 gm AD)	0.5 gm IV q12h	1-2 gm q12h
Cephalosporins, IV, 2nd gen									
Cefotetan	4	13-25	1-2 gm IV q12h	1-2 gm q12h	1-2 gm q24h	1-2 gm q48h	1-2 gm q24h (+ extra 1 gm AD)	1 gm q24h	750 mg q12h
Cefoxitin[4]	0.8	13-23	2 gm IV q8h	2 gm q8h	2 gm q8-12h	2 gm q24h	2 gm q24-48h (+ extra 1 gm AD)	1 gm q24h	2 gm q8-12h
Cefuroxime	1.5	17	0.75-1.5 gm IV q8h	0.75-1.5 gm q8h	0.75-1.5 gm q8-12h	0.75-1.5 gm q24h	0.75-1.5 gm q24h (give dialysis day dose AD)	0.75-1.5 gm q24h	0.75-1.5 gm q8-12h
Cephalosporins, IV, 3rd gen, non-antipseudomonal									
Cefotaxime[5]	1.5	15-35	2 gm IV q8h	2 gm q8-12h	2 gm q12-24h	2 gm q24h	2 gm q24h (+ extra 1 gm AD)	0.5-1 gm q24h	2 gm q12-24h
Ceftizoxime	1.7	15-35	2 gm IV q8h	2 gm q8-12h	2 gm q12-24h	2 gm q24h	2 gm q24h (+ extra 1 gm AD)	0.5-1 gm q24h	2 gm q12-24h
Ceftriaxone[5]	8	Unchanged	1-2 gm IV q12-24h	1-2 gm q12-24h	1-2 gm q12-24h	1-2 gm q12-24h	1-2 gm q12-24h	1-2 gm q12-24h	1-2 gm q12-24h
Cephalosporins, IV, antipseudomonal									
Cefepime	2	18	2 gm IV q8h	>60: 2 gm q8-12h	30-60: 2 gm q12h; 11-29: 2 gm q24h	1 gm q24h	1 gm q24h (+ extra 1 gm AD)	1-2 gm q48h	2 gm q12-24h
Ceftazidime	1.9	13-25	2 gm IV q8h	2 gm q8-12h	2 gm q12-24h	2 gm q24-48h	2 gm q24-48h (+ extra 1 gm AD)	1-2 gm q48h	1-2 gm q12-24h (depends on flow rate)
Ceftazidime/avibactam	ceftaz 2.8, avi 2.7	ceftaz 13-25	2.5 gm IV q8h	2.5 gm q8h	30-60: 1.25 gm q8h; 10-30: 0.94 gm q12h	0.94 gm q48h	0.94 gm q48h (give dialysis day dose AD)	No data	No data
Ceftolozane/tazobactam	ceftolozane 3.1	ceftolozane 40	1.5 gm IV q8h	1.5 gm q8h	30-50: 750 mg q8h; 15-30: 375 mg q8h	<15: see HD	750 mg x1, then 150 mg q8h (give dialysis day doses AD)	No data	No data
Cephalosporins, IV, anti-MRSA									
Ceftaroline	2.7	No data	600 mg (over 1 hr) IV q12h	600 mg q12h	30-50: 400 mg q12h; 15-30: 300 mg q12h	<15: 200 mg q12h	200 mg q12h	No data	No data
Ceftobiprole[NUS]	2.9-3.3	21	500 mg IV q8-12h	500 mg q8-12h	30-50: 500 mg q12h over 2 hr; 10-30: 250 mg q12h over 2 hr	No data	No data	No data	No data

TABLE 17A (4)

ANTIMICROBIAL	Half-life, hrs (renal function normal)	Half-life, hrs (ESRD)	Dose (renal function normal)	CrCl >50-90	CrCl 10-50	CrCl <10	Hemodialysis	CAPD	CRRT
Cephalosporins, oral, 1st gen									
Cefadroxil	1.5	20	1 gm po q12h	1 gm q12h	1 gm, then 500 mg q12-24h	1 gm, then 500 mg q36h	1 gm, then 1 gm AD	500 mg q12h	No data
Cephalexin	1	20	500 mg po q6h	500 mg q12h	500 mg q12h	250 mg q12h	250 mg q12h (give one of the dialysis day doses AD)	500 mg q12h	No data
Cephalosporins, oral, 2nd gen									
Cefaclor	0.8	3	500 mg q8h	500 mg q8h	500 mg q8h	500 mg q12h	500 mg q12h (give one of the dialysis day doses AD)	500 mg q12h	No data
Cefprozil	1.5	5-6	500 mg po q12h	500 mg q12h	500 mg q24h	250 mg q12h	250 mg q12h (give one of the dialysis day doses AD)	250 mg q24h	No data
Cefuroxime axetil	1.5	17	500 mg po q8h	500 mg q8h	500 mg q12h	500 mg q24h	500 mg q24h (give extra 250 mg AD)	500 mg q24h	No data
Cephalosporins, oral, 3rd gen									
Cefdinir	1.7	16	300 mg q12h	300 mg q12h	300 mg q12h	300 mg q24h	300 mg q24h (dose AD on dialysis days)	300 mg q24h	No data
Cefditoren pivoxil	1.6	5	400 mg q12h	400 mg q12h	400 mg q12h	200 mg 24h	200 mg q24h (dose AD on dialysis days)	200 mg q24h	No data
Cefixime	3	12	400 mg q24h	400 mg q24h	300 mg q24h	200 mg q24h	200 mg q24h (dose AD on dialysis days)	200 mg q24h	No data
Cefpodoxime proxetil	2.3	10	200 mg q12h	200 mg q12h	200 mg q12h	200 mg q24h	200 mg q24h (dose AD on dialysis days)	200 mg q24h	No data
Ceftibuten	2.5	13	400 mg q24h	400 mg q24h	200 mg q24h	100 mg q24h	100 mg q24h (dose AD on dialysis days)	100 mg po q24h	No data
Monobactams									
Aztreonam	2	6-8	2 gm IV q8h	2 gm q8h	1-1.5 gm q8h	500 mg q8h	500 mg q8h (give additional 250 mg AD)	500 mg q8h	1-1.5 gm q8h
Penicillins (natural)									
Penicillin G	0.5	6-20	0.5-4 million U IV q4h	0.5-4 million U q4h	0.5-4 million U q8h	0.5-4 million U q12h	0.5-4 million U q12h (give one of the dialysis day doses AD)	0.5-4 million U q12h	1-4 million U q6-8h
Penicillin V	0.5	4.1	250-500 mg po q6-8h	250-500 mg q6-8h	250-500 mg q6-8h	250-500 mg q6-8h	250-500 mg q6-8h (give one or more doses AD)	250-500 mg q6-8h	No data

TABLE 17A (5)

ANTIMICROBIAL	Half-life, hrs (renal function normal)	Half-life, hrs (ESRD)	Dose (renal function normal)	CrCl >50-90	CrCl 10-50	CrCl <10	Hemodialysis	CAPD	CRRT
Penicillins (amino)									
Amoxicillin	1.2	5-20	250-500 mg po q8h	250-500 mg q8h	250-500 mg q8-12h	250-500 mg q24h	250-500 mg q24h (give dialysis day dose AD)	250 mg q12h	250-500 mg q8-12h
Amoxicillin ER	1.2-1.5	?	775 mg po q24h	775 mg q24h	30: No data, avoid usage	No data, avoid usage	No data	No data	No data
Amoxicillin/Clavulanate [6]	amox 1.4, clav 1	amox 5-20, clav 4	500/125 mg po q8h	500/125 mg q8h	250-500 mg (amox component) q12h	250-500 mg (amox) q24h	250-500 mg (amox) q24h (give an extra dose AD on dialysis days)	No data	No data
Ampicillin	1.2	7-20	1-2 gm IV q4-6h	1-2 gm q4-6h	30-50: 1-2 gm q6-8h; 10-30: 1-2 gm q8-12h	1-2 gm q12h	1-2 gm q12h (give one of the dialysis day doses AD)	500 mg - 1 gm q12h	1-2 gm q8-12h
Ampicillin/Sulbactam	amp 1.4, sulb 1.7	amp 7-20, sulb 10	3 gm IV q6h	3 gm q6h	3 gm q8-12h	3 gm q24h	3 gm q24h (give AD on dialysis day)	3 gm q24h	3 gm q12h
Penicillins (penicillinase-resistant)									
Dicloxacillin	0.7	No change	125-500 mg po q6h	125-500 mg q6h	125-500 mg q6h	125-500 mg q6h			
Temocillin	4	No data	1-2 gm IV q12h	1-2 gm q12h	1-2 gm q24h	1 gm q48h	1 gm q48h (give AD on dialysis days)	1 gm q48h	No data
Penicillins (antipseudomonal)									
Piperacillin/Tazobactam (non-Pseudomonas dose)	pip 1, Tazo 2.8	pip 3-5, Tazo 2.8	3.375 gm IV q6h (over 30 min)	>40: 3.375 gm q6h	20-40: 2.25 gm q6h; <20: 2.25 gm q8h	2.25 gm q8h	2.25 gm q12h (+ extra 0.75 gm AD)	2.25 gm q12h	2.25 gm q6h
Piperacillin/Tazobactam (Pseudomonas dose)	pip 1, Tazo 1	pip 3-5, Tazo 2.8	4.5 gm IV q6h (over 30 min)	>40: 4.5 gm q6h	20-40: 3.375 gm q6h; <20: 2.25 gm q8h	2.25 gm q6h	2.25 gm q8h (+ extra 0.75 gm AD)	2.25 gm q8h	3.375 gm q6h
FLUOROQUINOLONES									
Ciprofloxacin po (not XR)	4	6-9	500-750 mg po q12h	500-750 mg q12h	250-500 mg q12h	500 mg q24h	500 mg q24h (dose AD on dialysis days)	500 mg q24h	250-500 mg q12h
Ciprofloxacin XR po	5-7	6-9	500-1000 mg po q24h	500-1000 mg q24h	30-50: 500-1000 mg q24h; 10-30: 500 mg q24h	500 mg q24h	500 mg q24h (dose AD on dialysis days)	500 mg q24h	No data

TABLE 17A (6)

ANTIMICROBIAL	Half-life, hrs (renal function normal)	Half-life, hrs (ESRD)	Dose (renal function normal)	CrCl >50-90	CrCl 10-50	CrCl <10	Hemodialysis	CAPD	CRRT
FLUOROQUINOLONES *(continued)*									
Ciprofloxacin IV	4	6-9	400 mg IV q12h	400 mg q12h	400 mg q24h	400 mg q24h	400 mg q24h (dose AD on dialysis days)	400 mg q24h	200-400 mg q12h
Gatifloxacin^NUS	7-8	11-40	400 mg po/IV q24h	400 mg q24h	400 mg, then 200 mg q24h	400 mg, then 200 mg q24h	200 mg q24h (give dialysis day dose AD)	200 mg q24h	400 mg, then 200 mg q24h
Gemifloxacin	7	>7	320 mg po q24h	320 mg q24h	160 mg q24h	160 mg q24h	160 mg q24h (give dialysis day dose AD)	160 mg q24h	No data
Levofloxacin	7	76	750 mg po/IV q24h	750 mg q24h	20-49: 750 mg q48h	<20: 750 mg x1, then 500 mg q48h	750 mg q24h	750 mg x1, then 500 mg q48h	750 mg x1, then 500 mg q48h
Norfloxacin	3-4	8	400 mg po q12h	400 mg q12h	30-49: 400 mg q12h; 10-30: 400 mg q24h	400 mg q24h	400 mg q24h	400 mg q24h	Not applicable
Ofloxacin	7	28-37	200-400 mg po q12h	200-400 mg q12h	200-400 mg po q24h	200 mg q24h	200 mg q24h (give dialysis day dose AD)	200 mg q24h	200-400 mg q24h
Prulifloxacin^NUS	10.6-12.1	No data	600 mg po q24h	No data	No data	No data	No data	No data	No data
GLYCOPEPTIDES, LIPOGLYCOPEPTIDES, LIPOPEPTIDES									
Dalbavancin	147-258 (terminal)	No data	1 gm IV x1, then 500 mg IV in 7 days	1 gm x1, then 500 mg in 7 days	30-49: 1 gm x1, then 500 mg in 7 days; <30, non-regular HD: 750 mg x1, then 375 mg in 7 days	30-49: 1 gm x1, then 500 mg in 7 days	Regularly scheduled HD: 1 gm x1, then 500 mg in 7 days	No data	No data
Daptomycin	8-9	30	4-6 mg/kg IV q24h	4-6 mg/kg q24h	30-49: 4-6 mg/kg q24h; <30: 6 mg/kg q48h	30-49: 4-6 mg/kg q24h; <30: 6 mg/kg q48h	6 mg/kg q48h (during or after q48h dialysis); if next planned dialysis is 72 hrs away, give 9 mg/kg (AAC 57:864, 2013; JAC 69:200, 2014)	6 mg/kg q48h	6 mg/kg q48h
Oritavancin	245 (terminal)	No data	1200 mg IV x1	1200 mg x1	<30: No data	No data	Not removed by hemodialysis	No data	No data
Teicoplanin^NUS	70-100	up to 230	6 mg/kg IV q24h	6 mg/kg q24h	30-50: 7.5mg/kg q24h; 10-30: 10mg/kg q48h	6 mg/kg q72h	6 mg/kg q72h (give AD on dialysis day)	6 mg/kg q72h	6 mg/kg q48h
Telavancin	8.1	17.9	10 mg/kg IV q24h	10 mg/kg q24h	30-50: 7.5mg/kg q24h; 10-30: 10mg/kg q48h	10 mg/kg q48h	No data	No data	No data

TABLE 17A (7)

ANTIMICROBIAL	Half-life, hrs (renal function normal)	Half-life, hrs (ESRD)	Dose (renal function normal)	CrCl >50-90	CrCl 10-50	CrCl <10	Hemodialysis	CAPD	CRRT
GLYCOPEPTIDES, LIPOGLYCOPEPTIDES, LIPOPEPTIDES *(continued)*									
Vancomycin [7]	4-6	200-250	15-30 mg/kg IV q12h	15-30 mg/kg q12h	15 mg/kg q24-96h	7.5 mg/kg q2-3 days	For trough conc of 15-20, give 15 mg/kg if next dialysis in 1 day, give 25 mg/kg if next dialysis in 2 days, give 35 mg/kg if next dialysis in 3 days (CID 53:124, 2011)	7.5 mg/kg q2-3 days	CAVH/CVVH: 500 mg q24-48h
MACROLIDES, AZALIDES, LINCOSAMIDES, KETOLIDES									
Azithromycin	68	Unchanged	250-500 mg IV/po q24h	250-500 mg q24h	250-500 mg q24h	250-500 mg q24h	250-500 mg q24h	250-500 mg q24h	250-500 mg q24h
Clarithromycin (not ER)	5-7	22	500 mg po q12h	500 mg q12h	500 mg q12-24h	500 mg q24h	500 mg q24h (dose AD on dialysis days)	500 mg q12-24h	500 mg q12-24h
Telithromycin [5]	10	15	800 mg po q24h	800 mg q24h	30-50: 800 mg 10-30: 600 mg q24h	600 mg q24h	600 mg q24h (give AD on dialysis days)	No data	No data
MISCELLANEOUS ANTIBACTERIALS									
Chloramphenicol [5]	4.1	Unchanged	50-100 mg/kg po/IV (divided q6h)	50-100 mg/kg/day (divided q6h)	50-100 mg/kg/day (divided q6h)	50-100 mg/kg/day (divided q6h)	50-100 mg/kg/day (divided q6h)	50-100 mg/kg/day (divided q6h)	50-100 mg/kg/day (divided q6h)
Fosfomycin po	5.7	50	3 gm po x1		Do not use (low urine concentrations)				
Fusidic acid [NUS, 5]	8.9-11	8.9-11	250-750 mg po q8-12h	250-750 mg q8-12h	250-750 mg q8-12h	250-750 mg q8-12h	250-750 mg q8-12h	250-750 mg q8-12h	250-750 mg q8-12h
Metronidazole [5]	6-14	7-21	7.5 mg/kg IV/po q6h	7.5 mg/kg q6h	7.5 mg/kg q6h	7.5 mg/kg q12h	7.5 mg/kg q12h (give one of the dialysis day doses AD)	7.5 mg/kg q12h	7.5 mg/kg q6h
Nitrofurantoin	1	-	100 mg q12h (Macrobid)	100 mg q12h (Macrobid)	Avoid use	Avoid use	Avoid use	Avoid use	Avoid use
Tinidazole [6]	13	No data	2 gm po q24h x 1-5 days	2 gm q24h x1-5 days	2 gm q24h x1-5 days	2 gm q24h x1-5 days	2 gm q24h x1-5 days (+ extra 1 gm AD)	No data	No data
Trimethoprim	8-15	20-49	100-200 mg po q12h	100-200 mg q12h	>30: 100-200 mg q12h; 10-30: 100-200 mg q18h	100-200 mg q24h	100-200 mg q24h (give dialysis day dose AD)	100-200 mg q24h	100-200 mg q18h

TABLE 11A (6)

ANTIMICROBIAL	Half-life, hrs (renal function normal)	Half-life, hrs (ESRD)	Dose (renal function normal)	CrCl >50-90	CrCl 10-50	CrCl <10	Hemodialysis	CAPD	CRRT
MISCELLANEOUS ANTIBACTERIALS (continued)									
TMP/SMX (treatment)	TMP 8-15, SMX 10	TMP 20-49, SMX 20-50	5-20 mg/kg/day po/IV (div q6-12h) base on TMP	5-20 mg/kg/day (divided q6-12h)	30-50: 5-20 mg/kg/day (div q6-12h); 10-29: 5-10 mg/kg/day (div q12h)	Not recommended (but if used: 5-10 mg/kg q24h)	Not recommended (but if used 5-10 mg/kg day dialysis day dose AD)	Not recommended (but if used: 5-10 mg/kg q24h)	5 mg/kg q8h
TMP/SMX (prophylaxis)	as above	as above	1 DS tab po q24h or 3x/week	1 DS tab q24h or 3x/week	1 DS tab q24h or 3x/week	1 DS tab q24h or 3x/week			
OXAZOLIDINONES									
Linezolid	5	6-8	600 mg po/IV q12h	600 mg q12h	600 mg q12h	600 mg q12h	600 mg q12h (give one of the dialysis day doses AD)	600 mg q12h	600 mg q12h
Tedizolid	12	Unchanged	200 mg po/IV q24h	200 mg q24h	200 mg q24h	200 mg q24h	200 mg q24h	200 mg q24h	200 mg q24h
POLYMYXINS									
Colistin (polymyxin E) Based on 105 patients (AAC 55:3284, 2011). All doses refer to colistin base in mg	6.3-12	≥48	Load: (2.5) x (2) x (pt wt in kg). Use lower of ideal or actual wt. Start maintenance 12 hrs later (see formula). Max daily dose: 340 mg	Daily maintenance dose = 2.5 x [(1.5 x CrCl) + 30] Divide and give q8-12h, max 475 mg daily. CrCln = CrCl x (pt BSA in m² divided by 1.73)		75 mg (divided q12h) (non-dialysis days); 112.5 mg (divided q12h) (dialysis days)	160 mg q24h	For Css of 2.5 µg/mL, total daily dose is 80 mg (divided q12h). This dose is necessarily high due to drug removal by the dialysis membrane. See AAC 55:3284, 2011
TETRACYCLINES, GLYCYLCYCLINES									
Tetracycline	6-12	57-108	250-500 mg po q6h	250-500 mg po q8-12h	250-500 mg q12-24h	250-500 mg q24h	250-500 mg q24h	250-500 mg q24h	250-500 mg q12-24h
ANTIMETABOLITES									
Flucytosine [a]	3-5	75-200	25 mg/kg po q6h	25 mg/kg q6h	25 mg/kg q12h	25 mg/kg q24h	25 mg/kg q24h (give dialysis day dose AD)	0.5-1 gm q24h	25 mg/kg q12h

TABLE 17A (9)

ANTIMICROBIAL	Half-life, hrs (renal function normal)	Half-life, hrs (ESRD)	Dose (renal function normal)	CrCl >50-90	CrCl 10-50	CrCl <10	Hemodialysis	CAPD	CRRT
ALLYLAMINES, AZOLES									
Fluconazole	20-50	100	100-400 mg po/IV q24h	100-400 mg q24h	50-200 mg q24h	50-200 mg q24h	100-400 mg q24h (give dialysis day dose AD)	50-200 mg q24h	200-400 mg q24h
Itraconazole (IV) [5]	35-40	Unchanged	200 mg IV q12h	200 mg q12h	Do not use IV itraconazole if CrCl <30 due to accumulation of cyclodextrin vehicle				
Itraconazole (oral solution) [5]	35-40	Unchanged	100-200 mg po q12h	100-200 mg q12h	100-200 mg q12h	50-100 mg q12h	100 q12-24h	100 mg q12-24h	100-200 mg q12h
Terbinafine	36	No data	250 mg q24h	250 mg q24h	Avoid use	Avoid use	Avoid use	Avoid use	Avoid use
Voriconazole (IV) [5]	dose-dependent	dose-dependent	6 mg/kg IV q12h x2 doses, then 4 mg/kg IV q12h	6 mg/kg q12h x2 doses, then 4 mg/kg q12h	If CrCl<50, IV vehicle (cyclodextrin) accumulates. Use oral or discontinue.			Avoid use	Avoid use
ANTIMYCOBACTERIALS **First line, tuberculosis**									
Ethambutol [9]	4	7-15	15-25 mg/kg po q24h	15-25 mg/kg q24h	CrCl 30-50: 15-25 mg/kg q24-36h; CrCl 10-30: 15-25 mg/kg q36-48h	15 mg/kg q48h	15 mg/kg q48h (administer AD on dialysis days)	15 mg/kg q48h	15-25 mg/kg q24h
Isoniazid (INH) [5]	0.7-4	8-17	5 mg/kg po q24h	5 mg/kg q24h	5 mg/kg q24h	5 mg/kg q24h	5 mg/kg q24h (administer AD on dialysis days)	5 mg/kg q24h	5 mg/kg q24h
Pyrazinamide	10-16	26	25 mg/kg (max 2.5 gm) po q24h	25 mg/kg q24h	CrCl 21-50: 25 mg/kg q24h; CrCl 10-20: 25 mg/kg q48h	25 mg/kg q48h	25 mg/kg q48h (administer AD on dialysis days)	25 mg/kg q24h	25 mg/kg q24h
Rifabutin [5]	32-67	Unchanged	300 mg po q24h	300 mg q24h	300 mg q24h	300 mg q24h	300 mg q24h	300 mg q24h	300 mg q24h
Rifampin [5]	1.5-5	up to 11	600 mg po q24h	600 mg q24h	300-600 mg q24h	300-600 mg	300-600 mg q24h	300-600 mg q24h	300-600 mg q24h
Rifapentine	13.2-14.1	Unchanged	600 mg po 1-2x/wk	600 mg 1-2x/wk	600 mg 1-2x/wk	600 mg 1-2x/wk	600 mg 1-2x/wk	600 mg 1-2x/wk	600 mg 1-2x/wk
Streptomycin [1,2]	2-3	30-70	15 mg/kg (max 1 gm) IM q24h	15 mg/kg q24h	15 mg/kg q24-72h	15 mg/kg q72-96h	15 mg/kg q72-96h (+ extra 7.5 mg/kg AD)	20-40 mg lost per L of dialysate/day	15 mg/kg q24-72h

TABLE 17A (10)

ANTIMICROBIAL	Half-life, hrs (renal function normal)	Half-life, hrs (ESRD)	Dose (renal function normal)	CrCl >50-90	CrCl 10-50	CrCl <10	Hemodialysis	CAPD	CRRT
ANTIMYCOBACTERIALS (continued)									
Second line, tuberculosis									
Bedaquiline	24-30 (terminal 4-5 mo)	No data	400 mg po q24h x2 wk, then 200 mg po 3x/wk x22 wk	400 mg q24h x2 wk, then 200 mg 3x/wk x22 wk	400 mg q24h x2 wk, then 200 mg 3x/wk x22 wk	Use with caution	Use with caution	Use with caution	Use with caution
Capreomycin	2-5	No data	15 mg/kg IM/IV q24h	15 mg/kg q24h	15 mg/kg q24h	15 mg/kg 3x/wk	15 mg/kg 3x/wk (give AD on dialysis days)	No data	No data
Cycloserine [10]	10	No data	250-500 mg po q12h	250-500 mg q12h	250-500 mg q12h-24h (dosing interval poorly defined)	500 mg q48h (or 3x/wk)	500 mg 3x/wk (give AD on dialysis days)	No data	No data
Ethionamide	2	9	500 mg po q12h	500 mg q12h	500 mg q12h	250 mg q12h	250 mg q12h	250 mg q12h	500 mg q12h
Kanamycin [1,2]	2-3	30-70	7.5 mg/kg IM/IV q12h	7.5 mg/kg q12h	7.5 mg/kg q24h	7.5 mg/kg q48h	7.5 mg/kg q48h (+ extra 3.25 mg/kg AD)	15-20 mg lost per L of dialysate/day	7.5 mg/kg q24h
Para-aminosalicylic acid (PAS)	0.75-1.0	23	4 gm po q12h	4 gm q12h	2-3 gm q12h	2 gm q12h	2 gm q12h (dose AD on dialysis days)	No data	No data
ANTIPARASITICS: **ANTIMALARIALS:**									
Artemether/lumefantrine (20 mg/120 mg)	art, DHA 1.6-2.2, lum 101-119	No data	4 tabs x1, 4 tabs in 8 hr, then 4 tabs q12h x2 days	4 tabs x1, 4 tabs in 8 hr, then 4 tabs q12h x2 days	4 tabs x1, then 4 tabs q12h x2 days	4 tabs x1, 4 tabs in 8 hr, then 4 tabs q12h x2 days	No data	No data	No data
Atovaquone	67	No data	750 mg po q12h	750 mg q12h	CrCl 30-50: 750 mg q12h; CrCl 10-30: use with caution	Use with caution	No data	No data	No data
Atovaquone/Proguanil (250 mg/100 mg)	atov 67, pro 12-21	No data	4 tabs po q24h x3 days	4 tabs q24h x3 days	CrCl <30: use with caution	Use with caution	No data	No data	No data
Chloroquine phosphate	45-55 days (terminal)	No data	2.5 gm po over 3 days	2.5 gm over 3 days	2.5 gm over 3 days	2.5 gm over 3 days (consider reducing dose 50%)	2.5 gm over 3 days (consider reducing dose 50%)	No data	No data

TABLE 17A (11)

ANTIMICROBIAL	Half-life, hrs (renal function normal)	Half-life, hrs (ESRD)	Dose (renal function normal)	CrCl >50-90	CrCl 10-50	CrCl <10	Hemodialysis	CAPD	CRRT
ANTIPARASITICS, ANTIMALARIALS *(continued)*									
Mefloquine	13-24 days	No data	750 mg po, then 500 mg po in 6-8 hrs	750 mg, then 500 mg in 6-8 hrs	750 mg, then 500 mg in 6-8 hrs	750 mg, then 500 mg in 6-8 hrs	No data	No data	No data
Quinine	9.7-12.5	up to 16	648 mg po q8h	648 mg q8h	648 mg q8-12h	648 mg q24h	648 mg q24h (give dialysis day dose AD)	648 mg q24h	648 mg q8-12h
OTHER									
Albendazole	8-12	No data	400 mg po q12-24h	400 mg q12-24h	400 mg q12-24h	400 mg q12-24h	No data	No data	No data
Dapsone	10-50	No data	100 mg po q24h	No data	No data	No data	No data	No data	No data
Ivermectin	20	No data	200 µg/kg/day x1-2 days	200 µg/kg/day x1-2 days	200 µg/kg/day x1-2 days	200 µg/kg/day x1-2 days	No data	No data	No data
Miltefosine	7-31 days	No data	50 mg po q8h	No data	No data	No data	No data	No data	No data
Nitazoxanide	tizoxanide 1.3-1.8	No data	500 mg po q12h	No data	No data	No data	No data	No data	No data
Pentamidine	3-12	73-118	4 mg/kg IM/IV q24h	4 mg/kg q24h	4 mg/kg q24h	4 mg/kg q24-36h	4 mg/kg q48h (give dialysis day dose AD)	4 mg/kg q24-36h	4 mg/kg q24h
ANTIVIRALS HEPATITIS B									
Adefovir	7.5	15	10 mg po q24h	10 mg q24h	10 mg q48-72h	10 mg q72h	10 mg weekly (dose AD on dialysis days)	No data	No data
Entecavir	128-149	?	0.5 mg po q24h	0.5 mg q24h	0.15-0.25 mg q24h	0.05 mg q24h	0.05 mg q24h (dose AD on dialysis days)	0.05 mg q24h	No data
Telbivudine	40-49	No data	600 mg po q24h	600 mg q24h	30-49: 600 mg q48h; 10-30: 600 mg q72h	600 mg q96h	600 mg q96h (dose AD on dialysis days)	No data	No data
HEPATITIS C (SINGLE AGENTS)									
Daclatasvir	12-15	No data	60 mg po q24h	60 mg q24h	60 mg q24h	60 mg q24h	No data	No data	No data
Ribavirin	44	No data	Depends on indication	No dosage adjustment	Use with caution	Use with caution	No data	No data	No data
Simeprevir	41	Unchanged	150 mg po q24h	150 mg q24h	Use with caution (no data for use in patients with CrCl<30)	Use with caution (no data for use in patients with CrCl<30)	No data	No data	No data
Sofosbuvir	sofosbuvir 0.50-0.75	Unchanged	400 mg po q24h	400 mg q24h	400 mg q24h	No data	No data	No data	No data

ANTIMICROBIAL	Half-life, hrs (renal function normal)	Half-life, hrs (ESRD)	Dose (renal function normal)	CrCl >50-90	CrCl 10-50	CrCl <10	Hemodialysis	CAPD	CRRT
HEPATITIS C (FIXED-DOSE COMBINATIONS)									
Harvoni (Ledipasvir, Sofosbuvir)	ledipasvir 47	No data	1 tab po q24h	1 tab q24h	Use with caution (no data for use in patients with CrCl <30)		No data	No data	No data
Technivie (Ombitasvir, Paritaprevir, RTV)	ombit 28-34, parita 5.8	No data	2 tabs po q24h	2 tabs q24h	2 tabs q24h	2 tabs q24h	No data	No data	No data
Viekira Pak (Dasabuvir, Ombitasvir, Paritaprevir, RTV)	dasabuvir 5-8	No data	2 Ombit/Parita/RTV tabs q24h, Dasa 250 mg q12h	2 Ombit/Parita/RTV tabs q24h, Dasa 250 mg q12h	2 Ombit/Parita/RTV tabs q24h, Dasa 250 mg q12h	2 Ombit/Parita/RTV tabs q24h, Dasa 250 mg q12h	No data	No data	No data
HERPESVIRUS [11]									
Acyclovir (IV) [11]	2.5-3.5	20	5-12.5 mg/kg IV q8h	5-12.5 mg/kg q8h	5-12.5 mg/kg q12-24h	2.5-6.25 mg/kg q24h	2.5-6.25 mg/kg q24h (dose AD on dialysis days)	2.5-6.25 mg/kg q24h	5-10 mg/kg q24h
Cidofovir (induction)	2.6	No data	5 mg/kg IV q-week x2 weeks	CrCl>55: 5 mg/kg q-week x2 weeks	Contraindicated in patients with CrCl of 55 ml/min or less	Contraindicated in patients with CrCl of 55 ml/min or less	Contraindicated	Contraindicated	Contraindicated
Cidofovir (maintenance)	2.6	No data	5 mg/kg IV every 2 weeks	CrCl>55: 5 mg/kg every 2 weeks	Contraindicated in patients with CrCl of 55 ml/min or less	Contraindicated in patients with CrCl of 55 ml/min or less	Contraindicated	Contraindicated	Contraindicated
Famciclovir	penciclovir 2-3	10-22	500 mg po q8h (VZV)	500 mg q8h	500 mg q12-24h	250 mg q24h	250 mg q24h (dose AD on dialysis days)	No data	No data
Ganciclovir (IV induction)	3.5	30	5 mg/kg IV q12h	CrCl 70-90, 5 mg/kg q12h; CrCl 50-69, 2.5 mg/kg q12h	CrCl 25-49, 2.5 mg/kg q24h; CrCl 10-24, 1.25 mg/kg q12h	1.25 mg/kg 3x/week	1.25 mg/kg 3x/week (dose AD on dialysis days)	1.25 mg/kg 3x/week	CVVHF: 2.5 mg/kg q24h (AAC 58:94, 2014)
Ganciclovir (IV maintenance)	3.5	30	5 mg/kg IV q24h	2.5-5 mg/kg q24h	0.625-1.25 mg/kg q24h	0.625 mg/kg 3x/week	0.625 mg/kg 3x/week (dose AD on dialysis days)	0.625 mg/kg 3x/week	No data
Ganciclovir (oral)	3.5	30	1 gm po q8h	0.5-1 gm q8h	0.5-1 gm q24h	0.5 gm 3x/week	0.5 gm 3x/week (dose AD on dialysis days)	0.5 gm q24h	No data
Valacyclovir	3	14	1 gm po q8h (VZV)	1 gm q8h	1 gm q12-24h	0.5 gm q24h	0.5 gm q24h (dose AD on dialysis days)	0.5 gm q24h	1 gm q12-24h
Valganciclovir	ganciclovir 4	ganciclovir 67	900 mg po q12h	900 mg q12h	450 mg q24-48h	Do not use	See prescribing information	No data	No data

TABLE 17A (13)

ANTIMICROBIAL	Half-life, hrs (renal function normal)	Half-life, hrs (ESRD)	Dose (renal function normal)	CrCl >50-90	CrCl 10-50	CrCl <10	Hemodialysis	CAPD	CRRT
			CrCl above 1.4 mL/min/kg (foscarnet only)	CrCl >1 to 1.4 mL/min/kg (foscarnet only)	CrCl >0.8 to 1.0 mL/min/kg (foscarnet only)	CrCl >0.6 to 0.8 mL/min/kg (foscarnet only)	CrCl >0.5 to 0.6 mL/min/kg (foscarnet only)	CrCl 0.4 to 0.5 mL/min/kg (foscarnet only)	CrCl <0.4 mL/min/kg (foscarnet only)
HERPESVIRUS *(continued)*									
Foscarnet (induction) special dosing scale	3 (terminal 18-88)	Very long	60 mg/kg IV q8h	45 mg/kg q8h	50 mg/kg q12h	40 mg/kg q12h	60 mg/kg q24h	50 mg/kg q24h	Not recommended
Foscarnet (maintenance) special dosing scale	3 (terminal 18-88)	Very long	90-120 mg/kg IV q24h	70-90 mg/kg q24h	50-65 mg/kg q24h	80-105 mg/kg q48h	60-80 mg/kg q48h	50-65 mg/kg q48h	Not recommended
INFLUENZA									
Amantadine	14.8	500	100 mg po q12h	100 mg q12h	100 mg q24-48h	100 mg weekly	100 mg weekly (give AD on dialysis days)	100 mg weekly	100 mg q24-48h
Oseltamivir [12]	carboxylate 6-10	carboxylate >20	75 mg po q12h	CrCl >60: 75 mg q12h	CrCl 31-60: 30 mg q12h; CrCl 10-30: 30 mg q24h	No recommendation unless HD	30 mg after each dialysis, no drug on non-HD days (see comments)	30 mg after a dialysis exchange	No data
Peramivir	20	No data	600 mg IV q24h	600 mg q24h	CrCl 31-49: 200 mg q24h; CrCl 10-30: 100 mg q24h	100 mg x1, then 15 mg q24h	100 mg x1, then 100 mg 2 hrs AD on dialysis days only	No data	No data
Rimantadine [5]	24-36	prolonged	100 mg po q12h	100 mg q12h	100 mg q12-24h	100 mg q24h			Use with caution
ANTIRETROVIRALS (NRTIs)									
Abacavir (ABC) [5]	1.5	No data	600 mg po q24h	600 mg q24h	600 mg q24h	600 mg q24h	No data	No data	No data
Didanosine enteric coated (ddI)	1.6	4.5	400 mg EC po q24h	400 mg EC q24h	125-200 mg EC q24h	Do not use	No data	No data	No data
Emtricitabine capsules (FTC)	10	>10	200 mg po q24h	200 mg q24h	CrCl 30-49: 200 mg q48h; CrCl 15-29: 200 mg q72h	CrCl <15: 200 mg q96h	200 mg q96h	No data	No data
Emtricitabine oral solution (FTC)	10	>10	240 mg po q24h	240 mg q24h	CrCl 30-49: 120 mg q24h; CrCl 15-29 80 mg q24h	CrCl <15: 60 mg q24h	60 mg q24h	No data	No data
Lamivudine (3TC)	5-7	15-35	300 mg po q24h (HIV dose)	300 mg q24h (HIV)	50-150 mg q24h (HIV)	25-50 mg q24h (HIV)	25-50 mg q24h (dose AD on dialysis days) (HIV)	25-50 mg po q24h (HIV)	100 mg first day, then 50 mg q24h (HIV)

TABLE 17A (4)

ANTIMICROBIAL	Half-life, hrs (renal function normal)	Half-life, hrs (ESRD)	Dose (renal function normal)	CrCl >50-90	CrCl 10-50	CrCl <10	Hemodialysis	CAPD	CRRT
ANTIRETROVIRALS (NRTIs) (continued)									
Stavudine (d4T)	1.2-1.6	5.5-8	30-40 mg po q12h	30-40 mg q12h	15-20 mg q12h	≥60 kg: 20 mg q24h; <60 kg, 15 mg q24h	≥60 kg: 20 mg q24h; <60 kg, 15 mg q24h (dose AD on dialysis days)	No data	30-40 mg q12h
Tenofovir (TDF)	17	Prolonged	300 mg po q24h	300 mg q24h	CrCl 30-49: 300 mg q48h; CrCl 10-29: 300 mg q72-96h	No data	300 mg AD every 3rd dialysis, or q7 days if no dialysis	No data	No data
Zidovudine (ZDV)	0.5-3	1.3-3	300 mg po q12h	300 mg q12h	300 mg q12h	100 mg q8h	100 mg q8h (dose AD on dialysis days)	No data	300 mg q12h
FUSION/ENTRY INHIBITORS									
Enfuvirtide (ENF, T20) [5]	3.8	Unchanged	90 mg sc q12h	90 mg q12h	Not studied in patients with CrCl <35, DO NOT USE		Avoid use	Avoid use	Avoid use
Maraviroc (MVC)	14-18	No data	300 mg po q12h	300 mg q12h	No data	No data	No data	No data	No data
FIXED-DOSE COMBINATIONS									
Atripla (EFV/FTC/TDF)	See components	See components	1 tab po q24h	1 tab q24h	Do not use	Do not use	Do not use	Do not use	Do not use
Combivir (3TC/ZDV)	See components	See components	1 tab po q12h	1 tab q12h	Do not use	Do not use	Do not use	Do not use	Do not use
Complera, Eviplera (RPV/FTC/TDF)	See components	See components	1 tab po q24h	1 tab q24h	Do not use	Do not use	Do not use	Do not use	Do not use
Dutrebis (3TC/RAL)	See components	See components	1 tab po q12h	1 tab q12h	Do not use	Do not use	Do not use	Do not use	Do not use
Epzicom, Kivexa (ABC/3TC)	See components	See components	1 tab po q24h	1 tab q24h	Do not use	Do not use	Do not use	Do not use	Do not use
Evotaz (ATV/cobi) [13]	See components	See components	1 tab po q24h	1 tab q24h	1 tab q24h	1 tab q24h	Do not use	No data	Do not use
Genvoya (EVG/FTC/TAF/cobi)	See components	See components	1 tab po q24h	1 tab po q24h	CrCl 30-49: 1 tab po q24h; do not use if CrCl <30	Do not use	Do not use	Do not use	Do not use
Prezcobix (DRV/cobi) [13]	See components	See components	1 tab po q24h	1 tab q24h	1 tab q24h	1 tab q24h	1 tab q24h	1 tab q24h	1 tab q24h

TABLE 17A (15)

ANTIMICROBIAL	Half-life, hrs (renal function normal)	Half-life, hrs (ESRD)	Dose (renal function normal)	CrCl >50-90	CrCl 10-50	CrCl <10	Hemodialysis	CAPD	CRRT
FIXED-DOSE COMBINATIONS (continued)									
Stribild (EVG/FTC/TDF/cobi)	See components	See components	1 tab po q24h	Do not use if CrCl <70	Do not use	Do not use	Do not use	Do not use	Do not use
Triumeq (DTG/ABC/3TC)	See components	See components	1 tab po q24h	1 tab q24h	Do not use	Do not use	Do not use	Do not use	Do not use
Trizivir (ABC/3TC/ZDV)	See components	See components	1 tab po q12h	1 tab q12h	Do not use	Do not use	Do not use	Do not use	Do not use
Truvada (FTC/TDF)	See components	See components	1 tab po q24h	1 tab q24h	CrCl 30-49: 1 tab q48h; do not use if CrCl <30	Do not use	Do not use	Do not use	Do not use

1 High flux HD membranes lead to unpredictable drug Cl; measure post-dialysis drug levels.
2 Check levels with CAPD, PK highly variable. Usual method w/CAPD: 2L dialysis fluid replaced qid (Example amikacin: give 8L x 20 mg lost/L = 160 mg amikacin IV supplement daily).
3 Gentamicin SLEDD dose: 6 mg/kg IV q48h beginning 30 min before start of SLEDD (AAC 54:3635, 2010)
4 May falsely increase Scr by interference with assay.
5 Dosage adjustment may be required in hepatic disease.
6 Clav cleared by liver; thus, as dose of combination is decreased, a clav deficiency may occur (JAMA 285:386, 2001). If CrCl≤30, do not use 875/125 or 1000/62.5.
7 New hemodialysis membranes increase vancomycin clearance; check levels.
8 Goal peak serum concentration: 25-100 μg/ml.
9 Monitor serum concentrations (if possible in dialysis patients.
10 Goal peak serum concentration: 20-35 μg/ml.
11 Rapid infusion can increase SCr.
12 Dosing for age >1 yr (dose after each hemodialysis): ≤15 kg, 7.5 mg. 16-23 kg, 10 mg. 24-40 kg, 15 mg. >40 kg, 30 mg (CID 50:127, 2010).
13 Do not use with tenofovir if CrCl <70.

TABLE 17B – NO DOSAGE ADJUSTMENT WITH RENAL INSUFFICIENCY BY CATEGORY

Antibacterials		Antifungals	Anti-TBc	Antivirals	
Azithromycin	Minocycline	Anidulafungin	Bedaquiline	Abacavir	
Ceftriaxone	Moxifloxacin	Caspofungin	Ethionamide	Atazanavir	Nelfinavir
Chloramphenicol	Nafcillin	Itraconazole oral solution	Isoniazid	Darunavir	Nevirapine
Ciprofloxacin XL	Oritavancin	Ketoconazole	Rifampin	Delavirdine	Raltegravir
Clindamycin	Polymyxin B	Micafungin	Rifabutin	Etavirenz	Ribavirin
Doxycycline	Pyrimethamine	Posaconazole, **po only**	Rifapentine	Enfuvirtide[1]	Saquinavir
Linezolid[ll]	Rifaximin	Voriconazole, **po only**		Fosamprenavir	Simeprevir[2]
	Tedizolid			Indinavir	Sofosbuvir[2]
	Tigecycline			Lopinavir	Tipranavir

[1] Enfuvirtide: Not studied in patients with CrCl <35 mL/min. DO NOT USE
[2] No data for CrCl <30 mL/min
[ll] Increased risk of bone marrow toxicity

TABLE 17C – ANTIMICROBIAL DOSING IN OBESITY

The number of obese patients is increasing. Intuitively, the standard doses of some drugs may not achieve effective serum concentrations. Pertinent data on anti-infective dosing in the obese patient is gradually emerging. Though some of the data needs further validation, the following table reflects what is currently known. **Obesity is defined as ≥ 20% over Ideal Body Weight (Ideal BW) or Body Mass Index (BMI) > 30. Dose = suggested body weight (BW) for dose calculation in obese patient, or specific dose if applicable.** In general, the absence of a drug in the table indicates a lack of pertinent information in the published literature.

Drug	Dose	Comments
Acyclovir	Use **Ideal BW** Example: for HSV encephalitis, give 10 mg/kg of Ideal BW q8h	Unpublished data from 7 obese volunteers (Davis, et al., ICAAC abstract, 1991).
Aminoglycosides	Use **Adjusted BW** Example: Critically ill patient, Gentamicin or Tobramycin (not Amikacin) 7 mg/kg of Adjusted BW IV q24h (See Comment)	Adjusted BW = Ideal BW + 0.4(Actual BW – Ideal BW). Ref: Pharmacother 27:1081, 2007. Follow levels so as to lower dose once hemodynamics stabilize.
Cefazolin (surgical prophylaxis)	No dose adjustment needed: 2 gm x 1 dose (repeat in 3 hours?)	Conflicting data; unclear whether dose should be repeated, or if an even higher dose is required. Patients with BMI 40-80 studied. Refs: Surg 136:738, 2004; Eur J Clin Pharmacol 67:985, 2011; Surg Infect 13:33, 2012.
Cefepime	Modest dose increase: 2 gm IV q8h instead of the usual q12h	Data from 10 patients (mean BMI 48) undergoing bariatric surgery; regimen yields free T > MIC of 60% for MIC of 8 μg/mL. Ref: Obes Surg 22:465, 2012.
Daptomycin	Use **Actual BW** Example: 4-12 mg/kg of Actual BW IV q24h	Data from a single-dose PK study in 7 obese volunteers. Ref: Antimicrob Ag Chemother 51:2741, 2007.
Flucytosine	Use **Ideal BW** Example: Crypto meningitis, give 25 mg/kg of Ideal BW po q6h	Date from one obese patient with cryptococcal disease. Ref: Pharmacother 15:251, 1995.
Levofloxacin	**No dose adjustment** required Example: 750 mg po/IV q24h	Data from 13 obese patients; variability in study findings renders conclusion uncertain. Refs: AAC 55:3240, 2011; JAC 66:1653, 2011. A recent PK study (requiring clinical validation) in patients with BMI of 40 or more suggests that higher doses may be necessary to achieve adequate drug exposure (Clin Pharmacokin 53:753, 2014).
Linezolid	**No dose adjustment required** Example: 600 mg po/IV q12h	Data from 20 obese volunteers up to 150 kg body weight suggest standard doses provide AUC values similar to nonobese subjects. In a recent case report, standard dosing in a 265 kg male with MRSA pneumonia seemed to have reduced clinical effectiveness. Refs: Antimicrob Ag Chemother 57:1144, 2013; Ann Pharmacother 47: e25, 2013.
Meropenem	**No dose adjustment required.** Example: 1 gm IV q8h.	PK data in ten hospitalized (non-ICU) patients similar to non-obese patients (Ann Pharmacother 48:178, 2014).

Ref. for NRTIs and NNRTIs: Kidney International 60:821, 2001

TABLE 17C (2)

Drug	Dose	Comments
Moxifloxacin	**No dose adjustment** required Example: 400 mg po/IV q24h	Data from 12 obese patients undergoing gastric bypass. Ref: *J Antimicrob Chemother 66:2330, 2011.*
Oseltamivir	**No dose adjustment** required Example: 75 mg po q12h	Data from 10 obese volunteers, unclear if applicable to patients >250 kg (OK to give 150 mg po q12h). Ref: *J Antimicrob Ag 41:52, 2013.*
Piperacillin-tazobactam	6.75 gm IV over 4 hours and dosed every 8 hours. No data for pt with impaired renal function	Data need confirmation. Based on 14 obese patients with actual BW >130 kg and BMI >40 kg/m². Ref: *Int J Antimicrob Ag 41:52, 2013.* High dose to optimize dose for pathogens with MIC ≤16 mcg/mL. May enhance bleeding propensity in uremic patients.
Telavancin	If weight is 30% or more over ideal BW, dose using adjusted BW as for aminoglycosides.	The correct dosing weight to use for Telavancin is unclear. Actual BW may overdose and increase nephrotoxicity, ideal BW may underdose (*JAC 67:723, 2012; JAC 67:1300, 2012*). Problematic because serum levels are not routinely available.
Vancomycin	Use **Actual BW** Example: in critically ill patient give 25-30 mg/kg of Actual BW load, then 15-20 mg/kg of Actual BW IV q8h-12h (infuse over 1.5-2 hr). No single dose over 2 gm. Check trough levels.	Data from 24 obese patients; Vancomycin half-life appears to decrease with little change in Vd. Ref: *Eur J Clin Pharmacol 54:621, 1998.*
Voriconazole po	**No dose adjustment** required Example: 400 mg po q12h x2 doses then 200 mg po q12h. Check trough concentrations (underdosing common with Voriconazole).	Data from a 2-way crossover study of oral voriconazole in 8 volunteers suggest no adjustment required, but data from one patient suggest use of adjusted BW. Recommended IV voriconazole dose based on actual BW (no supporting data). Refs: *Antimicrob Ag Chemother 55:2601, 2011; Clin Infect Dis 53:745, 2011.*

TABLE 18 – ANTIMICROBIALS AND HEPATIC DISEASE: DOSAGE ADJUSTMENT*

The following alphabetical list indicates antibacterials excreted/metabolized by the liver **wherein a dosage adjustment may be indicated** in the presence of hepatic disease. Space precludes details; consult the PDR or package inserts for details. List is **not** all-inclusive:

Antibacterials		Antifungals	Antivirals[§]	
Ceftriaxone	Nafcillin	Caspofungin	Abacavir	Indinavir
Chloramphenicol	Rifabutin	Itraconazole	Atazanavir	Lopinavir/ritonavir
Clindamycin	Rifampin	Voriconazole	Darunavir	Nelfinavir
Fusidic acid	Synercid**		Delavirdine	Nevirapine
Isoniazid	Telithromycin++		Efavirenz	Rimantadine
Metronidazole	Tigecycline		Enfuvirtide	Ritonavir
	Tinidazole		Fosamprenavir	Stribild

[§] Ref. on antiretrovirals: *CID 40:174, 2005*   ** Quinupristin/dalfopristin   ++ Telithro: reduce dose in renal & hepatic failure

TABLE 19 – TREATMENT OF CAPD PERITONITIS IN ADULTS*
(Periton Dial Intl 30:393, 2010)[1]

EMPIRIC Intraperitoneal Therapy: Culture Results Pending *(For MRSA see footnote[2])*

Drug		Residual Urine Output	
		<100 mL per day	>100 mL per day
(Cefazolin or Vanco) +	Can mix in same bag	1 gm per bag, q24h	20 mg per kg BW per bag, q24h
Ceftazidime		3 gm LD, then 1-2 gm IP q24h *(AAC 58:19, 2014)*	20 mg per kg BW per bag, q24h

Drug Doses for SPECIFIC Intraperitoneal Therapy—Culture Results Known. NOTE: Few po drugs indicated

Drug	Intermittent Dosing (once per day)		Continuous Dosing (per liter exchange)	
	Anuric	Non-Anuric	Anuric	Non-Anuric
Amphotericin B	NA	NA	MD 1.5 mg	NA
Ampicillin	250–500 mg po bid	ND	No LD, MD 125 mg	ND
Amp-sulbactam	2 gm q12h	ND	LD 1 gm, MD 100 mg	LD 1 gm, MD ↑ 25%
Cefazolin	15 mg per kg	20 mg per kg	LD 500 mg, MD 125 mg	LD 500 mg, ↑ MD 25%
Cefepime	1 gm in one exchange/day	1.25 gm	LD 500 mg, MD 125 mg	LD 500 mg, ↑ MD 25%
Ceftazidime	1000–2000 mg	ND	LD 500 mg, MD 125 mg	LD 500 mg; ↑ MD 25%
Ciprofloxacin	500 mg po bid	ND	LD 50 mg, MD 25 mg	ND
Daptomycin			LD 100 mg, MD 20 mg	LD 500 mg, ↑ MD 25%
Fluconazole	200 mg q24h	ND	200 mg q24h	ND
Gentamicin	0.6 mg per kg	↑ dose 25%	Not recommended	Not recommended
Imipenem	1 gm in one exchange q12h		LD 250 mg, MD 50 mg	LD 250 mg, ↑ MD 25%
Itraconazole	100 mg q12h	100 mg q12h	100 mg q12h	100 mg q12h
Metronidazole	250 mg po bid	ND	250 mg po bid	ND
TMP-SMX	160/800 mg po bid	ND	LD 320/1600 mg po, MD 80/400 mg po q24h	ND
Vancomycin	15–30 mg per kg q3–7 days	↑ dose 25%	LD 1 gm; MD 25 mg	LD 1 gm, ↑ MD 25%

CAPD = continuous ambulatory peritoneal dialysis
Indications for catheter removal: 1) Relapse with same organism within 1 mo; 2) Failure to respond clinically within 5 days; 3) Exit site and tunnel infection; 4) Fungal peritonitis; 5) Fecal flora peritonitis (suggests bowel perforation).

All doses IP unless indicated otherwise.
LD = loading dose, **MD** = maintenance dose, **ND** = no data; **NA** = not applicable—dose as normal renal function.
Anuric = <100 mL per day, **non-anuric** = >100 mL per day
[2] **Does not provide treatment for MRSA.** If gram-pos cocci on gram stain, include vanco.

TABLE 20A – ANTI-TETANUS PROPHYLAXIS, WOUND CLASSIFICATION, IMMUNIZATION

WOUND CLASSIFICATION

Clinical Features	Tetanus Prone	Non-Tetanus Prone
Age of wound	> 6 hours	≤ 6 hours
Configuration	Stellate, avulsion	Linear
Depth	> 1 cm	≤ 1 cm
Mechanism of injury	Missile, crush, burn, frostbite	Sharp surface (glass, knife)
Devitalized tissue	Present	Absent
Contaminants (dirt, saliva, etc.)	Present	Absent

IMMUNIZATION SCHEDULE

History of Tetanus Immunization	Dirty, Tetanus-Prone Wound		Clean, non-Tetanus-Prone Wound	
	Td[1,2]	Tetanus Immune Globulin	Td[1,2]	Tetanus Immune Globulin
Unknown or < 3 doses[3]	Yes	Yes	Yes	No
3 or more doses	No[4]	No	No[5]	No

Ref: *MMWR 60:13, 2011; MMWR 61:468, 2012; MMWR 62:131, 2013 (pregnancy).*

[1] Td = Tetanus & diphtheria toxoids, adsorbed (adult). For adult who has not received Tdap previously, substitute one dose of Tdap for Td when immunization is indicated *(MMWR 61::468, 2012).*
[2] For children < 7 years, use DTaP unless contraindicated; for persons ≥ 7 years, Td is preferred to tetanus toxoid alone, but single dose of Tdap can be used if required for catch-up series.
[3] Individuals who have not completed vaccine series should do so.
[4] Yes, if >5 years since last booster.
[5] Yes, if >10 years since last booster.

TABLE 20B – RABIES POSTEXPOSURE PROPHYLAXIS
All wounds should be cleaned immediately & thoroughly with soap & water.
This has been shown to protect 90% of experimental animals![1]

Animal Type	Evaluation & Disposition of Animal	Recommendations for Prophylaxis
Dogs, cats, ferrets	Healthy & available for 10-day observation	Don't start unless animal develops sx, then immediately begin HRIG + vaccine
	Rabid or suspected rabid	Immediate HRIG + vaccine
	Unknown (escaped)	Consult public health officials
Skunks, raccoons, bats,* foxes, coyotes, most carnivores	Regard as rabid	Immediate vaccination
Livestock, horses, rodents, rabbits; includes hares, squirrels, hamsters, guinea pigs, gerbils, chipmunks, rats, mice, woodchucks	Consider case-by-case	Consult public health officials. Bites of squirrels, hamsters, guinea pigs, gerbils, chipmunks, rats, mice, other small rodents, rabbits, and hares **almost never** require rabies post-exposure prophylaxis.

* Most recent cases of human rabies in U.S. due to contact (not bites) with silver-haired bats or rarely big brown bats but risk of acquiring rabies from non-contact bat exposure is exceedingly low (CID 48:1493, 2009). For more detail, see CID 30:4, 2000; JAVMA 219:1687, 2001; CID 37:96, 2003 (travel medicine advisory); Ln 363:959, 2004; EID 11:1921, 2005; MMWR 55 (RR-5), 2006.

Postexposure Rabies Immunization Schedule

IF NOT PREVIOUSLY VACCINATED

Treatment	Regimen[2]
Local wound cleaning	**All postexposure treatment should begin with immediate, thorough cleaning of all wounds with soap & water.**
Human rabies immune globulin (HRIG)	20 units per kg body weight given once on day 0. If anatomically feasible, the full dose should be infiltrated around the wound(s), the rest should be administered IM in the gluteal area. If the calculated dose of HRIG is insufficient to inject all the wounds, it should be diluted with normal saline to allow infiltration around additional wound areas. HRIG should **not** be administered in the **same syringe, or** into the **same anatomical site** as vaccine, or more than 7 days after the initiation of vaccine. Because HRIG may partially suppress active production of antibody, no more than the recommended dose should be given.[3]
Vaccine	Human diploid cell vaccine (HDCV), rabies vaccine adsorbed (RVA), or purified chick embryo cell vaccine (PCECV) 1 mL **IM (deltoid area[4])**, one each days 0, 3, 7, 14[5].

IF PREVIOUSLY VACCINATED[6]

Treatment	Regimen[2]
Local wound cleaning	All postexposure treatment should begin with immediate, thorough cleaning of all wounds with soap & water.
HRIG	HRIG should **not** be administered
Vaccine	HDCV or PCEC, 1 mL **IM (deltoid area[4])**, one each on days 0 & 3

CORRECT VACCINE ADMINISTRATION SITES

Age Group	Administration Site
Children & adults	**DELTOID[4]** only (**NEVER** in gluteus)
Infants & young children	Outer aspect of thigh (anterolateral thigh) may be used (**NEVER** in gluteus)

[1] From MMWR 48:RR-1, 1999; CID 30:4, 2000; B. T. Matyas, Mass. Dept. of Public Health. MMWR 57:1, 2008

[2] These regimens are applicable for all age groups, including children.

[3] In most reported post-exposure treatment failures, only identified deficiency was failure to infiltrate wound(s) with HRIG (CID 22:228, 1996). However, several failures reported from SE Asia in patients in whom WHO protocol followed (CID 28:143, 1999).

[4] The **deltoid** area is the **only** acceptable site of vaccination for adults & older children. For infants & young children, outer aspect of the thigh (anterolateral thigh) may be used. Vaccine should **NEVER** be administered in gluteal area.

[5] Note that this is a change from previous recommendation of 5 doses (days 0, 3, 7, 14 & 28) based on new data & recommendations from ACIP. Note that the number of doses for persons with altered immunocompetence remains unchanged (5 doses on days 0, 3, 7, 14 & 28) and recommendations for pre-exposure prophylaxis remain 3 doses administered on days 0, 7 and 21 or 28 (MMWR 59 (RR-2), 2010).

[6] Any person with a history of pre-exposure vaccination with HDCV, RVA, PCECV; prior post-exposure prophylaxis with HDCV, PCEC or rabies vaccine adsorbed (RVA); or previous vaccination with any other type of rabies vaccine & a documented history of antibody response to the prior vaccination.

TABLE 21 SELECTED DIRECTORY OF RESOURCES

ORGANIZATION	PHONE/FAX	WEBSITE(S)
ANTIPARASITIC DRUGS & PARASITOLOGY INFORMATION		
CDC Drug Line	Weekdays: 404-639-3670	http://www.cdc.gov/ncidod/srp/drugs/drug-service.htr
	Evenings, weekends, holidays: 404-639-2888	
DPDx: Lab ID of parasites		www.dpd.cdc.gov/dpdx/default.htm
Malaria	daytime: 770-488-7788	www.cdc.gov/malaria
	other: 770-488-7100	
	US toll free: 855-856-4713	
Expert Compound. Pharm.	800-247-9767/Fax: 818-787-7256	www.expertpharmacy.org
World Health Organization (WHO)		www.who.int
Parasites & Health		www.dpd.cdc.gov/dpdx/HTML/Para_Health.htm
BIOTERRORISM		
Centers for Disease Control & Prevention	770-488-7100	www.bt.cdc.gov
Infectious Diseases Society of America	703-299-0200	www.idsociety.org
Johns Hopkins Center Civilian Biodefense		www.jhsph.edu
Center for Biosecurity of the Univ. of Pittsburgh Med. Center		www.upmc-biosecurity.org
US Army Medical Research Institute of Inf. Dis.		www.usamriid.army.mil
HEPATITIS B		
Hepatitis B Foundation		www.hepb.org, www.natap.org
HEPATITIS C		
CDC		www.cdc.gov/ncidod/diseases/hepatitis/C
Individual		http://hepatitis-central.com
		www.natap.org
HCV Guidelines		www.hcvguidelines.org
HIV		
General		
HIV InSite		http://hivinsite.ucsf.edu
		www.natap.org
Drug Interactions		
Liverpool HIV Pharm. Group		www.hiv-druginteractions.org
Other		http://AIDS.medscape.com
Prophylaxis/Treatment of Opportunistic Infections; HIV Treatment		www.aidsinfo.nih.gov
IMMUNIZATIONS		
CDC, Natl. Immunization Program	404-639-8200	www.cdc.gov/vaccines/
FDA, Vaccine Adverse Events	800-822-7967	www.fda.gov/cber/vaers/vaers.htm
National Network Immunization Info.	877-341-6644	www.immunizationinfo.org
Influenza vaccine, CDC	404-639-8200	www.cdc.gov/vaccines/
Institute for Vaccine Safety		www.vaccinesafety.edu
OCCUPATIONAL EXPOSURE, BLOOD-BORNE PATHOGENS (HIV, HEPATITIS B & C)		
Clinicians Consultation Center	888-448-4911	www.ucsf.edu/hivcntr
PEPline (exposed clinicians)		
WARMline (clinicians of HIV pts)		
Perinatal HIV Hotline	888-448-8765	www.ucsf.edu/hivcntr
Q-T$_c$ INTERVAL PROLONGATION BY DRUGS		www.qtdrugs.org; www.crediblemeds.org
TRAVELERS' INFO: Immunizations, Malaria Prophylaxis, More		
Amer. Soc. Trop. Med. & Hyg.		www.astmh.org
CDC, general	877-394-8747	http://www.cdc.gov/travel/default.asp
CDC, Malaria:		www.cdc.gov/malaria
Prophylaxis		http://www.cdc.gov/travel/default.asp
MD Travel Health		www.mdtravelhealth.com
Pan American Health Organization		www.paho.org
World Health Organization (WHO)		www.who.int/home-page

TABLE 22A – ANTI-INFECTIVE DRUG-DRUG INTERACTIONS

Importance: ± = theory/anecdotal; + = of probable importance; ++ = of definite importance
To check for interactions between more than 2 drugs, *see:* http://www.drugs.com/drug_interactions.html;
http://www.healthline.com/druginteractions; www.medscape.com

ANTI-INFECTIVE AGENT (A)	OTHER DRUG (B)	EFFECT	IMPORT
bacavir	Methadone	↓ levels of B	++
mantadine (ymmetrel)	Alcohol	↑ CNS effects	+
	Anticholinergic and anti-Parkinson agents (ex. Artane, scopolamine)	↑ effect of B: dry mouth, ataxia, blurred vision, slurred speech, toxic psychosis	+
	Trimethoprim	↑ levels of A & B	+
	Digoxin	↑ levels of B	±
minoglycosides— arenteral (amikacin, entamicin, kanamycin, etilmicin, sisomicin, treptomycin, tobramycin)	Amphotericin B	↑ nephrotoxicity	++
	Cis platinum (Platinol)	↑ nephro & ototoxicity	+
	Cyclosporine	↑ nephrotoxicity	+
	Neuromuscular blocking agents	apnea or respiratory paralysis	+
	Loop diuretics (e.g., furosemide)	↑ ototoxicity	++
	NSAIDs	↑ nephrotoxicity	+
	Non-polarizing muscle relaxants	↑ apnea	+
	Radiographic contrast	↑ nephrotoxicity	+
	Vancomycin	↑ nephrotoxicity	+
minoglycosides— ral (kanamycin, neomycin)	**Warfarin**	↑ prothrombin time	+
mphotericin B and ampho lipid formulations	Antineoplastic drugs	↑ nephrotoxicity risk	+
	Digitalis	↑ toxicity of B if K⁺ ↓	+
	Nephrotoxic drugs: aminoglycosides, cidofovir, cyclosporine, foscarnet, pentamidine	↑ nephrotoxicity of A	++
mpicillin, amoxicillin	Allopurinol	↑ frequency of rash	++
rtemether-lumefantrine	CYP3A inhibitors: amiodarone, atazanavir, itraconazole, ritonavir, voriconazole	↑ levels of A; ↑ QTc interval	++
	CYP2D6 substrates: flecainide, imipramine, amitriptyline	↑ levels of B; ↑ QTc interval	++
tazanavir	*See protease inhibitors and Table 22B*		
tovaquone	Rifampin (perhaps rifabutin)	↓ serum levels of A; ↑ levels of B	+
	Metoclopramide	↓ levels of A	+
	Tetracycline	↓ levels of A	++

zole Antifungal Agents [Flu = fluconazole, **Itr** = itraconazole, **Ket** = ketoconazole, **Posa** = posaconazole **Vor** = voriconazole, **Isa** = Isavuconazole + = occurs; **blank space** = either studied & no interaction OR no data found (may be in pharm. co. databases)]

Flu	Itr	Ket	Posa	Vor	Isa	OTHER DRUG (B)	EFFECT	IMPORT
+	+					Amitriptyline	↓ levels of B	+
				+		Bupropion	↓ levels of B	++
+	+	+		+		Calcium channel blockers	↑ levels of B	++
	+					Carbamazepine (vori contraindicated)	↓ levels of A	++
+	+	+	+	+	+	Cyclosporine	↑ levels of B, ↑ risk of nephrotoxicity	+
	+	+				Didanosine	↓ absorption of A	+
	+					Digoxin	↑ levels of B	++
	+	+	+	+		Efavirenz	↓ levels of A, ↑ levels of B	++ (avoid)
+	+	+	+			H₂ blockers, antacids, sucralfate	↓ absorption of B	+
+	+	+	+	+		Hydantoins (phenytoin, Dilantin)	↑ levels of B, ↓ levels of A	++
	+	+				Isoniazid	↓ levels of B	+
	+	+	+	+	+	Lovastatin/simvastatin, atorvastatin	Rhabdomyolysis reported; ↑ levels of B	++
				+		Methadone	↑ levels of B	+
			+			Mycophenolate	↑ levels of B	++
+	+	+	+	+		Midazolam/triazolam, po	↑ levels of B	++
+	+	+	+	+		Warfarin	↑ effect of B	++
+	+	+	+			Oral hypoglycemics	↑ levels of B	++
			+	+		Pimozide	↑ levels of B—**avoid**	++
	+	+	+	+	+	Protease inhibitors, e.g., LPV	↑ levels of B	++
+	+	+	+	+		Proton pump inhibitors	↓ levels of A, ↑ levels of B	++
+	+	+	+	+	+	Rifampin/rifabutin (vori contraindicated)	↑ levels of B, ↓ serum levels of A	++
	+					Rituximab	Inhibits action of B	++
			+	+	+	Sirolimus (vori and posa contraindicated)	↑ levels of B	++
+		+	+	+	+	Tacrolimus	↑ levels of B with toxicity	++
+	+					Theophyllines	↑ levels of B	+
		+				Trazodone	↑ levels of B	++
+						Zidovudine	↑ levels of B	+

TABLE 22A (2)

ANTI-INFECTIVE AGENT (A)	OTHER DRUG (B)	EFFECT	IMPORT
Bedaquiline	Rifampin	↓ levels of A	++
	Ketoconazole	↑ levels of A	++
Caspofungin	Cyclosporine	↑ levels of A	++
	Tacrolimus	↓ levels of B	++
	Carbamazepine, dexamethasone, efavirenz, nevirapine, phenytoin, rifamycin	↓ levels of A; ↑ dose of caspofungin to 70 mg/d	++
Chloramphenicol	Hydantoins	↑ toxicity of B, nystagmus, ataxia	++
	Iron salts, Vitamin B12	↓ response to B	++
	Protease inhibitors—HIV	↑ levels of A & B	++
Clindamycin (Cleocin)	Kaolin	↓ absorption of A	++
	Muscle relaxants, e.g., atracurium, baclofen, diazepam	↑ frequency/duration of respiratory paralysis	++
	St John's wort	↓ levels of A	++
Cobicistat	*See Integrase Strand Transfer Inhibitors*		
Cycloserine	Ethanol	↑ frequency of seizures	+
	INH, ethionamide	↑ frequency of drowsiness/dizziness	+
Dapsone	Atazanavir	↓ levels of A - Avoid	++
	Didanosine	↓ absorption of A	+
	Oral contraceptives	↓ effectiveness of B	+
	Pyrimethamine	↑ in marrow toxicity	+
	Rifampin/Rifabutin	↓ serum levels of A	+
	Trimethoprim	↑ levels of A & B (methemoglobinemia)	+
	Zidovudine	May ↑ marrow toxicity	+
Daptomycin	HMG-CoA inhibitors (statins)	Consider DC statin while on dapto	++
Delavirdine (Rescriptor)	*See Non-nucleoside reverse transcriptase inhibitors (NNRTIs) and Table 22B*		
Didanosine (ddI) (Videx)	Allopurinol	↑ levels of A—AVOID	++
	Cisplatin, dapsone, INH, metronidazole, nitrofurantoin, stavudine, vincristine, zalcitabine	↑ risk of peripheral neuropathy	+
	Ethanol, lamivudine, pentamidine	↑ risk of pancreatitis	+
	Fluoroquinolones	↓ absorption 2° to chelation	+
	Drugs that need low pH for absorption: dapsone, indinavir, itra/ ketoconazole, pyrimethamine, rifampin, trimethoprim	↓ absorption	+
	Methadone	↓ levels of A	++
	Ribavirin	↑ levels ddI metabolite—avoid	++
	Tenofovir	↑ levels of A (reduce dose of A)	++
Dolutegravir	*See Integrase Strand Transfer Inhibitors*		
Doripenem	Probenecid	↑ levels of A	++
	Valproic acid	↓ levels of B	++
Doxycycline	Aluminum, bismuth, iron, Mg⁺⁺	↓ absorption of A	+
	Barbiturates, hydantoins	↓ serum t/2 of A	+
	Carbamazepine (Tegretol)	↓ serum t/2 of A	+
	Digoxin	↑ serum levels of B	+
	Warfarin	↑ activity of B	++
Efavirenz (Sustiva)	*See non-nucleoside reverse transcriptase inhibitors (NNRTIs) and Table 22B*		
Elvitegravir	*See Integrase Strand Transfer Inhibitors*		
Ertapenem (Invanz)	Probenecid	↑ levels of A	++
	Valproic acid	↓ levels of B	++
Ethambutol (Myambutol)	Aluminum salts (includes didanosine buffer)	↓ absorption of A & B	+
Etravirine	*See non-nucleoside reverse transcriptase inhibitors (NNRTIs) and Table 22B*		

Fluoroquinolones (**Cipro** = ciprofloxacin; **Gati** = gatifloxacin; **Gemi** = gemifloxacin; **Levo** = levofloxacin; **Moxi** = moxifloxacin; **Oflox** = ofloxacin)

NOTE: Blank space = either studied and no interaction OR no data found

Cipro	Gati	Gemi	Levo	Moxi	Oflox	OTHER DRUG (B)	EFFECT	IMPORT
+	+		+	+	+	**Antiarrhythmics (procainamide, amiodarone)**	↑ Q-T interval (torsade)	++
+	+		+	+	+	Insulin, oral hypoglycemics	↑ & ↓ blood sugar	++
+						Caffeine	↑ levels of B	+
+					+	Cimetidine	↑ levels of B	+
+					+	Cyclosporine	↑ levels of B	±
+			+		+	Didanosine	↓ absorption of A	++
+	+	+	+	+	+	**Cations: Al+++, Ca++, Fe++, Mg++, Zn++ (antacids, vitamins, dairy products), citrate/citric acid**	↓ absorption of A (some variability between drugs)	++
+						Methadone	↑ levels of B	++
+	+		+		+	**NSAIDs**	↑ risk CNS stimulation/seizures	++
+						Phenytoin	↑ or ↓ levels of B	+

Cipro	Gati	Gemi	Levo	Moxi	Oflox	OTHER DRUG (B)	EFFECT	IMPORT
						ANTI-INFECTIVE AGENT (A) — Fluoroquinolones *(continued)*	NOTE: Blank space = either studied and no interaction OR no data found	
+	+	+			+	Probenecid	↓ renal clearance of A	+
+						Rasagiline	↑ levels of B	+ +
				+		Rifampin	↓ levels of A *(CID 45:1001, 2007)*	+ +
+	+	+	+		+	**Sucralfate**	**↓ absorption of A**	+ +
+						Theophylline	↑ levels of B	+ +
+						Thyroid hormone	↓ levels of B	+ +
+						Tizanidine	↑ levels of B	+ +
			+	+	+	Warfarin	↑ prothrombin time	+

Ganciclovir (Cytovene) & Valganciclovir (Valcyte)

OTHER DRUG (B)	EFFECT	IMPORT
Imipenem	↑ risk of seizures reported	+
Probenecid	↑ levels of A	+
Zidovudine	↓ levels of A, ↑ levels of B	+

Gentamicin — See *Aminoglycosides—parenteral*

Imipenem & Meropenem

OTHER DRUG (B)	EFFECT	IMPORT
BCG	↓ effectiveness of B–avoid combination	+ +
Divalproex	↓ levels of B	+ +
Ganciclovir	↑ seizure risk	+ +
Probenecid	↑ levels of A	+ +
Valproic acid	↓ levels of B	+ +

Indinavir — See *protease inhibitors and Table 22B*

Integrase Strand Transfer Inhibitors (INSTI): Dolutegravir (**DTG**), Raltegravir (**RAL**), Elvitegravir (**ELV**)
NOTE: interactions involving Stribild (elvitegravir + cobicistat + emtricitabine + tenofovir) reflect one or more of its components (the specifics may not be known).

DTG	RAL	Stribild (ELV)	OTHER DRUG (B)	EFFECT	IMPORT
x	x	x	Antacids (polyvalent cations)	↓ levels of A—space dosing	+ +
		x	Antiarrhythmics, digoxin	↑ levels of B—monitor	+
	x		Atazanavir/RTV	↑ levels of A—monitor	±
		x	Atorvastatin	↑ levels of B—monitor	+
		x	Benzodiazepines	↑ levels of B—monitor	+
		x	Beta-blockers	↑ levels of B—monitor	+
		x	Bosentan	**↑ levels of B—adjust dose or avoid**	+ +
		x	Buprenorphine	↑ levels of B—monitor	+
		x	Buspirone	↑ levels of B—monitor	+
		x	Calcium channel blockers	↑ levels of B—monitor	+
x			Carbamazepine	**↓ levels of A—avoid**	+ +
		x	Carbamazepine	**↓ levels of A, ↑ levels of B—avoid**	+ +
		x	Clarithromycin	↑ levels of A and B—monitor	+
		x	Clonazepam	↑ levels of B—monitor	+
		x	Colchicine	↑ levels of B—adjust dose	+
		x	Cyclosporine	↑ levels of B—monitor	+
x			Dexamethasone	**↑ levels of B—avoid**	+ +
x			Dofetilide	**↑ levels of B—avoid**	+ +
x			Efavirenz	↓ levels of A—adjust dose	+ +
	x		Efavirenz	↓ levels of A—monitor	+
		x	Ethosuximide	↑ levels of B—monitor	+
x			Etravirine	**↓ levels of A—avoid**	+ +
	x		Etravirine	↓ levels of A—monitor	+
		x	Fluticasone	**↑ levels of B**	+ +
x			Fosamprenavir/RTV	↓ levels of A—adjust dose or avoid	+ +
x		x	Fosphenytoin/phenytoin	**↓ levels of A—avoid**	+ +
		x	Fluconazole	**↑ levels of A—avoid**	+ +
		x	Itraconazole	**↑ levels of A and B—adjust dose or avoid**	+ +
		x	Ketoconazole	↑ levels of A and B—adjust dose or avoid	+ +
x			Metformin	↑ levels of B—monitor	+ +
x			Nevirapine	**↓ levels of A—avoid**	+ +
	x		Omeprazole	↑ levels of A—monitor	±
		x	Oral contraceptives	↑ or ↓ levels of B—avoid	+ +
x		x	Oxcarbazepine	**↓ levels of A—avoid**	+ +

TABLE 22A (4)

Integrase Strand Transfer Inhibitors (INSTI) (continued)

DTG	RAL	Stribild (ELV)	OTHER DRUG (B)	EFFECT	IMPORT
x		x	Phenobarbital	↓ levels of A—avoid	++
		x	Phenothiazines	↑ levels of B—monitor	+
		x	Phosphodiesterase-5 inhibitors	↑ levels of B—adjust dose or avoid	++
x		x	Primidone	↓ levels of A—avoid	++
x	x	x	Rifampin, rifabutin, rifapentine	↓ levels of A—adjust dose or avoid	++
		x	Risperidone	↑ levels of B—monitor	+
		x	Salmeterol	↑ levels of B—avoid	++
		x	Sirolimus	↑ levels of B—monitor	+
x		x	St. John's wort	↓ levels of A—avoid	++
		x	SSRIs	↑ levels of B—monitor	+
x	x	x	Sucralfate	↓ levels of A—space dosing	++
		x	Tacrolimus	↑ levels of B—monitor	++
x			Tipranavir/RTV	↓ levels of A—adjust dose or avoid	++
	x			↓ levels of A—monitor	±
		x	Trazodone	↑ levels of B—monitor	+
		x	Tricyclic antidepressants	↑ levels of B—monitor	+
		x	Voriconazole	↑ levels of A and B—adjust dose or avoid	++
		x	Warfarin	↑ or ↓ levels of B—monitor	+
		x	Zolpidem ("Z" drugs)	↑ levels of B—monitor	+
Isoniazid			**Alcohol, rifampin**	**↑ risk of hepatic injury**	++
			Aluminum salts	↓ absorption (take fasting)	++
			Carbamazepine, phenytoin	↑ levels of B with nausea, vomiting, nystagmus, ataxia	++
			Itraconazole, ketoconazole	↓ levels of B	+
			Oral hypoglycemics	↓ effects of B	+
Lamivudine			Zalcitabine	**Mutual interference—do not combine**	++
Linezolid (Zyvox)			Adrenergic agents	Risk of hypertension	++
			Aged, fermented, pickled or smoked foods — ↑ tyramine	Risk of hypertension	+
			Clarithromycin	↑ levels of A	++
			Meperidine	Risk of serotonin syndrome	++
			Rasagiline (MAO inhibitor)	Risk of serotonin syndrome	+
			Rifampin	↓ levels of A	++
			Serotonergic drugs (SSRIs)	Risk of serotonin syndrome	++
Lopinavir			See protease inhibitors		

Macrolides [**Ery** = erythromycin; **Azi** = azithromycin; **Clr** = clarithromycin; **+** = occurs; **blank space** = either studied and no interaction OR no data]

Ery	Azi	Clr			
	+		Calcium channel blockers	↑ serum levels of B	++
+		+	Carbamazepine	↑ serum levels of B, nystagmus, nausea, vomiting, ataxia	++ (avoid w/ erythro)
+		+	Cimetidine, **ritonavir**	↑ levels of B	+
+			Clozapine	↑ serum levels of B, CNS toxicity	+
		+	Colchicine	↑ levels of B (potent, fatal)	++ (avoid)
+			Corticosteroids	↑ effects of B	+
+	+	+	Cyclosporine	↑ serum levels of B with toxicity	+
+	+	+	Digoxin, digitoxin	↑ serum levels of B (10% of cases)	+
		+	Efavirenz	↓ levels of A	++
+		+	Ergot alkaloids	↑ levels of B	++
		+	Linezolid	↑ levels of B	++
+		+	Lovastatin/simvastatin	↑ levels of B; rhabdomyolysis	++
+		+	Midazolam, triazolam	↑ levels of B, ↑ sedative effects	+
+		+	Phenytoin	↑ levels of B	+
+	+	+	Pimozide	**Q-T interval**	++
+		+	Rifampin, rifabutin	↓ levels of A	+
+		+	Tacrolimus	↑ levels of B	++
+		+	Theophylline	↑ serum levels of B with nausea, vomiting, seizures, apnea	++
+		+	Valproic acid	↑ levels of B	+
+			Warfarin	May ↑ prothrombin time	+
		+	Zidovudine	↓ levels of B	+

TABLE 22A (5)

ANTI-INFECTIVE AGENT (A)	OTHER DRUG (B)	EFFECT	IMPORT
Maraviroc	Clarithromycin	↑ serum levels of A	++
	Delavirdine	↑ levels of A	++
	Itraconazole/ketoconazole	↑ levels of A	++
	Nefazodone	↑ levels of A	++
	Protease Inhibitors (not tipranavir/ritonavir)	↑ levels of A	++
	Anticonvulsants: carbamazepine, phenobarbital, phenytoin	↓ levels of A	++
	Efavirenz	↓ levels of A	++
	Rifampin	↓ levels of A	++
Mefloquine	ß-adrenergic blockers, calcium channel blockers, quinidine, quinine	↑ arrhythmias	+
	Divalproex, valproic acid	↓ level of B with seizures	++
	Halofantrine	Q-T prolongation	++ (avoid)
	Calcineurin inhibitors	Q-T prolongation (avoid)	++
Meropenem	See Imipenem		
Methenamine mandelate or hippurate	Acetazolamide, sodium bicarbonate, thiazide diuretics	↓ antibacterial effect 2° to ↑ urine pH	++
Metronidazole /Tinidazole	**Alcohol**	Disulfiram-like reaction	+
	Cyclosporin	↑ levels of B	++
	Disulfiram (Antabuse)	Acute toxic psychosis	+
	Lithium	↑ levels of B	++
	Warfarin	↑ anticoagulant effect	++
	Phenobarbital, hydantoins	↓ levels of B	++
Micafungin	Nifedipine	↑ levels of B	+
	Sirolimus	↑ levels of B	+
Nafcillin	Warfarin	↓ Warfarin effect	++
Nelfinavir	See protease inhibitors and Table 22B		
Nevirapine (Viramune)	See non-nucleoside reverse transcriptase inhibitors (NNRTIs) and Table 22B		
Nitrofurantoin	Antacids	↓ absorption of A	+

Non-nucleoside reverse transcriptase inhibitors (NNRTIs): For interactions with protease inhibitors, see Table 22B.
Del = delavirdine; **Efa** = efavirenz; **Etr** = etravirine; **Nev** = nevirapine

Del	Efa	Etr	Nev	Co-administration contraindicated (See package insert):		
+		+		Anticonvulsants: carbamazepine, phenobarbital, phenytoin		++
+		+		Antimycobacterials: rifabutin, rifampin		++
+				Antipsychotics: pimozide		++
+	+	+		Benzodiazepines: alprazolam, midazolam, triazolam		++
+	+			Ergotamine		++
+	+	+		HMG-CoA inhibitors (statins): lovastatin, simvastatin, atorvastatin, pravastatin		++
+	+	+		St. John's wort		++
				Dose change needed:		
+			+	Amphetamines	↑ levels of B—**caution**	++
+		+	+	Antiarrhythmics: amiodarone, lidocaine, others	↓ or ↑ levels of B—**caution**	++
+	+	+	+	Anticonvulsants: carbamazepine, phenobarbital, phenytoin	↓ levels of A and/or B	++
+	+	+	+	Antifungals: itraconazole, ketoconazole, voriconazole, posaconazole	Potential ↓ levels of B, ↑ levels of A	++ (avoid)
+				Antirejection drugs: cyclosporine, rapamycin, sirolimus, tacrolimus	↑ levels of B	++
+				Calcium channel blockers	↑ levels of B	++
+		+	+	Clarithromycin	↓ levels of B metabolite, ↑ levels of A	++
+	+	+		Cyclosporine	↑ levels of A	++
+				Dexamethasone	↓ levels of A	++
+	+	+		Sildenafil, vardenafil, tadalafil	↑ levels of B	++
+				Fentanyl, methadone	↑ levels of B	++
+				Gastric acid suppression: antacids, H-2 blockers, proton pump inhibitors	↓ levels of A	++
	+		+	Mefloquine	↓ levels of B	++
	+	+	+	Methadone, fentanyl	↓ levels of B	++
	+		+	Oral contraceptives	↑ or ↓ levels of B	++
				Protease inhibitors—see Table 22B		
+	+	+	+	**Rifabutin, rifampin**	↑ or ↓ levels of rifabutin; ↓ levels of A—**caution**	++
+	+	+	+	St. John's wort	↓ levels of B	
+	+	+	+	Warfarin	↑ levels of B	++
Oritavancin				Warfarin	↑ levels of B	++
Pentamidine, IV				Amphotericin B	↑ risk of nephrotoxicity	+
				Pancreatitis-assoc drugs, eg, alcohol, valproic acid	↑ risk of pancreatitis	+
PIP-TZ				Methotrexate	↑ levels of B	++
Polymyxin B				Curare paralytics	Avoid: neuromuscular blockade	++

TABLE 22A (6)

ANTI-INFECTIVE AGENT (A)	OTHER DRUG (B)	EFFECT	IMPOR*
Polymyxin E (Colistin)	Curare paralytics	Avoid: neuromuscular blockade	++
	Aminoglycosides, Ampho B, Vanco	↑ nephrotoxicity risk	++
Primaquine	Chloroquine, dapsone, INH, probenecid, quinine, sulfonamides, TMP/SMX, others	↑ risk of hemolysis in G6PD-deficient patients	++

Protease Inhibitors—Anti-HIV Drugs. (**Atazan** = atazanavir; **Darun** = darunavir; **Fosampren** = fosamprenavir; **Indin** = *indinavir*; **Lopin** = lopinavir; **Nelfin** = nelfinavir; **Saquin** = saquinavir; **Tipran** = tipranavir. For interactions with antiretrovirals, see *Table 22B* **Only a partial list—check package insert**

Also see http://aidsinfo.nih.gov
To check for interactions between more than 2 drugs, see:
http://www.drugs.com/drug_interactions.html and http://www.healthline.com/druginteraction

Atazan	Darun	Fosampren	Indin	Lopin	Nelfin	Saquin	Tipran	OTHER DRUG (B)	EFFECT	IMPOR
								Analgesics:		
							+	1. Alfentanil, fentanyl, hydrocodone, tramadol	↑ levels of B	+
	+			+		+	+	2. Codeine, hydromorphone, morphine, methadone	↓ levels of B (*JAIDS 41:563, 2006*)	+
+	+	+	+	+			+	**Anti-arrhythmics: amiodarone, lidocaine, mexiletine, flecainide**	↑ levels of B; **do not co-administer or use caution** (*See package insert*)	++
	+	+		+		+	+	**Anticonvulsants: carbamazepine, clonazepam, phenobarbital**	↓ levels of A, ↑ levels of B	++
+		+	+				+	Antidepressants, all tricyclic	↑ levels of B	++
+	+	+					+	Antidepressants, all other	↑ levels of B; do not use pimozide	++
	+							Antidepressants, SSRIs	↓ levels of B - avoid	++
							+	Antihistamines	**Do not use**	++
+	+	+	+	+		+		**Benzodiazepines, e.g., diazepam, midazolam, triazolam**	↑ **levels of B—do not use**	++
+	+			+				Boceprevir	↓ levels of A & B	++
+	+		+	+	+	+	+	Calcium channel blockers (all)	↑ levels of B	++
+	+		+	+		+		Clarithro, erythro	↑ levels of B if renal impairment	+
+	+		+	+				Contraceptives, oral	↓ levels of A & B	++
	+	+	+	+		+		Corticosteroids: prednisone, dexamethasone	↓ levels of A, ↑ levels of B	+
+	+	+	+	+		+	+	Cyclosporine	↑ levels of B, monitor levels	+
							+	Digoxin	↑ levels of B	++
+	+	+	+	+		+	+	Ergot derivatives	↑ **levels of B—do not use**	++
		+	+			+	+	Erythromycin, clarithromycin	↑ levels of A & B	+
			+			+	+	Grapefruit juice (>200 mL/day)	↓ indinavir & ↑ saquinavir levels	++
+	+	+	+					H2 receptor antagonists	↓ levels of A	++
+	+	+	+	+		+	+	**HMG-CoA reductase inhibitors (statins): lovastatin, simvastatin**	↑ **levels of B—do not use**	++
+								Irinotecan	↑ **levels of B—do not use**	++
+	+	+	+	+		+	+	Ketoconazole, itraconazole, ? vori.	↑ levels of A & B	+
	+	+	+	+	+	+	+	Posaconazole	↑ levels of A, no effect on B	++
							+	Metronidazole	Poss. disulfiram reaction, alcohol	+
			+					Phenytoin (*JAIDS 36:1034, 2004*)	↓ levels of A & B	++
+	+	+	+	+	+	+	+	**Pimozide**	↑ **levels of B—do not use**	++
+	+		+			+	+	Proton pump inhibitors	↓ levels of A	++
+	+	+	+	+	+	+	+	Rifampin, rifabutin	↓ levels of A, ↑ levels of B **(avoid)**	++
+	+	+	+	+	+	+	+	Sildenafil (Viagra), tadalafil, vardenafil	Varies, some ↑ & some ↓ levels of B	++
+	+	+	+	+	+	+	+	**St. John's wort**	↓ **levels of A—do not use**	++
+	+	+	+	+	+	+	+	**Sirolimus, tacrolimus**	↑ **levels of B**	++
+								Tenofovir	↓ levels of A—add ritonavir	++
	+	+	+	+				Theophylline	↓ levels of B	+
+		+					+	Warfarin	↓ levels of B	+
Pyrazinamide								INH, rifampin	May ↑ risk of hepatotoxicity	±
Pyrimethamine								Lorazepam	↑ risk of hepatotoxicity	+
								Sulfonamides, TMP/SMX	↑ risk of marrow suppression	+
								Zidovudine	↑ risk of marrow suppression	+
Quinine								Digoxin	↑ digoxin levels; ↑ toxicity	++
								Mefloquine	↑ arrhythmias	+
								Warfarin	↑ prothrombin time	++
Quinupristin- dalfopristin (Synercid)								Anti-HIV drugs: NNRTIs & PIs	↑ levels of B	++
								Antineoplastic: vincristine, docetaxel, paclitaxel	↑ levels of B	++
								Calcium channel blockers	↑ levels of B	++
								Carbamazepine	↑ levels of B	++
								Cyclosporine, tacrolimus	↑ levels of B	++

TABLE 22A (7)

TI-INFECTIVE AGENT (A)	OTHER DRUG (B)	EFFECT	IMPORT
inupristin-dalfopristin (nercid) (continued)	Lidocaine	↑ levels of B	++
	Methylprednisolone	↑ levels of B	++
	Midazolam, diazepam	↑ levels of B	++
	Statins	↑ levels of B	++
itegravir	See Integrase Strand Transfer Inhibitors		
avirin	Didanosine	↑ levels of B → toxicity—avoid	++
	Stavudine	↓ levels of B	++
	Zidovudine	↓ levels of B	++
amycins	Al OH, ketoconazole, PZA	↓ levels of A	+
ampin, rifabutin)	Atovaquone	↑ levels of A, ↓ levels of B	+
	Beta adrenergic blockers (metoprolol, propranolol)	↓ effect of B	+
.: ArIM 162:985, 2002	Caspofungin	↓ levels of B—increase dose	++
	Clarithromycin	↑ levels of A, ↓ levels of B	++
e following is a partial	Corticosteroids	↑ replacement requirement of B	++
of drugs with rifampin-	Cyclosporine	↓ effect of B	++
uced ↑ metabolism	Delavirdine	↑ levels of A, ↓ levels of B—avoid	++
d hence lower than	Digoxin	↓ levels of B	++
icipated serum levels:	Disopyramide	↓ levels of B	++
E inhibitors, dapsone,	Fluconazole	↑ levels of A	+
azepam, digoxin,	Amprenavir, indinavir, nelfinavir, ritonavir	↓ levels of A (↓ dose of A), ↓ levels of B	++
iazem, doxycycline,	INH	Converts INH to toxic hydrazine	++
conazole, fluvastatin,	Itraconazole, ketoconazole	↓ levels of B, ↑ levels of A	++
operidol, moxifloxacin,	Linezolid	↓ levels of B	++
edipine, progestins,	Methadone	↓ serum levels (withdrawal)	+
azolam, tricyclics,	Nevirapine	↓ levels of B—avoid	++
riconazole, zidovudine	Warfarin	Suboptimal anticoagulation	++
in Pharmacokinetic	Oral contraceptives	↓ effectiveness; spotting, pregnancy	+
819, 2003).	Phenytoin	↓ levels of B	+
	Protease inhibitors	↓ levels of A, ↑ levels of B—CAUTION	++
	Quinidine	↓ effect of B	+
	Raltegravir	↓ levels of B	++
	Sulfonylureas	↓ hypoglycemic effect	+
	Tacrolimus	↓ levels of B	++
	Theophylline	↑ levels of B	+
	TMP/SMX	↑ levels of A	+
	Tocainide	↓ effect of B	+
mantadine	See Amantadine		
onavir	See protease inhibitors and Table 22B		
quinavir	See protease inhibitors and Table 22B		
avudine	Ribavirin	↓ levels of A—AVOID	++
	Zidovudine	Mutual interference—do not combine	++
and Transfer Integrase ibitors (INSTI)	See Integrase Strand Transfer Inhibitors		
lfonamides	Beta blockers	↑ levels of B	++
	Cyclosporine	↓ cyclosporine levels	+
	Methotrexate	↑ antifolate activity	+
	Warfarin	↑ prothrombin time; bleeding	+
	Phenobarbital, rifampin	↓ levels of A	+
	Phenytoin	↑ levels of B; nystagmus, ataxia	+
	Sulfonylureas	↑ hypoglycemic effect	+
lithromycin (Ketek)	Carbamazepine	↓ levels of A	++
	Digoxin	↑ levels of B—do digoxin levels	++
	Ergot alkaloids	↑ levels of B—avoid	++
	Itraconazole; ketoconazole	↑ levels of A; no dose change	+
	Metoprolol	↑ levels of B	++
	Midazolam	↑ levels of B	++
	Warfarin	↑ prothrombin time	+
	Phenobarbital, phenytoin	↓ levels of A	++
	Pimozide	↑ levels of B; QT prolongation—AVOID	++
	Rifampin	↓ levels of A—avoid	++
	Simvastatin & other "statins"	↑ levels of B (↑ risk of myopathy)	++
	Sotalol	↓ levels of B	++
	Theophylline	↑ levels of B	++

TABLE 22A (8)

ANTI-INFECTIVE AGENT (A)	OTHER DRUG (B)	EFFECT	IMPOR
Tenofovir	Atazanavir	↓ levels of B—add ritonavir	++
	Didanosine (ddI)	**↑ levels of B (reduce dose)**	++
Terbinafine	Cimetidine	↑ levels of A	+
	Phenobarbital, rifampin	↓ levels of A	+
Tetracyclines	See *Doxycycline, plus:*		
	Atovaquone	↓ levels of B	+
	Digoxin	↑ toxicity of B (may persist several months—up to 10% pts)	++
	Methoxyflurane	↑ toxicity; polyuria, renal failure	+
	Sucralfate	↓ absorption of A (separate by ≥2 hrs)	+
Thiabendazole	Theophyllines	↑ serum theophylline, nausea	+
Tigecycline	Oral contraceptives	↓ levels of B	++
Tinidazole (Tindamax)	See *Metronidazole—similar entity, expect similar interactions*		
Tobramycin	See *Aminoglycosides*		
Trimethoprim	Amantadine, dapsone, digoxin, methotrexate, procainamide, zidovudine	↑ serum levels of B	++
	Potassium-sparing diuretics	↑ serum K⁺	++
	Repaglinide	↑ levels of B (hypoglycemia)	++
	Thiazide diuretics	↓ serum Na⁺	+
Trimethoprim-Sulfamethoxazole	Ace inhibitors	↑ serum K+	++
	Amantadine	↑ levels of B (toxicity)	++
	Azathioprine	Reports of leukopenia	+
	Cyclosporine	↓ levels of B, ↑ serum creatinine	+
	Loperamide	↑ levels of B	+
	Methotrexate	Enhanced marrow suppression	++
	Oral contraceptives, pimozide, and 6-mercaptopurine	↓ effect of B	+
	Phenytoin	↑ levels of B	+
	Rifampin	↑ levels of B	+
	Spironolactone, sulfonylureas	↑ levels K+	++
	Warfarin	↑ activity of B	+
Valganciclovir (Valcyte)	See *Ganciclovir*		
Vancomycin	Aminoglycosides	↑ frequency of nephrotoxicity	++
Zalcitabine (ddC) (HIVID)	Valproic acid, pentamidine (IV), alcohol, lamivudine	↑ pancreatitis risk	+
	Cisplatin, INH, metronidazole, vincristine, nitrofurantoin, d4T, dapsone	↑ risk of peripheral neuropathy	+
Zidovudine (ZDV) (Retrovir)	Atovaquone, fluconazole, methadone	↑ levels of A	+
	Clarithromycin	↓ levels of A	±
	Indomethacin	↑ levels of ZDV toxic metabolite	+
	Nelfinavir	↓ levels of A	++
	Probenecid, TMP/SMX	↑ levels of A	+
	Rifampin/rifabutin	↓ levels of A	++
	Stavudine	**Interference—DO NOT COMBINE!**	++
	Valproic Acid	↑ levels of A	++

TABLE 22B – DRUG-DRUG INTERACTIONS BETWEEN NON-NUCLEOSIDE REVERSE TRANSCRIPTASE INHIBITORS (NNRTIS) AND PROTEASE INHIBITORS
(Adapted from Guidelines for the Use of Antiretroviral Agents in HIV-Infected Adults & Adolescents; see www.aidsinfo.nih.gov)

NAME (Abbreviation, Trade Name)	Atazanavir (ATV, Reyataz)	DARUNAVIR (DRV, Prezista)	Fosamprenavir (FOS-APV, Lexiva)	Indinavir (IDV, Crixivan)	Lopinavir/Ritonavir (LP/R, Kaletra)	Nelfinavir (NFV, Viracept)	Saquinavir (SQV, Invirase)	Tipranavir (TPV)
Delavirdine (DLV, Rescriptor)	No data	No data	Co-administration not recommended	IDV levels ↑ 40%. Dose: IDV 600 mg q8h; DLV standard	Expect LP levels to ↑. No dose data	NFV levels ↑ 2X; DLV levels ↓ 50%. Dose: No data	SQV levels ↑ 5X. Dose: SQV 800 mg q8h; DLV standard	No data
Efavirenz (EFZ, Sustiva)	ATV AUC ↓ 74%. Dose: EFZ standard; ATA/RTV 300/100 mg q24h with food	Standard doses of both drugs	FOS-APV levels ↓. Dose: EFZ standard; FOS-APV 1400 mg + RTV 300 mg q24h or 700 mg FOS-APV + 100 mg RTV q12h	Levels: IDV ↓ 31%. Dose: IDV 1000 mg q8h. EFZ standard	Level of LP ↓ 40%. Dose: LP/R 533/133 mg q12h, EFZ standard	Standard doses	Level: SQV ↓ 62%. Dose: SQV 400 mg + RTV 400 mg q12h	No dose change necessary
Etravirine (ETR, Intelence)	↑ ATV & ↑ ETR levels.	Standard doses of both drugs	↑ levels of FOS-APV.	↓ level of IDV.	↑ levels of ETR, ↓ levels of LP/R.	↑ levels of NFV.	↓ ETR levels 33%, SQV/Rt no change Standard dose of both drugs.	↓ levels of ETR, ↑ levels of TPV & RTV Avoid combination.
Nevirapine (NVP, Viramune)	Avoid combination. ATZ increases NVP concentrations > 25%; NVP decreases ATZ AUC by 42%	Standard doses of both drugs	Use with caution. NVP AUC increased 14% (700/100 Fos/rit; NVP AUC inc 29% (Fos 1400 bid)	IDV levels ↓ 28%. Dose: IDV 1000 mg q8h or combine with RTV; NVP standard	LP levels ↓ 53%; Dose: LP/R 533/133 mg q12h; NVP standard	Standard doses	Dose: SQV + RTV 400/400 mg, both q12h	Standard doses

TABLE 23 – LIST OF GENERIC AND COMMON TRADE NAMES

GENERIC NAME: TRADE NAMES	GENERIC NAME: TRADE NAMES	GENERIC NAME: TRADE NAMES
Abacavir: Ziagen	Elvitegravir: Vitekta	Paritaprevir, ritonavir, ombitasvir:
Abacavir + Lamivudine: Epzicom	Elvitegravir + Cobicistat + Emtricitabine	Technivie
Abacavir + Lamivudine +	+ Tenofovir: Stribild	Paritaprevir, ritonavir, ombitasvir,
Dolutegravir: Triumeq	Emtricitabine: Emtriva	dasabuvir: Viekira Pak
Abacavir + Lamivudine + Zidovudine:	Emtricitabine + tenofovir: Truvada	Paromomycin: Humatin
Trizivir	Emtricitabine + tenofovir + rilpivirine:	Pentamidine: NebuPent, Pentam 300
Acyclovir: Zovirax	Complera	Peramivir: Rapivab
Adefovir: Hepsera	Enfuvirtide (T-20): Fuzeon	Piperacillin/tazobactam: Zosyn,
Albendazole: Albenza	Entecavir: Baraclude	Tazocin
Amantadine: Symmetrel	Ertapenem: Invanz	Piperazine: Antepar
Amikacin: Amikin	Etravirine: Intelence	Podophyllotoxin: Condylox
Amoxicillin: Amoxil, Polymox	Erythromycin(s): Ilotycin	Polymyxin B: Poly-Rx
Amoxicillin extended release: Moxatag	*Ethyl succinate*: Pediamycin	Posaconazole: Noxafil
Amox./clav.: Augmentin, Augmentin	*Glucoheptonate*: Erythrocin	Praziquantel: Biltricide
ES-600: Augmentin XR	*Estolate*: Ilosone	Primaquine: Primachine
Amphotericin B: Fungizone	Erythro/sulfisoxazole: Pediazole	Proguanil: Paludrine
Ampho B-liposomal: AmBisome	Ethambutol: Myambutol	Pyrantel pamoate: Antiminth
Ampho B-lipid complex: Abelcet	Ethionamide: Trecator	Pyrimethamine: Daraprim
Ampicillin: Omnipen, Polycillin	Famciclovir: Famvir	Pyrimethamine/sulfadoxine: Fansidar
Ampicillin/sulbactam: Unasyn	Fidaxomicin: Dificid	Quinupristin/dalfopristin: Synercid
Artemether-Lumefantrine: Coartem	Fluconazole: Diflucan	Raltegravir: Isentress
Atazanavir: Reyataz	Flucytosine: Ancobon	Retapamulin: Altabax
Atovaquone: Mepron	Fosamprenavir: Lexiva	Ribavirin: Virazole, Rebetol
Atovaquone + proguanil: Malarone	Foscarnet: Foscavir	Rifabutin: Mycobutin
Azithromycin: Zithromax	Fosfomycin: Monurol	Rifampin: Rifadin, Rimactane
Azithromycin ER: Zmax	Fusidic acid: Taksta	Rifapentine: Priftin
Aztreonam: Azactam, Cayston	Ganciclovir: Cytovene	Rifaximin: Xifaxan
Bedaquiline: Sirturo	Gatifloxacin: Tequin	Rilpivirine: Edurant
Boceprevir: Victrelis	Gemifloxacin: Factive	Rimantadine: Flumadine
Caspofungin: Cancidas	Gentamicin: Garamycin	Ritonavir: Norvir
Cefaclor: Ceclor, Ceclor CD	Griseofulvin: Fulvicin	Saquinavir: Invirase
Cefadroxil: Duricef	Halofantrine: Halfan	Spectinomycin: Trobicin
Cefazolin: Ancef, Kefzol	Idoxuridine: Dendrid, Stoxil	Stavudine: Zerit
Cefdinir: Omnicef	INH + RIF: Rifamate	Stiboglucuonate: Pentostam
Cefditoren pivoxil: Spectracef	INH + RIF + PZA: Rifater	Silver sulfadiazine: Silvadene
Cefepime: Maxipime	Interferon alfa: Intron A	Simeprevir: Olysio
Cefixime[NUS]: Suprax	Interferon, pegylated: PEG-Intron,	Sofosbuvir: Solvadi
Cefoperazone-sulbactam:	Pegasys	Sulfamethoxazole: Gantanol
Sulperazon[NUS]	Interferon + ribavirin: Rebetron	Sulfasalazine: Azulfidine
Cefotaxime: Claforan	Imipenem + cilastatin: Primaxin,	Sulfisoxazole: Gantrisin
Cefotetan: Cefotan	Tienam	Tedizolid: Sivextro
Cefoxitin: Mefoxin	Imiquimod: Aldara	Telaprevir: Incivek
Cefpodoxime proxetil: Vantin	Indinavir: Crixivan	Telavancin: Vibativ
Cefprozil: Cefzil	Isavuconazole: Cresemba	Telbivudine: Tyzeka
Ceftaroline: Teflaro	Itraconazole: Sporanox	Telithromycin: Ketek
Ceftazidime: Fortaz, Tazicef, Tazidime	Iodoquinol: Yodoxin	Temocillin: Negaban, Temopen
Ceftazidime-avibactam: Avycaz	Ivermectin: Stromectol, Sklice	Tenofovir: Viread
Ceftibuten: Cedax	Ketoconazole: Nizoral	Terbinafine: Lamisil
Ceftizoxime: Cefizox	Lamivudine: Epivir, Epivir-HBV	Thalidomide: Thalomid Thiabendazole:
Ceftobiprole: Zeftera	Lamivudine + abacavir: Epzicom	Mintezol
Ceftolozane-tazobactam: Zerbaxa	Levofloxacin: Levaquin	Tigecycline: Tygacil
Ceftriaxone: Rocephin	Linezolid: Zyvox	Tinidazole: Tindamax
Cefuroxime: Zinacef, Ceftin	Lomefloxacin: Maxaquin	Tipranavir: Aptivus
Cephalexin: Keflex	Lopinavir/ritonavir: Kaletra	Tobramycin: Nebcin
Cephradine: Anspor, Velosef	Loracarbef: Lorabid	Tretinoin: Retin A
Chloroquine: Aralen	Mafenide: Sulfamylon	Trifluridine: Viroptic
Cidofovir: Vistide	Maraviroc: Selzentry	Trimethoprim: Primsol
Ciprofloxacin: Cipro, Cipro XR	Mebendazole: Vermox	Trimethoprim/sulfamethoxazole:
Clarithromycin: Biaxin, Biaxin XL	Mefloquine: Lariam	Bactrim, Septra
Clindamycin: Cleocin	Meropenem: Merrem	Valacyclovir: Valtrex
Clofazimine: Lamprene	Mesalamine: Asacol, Pentasa	Valganciclovir: Valcyte
Clotrimazole: Lotrimin, Mycelex	Methenamine: Hiprex, Mandelamine	Vancomycin: Vancocin
Cloxacillin: Tegopen	Metronidazole: Flagyl	Voriconazole: Vfend
Colistimethate: Coly-Mycin M	Micafungin: Mycamine	Zalcitabine: HIVID
Cycloserine: Seromycin	Minocycline: Minocin	Zanamivir: Relenza
Daclatasvir: Daklinza	Moxifloxacin: Avelox	Zidovudine (ZDV): Retrovir
Daptomycin: Cubicin	Mupirocin: Bactroban	Zidovudine + 3TC: Combivir
Dalbavancin: Dalvance	Nafcillin: Unipen	Zidovudine + 3TC + abacavir: Trizivir
Darunavir: Prezista	Nelfinavir: Viracept	Abelcet: Ampho B-lipid complex
Delavirdine: Rescriptor	Nevirapine: Viramune	Albenza: Albendazole
Dicloxacillin: Dynapen	Nitazoxanide: Alinia	Aldara: Imiquimod
Didanosine: Videx	Nitrofurantoin: Macrobid, Macrodantin	Alinia: Nitazoxanide
Diethylcarbamazine: Hetrazan	Nystatin: Mycostatin	Altabax: Retapamulin
Diloxanide furoate: Furamide	Ofloxacin: Floxin	AmBisome: Ampho B-liposomal
Dolutegravir: Tivicay	Olysio: Simeprevir	Amikin: Amikacin
Doripenem: Doribax	Oritavancin: Orbactiv	Amoxil: Amoxicillin
Doxycycline: Vibramycin	Oseltamivir: Tamiflu	Ancef: Cefazolin
Efavirenz: Sustiva	Oxacillin: Prostaphlin	Ancobon: Flucytosine
Efavirenz/Emtricitabine/Tenofovir:	Palivizumab: Synagis	Anspor: Cephradine
Atripla		

TABLE 23 (2)
LIST OF COMMON TRADE AND GENERIC NAMES

TRADE NAME: GENERIC NAME	TRADE NAME: GENERIC NAME	TRADE NAME: GENERIC NAME
Antepar: Piperazine	Isentress: Raltegravir	Stromectol: Ivermectin
Antiminth: Pyrantel pamoate	Kantrex: Kanamycin	Sulfamylon: Mafenide
Aptivus: Tipranavir	Kaletra: Lopinavir/ritonavir	Sulperazon[N,6]: Cefoperazone-sulbactam
Aralen: Chloroquine	Keflex: Cephalexin	Suprax: Cefixime[N,6]
Asacol: Mesalamine	Ketek: Telithromycin	Sustiva: Efavirenz
Atripla: Efavirenz/emtricitabine/tenofovir	Lamisil: Terbinafine	Symmetrel: Amantadine
Augmentin, Augmentin ES-600	Lamprene: Clofazimine	Synagis: Palivizumab
Augmentin XR: Amox./clav.	Lariam: Mefloquine	Synercid: Quinupristin/dalfopristin
Avelox: Moxifloxacin	Levaquin: Levofloxacin	Taksta: Fusidic acid
Avycaz: Ceftazidime-avibactam	Lexiva: Fosamprenavir	Tamiflu: Oseltamivir
Azactam: Aztreonam	Lorabid: Loracarbef	Tazicef: Ceftazidime
Azulfidine: Sulfasalazine	Macrodantin, Macrobid: Nitrofurantoin	Technivie: Paritaprevir, ritonavir, ombitasvir
Bactroban: Mupirocin	Malarone: Atovaquone + proguanil	Teflaro: Ceftaroline
Bactrim: Trimethoprim/sulfamethoxazole	Mandelamine: Methenamine mandel	Tegopen: Cloxacillin
Baraclude: Entecavir	Maxaquin: Lomefloxacin	Tequin: Gatifloxacin
Biaxin, Biaxin XL: Clarithromycin	Maxipime: Cefepime	Thalomid: Thalidomide
Biltricide: Praziquantel	Mefoxin: Cefoxitin	Tienam: Imipenem
Cancidas: Caspofungin	Mepron: Atovaquone	Tinactin: Tolnaftate
Cayston: Aztreonam (inhaled)	Merrem: Meropenem	Tindamax: Tinidazole
Ceclor, Ceclor CD: Cefaclor	Minocin: Minocycline	Tivicay: Dolutegravir
Cedax: Ceftibuten	Mintezol: Thiabendazole	Trecator SC: Ethionamide
Cefizox: Ceftizoxime	Monocid: Cefonicid	Triumeq: Abacavir + Lamivudine + Dolutegravir
Cefotan: Cefotetan	Monurol: Fosfomycin	Trizivir: Abacavir + ZDV + 3TC
Ceftin: Cefuroxime axetil	Moxatag: Amoxicillin extended release:	Trobicin: Spectinomycin
Cefzil: Cefprozil	Myambutol: Ethambutol	Truvada: Emtricitabine + tenofovir
Cipro, Cipro XR: Ciprofloxacin & extended release	Mycamine: Micafungin	Tygacil: Tigecycline
Claforan: Cefotaxime	Mycobutin: Rifabutin	Tyzeka: Telbivudine
Coartem: Artemether-Lumefantrine	Mycostatin: Nystatin	Unasyn: Ampicillin/sulbactam
Coly-Mycin M: Colistimethate	Nafcil: Nafcillin	Unipen: Nafcillin
Combivir: ZDV + 3TC	Nebcin: Tobramycin	Valcyte: Valganciclovir
Complera: Emtricitabine + tenofovir + rilpivirine	NebuPent: Pentamidine	Valtrex: Valacyclovir
Cresemba: Isavuconazole	Nizoral: Ketoconazole	Vancocin: Vancomycin
Crixivan: Indinavir	Norvir: Ritonavir	Vantin: Cefpodoxime proxetil
Cubicin: Daptomycin	Noxafil: Posaconazole	Velosef: Cephradine
Daklinza: Daclatasvir	Olysio: Simeprevir	Vermox: Mebendazole
Cytovene: Ganciclovir	Omnicef: Cefdinir	Vfend: Voriconazole
Dalvance: Dalbavancin	Omnipen: Ampicillin	Vibativ: Telavancin
Daraprim: Pyrimethamine	Orbactiv: Oritavancin	Vibramycin: Doxycycline
Dificid: Fidaxomicin	Pediamycin: Erythro. ethyl succinate	Victrelis: Boceprevir
Diflucan: Fluconazole	Pediazole: Erythro. ethyl succinate + sulfisoxazole	Videx: Didanosine
Doribax: Doripenem	Pegasys, PEG-Intron: Interferon, pegylated	Viekira Pak: Paritaprevir, ritonavir, ombitasvir, dasabuvir
Duricef: Cefadroxil	Pentam 300: Pentamidine	Viracept: Nelfinavir
Dynapen: Dicloxacillin	Pentasa: Mesalamine	Viramune: Nevirapine
Edurant: Rilpivirine	Polycillin: Ampicillin	Virazole: Ribavirin
Emtriva: Emtricitabine	Polymox: Amoxicillin	Viread: Tenofovir
Epivir, Epivir-HBV: Lamivudine	Poly-Rx: Polymyxin B	Vistide: Cidofovir
Epzicom: Lamivudine + abacavir	Prezista: Darunavir	Vitekta: Elvitegravir
Factive: Gemifloxacin	Priftin: Rifapentine	Xifaxan: Rifaximin
Famvir: Famciclovir	Primaxin: Imipenem + cilastatin	Yodoxin: Iodoquinol
Fansidar: Pyrimethamine + sulfadoxine	Primsol: Trimethoprim	Zerit: Stavudine
Flagyl: Metronidazole	Prostaphlin: Oxacillin	Zeftera: Ceftobiprole
Floxin: Ofloxacin	Rapivab: Peramivir	Zerbaxa: Ceftolozane-tazobactam
Flumadine: Rimantadine	Rebetol: Ribavirin	Ziagen: Abacavir
Foscavir: Foscarnet	Rebetron: Interferon + ribavirin	Zinacef: Cefuroxime
Fortaz: Ceftazidime	Relenza: Zanamivir	Zithromax: Azithromycin
Fulvicin: Griseofulvin	Rescriptor: Delavirdine	Zmax: Azithromycin ER
Fungizone: Amphotericin B	Retin A: Tretinoin Retrovir: Zidovudine (ZDV)	Zovirax: Acyclovir
Furadantin: Nitrofurantoin	Reyataz: Atazanavir	Zosyn: Piperacillin/tazobactam
Fuzeon: Enfuvirtide (T-20)	Rifadin: Rifampin	Zyvox: Linezolid
Gantanol: Sulfamethoxazole	Rifamate: INH + RIF	
Gantrisin: Sulfisoxazole	Rifater: INH + RIF + PZA	
Garamycin: Gentamicin	Rimactane: Rifampin	
Halfan: Halofantrine	Rocephin: Ceftriaxone	
Hepsera: Adefovir	Selzentry: Maraviroc	
Herplex: Idoxuridine	Septra: Trimethoprim/sulfa	
Hiprex: Methenamine hippurate	Seromycin: Cycloserine	
HIVID: Zalcitabine	Silvadene: Silver sulfadiazine	
Humatin: Paromomycin	Sirturo: Bedaquiline	
Ilosone: Erythromycin estolate	Sivextro: Tedizolid	
Ilotycin: Erythromycin	Sklice: Ivermectin lotion	
Incivek: Telaprevir	Solvadi: Sofosbuvir	
Intron A: Interferon alfa	Spectracef: Cefditoren pivoxil	
Invanz: Ertapenem	Sporanox: Itraconazole	
Invirase: Saquinavir	Stoxil: Idoxuridine	
	Stribild: Elvitegravir + Cobicistat + Emtricitabine + Tenofovir